Eat, Move, Sleep, Repeat

PROFESSOR MICHAEL GLEESON

EAT, MOVE, SLEEP, REPEAT

A Healthy Lifestyle Guidebook

Diet & Fitness for Living Long & Healthy

Meyer & Meyer Sport

British Library Cataloguing in Publication Data
A catalogue record for this book is available from the British Library

Eat, Move, Sleep, Repeat
Maidenhead: Meyer & Meyer Sport (UK) Ltd., 2020
ISBN: 978-1-78255-187-4

Aachen, Auckland, Beirut, Cairo, Cape Town, Dubai, Hägendorf, Hong Kong, Indianapolis, Manila, New Delhi, Singapore, Sydney, Tehran, Vienna

 Member of the World Sport Publishers' Association (WSPA)

Printed by: C-M Books, Ann Arbor, MI
ISBN: 978-1-78255-187-4
Email: info@m-m-sports.com
www.thesportspublisher.com

CONTENTS

Chapter 1

Optimizing Health, Fitness, and Well-Being Throughout the Lifespan

Objectives

After studying this chapter, you should:

- Understand the scope of this book

- Know something about the author

- Have a basic understanding of how particular aspects of your lifestyle and behavior can have a negative or positive impact on your health

- Appreciate the potential long-term health problems caused by being overweight

- Understand the concept of optimal health

- Appreciate how our genetics influences our susceptibility to gaining or losing body fat in response to dietary energy intake and exercise

- Appreciate the concept of relative risk

INTRODUCTION

Firstly, I want to thank you for buying this book and congratulate you on your decision. The title indicates that this is a guidebook that can direct you to a healthier lifestyle. Well, the aim of any guidebook, in my opinion, should be to explain exactly how to achieve your desired goals, and this is just what my book does. But it doesn't only provide advice and recommendations about appropriate eating, exercising, and sleeping behaviors, it also explains the scientific reasons for this guidance in a way that any reasonably intelligent person can understand. In this book I use my extensive experience of working with elite athletes and games players to help you, the general public, learn how to safely and effectively lose weight, get fitter, sleep better, avoid illness and live healthily for longer. You can trust the advice I give as it is all based on the latest scientific evidence. I do not promote any fad diets or exercise regimens, just ones that have been proven to be safe and effective. From me you will learn the principles of healthy eating and what you can do to make your health optimal...that is as good as it can be. Essentially, this book describes what you should eat and how you can make informed choices about your food selections based on what is healthy and what your personal preferences are. It explains exactly how you can take control of managing your appetite and how to lose weight (and more importantly body fat) by dieting or doing more exercise. It explains the basis of many different weight loss diets and informs you of the outcomes of scientific studies that have evaluated their efficacy: in other words, whether or not they work and just how effective they actually are.

In this book, I also explore how exercise can be used to achieve weight loss, what the best form of exercise is for fat burning, and the basis for the health benefits of regular exercise that you will have heard about. You will also discover the new evidence that tells us that sleep quantity and quality are also important for our health and how you can improve your own sleep quality. You will also learn about nutrition and lifestyle behavior strategies that will help you avoid common illnesses such as the common cold and tummy upsets as well as practical advice about maintaining healthy senses (eyesight and hearing), tissues and organs (teeth and gums, gut, bones, muscles, skin, heart, lungs, bladder, reproductive system, brain, etc.). Finally, you will be provided with a novel weight loss plan that can be personalized to your own preferences and incorporates multiple weight loss diets (avoiding the boredom of sticking to just one type of diet), combined with some daily moderate exercise that will leave you invigorated rather than exhausted.

Exercise and nutrition programs designed to achieve weight loss and improved health or fitness have continued to receive considerable attention in recent decades, and a large number of books have been published on the subject by authors, including nutritionists, dieticians, medics, sport scientists, personal trainers, and media celebrities. The vast majority of these books focus on the latest fad diet (e.g., Atkins, Intermittent Fast, Sugarbusters, Noncombination, Zone, Paleo, Macrobiotic, Alkaline, Dukan, etc.) usually alone or sometimes in combination with the latest fad exercise regimen (e.g., Aerobics, Stepping, Spinning, High Intensity Interval Exercise) but rarely provide a scientific evidence-based rationale for their use, except in very simplistic terms, nor indicate the range of other options available. People are very different in their goals, physical capabilities, and occupations, and this is often not taken into account; some of these fad diets and exercise regimens are only suitable or effective for a limited number of people. My book is different. It provides both a scientific evidence-based rationale for selecting certain diets and forms of physical activity that can help to achieve effective loss of body fat, explains how to develop a personalized weight loss plan, gives guidelines for a healthy balanced diet, provides advice on how to improve sleep quality, avoid common illnesses, and how much and what type of exercise is needed to see health benefits. As the title suggests, this book aims to provide a set of evidence-based guidelines on how to establish a healthy lifestyle that will promote a better quality of life with reduced risk of chronic disease (e.g., coronary heart disease, type 2 diabetes, cancer, dementia, etc.) throughout the lifespan and extend longevity. In simpler terms, it can help you to live a more satisfying, healthier, and longer life. I hope that by reading this book you will be motivated and better able to implement the changes to your lifestyle that you need to make to make your life healthier and better. Let me begin by telling you something about myself and what is different about my book.

WHO AM I?

I am a recently retired university professor who has spent the last 40 years of his life teaching and researching in the field of exercise physiology, metabolism, immunology, and health with a particular interest in sport nutrition. My last two academic positions were at the University of Birmingham and Loughborough University, two of the top universities in the world for sport, exercise, and health science. I have coauthored several books on the biochemistry of exercise and training, immune function in sport and exercise, and nutrition for sport, and contributed chapters to more than 30 other books. I have published over 200 research papers in the scientific and medical literature, and much of this has been focused on the well-being of athletes and the factors influencing their performance. Now, as an aging member of the general public, I have turned my attention to the issue of living a healthy lifestyle (in part, to improve my own quality of life and longevity) and have spent the last couple of years formulating the ideas for this new book. Some people have called me "the second most famous professor from Chadderton" (my hometown in the county of Lancashire, England). The most (and far more) famous professor from Chadderton is, of course, the physicist Brian Cox, (who actually grew up on the same street as me) and can so engagingly explain the workings of the universe on television and in his books as well as happening to be an ex-rock star! Well, I can't compete with that, but I do hope you will enjoy reading this book. I have tried to emulate Brian's writing style by attempting to explain the science in a way that the average person can understand, learn from, and enjoy. I suggest that you read this book slowly, just as you would savor a fine meal, take time to digest the information (pardon the pun!), and use it to change the way you live to make you and your loved ones both healthier and happier.

WHAT IS DIFFERENT ABOUT THIS BOOK?

A lot of people equate being healthy with being slim, and as the majority of the population in the Western world is overweight there is much emphasis on how weight loss can be achieved. There are so many books out there on dieting to lose weight, and some of those books also mention exercises that can help with weight loss. Most of these books spend a few pages explaining the scientific basis of some new diet (though often only using selected evidence that favors the new idea and ignoring evidence that does not), and some may briefly cover the health benefits of weight loss, but almost invariably the rest of the book will contain pictures of appetizing dishes and recipes. In fact, the difference between these books and the seemingly ever popular cook books by celebrity chefs is really often rather small.

The books that focus more on exercise may provide a list of health benefits and suggest which type of exercise is best for fitness and weight loss, but again the majority of the pages will mostly be filled with pictures; usually these will illustrate a series of supposedly suitable exercises being performed by a young, slim, attractive person in minimal clothing! That is why I decided to write this book with a very different approach, with more emphasis on the science, and limiting recommendations and guidelines to those that are evidence-based. As my 40-year career has been as an educator of university students, I wanted to apply what I know about exercise and nutrition to the issue of weight loss and explain the science behind a healthy lifestyle. It is my firm belief that if people gain a better understanding of the principles underlying the health consequences of overeating, not exercising, and not getting good, quality sleep, and learn how these poor lifestyle habits can be easily remedied to improve their long-term health, quality of life, and longevity, they are much more likely to decide (and stick with it) to change their behaviors to the benefit of their health and enjoyment of life. It is about understanding the reasons for the expert advice and recommendations and realizing that it is relatively simple to change bad habits to good ones without big changes to daily routines and personal preferences.

So, this book is written with the aim of teaching the average, reasonably intelligent person about the nature of the food we eat (chapter 2), why some foods are essential to our health and some are not (chapter 3), the potentially harmful consequences of eating too much or too little of certain **nutrients**, and the basis of a healthy balanced diet (chapter 4). The concept of **energy balance (calories** in versus calories out) is clearly explained in chapter 5, and you will also learn in chapter 6 about the factors that influence **appetite** and **satiety** (i.e., what controls our hunger and what makes us feel full after a good meal). Because many people are overweight (or overfat), chapters are devoted to different diet and exercise strategies to lose body fat. You will also learn about all the benefits of exercise, and the importance of getting sufficient amounts of good quality sleep. For example, did you know that both these aspects of our daily lives have important influences on our risk of developing **chronic diseases** such as cardiovascular disease, **type 2 diabetes**, **dementia**, and **cancer** later in life, and also on our current risk of infections? The reasons are explained in this book, and I have also included a chapter on how to maintain a robust **immune system**, with practical advice on how to avoid common infections. In this paragraph you will have noticed that some words are in **bold** font. Any word that appears in **bold** font in this book is defined in the glossary which you will find at the end of the book. I have tried to identify some of the key words or terms as well as words that may be unfamiliar to some readers and some other words that it is just useful to know the exact meaning of.

Finally, you will learn about an effective weight loss plan I have devised that is achievable for any moderately overweight but mobile adult who is between 18 and 70 years of age. This does not require sticking to the same boring diet for several months. In fact, the plan incorporates multiple diets that can be changed every week and combines this with exercise so that you will lose fat, not lean muscle. With this moderate but effective weight loss plan you can lose on average 100 g (4 oz) of body fat per day which means you can lose about 7 kg (15 lbs.) of fat in just 10 weeks.

WHAT DO YOU NEED TO BE HEALTHY?

When I have asked different people the question "what do you think you need to do to be healthy?", almost all mention "not overeating" and "not smoking" which is entirely correct, but not many will mention "eating well" or "eating healthy foods". Some will include "doing some regular exercise" or "avoiding excess **alcohol**" in their reply. Very few will mention "not being overweight", "not having too much abdominal fat", or "getting sufficient sleep". Yet all of the above are important to health. And by health I not only mean remaining free from illness, but guarding against the risks of **chronic disease**, reduced mobility, and dementia later in life.

Let's think about what our everyday lives involve: At the most basic level we eat, we move, and we sleep. All these actions are needed for basic survival. Without appropriate foods supplying energy and essential nutrients we would waste away, become ill, and die. Without exercise, our immobilized muscles would wither away making us weak and unable to perform basic tasks needed for normal living. With insufficient sleep, we would feel tired, lethargic, and irritable, and life would become a chore. So, we must satisfy the body's needs for nutrition, physical activity, and sleep, but why stop there. Let's rephrase the original question. We should really be asking "what do we need to do to achieve and maintain **optimal health** throughout the lifespan?" because this is what can give us the best quality of life. Optimal health should be considered as a state of complete physical, mental, and social well-being and not merely the absence of illness, disease, or infirmity. The key word here is "optimal"; it is not just what we need to survive, but what we can do to attain the best possible health outcomes and enable us to improve our quality of life, not only in the present but also in the future. You will realize and appreciate the importance of this as you get older, just as I have! By being healthier, fitter, stronger, and more robust, we can lead more fulfilling and enjoyable lives, live independently for longer, and actually live longer.

THE OBESITY PROBLEM: IT'S NOT ALL ABOUT GENETICS

One of the major problems in developed countries is the **obesity** epidemic. In the USA, two in three people are now classed as being overweight or obese; in fact, almost 38% of the adult population are classed as obese, a trend that has been growing for the past three decades. The UK has the highest proportion of obese people in Europe at 27%. Being obese or just overweight increases the risk of developing chronic metabolic and cardiovascular diseases and dying at an earlier age. Being overweight is the major cause of type 2 diabetes and is also an important risk factor for coronary heart disease, **peripheral vascular disease**, dementia, and cancer. The **metabolic syndrome** is a term used by clinicians and scientists to describe the co-occurrence of several known cardiovascular disease risk factors, including insulin resistance, obesity, high blood cholesterol, and high blood pressure **(hypertension)**. All these risk factors are more prevalent in people who are carrying too much weight or an excess of fat, particularly around the waist (called **visceral fat**).

What the Science Tells Us About the Genetics of Obesity

To study the influence of genetics on the effects of overfeeding, identical twins were investigated. In one study, identical (monozygotic) twins were submitted to an energy surplus of 1,000 **kcal**/day (4.2 **MJ**/day) six days per week for 100 days. The excess energy intake over the entire period was 84,000 kcal (353 MJ). The average gain in body mass was 8.1 kg, but considerable variation between individuals was evident. The range of weight gain was 4.3 to 13.3 kg, and the variation between 12 different pairs of twins was more than three times greater than the variation within pairs (which averaged 1.8 kg), suggesting an important genetic component (figure 1.1a). The variation between pairs was even greater for changes in visceral fat, indicating that the site of storage is also partly genetically determined.

Similarly, when seven pairs of identical twins completed a weight loss protocol by exercising over a period of 93 days without increasing energy intake, more variation occurred between pairs than within pairs. The energy deficit was estimated to be 58,000 kcal (244 MJ), and the mean body-weight loss was 5.0 kg. The range of weight loss, however, was 1.0 to 8.0 kg whereas the average difference within pairs was only 1.4 kg as illustrated in figure 1.1b.

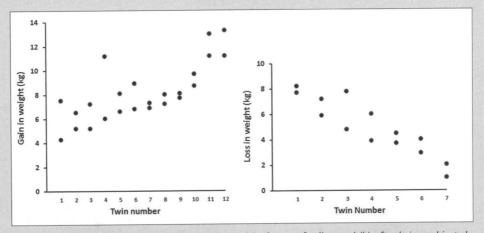

Figure 1.1: Changes in body mass in identical twins (a) after overfeeding and (b) after being subjected to a negative energy balance by exercise. Considerably more variation occurred between pairs than within pairs, strongly suggesting a genetic component in the regulation of body mass. Data from Bouchard et al. (1990) and Bouchard et al. (1994).

Our tendency to put on weight is partly due to our behaviors with regard to eating too much, exercising too little, and not getting good quality sleep, but a significant portion of the variation in body-fat levels between individuals is genetically determined, though not quite as much as you might think. Perhaps 25% to 40% of the fat stored in our body is the result of our genes that influence both our metabolic efficiency and, at least to some degree, our preferred behaviors (e.g., whether we enjoy or hate exercise, whether we need relatively little or lots of sleep to function well, and whether we are "night owls" or "morning people"). Genetic factors also determine the susceptibility to gaining or losing body fat in response to dietary energy intake and exercise.

Several classic early studies (see the sidebar) have demonstrated a genetic factor in the development of obesity. This link has been confirmed by large scale studies that have analyzed the contribution of potential genetic and environmental risk factors, identified at the molecular level, to the patterns and causes of obesity in defined populations (known as **molecular epidemiology studies**), and now more than 250 **genes** are believed to have the potential to influence body fatness.

Several of the risk factors known to be associated with weight gain, such as a low **resting metabolic rate**, high reliance on **carbohydrate** metabolism, and a lower level of spontaneous physical activity, almost certainly have a genetic basis. But the relative contribution of genetic versus environmental (lifestyle-related) factors is still a subject of debate. You can't do anything to modify your genes, but you can decide to adopt behaviors that will reduce your risk of becoming overweight. These behaviors include your eating, exercising, and sleeping habits (figure 1.2) as will be explained in detail later in this book.

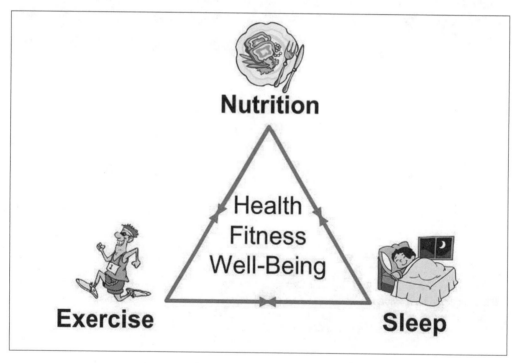

Figure 1.2: Our nutrition, exercise, and sleep behaviors have important influences on our health, well-being, and longevity. Note the bidirectional arrows in the triangle indicating that (a) nutrition and sleep affect our ability to exercise, (b) nutrition and exercise affect how we sleep and (c) exercise and sleep influence our nutrition (appetite and food choices).

TAKING CONTROL

So, we can't control our genetics, but we can control how we live and what we eat. Nourishing our bodies by eating a healthy diet, maintaining an equal balance between energy intake and energy expenditure, not smoking, and doing some form of regular exercise are the most important things you can do to prevent the accumulation of body fat and the development of chronic health conditions like type 2 diabetes, heart disease, cancer, and dementia. Getting sufficient amounts of good quality sleep is also now recognized as having an important influence on our eating habits, our risk of chronic diseases, as well as our mood, and mental health.

Research shows that in order to maintain a healthy weight, eating appropriate amounts of a healthy diet is very important. After all, you can take in calories from food and beverages much faster than you can burn them off with metabolism and exercise! The US Office of Disease Prevention and Health Promotion recommends eating a variety of fruits and vegetables, whole grains, low-fat dairy, and lean sources of protein, while limiting sodium, added sugars, alcohol and fats, particularly saturated and trans fats. This is sound advice, but the devil is in the details; for example, do you know what *trans* fats are, or what the main sources of sodium in the diet are, or what amounts of sugar or alcohol are considered to be too much? After all, in reality we eat foods, not nutrients. Knowing what you are eating and understanding the consequences of consuming excess amounts of certain nutrients or food groups can empower you in selecting foods from the myriad of options displayed on the supermarket shelves. These important issues are covered in the next three chapters.

Regular physical activity can also help with weight control and allow us to enjoy eating well without going over the calorie limit, which would lead to putting on body fat and body weight. Exercise itself brings health benefits that will enhance your quality of life and reduce the risk of many health problems and potential disabilities that can develop as we get older. Another problem with aging is that we tend to lose muscle mass (the medics call this **sarcopenia**), which means that we become weaker and at some point may be no longer able to function independently (for example, you need a certain amount of leg strength just to get up from an armchair or the toilet!). Regular exercise, and in particular **resistance exercise**, together with appropriate ingestion of dietary protein, can help to maintain muscle mass across the lifespan. Chapter 9 describes how your body adapts to doing regular moderate exercise, and the various health benefits that ensue. In short, some regular moderate exercise in combination with good nutrition can help you stay healthy, live longer, and be happier. Knowing what types of exercise are best, and understanding how your body adapts to exercise, how much is needed for health benefits, and just how many calories you are burning in different activities will allow you to decide what is best for you and what is easiest to fit into your normal daily routine.

Poor sleep quality (e.g., regular awakenings during the night, sleeping lightly or sleeping for less than seven hours per night) can be detrimental to both your short-term and long-term health. Poor sleep quality will make you feel tired during the day time, will negatively affect your mood, and contribute to the development of mental health problems. But don't despair; there are several things you can do to help you sleep better, and these are explained in chapter 10.

Another very important aspect of a healthy lifestyle is having good mental well-being. This is sometimes taken to mean that you are simply free from depression or mental illness, but again, just like with health in general, we should be aiming to have optimal mental well-being (i.e., feeling as good as we can be) as part of our overall aim to have optimal health. Having good mental well-being can be said to underpin all aspects of living healthily and not just managing and recovering from illness or coping with living with long-term illness conditions. Mental well-being encompasses our emotional, psychological, and social well-being, and it affects how we think, feel, and act. It also influences how we react to stress and cope with problems, how we communicate with others, and the decisions and choices that we make in our daily lives. Nurturing our brains through things that stimulate us to think, understand, solve problems, and promote our enjoyment of life (e.g., listening to music, watching a theater show or movie, reading a book, or playing a favorite sport) can also help us combat or prevent depression and other mental health problems that are sometimes associated with a chronic physical illness and aging. In some cases, good mental well-being can even prevent the onset or relapse of a physical or mental illness. For example, it is known that being able to cope well with stress can have a positive impact on delaying coronary heart disease and stroke. Being happy provides a great boost to mental well-being. For many people, happiness comes from knowing you are loved, valued, respected, or cared for by others and the enjoyment that comes from doing things we like such as being outdoors in good weather, going on holidays, playing with children or pets. Just being nice to others can make us feel good, too. More information about keeping our brains active and healthy can be found in chapter 12. Figure 1.3 summarizes the various components of a healthy lifestyle, and much of the content of this book is devoted to explaining how we can ensure that we include them in our lives to get as close as we can to the ideal of optimal health.

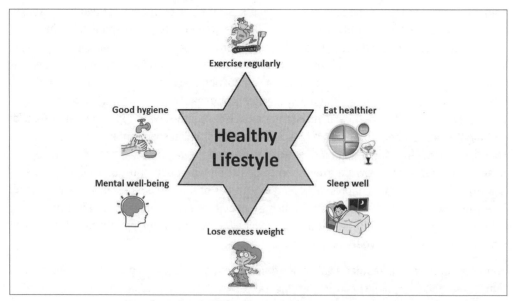

Figure 1.3: Components of a healthy lifestyle that can reduce our risk of disease and extend our longevity. If any of these components is missing, it is unlikely that we will attain optimal health (i.e., as good as it can be). This is not a comprehensive list. For example, avoiding drinking excess alcohol, practicing safe sex, and keeping well hydrated by drinking plenty of water could also be included.

Reading this book will help you to understand the science that underpins the advice and recommendations about a healthy lifestyle. Many people are at least slightly overweight and want to know how to lose weight effectively but with as little disruption to their normal lifestyle as possible. This book can help you with that too. Chapters 7 and 8 discuss the various ways in which you can lose body fat by dieting and exercising, respectively. Chapter 13 provides all the information you need to develop your own personalized weight loss plan involving a combination of multiple diets with a selection of suitable exercises that should see you lose about 7 kg (15 lbs.) of body fat in just 10 weeks. Example meal plans for the different weight loss diets are provided in chapter 14. Chapter 11 explains how to minimize your risk of picking up infections, and chapter 12 provides useful tips on how to maintain the health of your senses, tissues, and organs throughout your lifespan.

Each of the chapters that follow begins with a list of objectives that explain what you should learn from the chapter. These objectives can be used to preview the chapter and to check whether you have achieved the objectives after reading the chapter. As mentioned previously, key terms (in **bold**) are defined in the text, and these, as well as many other terms that may not be familiar to readers without a science background, are defined in the glossary. Chapters are organized to promote learning of concepts and ideas rather than simple memorization of facts and figures. The illustrations and tables used in each chapter help accomplish this goal, as do occasional sidebars, which provide more detailed, in-depth coverage of selected topics, or summarize some important guidelines. At the end of every chapter, a list of the key points reemphasizes the important messages that you should take away from each chapter. In-text citations (i.e., references to the published scientific literature) are not included so as not to interrupt the flow of the writing, but at the end of the book there is a list of selected reference sources that I have used to compile this book and for the reader who wants to delve into more detail. The appendices provide at-a-glance information on the **recommended dietary allowances** (RDAs) or their equivalents for adults in North America, the UK, Australia and New Zealand.

A NOTE ABOUT RELATIVE RISK

In this book you will read about many scientific studies that report the relative health risks of certain lifestyle behaviors, such as being sedentary, eating too much sugar and fat, smoking, drinking alcohol, etc. It is important to realize that the comparisons of risk are made relative to the average person who, for example does some exercise, consumes an average amount of sugar or fat, does not smoke or does not drink alcohol. It is not to say that the risk of health problems in these people with healthy habits is zero. Everyone has a certain degree of risk for a particular health problem like heart disease, type 2 diabetes, or cancer, but the risk of some diseases can be increased above the average by unhealthy lifestyle behaviors. Let's take alcohol as an example. A massive global study published in the Lancet in 2018 concluded that there is no safe level of alcohol consumption. In other words, drinking even one glass of wine or beer per day increases the risk of health problems such as cancer, injuries, and infectious diseases (see chapter 4 for an in-depth discussion of this topic). But the increased risk to health of having just one alcoholic beverage per day is only 0.5% and this would probably not dissuade people from having a daily glass of wine with their meal. Indeed, Prof David Spiegelhalter, Winton Professor for the Public Understanding of Risk at the University of Cambridge, UK, has sounded a note of caution about such findings. He has said, "Given the pleasure presumably associated with moderate drinking, claiming there is no safe level *(of drinking)* does not seem an argument for abstention." He added, "There is no safe level of driving, but the government does not recommend that people avoid driving." He finished with the comment, "Come to think of it, there is no safe level of living, but nobody would recommend abstention." Bear his comments in mind when you read about relative risk in this book. Of course, this does not apply to all potentially unhealthy lifestyle behaviors. Take smoking for example. Having just one cigarette per day has been reported to increase the risk of **coronary heart disease (CHD)** by over 50%, and that should be interpreted as a very good reason for not smoking at all. Some risks are bigger than others, and what decisions you make about changes to your current lifestyle should be well-informed ones that take into account the magnitude of any relative risk.

Key Points

- By being healthier, fitter, and stronger we can lead more fulfilling and enjoyable lives, live independently for longer, and actually live longer.

- Being obese or just overweight increases the risk of developing chronic metabolic and cardiovascular diseases and dying at an earlier age.

- Optimal health is a state of complete physical, mental, and social well-being and not merely the absence of illness, disease, or infirmity. Optimal health is not just what we need to survive but what we can do to attain the best possible health outcomes that will enable us to improve our quality of life, not only in the present, but also in the future.

- Our tendency to put on weight is partly due to our behaviors with regard to eating, exercising, and sleeping, but a significant portion of the variation in body-fat levels between individuals is genetically determined. We can't control our genetics, but we can control how we live and what we eat.

- Nourishing our bodies by eating a healthy diet, maintaining an equal balance between energy intake and energy expenditure, not smoking, and doing some form of regular exercise are the most important things you can do to reduce your risk of accumulating body fat, and developing chronic health conditions like type 2 diabetes, heart disease, cancer, and dementia.

- Exercise brings a variety of health benefits that will enhance your quality of life as you get older and reduce the risk of many health problems and potential disabilities. It may well help you live independently and healthily for longer.

- Getting sufficient amounts of good quality sleep also has an important influence on your eating habits and risk of chronic diseases as well as your mood and mental health.

- In addition to regular exercise, a healthy diet, good sleep quality, and other lifestyle behaviors can be employed to help maintain the health of your senses, tissues, and organ systems throughout the lifespan.

Chapter 2

Know What You Eat

Objectives

After reading this chapter, you should:

- Know the main components of a normal Western diet

- Know the main classes of nutrients

- Understand the different types of carbohydrates (monosaccharides, disaccharides, polysaccharides, and dietary fiber) and their main functions in the body

- Understand the functions of fats (lipids), the differences between saturated and unsaturated fatty acids, and the differences between *cis* and **trans** fatty acids

- Know the functions of protein in the body

- Understand the general role of water in the human body

- Know the different classes and the general role of micronutrients in the human body

If you want to have a healthy diet and before you even think about restricting dietary energy intake to lose weight, it helps to know something about the nature of the food you eat. This will help you to decide which type of diet is best for you. It will also help to ensure that you choose healthy options and understand why you should never cut out any major food group or major nutrient from your diet whether trying to lose weight or simply maintain your current weight. It should also help you understand why "a healthy diet" is not just about the number of calories you eat, and that other aspects of the diet, such as the amount and quality of protein, the amount and type of fat you consume, and vitamin and mineral needs must also be considered in order to eat healthily.

WHAT ARE NUTRIENTS?

The food that we eat contains **nutrients** and is part of our **nutrition**. Nutrition is often defined as the total of the processes of ingestion (eating and drinking), **digestion** (breaking down), **absorption** (moving nutrients from the gut into the blood), and metabolism (processing) of food, and the subsequent assimilation of nutrient materials into the **tissues** and organs. A **nutrient** is a substance found in food that performs one or more specific functions in the body.

The body requires substantial amounts of certain nutrients every day, whereas other nutrients may be ingested only in small amounts. Nutrients for which the daily intake is more than a few grams are usually referred to as **macronutrients**. Macronutrients are carbohydrates, fats, proteins, and water. Nutrients that are needed in only small amounts (less than 1 g/day) are referred to as **micronutrients**. Most nutrients are micronutrients, and they consist of **vitamins**, **minerals**, and **trace elements**. Many micronutrients (including all of the vitamins) are essential for our health, and deficiencies result in disease states (e.g., **scurvy** when vitamin C intake is inadequate, and **anemia** when iron intake is inadequate). There are also some plant-derived micronutrients that are called **phytonutrients**, and although not considered **essential nutrients**, many may be needed for optimal health. The latter is a term that is referred to repeatedly in this book and for good reason. Everyone's aim should be to have the best health that is achievable, and this is more than just aiming to avoid diseases caused by inadequate or excessive intake of certain nutrients.

This chapter discusses the properties and functions of various components of the diet – including the macronutrients, micronutrients and phytonutrients – and the subsequent chapter explains why we have **recommended daily intakes** of various nutrients and what these are.

FUNCTIONS OF NUTRIENTS

Food provides nutrients that have one or more physiological or biochemical functions in the body. Nutrients are usually divided into six different categories: carbohydrates, fats, proteins, water, vitamins, and minerals.

The functions of nutrients are often divided into three main categories:

- *Promotion of growth and development.* This function is mainly performed by **proteins**. Muscle, soft tissues, and organs consist largely of protein, and protein is required for any tissue growth or repair (e.g., following injury or illness). In addition, calcium and phosphorus are important building blocks for the bones and teeth.

- *Provision of energy.* This function is predominantly performed by **carbohydrates** and **fats**. Although protein can also function as a fuel, its contribution to energy expenditure is usually small, and energy provision is not a primary function of protein.

- *Regulation of metabolism.* Nutrients used in this function are vitamins, minerals, trace elements, and proteins. **Enzymes** are proteins that play an important role as **catalysts**, allowing metabolic reactions to proceed at much faster rates than they would spontaneously. An example of an enzyme is lipase, which breaks down the storage form of fat (known as **triglyceride**) in white **adipose tissue** and muscles. Another important protein, though not an enzyme, is **hemoglobin**, which is found in **erythrocytes** (red blood **cells**). Erythrocytes are essential for the transport of oxygen from the lungs to the tissues, and the hemoglobin **molecule** acts as an oxygen carrier. The hemoglobin molecule is a complex of protein (**polypeptide** chains) and nonprotein groups (in this case porphyrin rings) that hold iron (to which oxygen molecules can be bound). For the synthesis of this complex, other enzymes, minerals and vitamins are required. Thus, the interaction between vitamins, minerals, and proteins in the regulation of metabolism can be quite complicated.

Categories of Nutrients

Macronutrients are present in relatively large amounts in the human diet, whereas micronutrients are present in minuscule amounts.

The macronutrients are:

- Carbohydrate

- Fat

- Protein

- Water

The micronutrients are:

- Vitamins

- Minerals (including the trace elements)

CARBOHYDRATE

The name carbohydrate indicates molecules built of carbon (carbo, C) and hydrogen (hydrate; water, H_2O). The general formula of a carbohydrate molecule is CH_2O. In other words, the ratio of carbon, hydrogen, and oxygen is 1:2:1 in all carbohydrates. A carbohydrate can be one or a combination of many of these CH_2O units, and this is often written as $(CH_2O)n$, where n is the number of CH_2O units. For example, in **glucose** (which is the sugar in our blood), n = 6; indicating that a molecule of glucose contains 6 carbon **atoms**, 12 hydrogen atoms, and 6 oxygen atoms and has the chemical formula $C_6H_{12}O_6$. Sugars like glucose, **fructose** (fruit sugar) and **sucrose** (cane sugar) are collectively known as **saccharides** meaning "sugar" or "sweet". The chemical structure of glucose is depicted in figure 2.1. Glucose is formed during photosynthesis in plants, and we obtain almost all our carbohydrates from plants. Carbohydrates, however, can be found in all living cells and are an important source of energy. In plants, the main storage form of carbohydrate is a glucose polymer called starch, whereas in animals its equivalent is called **glycogen** (both are illustrated in figure 2.1). These large molecules which may contain thousands of linked glucose molecules are called **polysaccharides**.

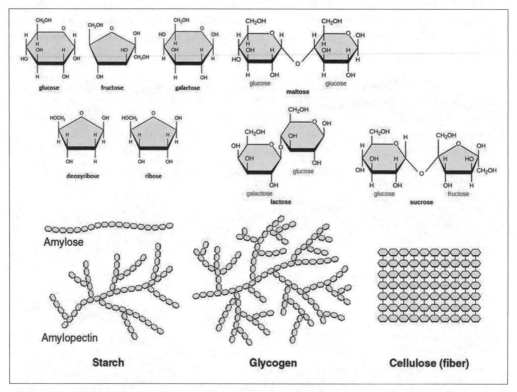

*Figure 2.1: Carbohydrates and their structures. Human nutrition includes three 6-carbon **monosaccharides** (glucose, fructose, and galactose), two 5-carbon monosaccharides (deoxyribose and ribose which found in DNA and RNA, respectively) and three **disaccharides** (maltose, sucrose, and lactose). Glucose polymers (polysaccharides), starch, glycogen and cellulose (an indigestible plant fiber) are a series of coupled glucose molecules in the form of long single chains or larger branched, tree-like structures.*

Carbohydrate-rich foods include bread, cereals, corn, grains, potatoes, pasta, and rice, which contain mostly starches and fiber, but a large percentage of carbohydrate intake in the Western world comes from sugar (for examples of carbohydrate sources see table 2.1 and photo 2.1). The most important carbohydrates in our diet are glucose, fructose, sucrose, short-chain glucose polymers **(maltodextrins)**, and starch **(amylopectin)**. Carbohydrates are typically divided into monosaccharides, disaccharides, polysaccharides, and **fiber**. The different classes of carbohydrate and some typical examples are shown in table 2.2.

Table 2.1: Types of carbohydrates and their food sources

Carbohydrate	Carbohydrate-rich foods
Sugars (simple carbohydrates)	Fruit juices, fruits, sweetened cereals and baked goods, candy, sweets, soft drinks, energy drinks, sports drinks, beet and cane sugar, brown sugar, table sugar, maple syrup, honey, treacle
Starches	Cereal products, corn, potatoes, sweet potatoes, pasta, macaroni, rice, bread
Fiber	Whole-grain cereals and breads, oats, dried beans and peas, fruits, and vegetables such as cabbage, zucchini (courgette), celery, spinach and salad leaves

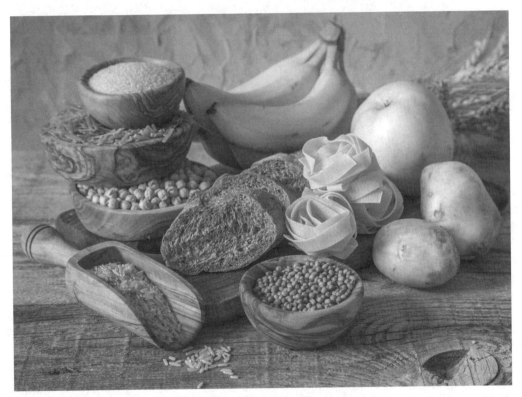

Photo 2.1: A variety of high-carbohydrate foods

Table 2.2: Classes of carbohydrates

Carbohydrate	Examples and common sources
Monosaccharides	Glucose (grape sugar, blood sugar)
	Fructose (fruit sugar)
	Galactose (brain sugar)
Disaccharides	Maltose (malt sugar)
	Sucrose (table sugar, cane sugar, or beet sugar)
	Lactose (milk sugar)
	Trehalose (mushroom sugar, shrimp and insect sugar)
	Isomaltulose (sucrose substitute; small amounts found in honey)
Polysaccharides	Maltodextrin (sports drinks)
	Oligosaccharides (most vegetables)
	Starch (main plant polysaccharide)
	Amylose
	Amylopectin
	Glycogen (liver, muscle; main animal polysaccharide)
Fiber	Cellulose
	β-glucans
	Gums
	Pectins
	Hemicellulose
	Resistant starch (some forms)

THE SIMPLE SUGARS: MONOSACCHARIDES AND DISACCHARIDES

The monosaccharides represent the basic unit of a carbohydrate, and three monosaccharides—glucose, fructose, and galactose—are present in our diet. Glucose is often called dextrose or grape sugar, and fructose is commonly referred to as fruit sugar. Galactose is usually present in only small amounts in our diet, but relatively large amounts are released after the digestion of the disaccharide milk sugar (lactose). The monosaccharides glucose, fructose, and galactose have a similar structure, the same chemical formula ($C_6H_{12}O_6$), and an identical number of carbon, hydrogen, and oxygen atoms, but slightly different carbon–hydrogen–oxygen linkages (see figure 2.1) give these molecules different biochemical characteristics. Glucose is the only carbohydrate that can be oxidized in the cells of the body. Fructose and galactose must be converted into glucose before they can be oxidized. The conversion of fructose and galactose into glucose occurs in the liver at relatively slow rates.

Disaccharides are a combination of two monosaccharides. Disaccharides and monosaccharides are collectively called sugars, simple sugars, or simple carbohydrates. The most important disaccharides are sucrose, **lactose**, and **maltose (figure 2.1)**. Sucrose, which is mainly derived from cane or beet, is by far the most abundant dietary disaccharide and currently provides about 20% to 25% of the daily energy intake in the Western world. Sucrose is composed of a glucose molecule linked to a fructose molecule. Foods that contain sucrose include beet and cane sugar, brown sugar, table sugar, maple syrup, treacle, and honey. Lactose, or milk sugar, is found in milk and consists of glucose and galactose. Maltose, or malt sugar, is present in beer, cereals, and germinating seeds and consists of two linked glucose molecules. Maltose is present in only relatively small amounts in our diet.

THE COMPLEX CARBOHYDRATES: OLIGOSACCHARIDES AND POLYSACCHARIDES

Oligosaccharides are three to nine monosaccharides combined and can be found in most vegetables. Polysaccharides contain 10 or more monosaccharides combined in one molecule. Polysaccharides can contain 10 to 20 monosaccharides (often referred to as glucose polymers, or maltodextrins) or up to thousands of monosaccharides (starch, glycogen, or cellulose, and other forms of fiber). Starch, glycogen, and cellulose (figure 2.1) are the predominant forms of polysaccharides. Starch and glycogen are the storage forms of carbohydrate in plants and animals, respectively, whereas cellulose is a structural component of plant cell walls.

Starch, or **complex carbohydrate**, is present in seeds, rice, corn, and various grains that are used to make bread, breakfast cereals, pasta, and pastries. Starch is the storage form of carbohydrates in plants. There are two structurally different forms of starch known as amylopectin and **amylose**. Amylopectin is a highly branched molecule consisting of a large number of glucose molecules, whereas amylose is a long chain of glucose molecules (200–4,000) twisted into a coil. Starches with a relatively large amount of amylopectin are rapidly digested and absorbed, whereas those with high amylose content are digested more slowly. Most starches contain both amylose and amylopectin, and the relative contribution determines the properties of the food. For example, the quantity of amylose in rice kernels has a big effect on the properties of cooked rice kernels. That is, boiled or fried rice with little amylose will be sticky and soft, whereas rice with a large amount of amylose will be harder and much less sticky. Approximately 50% of our total daily carbohydrate intake is in the form of starch.

Glycogen is the storage form of carbohydrate in animals, including humans. It is stored mostly in the liver (80 to 100 g) and in skeletal muscles (300 to 900 g), and its structure is similar to amylopectin. It is very important as a fuel for prolonged, intensive exercise. However, it is not an important source of carbohydrate in our diet.

Fiber used to be known as roughage. It comprises the edible parts of plants that are not broken down and absorbed in the human **gastrointestinal tract**. Fiber consists of structural plant polysaccharides such as **cellulose**. The human small intestine has no enzymes to break down these polysaccharides (and so they cannot be digested here; some digestion can occur, however, in the large intestine due to the presence of large numbers of bacteria). Although cellulose may be the most common type of fiber, there are many other types of fiber including gums, hemicellulose, β-glucans, and pectin.

Dietary fiber is also often divided into soluble and **insoluble fiber**. **Soluble fiber** dissolves well in **water**, whereas insoluble does not. Both types of fiber are present in plant foods. Some plants contain more soluble fiber, and others have more insoluble fiber. For example, plums have a thick skin covering a juicy pulp. The skin is an example of an insoluble fiber source, whereas the pulp contains soluble fiber sources. Soluble fiber undergoes metabolic processing through fermentation by bacteria that are present in our large intestine, yielding end products such as **short-chain fatty acids** that can be absorbed and have broad, significant health effects. Good sources of fiber are listed in table 2.3, and several can be seen in photo 2.2.

Table 2.3: Dietary fiber and food sources

Type of fiber	Food sources
Soluble fiber	Legumes (peas, soybeans, and other beans)
	Oats, rye, and barley
	Some fruits and fruit juices (particularly prune juice, plums, and berries)
	Certain vegetables such as broccoli and carrots
	Root vegetables such as potatoes, sweet potatoes, and onions (the skins of these vegetables are sources of insoluble fiber)
Insoluble fiber	Whole-grain foods
	Bran
	Nuts and seeds
	Vegetables such as green beans, cabbage, cauliflower, zucchini (courgette), and celery
	Skins of some fruits, including grapes, plums, and tomatoes

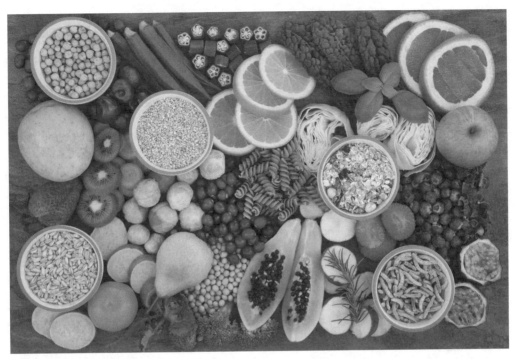

Photo 2.2: A variety of high-fiber foods

FUNCTIONS OF CARBOHYDRATE

All carbohydrates contain about 4 kilocalories (kcal) or 17 kilojoules (kJ) of energy per gram and they play an important role in energy provision for many cells of the body but particularly for those in the brain, nerves, muscles, and blood. Energy is considered in detail in chapter 5. Carbohydrates are the predominant fuel used during moderate to high intensity exercise. Carbohydrate is stored in relatively small amounts as glycogen in muscle and liver and can become completely depleted after prolonged strenuous exercise. This can result in fatigue, and in marathon running it is commonly referred to as "hitting the wall". Ingestion of carbohydrate will rapidly replenish carbohydrate stores, and excess carbohydrate from food is converted into fat and stored in adipose tissue.

In normal conditions, blood glucose is the only fuel used by the nerve cells of the brain and spinal cord (known collectively as the central nervous system). After prolonged **fasting** (about three days), **ketone bodies** are produced by the liver (from **fatty acids**), which can serve as an alternative fuel for the central nervous system. The central nervous system functions optimally when the blood glucose concentration is maintained above 4 **millimoles** per liter (mmol/L). Normal blood glucose concentration is about 5 mmol/L (equivalent to 0.9 g/L). At concentrations below 3 mmol/L, symptoms of **hypoglycemia** (low blood sugar) may develop, including weakness, hunger, dizziness, and shivering. Prolonged and severe hypoglycemia can result in unconsciousness, coma, and irreversible brain damage. Therefore, tight control of blood glucose concentration is crucial. Blood glucose also provides fuel for the red and **white blood cells**. New dietary guidelines for children and adults state that an intake of at least 130 g of carbohydrate each day should be achieved. This recommendation is based on the minimum amount of carbohydrate needed to produce sufficient glucose for the brain to function. Most people, however, consume far more than 130 g per day, and excessive carbohydrate intake contributes to the development of obesity.

The functions of fiber are determined by whether the fiber is classified as soluble or insoluble. Insoluble fiber has its effects mainly in the large intestine or **colon**, where it adds bulk and helps to retain water, resulting in a softer and larger stool. Fiber decreases the **transit time** of fecal matter through the intestines. So, a diet high in insoluble fiber is most often used in treatment of constipation resulting from poor dietary habits and is known to promote bowel regularity. On the other hand, soluble fiber lowers blood cholesterol concentrations and normalizes blood glucose and both of these actions are good for our health.

In addition, most soluble fiber is highly fermentable, and fermentable fibers help maintain healthy populations of friendly bacteria (our gut normally contains at least 1 kg of bacteria). Besides producing necessary short-chain fatty acids, these bacteria play an important role in tandem with the immune system by preventing pathogenic (disease-causing) bacteria from surviving in the intestinal tract. Fiber also has several effects on nutrient digestion and absorption. It reduces the rate of gastric emptying and can influence the absorption of various micronutrients. Fiber increases food bulk, which increases satiety (the sensation of feeling full and satisfied after a meal), and it can reduce energy intake by 100 to 200 kcal/day (400 to 800 kJ/day). Fiber is associated with various health effects that will be discussed in more detail in chapter 4. For most people, the recommended intake would be 20 to 35 g of fiber per day, but the average fiber intake in Western countries is only 10 to 15 g per day.

FAT

Fats or **lipids** are compounds that are soluble in organic liquids such as acetone, ether, and chloroform but have very poor solubility in water. The term *lipid*, derived from the Greek word *lipos* (meaning fat), is a general name for oils, fats, waxes, and related compounds. Oils are liquid at room temperature, whereas fats are solid. For simplicity, and to avoid confusion, the term "fat" is used throughout this book. Fat molecules contain the same structural elements as carbohydrates, namely: carbon, hydrogen, and oxygen but fats have little oxygen relative to carbon and hydrogen. For example, a common fat in the body is the **triglyceride** called tripalmitin which has the chemical formula $C_{51}H_{98}O_6$ meaning it contains 51 carbons, 98 hydrogens, and only 6 oxygens.

The three classes of fats most commonly recognized are simple fats, compound fats, and derived fats (see table 2.4). An overview of various fats and their structure is provided in figure 2.2.

Table 2.4: The three main classes of fats

Fat class	Fat type	Examples
Simple fats	Neutral fat	Triglyceride (triacylglycerol)
	Waxes	Beeswax
Compound fats	Phospholipids	Cephalins, lecithins, lipositols
	Glycolipids	Cerebrosides, gangliosides
	Lipoproteins	Chylomicrons, low-density lipoproteins (LDL), high-density lipoproteins (HDL)
Derived fats	Fatty acids	Linoleic acid, palmitic acid, oleic acid, stearic acid
	Steroids	Bile acids, cholesterol, cortisol, estrogen, testosterone, vitamin D
	Hydrocarbons	Terpenes

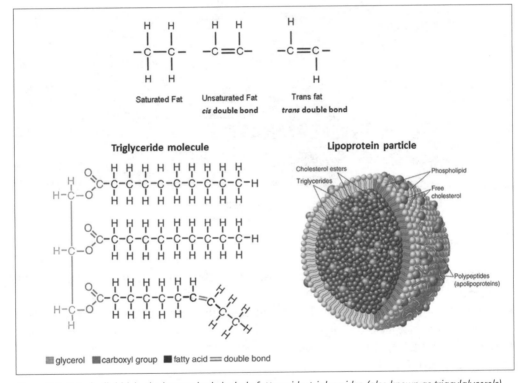

Figure 2.2: Fats (or lipids) in the human body include fatty acids, triglycerides (also known as triacylglycerols), lipoproteins, and phospholipids. Fatty acids differ in their chain length (number of carbons) and the number and location of double bonds. In a triglyceride molecule, three fatty acids are linked to a molecule of glycerol via their carboxylic acid groups. The upper part of the figure illustrates the bonding arrangements in the hydrocarbon chains of saturated, unsaturated, and trans fats.

TRIGLYCERIDES AND FATTY ACIDS

Triglycerides, also known as **triacylglycerols**, are the most abundant dietary fats consumed by humans. Common food sources include fatty cuts of meat (e.g., beef, pork, lamb) and poultry (e.g., chicken, duck, goose), animal liver, oily fish like mackerel and salmon, egg yolk, cream, cheese, butter, margarine, oils, nuts, and avocado. Many processed foods including ready meals and sauces plus any foods cooked in oil like French fries and fish in batter tend to be high in fat. Some of the less healthy high-fat foods (often called junk food) are shown in photo 2.3, and some healthier sources of dietary fat can be seen in photo 2.4.

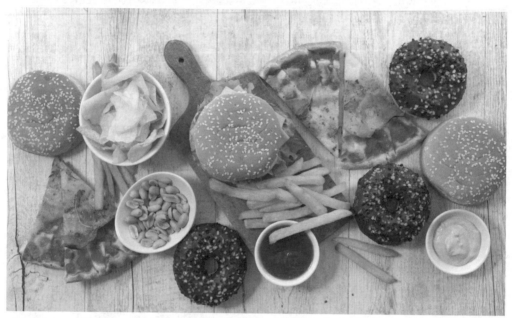

Photo 2.3: A variety of not-so-healthy high-fat foods (junk foods)

Triglycerides are composed of a three-carbon glycerol backbone linked to three **fatty acids**. Fatty acids have a **carboxylic acid group** (COOH) at one end of the molecule and a methyl **group (CH$_3$)** at the other end, separated by a hydrocarbon chain of repeating CH$_2$ units that can vary in length. The carboxylic acid group can bind to the 3-carbon molecule **glycerol** ($C_3H_8O_3$) to form a mono-, di-, or triglyceride (see figure 2.2). Simple triglycerides are those in which the molecule of glycerol is combined with three molecules of one particular fatty acid. For example, the triglyceride called tripalmitin, $C_3H_5(OCOC_{15}H_{31})_3$ is composed of a glycerol backbone linked to three molecules of palmitic acid, $C_{15}H_{31}COOH$.

Triglycerides differ in their fatty acid composition. In humans, the chain length of the fatty acids typically varies from C14 to C24, although shorter or longer chains may occur. Fatty acids with a chain length of C8 or C10 are **medium-chain fatty acids (MCFAs)**, and those with a chain length of C6 or less are **short-chain fatty acids (SCFAs)**. The most abundant fatty acids are the long-chain fatty acids (LCFAs), which have a chain length of C12 or more. Of the long-chain fatty acids, **palmitic acid** (C16) and **oleic acid** (C18, one double bond) are the most abundant. Fatty

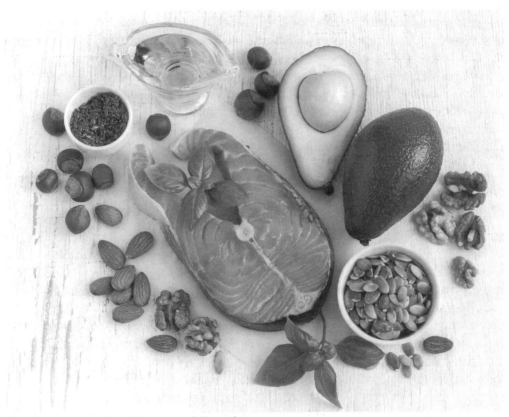

Photo 2.4: A variety of healthier sources of dietary fat

acids with no double bonds in their hydrocarbon chains are called **saturated fatty acids** (SFAs). Those with one or more double bonds are **unsaturated fatty acids (UFAs)**.

Monounsaturated fatty acids (MUFAs) have one double bond within the hydrocarbon chain. Typically, plant sources rich in monounsaturated fatty acids (e.g., canola oil, olive oil, and safflower and sunflower oils) are liquid at room temperature. Monounsaturated fatty acids, including the most common one, oleic acid, are important components of cell membranes.

The **polyunsaturated fatty acids** (PUFAs) have two or more double bonds and can be roughly divided into two categories: *n*-3 and *n*-6 fatty acids (also known as omega-3 and omega-6 fatty acids because they always have one double bond located three and six carbon atoms away from the methyl end of the fatty acid molecule, respectively). *n*-3 PUFAs tend to be highly unsaturated and include α-linolenic acid, eicosapentaenoic acid, docosapentaenoic acid, and docosahexaenoic acid. Humans cannot synthesize α-**linolenic acid**, and it is considered to be an essential nutrient as a lack of it results in neurological abnormalities and poor growth. It is also the precursor for synthesis of eicosapentaenoic acid (EPA) and docosahexaenoic acid (DHA). EPA is the precursor of *n*-3 eicosanoids, which are signaling molecules that have been shown to have beneficial effects in limiting **inflammation** and preventing coronary heart disease, arrhythmias, and thrombosis. The most important *n*-6 PUFAs are linoleic acid, γ-linolenic acid, and arachidonic acid. Humans cannot synthesize **linoleic acid**, and a lack of it results in the development of a scaly skin rash and reduced growth. Linoleic acid is also the precursor to arachidonic acid, which is used to produce many different **eicosanoids** that influence inflammation, allergy, fever, immune function, pain perception, cell growth, blood pressure, and tissue blood flow. Linoleic acid is also a component of cell membranes and is important in intracellular signaling pathways. n-6 PUFAs also play critical roles in the normal functions of the epithelial cells that line the gut, respiratory and genitourinary tracts. All the fatty acids mentioned above have a so-called *cis* configuration, which refers to the arrangement of the double bond (see figure 2.2). Fatty acids that have a *trans* configuration are called the *trans fatty* acids.

Trans Fats

Trans fats are fats that contain unsaturated fatty acids and that have at least one double bond in the *trans* configuration rather than the usual *cis* configuration. The difference between *cis* and *trans* is that the two H atoms are on the same side of the double bond *(cis)*, compared to being on opposite sides *(trans)* as illustrated in figure 2.2. This may not seem like much of a difference, but it affects the shapes of the molecules. In turn, this makes the chemical properties of *trans* fatty acids more similar to that of saturated fatty acids rather than that of *cis* unsaturated, double-bond-containing fatty acids. Fatty acids containing a *trans* double bond have the potential for closer packing together, and when incorporated into membranes, it results in decreased mobility and fluidity which can impair some cell functions. The *trans* fatty acid content in foods tends to be higher in foods containing hydrogenated oils. Production of hydrogenated oils and fats increased steadily until the 1960s as processed vegetable fats replaced animal fats in the United States and other Western countries. These more saturated fats have a higher melting point, which makes them attractive for baking and extends their shelf life. Unlike other dietary fats, *trans* fats are neither essential nor salubrious and, in fact, the consumption of *trans* fats increases the risk of coronary heart disease. Current dietary guidelines recommend keeping the intake of *trans* fats to a minimum (see chapter 4 for further details).

CHOLESTEROL, PHOSPHOLIPIDS, AND LIPOPROTEINS

Cholesterol is a type of fat found in the cell membranes of all animal tissues, and it is transported in the blood **plasma**. Cholesterol also aids in the manufacture of bile (which is stored in the gallbladder and helps digest fats), is important for the metabolism of fat soluble vitamins, and is the major precursor for the synthesis of vitamin D and various steroid hormones (e.g., cortisol, testosterone, estrogen). Most of the cholesterol in our bodies is synthesized in the liver with a relatively small proportion coming from the diet. Most cholesterol in the blood is found in lipoprotein particles. Total levels of cholesterol in the blood plasma are normally about 5 mmol/L. More than this is considered unhealthy as it increases the risk of coronary heart disease. Blood cholesterol can be lowered by changes to diet and exercise habits and by drugs called statins, which inhibit the synthesis of cholesterol by the liver.

Phospholipids are a class of fats that are a major component of all cell membranes. They can line up and arrange themselves into two parallel layers, called a phospholipid bilayer. This layer makes up your cell membranes and is critical to a cell's ability to function. Each phospholipid molecules generally consists of two hydrophobic (water hating) fatty acid "tails" and a hydrophilic (water loving) "head" containing a phosphate (PO_4) group. Phospholipids are also found in lipoprotein particles, and it is their presence that allows the particles to be soluble in water

Triglycerides found in the blood plasma are usually incorporated into the core of a lipoprotein (figure 2.2) with phospholipids, cholesterol, and **apolipoproteins** surrounding it. Apoprotein is a general name given to a protein that is combined with another type of molecule, and apolipoproteins are proteins that combine with lipids (fats) to form a complex as in the various lipoprotein particles. Various plasma lipoproteins differ in their density, triglyceride content, and cholesterol content, but they also fulfill different functions. Examples of such lipoproteins are **chylomicrons** (these are produced as fats and are absorbed from the gut after eating a fatty meal), low-density lipoproteins (LDLs), and high-density lipoproteins (HDLs). The LDLs are larger particles than the HDLs and contain a higher proportion of triglyceride and cholesterol and a smaller proportion of protein. LDL is usually referred to as "bad" cholesterol because it deposits its cholesterol on the walls of arteries contributing to the development of **arteriosclerosis** (also known as atherosclerosis) and **coronary heart disease**. In contrast, an important function of HDL is to remove such fatty deposits from blood vessel walls. Therefore, a useful measure of a healthy blood lipid profile is the HDL/LDL ratio (this is simply the plasma concentration of HDL divided by the concentration of LDL). A high value is good, but a low value is a risk factor for cardiovascular disease.

FUNCTIONS OF FATS

Fats contain approximately 9 kcal of energy per gram (37 kJ/g), making it the most energy dense of the macronutrients. Fats are an important energy source for many cells of the body, but especially for muscle fibers during prolonged exercise. Large amounts of fat can be stored as triglyceride in the body, mainly around the organs (visceral fat) and directly below the skin (subcutaneous fat), from which it is mobilized and transported as fatty acids in the blood to the tissues and organs that use it. These storage depots of fat are known collectively as white adipose tissue with each cell (adipocyte) containing a large globule of triglyceride fat surrounded by a thin layer of **cytoplasm**. Skeletal muscle also contains its own directly accessible store of fat (intramuscular triglyceride) which is used as a fuel for exercise. Fats have many other important functions, including the following:

- Some body fat is essential for physiological functioning. It is found in bone marrow, the heart, kidneys, intestines, liver, lungs, muscles, spleen, and fat-rich tissues of the central nervous system. Essential fat for men and women (as a percentage of body weight) is approximately 3% and 12%, respectively. In women, essential fat is higher because it includes fat in the breasts, hips and pelvis for reproduction. Fat protects vital organs such as the heart, liver, spleen, kidneys, brain, and spinal cord. A layer of adipose tissue covers these organs to protect them against trauma.

- The intake of fat-soluble vitamins A, D, E, and K and carotenoids depends on daily fat intake, and fats provide the transport medium in the body.

- Phospholipids and cholesterol are important constituents of cell membranes.

- Cholesterol is also an important precursor in the formation of bile and is itself an important component of bile.

- Cholesterol is a precursor for important hormones, in particular steroids such as testosterone and estrogen.

- Linoleic acid plays an important role in the formation of eicosanoids, hormone-like substances formed in cells with a regulatory function. Eicosanoids play a role in the control of many bodily functions including blood pressure, inflammation, immune function and cell growth.

- Fat often makes food tastier and more attractive. It carries many aromatic substances and makes food creamier and more appetizing.

FATS AS FUEL

Stored fat is the body's main form of energy reserves. Fat is accumulated for later use when excess dietary energy is consumed, and fat decreases when more energy is burned than is consumed. Visceral fat wraps around organs like a blanket, and when in excess it becomes infiltrated with white blood cells, which contributes to inflammation. This inflammation is associated with higher risk for several chronic metabolic and cardiovascular diseases.

Only some types of fat in the body can be used as fuel. The main oxidizable fats include fatty acids (derived from the breakdown of adipose tissue triglyceride), intramuscular triglycerides (IMTG), and circulating plasma triglycerides in the form of chylomicrons and very low density lipoproteins. In addition, fat-derived compounds such as ketone bodies (acetoacetate and β-hydroxybutyrate) can serve as a fuel, particularly during periods of starvation or low-carbohydrate availability, and glycerol (also produced as a result of triglyceride breakdown) can be converted into glucose in the liver and subsequently used to help maintain the blood glucose concentration when dietary carbohydrate intake is low.

PROTEIN

Amino acids are the building blocks of all proteins. Each amino acid consists of a carbon atom bound to four chemical groups: a hydrogen atom; an amino group (NH_2), which contains nitrogen; a carboxylic acid group (COOH); and a fourth group called an organic side chain, which varies in length and structure (see figure 2.3). Different side chains give different properties to the amino acid. Amino acids can form chains with each amino acid bound to the next one by so-called **peptide bonds**, and once connected they are called a **peptide**. Most proteins are polypeptides combining up to 300 amino acids, and in some proteins there may be more than one polypeptide chain (e.g., in hemoglobin there are four). Proteins have many important roles to play, as enzymes, which are catalysts of metabolic reactions, oxygen carriers (e.g., hemoglobin), membrane transporters and receptors, hormones (e.g., **insulin**), **cytokines** or as functional and structural components such as actin and myosin, which are part of the contractile apparatus in muscles. Because muscle is 20-25% protein, meat is a good source of protein. Up to 20 different amino acids (their structures are shown in figure 2.4) can be found in proteins.

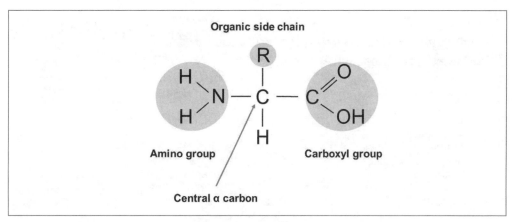

Figure 2.3: General structure of an amino acid

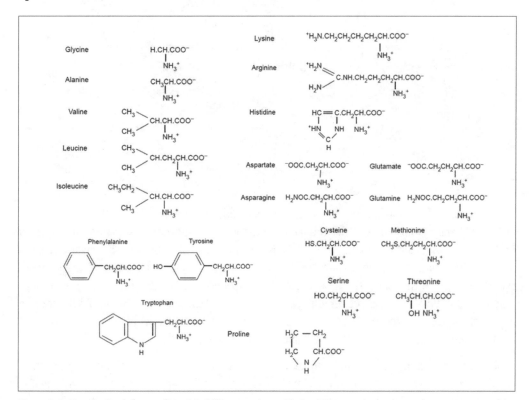

Figure 2.4: Chemical structures of the 20 different amino acids found in proteins

Of the 20 amino acids found in proteins, humans can synthesize 11- these are called **nonessential amino acids**. There are nine other amino acids which the human body cannot manufacture called **essential amino acids** (see the following sidebar). These must be obtained from the diet.

Amino acids have central roles in the metabolism of many organs and tissues. Amino acids are not only precursors for the synthesis of body proteins but also precursors of important metabolic compounds with a regulatory biological activity including **neurotransmitters**, hormones, and the nucleic acids (DNA and RNA).

Dispensable (Nonessential) Amino Acids and Indispensable (Essential) Amino Acids

Dispensable (nonessential) amino acids:

- Alanine
- Arginine
- Asparagine
- Aspartate
- Cysteine
- Glutamate
- Glutamine
- Glycine
- Proline
- Serine
- Tyrosine

Indispensable (essential) amino acids:

- Histidine
- Isoleucine
- Leucine
- Lysine
- Methionine
- Phenylalanine
- Threonine
- Tryptophan
- Valine

Proteins provide structure to all cells in the human body. They are an integral part of the cell membrane, the cytoplasm, and the organelles. Muscle, skin, and hair are composed largely of protein. Bones and teeth are composed of minerals embedded in a protein framework. When a diet is deficient in protein, these structures break down, resulting in reduced muscle mass, loss of skin elasticity, and thinning hair. Many proteins are enzymes that increase the rate of metabolic reactions. Protein contains 5 kcal of energy per gram (23 kJ/g) but only 4 kcal (17 kJ) per gram is available to use in the body and it is not normally used as an energy source except when carbohydrate (glycogen) stores become depleted and during periods of starvation.

Unlike fat and carbohydrate, a high intake of protein is not usually linked with diseases such as cancer, tooth decay, or arteriosclerosis. For this reason, protein is often associated with health, and many companies use this association in their marketing strategies (e.g., protein shampoo).

Indeed, in the developed world, where protein deficiency is uncommon, dietary protein intake is less critical and not related to disease. Prolonged deficiencies of dietary protein, however, have devastating consequences for health that result in severely impaired immunity with a high risk of infection, fluid accumulation in the abdomen and limb extremities (known as edema), and muscle wasting; ultimately, organ failure will result in death. Large excess intakes of protein are relatively rare, and it is not considered to be a health issue except for people with impaired kidney function.

The recommended daily protein intake is usually a minimum of 0.8 g protein per kg of body weight (so about 56 g for a person weighing 70 kg). Protein intake in the Western world is usually well in excess of the recommendations, averaging about 80 to 100 g/day with protein providing 10% to 15% of the total daily energy intake. Several foods with high-protein content are shown in photo 2.5. Because meat, poultry, and fish are the most common sources of protein, **vegetarians** and **vegans** could be at risk for marginal protein intake. Vegetarians often compensate by eating more grains and **legumes** (photo 2.6), which both are excellent protein sources. But grains and legumes do not contain all essential amino acids. Grains (e.g., wheat, rice, oats, cornmeal, barley) lack the essential amino acid lysine, and legumes (e.g., peas, beans, chickpeas, lentils) lack methionine. An exception may be well-processed soybean protein, which is a high-quality protein comparable to protein from animal sources. For vegetarians who might lack certain essential amino acids in their diet, the problem can be solved by not eating grains and legumes in isolation but combining both grains and legumes in their meals (together with other protein sources such as cheese or egg). Some people prefer to follow a semi-vegetarian diet – also called a **flexitarian diet** – which is primarily a plant-based diet but includes meat, dairy, eggs, poultry, and fish on occasion or in small quantities. This option can be a very healthy diet.

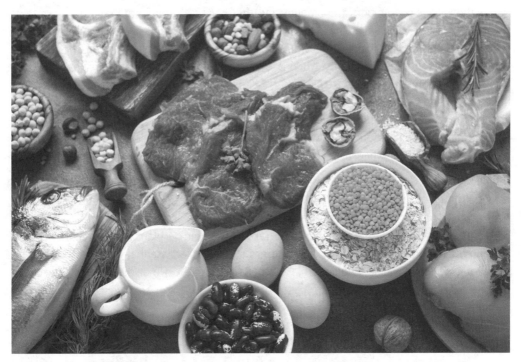

Photo 2.5: A variety of high-protein foods

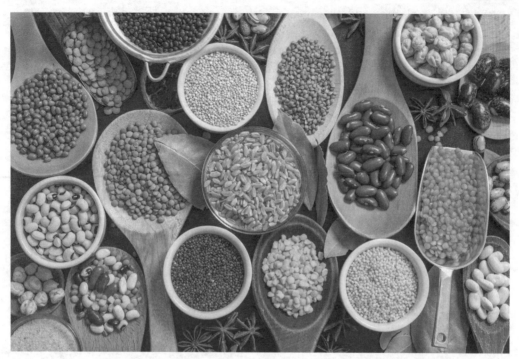

Photo 2.6: A variety of legumes (e.g., peas, beans, chickpeas, lentils) that are among the best sources of protein from plants.

As mentioned previously, both the amount and the quality of protein are important. Proteins that contain all the essential amino acids are called **complete proteins** or **high-quality proteins**. Proteins that are deficient in one or more amino acids are called incomplete proteins, and they are commonly referred to as low-quality proteins. Incomplete proteins are unable to support human life and growth. Animal proteins are generally of higher quality than plant proteins, although the individual amino acids found in animal proteins and plant proteins are identical and of equal quality. The quality of the protein therefore depends purely on the kinds of amino acids present in the protein. Animal protein is considered of higher quality not only because all essential amino acids are present but also because they are present in larger quantities and in proper proportion.

All nine essential amino acids must be obtained by dietary intake. Even a short supply of any essential amino acid can interfere with normal protein synthesis. An appropriate selection of plant protein sources can provide an adequate supply of amino acids, but consumption of animal protein is more likely to ensure a balanced intake. By combining plant foods such as rice and beans, obtaining a balanced intake of amino acids is possible. Essential amino acids that are deficient in one food can be obtained from another, so that in the overall diet, all amino acids are obtained. Proteins from sources that balance the amino acid intake are called **complementary proteins**.

Quality of Proteins

The quality of a protein relates to the degree to which that protein contributes to daily requirements. Proteins that contain all the essential amino acids are called complete proteins or high-quality proteins. Proteins that are deficient in one or more amino acids are called incomplete proteins, and they are commonly referred to as low-quality proteins.

WATER

Water (H_2O), the most abundant molecule on the surface of the Earth, is essential for the survival of all known forms of life. One molecule of water has two hydrogen atoms bonded to a single oxygen atom. The adult body is about 60% water by weight, so a 70 kg person consists of approximately 40 kg of water. The percentage of water is highest in infants and generally decreases with age. Water content varies among different tissues of the body. Blood is about 90% water, muscle is about 75%, bone is about 25%, and adipose tissue is about 5%. The proportion of water in various body compartments also varies. About two-thirds of body water is found inside cells as **intracellular fluid** (also known as cytoplasm). The remaining one-third is found outside cells as **extracellular fluid**. Extracellular fluid includes water in the blood plasma, lymph, and **cerebrospinal fluid** as well as the fluid found between cells (called **interstitial fluid**).

Water transports nutrients, provides protection, helps regulate body temperature, participates in biochemical reactions, and provides the medium in which these reactions take place. The transport function of water is exemplified by the blood circulation which transports nutrients and oxygen to the tissues and transports carbon dioxide and waste products away from the tissues. The lymphatic system is responsible for the removal and filtration of excess interstitial fluid from tissues, absorbs and transports fatty acids and fats as chylomicrons from the digestive system into the blood, and transports many of the cells involved in immune system function via the watery lymph fluid. Water in **urine** transports waste products such as **urea**, ammonia, excess ketone bodies, and **salt** out of the body.

The protective functions of water are lubrication, cleansing, and cushioning. Tears lubricate the eyes and wash away dirt. Synovial fluid lubricates the joints. Saliva lubricates the mouth, making chewing and swallowing food possible. Water inside the eyeballs acts as a cushion against shock. During pregnancy, water in the amniotic fluid provides a protective cushion for the fetus. Water also acts in the body as a **solvent**, a fluid in which substances dissolve to form a solution.

An important role of water during heat exposure and exercise is regulating body temperature. When body temperature starts to rise above the normal temperature of around 37 °C (98.6 °F), the blood vessels in the skin open up, causing blood to flow close to the surface of the body and release some of the heat. This release occurs with fever, with an increase in the environmental temperature, and with hard exercise. In a cold environment, blood vessels in the skin constrict, restricting blood flow near the surface and conserving body heat. Perhaps the most obvious way that water helps regulate body temperature is through sweating. When body temperature increases, the sweat glands in the skin secrete sweat onto the skin surface. As the sweat evaporates, heat is removed from the body surface. Some people can lose up to three liters of sweat per hour during exercise in the heat.

As with all other nutrients, a regular and sufficient water intake is required to maintain health and good physical performance. The **hydration status** of the body is determined by the balance between water intake and water loss. Loss of water (through **diarrhea** or sweating) may result in dehydration; a failure to drink fluid for more than only a few days can result in death. When water loss exceeds about 3% of total body weight, blood volume decreases and exercise performance deteriorates. A 5% loss can result in confusion and disorientation, and a loss greater than 10% can be life threatening.

Water intake of an adult is typically 2.0 to 2.8 L/day. Because water requirements are highly dependent on sweat rates, and sweat rates are dependent on energy expenditure, as a rule of thumb, fluid requirements are 1 mL for every 1 kcal (4 kJ) of energy expended. Of the daily 2.0 to 2.8 L consumed, 1.0 to 1.5 L is usually in the form of beverages and the remainder is obtained from foods.

ALCOHOL

Alcohol (ethanol) can also be considered as a macronutrient but is not essential in our diet. Alcohol is usually consumed as a beverage in beers, wines, and spirits and provides 7 kcal of energy per gram (28 kJ/g). Most of it gets converted to fat. Although some alcoholic drinks (particularly red wine) may have health benefits when ingested in moderation, excessive consumption impairs brain function and has other detrimental effects on long term health (see chapter 4 for further details).

VITAMINS, MINERALS, AND TRACE ELEMENTS

Vitamins are organic compounds, and minerals and trace elements are inorganic compounds. Collectively known as micronutrients, these essential compounds have many biological functions. Vitamins and minerals are needed in the body for several important processes, including the growth and repair of body tissues, as cofactors in enzyme catalyzed metabolic reactions, for oxygen transport and oxidative metabolism, for immune function, and as antioxidants. Any sustained deficiency of an essential vitamin or mineral will cause ill health. People often consider vitamin intake synonymous with good health (e.g., folic acid prevents birth defects, vitamin E protects the heart, and vitamin A prevents cancer), and some minerals are reputed to have strong relations to health (e.g., calcium helps to prevent **osteoporosis** and iron helps to prevent anemia).

All of the 13 known vitamins that are essential for human health have important functions in most metabolic processes in the body. Vitamins must be obtained from the diet, except vitamin D, which can also be synthesized in the skin from sunlight, and vitamin K, which is synthesized by bacteria in the intestine. When a vitamin becomes unavailable in the diet, a deficiency may develop within three to four weeks. Vitamins are either water soluble or fat soluble (see tables 2.5 and 2.6). Water-soluble vitamins dissolve in water; fat-soluble vitamins dissolve in organic solvents and are usually ingested with fats.

Although vitamins do not directly contribute to energy supply, they play an important role in regulating metabolism, acting as reusable **coenzymes** (or cofactors) and are essential for the proper functioning of some important enzymes in metabolism. A deficiency of some of the B-group vitamins, which act as cofactors of enzymes in carbohydrate (e.g., niacin [B3], pyridoxine [B6], and thiamin [B1]), fat (e.g., riboflavin [B2], thiamin [B1], pantothenic acid [B5], and biotin [B7]), and protein (pyridoxine [B6]) metabolism, results in feelings of tiredness and an inability to sustain exercise (table 2.5). Other vitamins play a role in red and white blood cell production (folic acid [B9] and cobalamin [B12]) or assist in the formation of bones, connective tissue, and cartilage (e.g., vitamins C and D). Vitamin C is also an **antioxidant**. The fat-soluble vitamins are A (retinol), D (calciferol), E (tocopherol), and K (menadione). Of these vitamins, only vitamin E has a probable role in energy metabolism but the other three have other important functions (table 2.6). In addition, β-carotene (provitamin A) and vitamin E have antioxidant properties. Vitamin K is required for the addition of sugar molecules to proteins to form **glycoproteins** and is essential for normal blood clotting.

Table 2.5: Major functions of water-soluble vitamins, effects of dietary deficiency and main food sources

Vitamin	Major roles in body	Effects of deficiency	Main food sources
B1 (thiamin)	Forms coenzyme involved in carbohydrate metabolism and central nervous system function	Loss of appetite, apathy, depression, beriberi, and pain in calf muscles	Whole-grain cereal products, fortified bread, pulses, potatoes, legumes, nuts, pork, ham and liver
B2 (riboflavin)	Forms coenzymes involved in carbohydrate and fat oxidation; maintains healthy skin	Dermatitis, lip and tongue sores, and damage to cornea of eyes	Dairy products, meat, liver, eggs, green leafy vegetables and beans
B3 (niacin)	Forms coenzymes involved in anaerobic glycolysis, carbohydrate and fat oxidation, and fat synthesis; maintains healthy skin	Weakness, loss of appetite, skin lesions, gut and skin problems, and pellegra	Meat, liver, poultry, fish, whole-grain cereal products, lentils and nuts
B5 (pantothenic acid)	Forms coenzyme A needed for energy metabolism, carbohydrate and fat oxidation and fat synthesis	Nausea, fatigue, depression, and loss of appetite	Liver, meat, dairy products, eggs, whole-grain cereal products, legumes and most vegetables
B6 (pyridoxine)	Forms coenzyme involved in protein metabolism, formation of hemoglobin and red blood cells, and glycogen breakdown	Irritability, convulsions, anemia, dermatitis, and tongue sores	Meat, liver, poultry, fish, whole-grain cereal products, potatoes, legumes, green leafy vegetables, dairy products, bananas and nuts
B7 (biotin)	Forms coenzyme involved in carbohydrate, fat, and protein metabolism	Nausea, fatigue, and skin rashes	Meat, milk, egg yolk, whole-grain cereal products, legumes and most vegetables
B9 (folic acid)	Forms coenzyme involved in production of DNA and RNA; promotes formation of hemoglobin and red and white blood cells; maintains gut	Anemia, fatigue, diarrhea, gut disorders, and infections	Meat, liver, green leafy vegetables, whole-grain cereal products, potatoes, legumes, nuts and fruit
B12 (cobalamin)	Forms coenzyme involved in production of DNA and RNA; promotes formation of red and white blood cells; maintains nerve, gut, and skin tissue	Pernicious anemia, fatigue, nerve damage, paralysis, and infections	Meat, fish, shellfish, poultry, liver, eggs, dairy products and fortified breakfast cereals
C (ascorbic acid)	Antioxidant; promotes collagen formation and development of connective tissue. Also promotes catecholamine and steroid hormone synthesis and iron absorption	Weakness, slow wound healing, infections, bleeding gums, anemia, scurvy	Citrus fruits, green leafy vegetables, blackcurrants, broccoli, kiwi fruit, melon, papaya, potatoes, peppers and strawberries

Table 2.6: Major functions of fat-soluble vitamins, the effects of dietary deficiency, and main food sources

Vitamin	Major roles in body	Effects of deficiency	Main food sources
A (retinol)	Maintains epithelial tissues in skin, mucous membranes, and visual pigments of eye; promotes bone development and immune function	Night blindness, infections, impaired growth, and impaired wound healing	Liver, fish, dairy products, eggs, margarine; formed in body from carotenoids in carrots, dark green leafy vegetables, tomatoes and oranges
D (calciferol)	Increases calcium absorption in gut and promotes bone formation. Also important for muscle and immune function	Weak bones (rickets in children and osteomalacia in adults). Suboptimal muscle function. Increased susceptibility to infections	Liver, fish, eggs, fortified dairy products, oils, and margarine; formed by action of sunlight on the skin
E (α-tocopherol)	Defends against free radicals; protects cell membranes	Hemolysis and anemia	Liver, eggs, whole-grain cereal products, vegetable oils, seed oils, margarine and butter
K (menadione)	Forms blood-clotting factors	Bleeding and hemorrhage	Liver, eggs, green leafy vegetables, cheese and butter; formed in large intestine by bacteria

Minerals can be divided into **macrominerals** and **microminerals** (or **trace elements**). Macrominerals are required in daily intakes of more than 100 mg or are present in the body in amounts greater than 0.01% of the body weight. The macrominerals include calcium, chlorine, magnesium, potassium, phosphorus, and sodium and just like the vitamins, they play important roles in bodily functions (table 2.7). Several of the macrominerals are classed as **electrolytes** which are minerals that can conduct electrical impulses in the body. Common electrolytes are calcium, chloride, potassium, and sodium. Electrolytes control the fluid balance of the body and are important in muscle contraction, energy generation, and many biochemical reactions in the body. The microminerals **(trace elements)** are required in daily intakes of less than 100 mg or are present in the body in amounts less than 0.01% of body weight. Despite the small amounts needed, they play essential roles in a variety of bodily functions (table 2.8). The microminerals include cobalt, copper, fluorine, iodine, iron, manganese, molybdenum, selenium, and zinc. Some of the microminerals such as iron and zinc form part of **metalloenzymes** which are enzymes in which the metal is bonded within the protein structure and functions as a cofactor that is necessary for the action of the enzyme.

Table 2.7: Major functions of macrominerals, effects of dietary deficiency, and main food sources

Macromineral	Major roles in the body	Effects of deficiency	Main Food Sources
Calcium	Promotes bone and teeth formation, muscle contraction and nerve impulse transmission; regulates enzyme activity	Osteoporosis, brittle bones, impaired muscle contraction and muscle cramps	Dairy products, egg yolk, beans and peas, dark green vegetables, and cauliflower
Chlorine	Promotes nerve impulse conduction and hydrochloric acid formation in the stomach	Convulsions	Meat, fish, bread, canned foods, table salt, beans and milk
Magnesium	Promotes protein synthesis and cofactor for important enzymes involved in muscle contraction and is a component of bone	Muscle weakness, fatigue, apathy, muscle tremor and cramps	Seafood, nuts, green leafy vegetables, fruits, whole-grain products, milk and yogurt
Potassium	Promotes nerve impulse generation, muscle contraction, and acid-base balance	Muscle cramps, apathy, loss of appetite and irregular heart beat	Meat, fish, milk, yogurt, fruit, vegetables and bread
Phosphorus	Promotes bone formation; buffer in muscle contraction; component of ATP, DNA, RNA, and cell membranes	Osteoporosis, brittle bones, muscle weakness and muscle cramps	Meat, eggs, fish, milk, cheese, beans, peas, whole-grain products and soft drinks
Sodium	Maintenance of blood volume, nerve impulse generation, muscle contraction, acid-base balance	Dizziness, coma, muscle cramps, nausea, vomiting, loss of appetite and seizures	Meat, fish, bread, canned foods, table salt, sauces and pickles
Sulfur	Acid-base balance; liver function	Unknown and extremely unlikely to occur	Bok choi, broccoli, cabbage, cauliflower, horseradish, kale, kohlrabi, mustard leaves, radish, turnips, watercress, coconut milk, milk, eggs, legumes and beans, meat and fish, nuts, onions, leeks, wine and grape juice

Table 2.8: Major functions of microminerals (trace elements), effects of dietary deficiency, and main food sources

Micromineral	Major roles in body	Effects of deficiency	Main food sources
Chromium	Increases insulin action	Glucose intolerance and impaired fat metabolism	Liver, kidney, meat, oysters, cheese, whole-grain products, beer, asparagus, mushrooms, nuts and stainless steel cookware
Cobalt	Forms component of vitamin B12 needed for red blood cell development	Pernicious anemia	Meat, liver, and milk
Copper	Promotes normal iron absorption, oxidative metabolism, connective tissue formation, and hemoglobin synthesis	Anemia, impaired immune function and bone demineralization	Liver, kidney, shellfish, meat, fish, poultry, eggs, bran cereals, nuts, legumes, broccoli, banana, avocado and chocolate
Fluorine	Promotes bone and teeth formation	Dental caries (tooth decay)	Milk, egg yolk, seafood, and drinking water
Iodine	Forms component of thyroid hormones	Goiter and reduced metabolic rate	Iodized salt, seafood, and vegetables
Iron	Transports oxygen as hemoglobin and myoglobin; forms cytochromes and metalloenzymes; promotes immune function	Anemia, fatigue, and increased infections	Liver, kidney, eggs, red meats, seafood, oysters, bread, flour, molasses, dried legumes, nuts, leafy green vegetables, broccoli, figs, raisins, and cocoa
Manganese	Forms cofactor with energy metabolism enzymes; promotes bone formation and fat synthesis	Poor growth	Whole grains, peas and beans, leafy vegetables, and bananas
Molybdenum	Forms cofactor with riboflavin in carbohydrate and fat metabolism enzymes	No known deficiency effects	Liver, kidney, whole-grain products, beans, and peas
Selenium	Forms cofactor with glutathione peroxidase an important antioxidant enzyme	Cardiomyopathy, cancer, heart disease, impaired immune function and red blood cell fragility	Meat, liver, kidney, poultry, fish, dairy products, seafood, whole grains, and nuts
Zinc	Forms metalloenzymes; promotes protein synthesis, immune function, tissue repair, energy metabolism, and antioxidant activity	Impaired growth, impaired healing, and increased number of infections	Oysters, shellfish, beef, liver, poultry, dairy products, whole grains, vegetables, asparagus, and spinach

PHYTONUTRIENTS

Another component of foods are the **phytonutrients**. Phytonutrients (*phyto* is Greek for plant) are certain organic components of plants that are thought to promote human health, but unlike vitamins, they are not considered an essential nutrient, meaning that without them people will not develop a nutritional deficiency. However, if they are absent from the diet, or present in only low amounts, health may not be optimal.

The many types of phytonutrients can be divided into different classes (see the sidebar). The most well known and most researched of these are probably the carotenoids which are found in carrots, broccoli, leafy green and yellow vegetables, and other vegetables.

Carotenoids are the red, orange, and yellow pigments in fruits and vegetables. The carotenoids most commonly found in vegetables are listed in table 2.9 along with common sources of these compounds. Fruits and vegetables high in carotenoids appear to protect humans against certain cancers, heart disease, and age-related macular degeneration (an eye condition which affects the central part of your retina called the macula. It causes changes to your central vision which can make some everyday tasks difficult).

Table 2.9: Carotenoids and their food sources

Carotenoid	Common food source
α-carotene	Carrots, pumpkin, squash
β-carotene	Leafy green and yellow vegetables (e.g., broccoli, carrots, pumpkin, swede, sweet potato)
β-cryptoxanthin	Citrus fruits, apricots, peaches
Lutein	Leafy greens such as kale, spinach, cabbage, spring greens
Lycopene	Guava, tomato products, pink grapefruit, watermelon
Zeaxanthin	Green vegetables, eggs, citrus fruits

Common Classes of Phytonutrients

Carotenoids

Flavonoids (polyphenols) including isoflavones (phytoestrogens)

Inositol phosphates (phytates)

Isothiocyanates and indoles

Lignans (phytoestrogens)

Phenols and cyclic compounds

Saponins

Sulfides and thiols

Terpenes

Other important phytonutrients include the polyphenols which are natural components of a wide variety of plants. Food sources rich in **polyphenols** include onions, apples, tea, red wine, red grapes, grape juice, strawberries, raspberries, blueberries, cranberries, and certain nuts (table 2.10). The average polyphenol intake in most countries has not been determined with precision, largely because no food database currently exists for these compounds. Polyphenols can be classified as nonflavonoids and flavonoids (table 2.6). It has been estimated that in the Dutch diet a subset of flavonoids (flavonols and flavones) provide 23 mg per day. These small amounts, however, may have significant effects.

Table 2.10: Polyphenols and their food sources

Nonflavonoids	Sources
Ellagic acid	Blueberries, raspberries, strawberries
Coumarins	Bell peppers, bok choi, broccoli, cereal grains
Flavonoids	Sources
Anthocyanins	Fruits
Catechins	Tea (black or green), wine
Flavanones	Citrus fruits
Flavones	Fruits and vegetables
Flavonols	Cocoa products, fruits, vegetables, tea, wine
Isoflavones	Soybeans

So now you know something about the various nutrients that are contained in the foods we eat, their properties, functions, and in which foods they are most abundant. In the next chapter we will learn how much of these nutrients we need to consume to stay healthy.

Key points

- Food provides nutrients that have one or more physiological or biochemical functions in the body.

- Nutrients are usually divided into six different categories: carbohydrates, fats, proteins, vitamins, minerals, and water.

- Functions of nutrients include promotion of growth and development, provision of energy, and regulation of metabolism.

- Among the several different classes of carbohydrates are sugars, starches, and fiber.

- Fiber, although it is not absorbed, has several important functions including maintaining normal gut function.

- There are several classes of fats, including fatty acids, triglycerides, and lipoproteins. Triglyceride (or triacylglycerol) is the main storage form.

- Amino acids are the building blocks of proteins. Of the 20 amino acids normally found in dietary protein, humans can synthesize 11. Those that can be synthesized are called nonessential amino acids. Those that cannot be synthesized and must be derived from the diet are called the essential amino acids.

- Proteins that contain all the essential amino acids are called complete proteins or high-quality proteins. Proteins that are deficient in one or more amino acids are called incomplete proteins, and they are commonly referred to as low-quality proteins.

- Water is an extremely important nutrient. The adult body is about 60% water by weight. Two-thirds of the water is intracellular fluid and the remaining one-third is extracellular fluid.

- Vitamins, minerals, and trace elements are micronutrients. Vitamins are organic compounds whereas minerals and trace elements are inorganic compounds. A deficiency of any essential vitamin or mineral results in ill health.

- Phytonutrients are certain organic components of plants which are thought to promote human health but are not considered to be essential nutrients. They differ from vitamins in that respect because a lack of phytonutrients will not cause a deficiency disease. However, they are required for optimal health.

Chapter 3

Recommended Intakes of Nutrients and How to Read Food Labels

Objectives

After reading this chapter, you should:

- Be able to explain the differences between essential and nonessential nutrients

- Understand the basis of recommended daily intakes of nutrients

- Understand the regulations regarding food labelling and health claims

- Know how to read a food label

- Know what the so-called superfoods are

- Understand why supplements are generally unnecessary

- Understand why vitamin D is different from all the other vitamins

In the previous chapter, the various nutrients and their functions were explained. In this chapter, the amounts of these nutrients that we are recommended to consume in order to stay healthy will be described. As mentioned earlier, nutrients can be divided into **nonessential nutrients** and **essential nutrients**; the former can be synthesized within the body and the latter cannot.

ESSENTIAL NUTRIENTS

In ancient times, people were already aware that certain food components could prevent disease or be used to treat diseases. However, it is only during the past two centuries that some specific nutrients have been identified and recognized as essential for human life. Until the mid-18th century, scurvy was a disease common among sailors and others aboard ships at sea longer than perishable fruits and vegetables could be stored. The typical characteristics of the condition were general weakness, anemia, gum disease, and dry, scaly, and bruised skin. In 1740 a Scottish surgeon named James Lind who served in the British navy discovered that the consumption of citrus fruits by sailors could prevent and cure scurvy. Other foods and medicine that were available on the ship did not have this effect. In 1757, Lind conducted the world's first clinical trial, proving lemon or lime juice prevented scurvy and subsequently the Royal Navy was persuaded to issue lime juice in its official grog ration, and British seamen became the healthiest in the world (for the time). Although scurvy was not attributed to a deficiency in vitamin C at that time, the essentiality of certain foods containing essential nutrients for the maintenance of health was established. The term 'lime-juicers', considered hilarious by Australians, New Zealanders, and South Africans, gradually became 'limeys', describing British land-lubbers as well as sailors and, eventually lost any connection with the sea. The term was also adopted by the Americans in the early 20th century.

On a more serious and disturbing note, tragic studies with prisoners in Nazi death camps have revealed the importance of various vitamins and minerals for human health. The prisoners were purposefully provided with a diet deficient in a certain vitamin or mineral, and their health status was recorded over the following months. With diets deficient in certain nutrients, specific diseases developed in the unfortunate prisoners and often ultimately resulted in death. For example, deficiency of vitamin B1 (thiamin) was shown to cause **beriberi** disease characterized mainly by damage to peripheral nerves, wasting, and congestive heart failure. In early experimental studies with animals (mostly rats and mice), diets that were formulated to be deficient in one or more nutrients retarded growth, and the animals experienced specific disease symptoms. When the animals were subsequently fed with the missing nutrient, their growth and illness symptoms improved, and they eventually recovered their health completely. The nutrients that exhibited these health effects were classified as essential. Nowadays, a nutrient is considered essential if it meets the following criteria:

- The substance is required in the diet for growth, health, and survival.

- Absence of the substance from the diet or inadequate intake results in characteristic signs of a deficiency disease and ultimately death.

- Growth failure and characteristic signs of deficiency are prevented only by the nutrient or a specific precursor of it and not by other substances.

- Below some critical level of intake of the nutrient, growth response and severity of signs of deficiency are proportional to the amount consumed.

- The substance is not synthesized in the body and is therefore required for some critical function throughout life.

Some nutrients are classified as **conditionally essential**, a term that was introduced in 1984 because some nutrients that normally are not essential seemed to become essential under certain conditions. Conditionally essential nutrients must be supplied in the diet or as a supplement to specific populations that do not synthesize them in adequate amounts. The deficiency can be the result of a defect in the synthesis of a certain nutrient or a temporarily increased need for that nutrient. An example of a defect in synthesis is the genetic defect in the synthesis of carnitine, a compound involved in fat burning in muscle. Sufferers of this condition experience muscle-wasting disease (myopathy), but when carnitine is supplemented, the condition is corrected. An example of a transiently increased need may occur in surgical patients in an intensive care unit who usually have lower than normal plasma and muscle glutamine concentrations. Glutamine is an amino acid, but it is not normally one of the essential ones. However, insufficient glutamine availability results in decreased protein synthesis and increased protein breakdown, resulting in muscle wasting and poor wound repair. The patients improve when glutamine is supplemented either orally or intravenously. Thus, glutamine is classified as conditionally essential.

Essential Nutrients

Amino acids:

- Histidine
- Isoleucine
- Leucine
- Lysine
- Methionine
- Phenylalanine
- Threonine
- Tryptophan
- Valine

Fatty acids:

- Linoleic acid
- α-Linolenic acid

Minerals:

- Calcium
- Iron
- Magnesium
- Phosphorus

Trace elements:

- Chromium
- Copper
- Iodine
- Manganese
- Molybdenum
- Selenium
- Zinc

Electrolytes:

- Chloride
- Potassium
- Sodium

Vitamins:

- Vitamin A
- Vitamin C (ascorbic acid)
- Vitamin D
- Vitamin E
- Vitamin K
- Biotin (B7)

- Folic acid (B9)
- Niacin (B3)
- Pantothenic acid (B5)
- Riboflavin (B2)
- Thiamin (B1)
- Vitamin B6 (pyridoxine)
- Vitamin B12 (cobalamin)

Ultra-Trace elements:

- Boron
- Cobalt
- Nickel
- Silicon
- Vanadium

Water

DEVELOPMENT OF RECOMMENDED INTAKES

Nowadays, the list of nutrients classified as essential is quite extensive (see the sidebar). More than 40 nutrients meet the criteria. In 1941, the first Food and Nutrition Board was formed in the United States, and two years later the first official dietary standards for evaluating nutritional intakes of large populations and for planning of agricultural production were published. Since then, the guidelines have been revised several times. Initially, reference values for only 10 nutrients were established, but this number has increased over the years such that current guidelines in the USA and Canada now cover 46 nutrients.

When the first set of recommended intakes of specific nutrients – called the **recommended dietary allowance** (RDA) – was created in 1941, its primary goal was to prevent known diseases caused by nutrient deficiencies. The RDAs were originally intended to be used to help evaluate and plan for the nutritional adequacy of large groups of people, for example, the armed forces and children in school lunch programs, rather than to determine the nutrient needs of individuals.

But because the RDAs were essentially the only nutrient values available, they began to be used in ways other than the intended use. Health professionals often used RDAs to judge the diets of individual patients or clients. Statistically speaking, RDAs would prevent deficiency diseases in 97% of a population, but there was no scientific basis that RDAs would meet the needs of a single specific person.

It was evident that the RDAs were not addressing individual needs, and new science needed to be included. Therefore, the Food and Nutrition Board sought to redefine nutrient requirements according to gender and age so that specific nutrient recommendations for individuals could be given. Along with these changes, concepts such as tolerable **upper intakes** (to help avoid potentially toxic intakes of some nutrients, particularly micronutrients as vitamin and mineral supplements rose in popularity) and **adequate intakes** (when an RDA could not be accurately determined) were developed to meet individuals' needs. A more recent development has been the publication of **acceptable macronutrient distribution ranges** (i.e., a recommended range of intake for specific macronutrients like carbohydrate, fat, and protein) that are associated with reduced risk of chronic metabolic and cardiovascular disease while providing sufficient essential nutrients (table 3.1). Thus, for the first time, the RDAs and various national dietary guidelines are no longer focused only on preventing deficiency diseases such as scurvy or beriberi. Now they are also aimed at reducing the risk of diet-related chronic conditions such as heart disease, type 2 diabetes, hypertension, and osteoporosis. After the initial guidelines were formulated, guidelines have also become more specific and have been developed for both males and females and various age groups (and also for pregnant and lactating women).

Definitions of Terms Related to Nutrient Requirements

Dietary Reference Intake (DRI)

The **dietary reference intake** (DRI) represents the new standards for nutrient recommendations that can be used to plan and assess diets for healthy people. Think of DRI as the umbrella term that includes all the following values:

Estimated Average Requirement (EAR)

The **estimated average requirement** (EAR) is a nutrient intake value that is estimated to meet the requirement of half of the healthy individuals in a group. It is used to assess nutritional adequacy of intakes of population groups. In addition, EARs are used to calculate RDAs.

Recommended Dietary Allowance (RDA)

This value is a goal for individuals and is based on the EAR. It is the daily dietary intake level that is sufficient to meet the nutrient requirement of 97 to 98% of all healthy people in a group. If an EAR cannot be set, no RDA value can be proposed. RDAs are available for most minerals and vitamins and a full list can be found in the appendix.

Adequate Intake (AI)

This value is used when an RDA cannot be determined. A recommended daily intake level is based on an observed or experimentally determined approximation of nutrient intake for a group (or groups) of healthy people. Examples of nutrients for which the AI is used include biotin, pantothenic acid, chromium, manganese, potassium, and sodium.

Tolerable Upper Intake Level (UL)

The UL is the highest level of daily nutrient intake that is likely to pose no risks of adverse health effects to almost all individuals in the general population. As intake increases above the UL, the risk of adverse effects increases. Some examples of ULs include niacin 35 mg/day, vitamin C 2 g/day, Vitamin D 100 micrograms (μg)/day equivalent to 4,000 International Units (IU)/day, calcium 2.5 g/day, iron 45 mg/day, and magnesium 350 mg/day.

Acceptable Macronutrient Distribution Ranges (AMDR)

The acceptable macronutrient distribution range (AMDR) is the range of intake for a particular energy source (i.e., carbohydrate, fat, and protein) that is associated with reduced risk of chronic disease while providing intakes of essential nutrients. If an individual's intake is outside of the AMDR, there is a potential of increasing the risk of chronic diseases and/or insufficient intakes of essential nutrients. The AMDR is expressed as a percentage of total energy intake (table 3.1). A key feature of each AMDR is that it has a lower and upper boundary. For example, the AMDR for carbohydrates ranges from 45 to 65 percent of total energy intake. Intakes that fall below or above this range increase the potential for an elevated risk of chronic diseases. Intakes outside of the range also raise the risk of inadequate consumption of essential nutrients.

Table 3.1: Acceptable Macronutrient Distribution Ranges (AMDR)

Nutrient	Range in nutritionally adequate diet (% of total dietary energy intake)
Carbohydrate	45–65
Cholesterol	As low as possible
Fat	20–35
α-Linolenic acid	0.6–1.2
Linoleic acid	5–10
Saturated fatty acids	As low as possible
Trans fatty acids	As low as possible
Protein	10–35
Sugar	<10

Data from Food and Nutrition Board (2005). *Dietary Reference Intakes for Energy, Carbohydrate. Fiber, Fat, Fatty Acids, Cholesterol, Protein, and Amino Acids* (2002/2005).

Dietary Reference Intakes (DRIs) have now been developed (see sidebar). These are reference values that are quantitative estimates of nutrient intakes to be used for planning and assessing diets for healthy people. Specifically, a diet should aim to meet any RDA (or Adequate Intake, AI, which is a recommended value for those nutrients where an RDA has not been established) set and not exceed the Upper Intake Level (UL). DRIs are based on averages of large populations and thus are not designed to detect nutrient deficiencies in individuals. So, someone below the recommendations for a particular nutrient may not actually be deficient in that nutrient. Only a clinical and biochemical examination can determine whether an individual has a nutritional deficiency. Comparison of an individual's intake to the RDA, however, can help determine whether the person is at risk for a deficiency. Full listings of the RDAs (or AIs) for various nutrients are shown in the appendix for North America, the UK, Australia, and New Zealand. To determine whether an individual's nutrient intake meets the RDA, it should be calculated from a detailed record of food intake with accurate portion sizes and using comprehensive food composition tables, over a period of about one week. A person whose diet does not contain the full RDA on one day is not necessarily at risk for deficiencies because the inadequacy can be compensated for on the next day. Note that the RDA does not reflect the absolute minimum requirements but a safe margin of excess intake.

Of course, people who consistently take in less than the RDA for one or more nutrients have a chance of becoming deficient over time. In the case of vitamin D, requirements have been determined on the basis of bone health although it is now recognized that the requirement may be higher than this for optimal immune function. Another issue with vitamin D is that, unlike all the other vitamins, it (specifically vitamin D3 or cholecalciferol) can be synthesized in the skin, from cholesterol, when exposure from sunlight ultraviolet B radiation is adequate. The synthesis of vitamin D from sunlight exposure is regulated by a mechanism that prevents toxicity, but because of uncertainty about the cancer risk from overexposure to sunlight, currently no recommendations are issued by national bodies regarding the amount of sunlight exposure required to meet vitamin D requirements. Accordingly, the RDA of vitamin D for adults (5 micrograms or 200 IU in the European Union, 10 micrograms or 400 IU in the UK, and 15 micrograms or 600 IU in the USA) assumes that no synthesis occurs, and all of a person's vitamin D is from food intake, although that will rarely occur in practice. Recent studies indicate that in the winter months, many individuals can become deficient in vitamin D, and that this may, at least in part, be responsible for the observed higher incidence of colds and flu during the winter months. Some countries, including the UK, now advise a daily vitamin D intake of up to 25 micrograms or 1,000 IU during wintertime and several countries in Europe as well as the USA encourage fortification of selected foods (usually milk, margarine, and cereal products).

RDAs do not account for unusual requirements caused by disease, environmental stress or very high levels of physical activity. Therefore, the RDAs may not be an accurate means of evaluating the nutritional needs of people engaged in regular strenuous exercise such as athletes, the military, and those in highly physical occupations.

Although recommendations like the DRI may provide guidance on nutrient requirements, they are not a practical way of informing people about appropriate food choices. For example, how does someone know whether he or she is consuming about 0.8 g/kg of body weight of protein per day or meeting the RDI for calcium, vitamin A, and other essential minerals and vitamins? A healthy diet is often referred to as a balanced diet that stresses variety and moderation. But how do we achieve a balanced diet? These questions are addressed in chapter 4.

WHAT INFORMATION IS PROVIDED ON FOOD LABELS?

The reference values used to determine RDAs are specific for both age and gender, and for food-labeling purposes, an additional set of more general reference values that could apply to most children as well as men and women of any age had to be produced. Because the information on food packages had to be the same for all people (with the exception of babies and young infants) the RDA values had to be condensed into a "one size fits all" recommendation for all groups. The US Food and Drug Administration developed these recommendations and usually picked the highest RDA level needed by age or gender group to determine them; they are now called the **daily value** (DV). The DVs are the US Food and Drug Administration's version of the Institute of Medicine's recommended intakes for vitamins and minerals. The Institute of Medicine and its Food and Nutrition Board are part of the National Academy of Sciences. The Institute of Medicine has been releasing new reports called Dietary Reference Intakes (DRIs). The report sets recommended dietary allowance (RDA), adequate intake (AI) and upper intake levels (UL) for vitamins and minerals. So far, the Food and Drug Administration (FDA) has not revised the Daily Values to reflect any of these changes, and it is only the DVs that are used on food and supplement labels to provide information to consumers.

The DV is based on two sets of references: (1) the **reference daily intake**, or RDI, which makes up most of the DVs and provides a set of dietary references for essential vitamins and minerals, and (2) the **daily reference value** (DRV), a standard for proteins and various dietary components that have no RDA or other established nutrient standard (e.g., cholesterol, total fat, carbohydrate, dietary fiber, sodium, and potassium) (see table 3.2). On food labels, all reference values are listed as DV although they can be either DRV or RDI. On current food labeling, the **% Daily Value** is the percentage of RDI or DRV available in a single serving.

Table 3.2: Daily Reference Values (DRV)

Food component	DRV
Total fat	Less than 65 g (30% of energy intake)
Saturated fat	Less than 20 g (10% of energy intake)
Cholesterol	Less than 300 mg
Total carbohydrate	300 g (60% of energy intake)
Sugars	Less than 10% of energy intake
Dietary fiber	28 g
Sodium	Less than 2,400 mg
Potassium	3,500 mg
Protein	50 g (10% of energy intake)

DRV based on a daily energy intake of 2,000 kcal (8.4 MJ). From US Food and Drug Administration, https://www.fda.gov/food/resourcesforyou/consumers/ucm274593.htm

DIFFERENCES BETWEEN COUNTRIES

Some countries have formulated recommendations with respect to the amount of each nutrient that should be consumed. Therefore, the RDA values differ slightly in different countries (see appendix). The United Nations and the European Union have formulated their own reference intakes, as have many individual countries. In the UK and Germany, the RDA has been redefined as the **reference nutrient intake** (RNI), and in Australia it has been redefined as the recommended daily intake (RDI). Canada now uses the same system as the USA.

In the UK and EU, the **Nutrient Reference Value** (NRV) has replaced the RDA, but the values are exactly the same. Labels on some foods (e.g., breakfast cereals) in the UK and EU include the %NRV for selected vitamins (e.g., vitamin D, vitamin B12, folic acid) and minerals (e.g., iron).

UNDERSTANDING THE INFORMATION ON FOOD LABELS FOR DIET PLANNING

The development of the nutrient recommendations described above may appear rather complicated, but the information now provided on food labels is a very useful tool for diet planning or nutritional assessment (see figure 3.1). Food labels help consumers make choices by providing detailed information about the nutrient content of food and the way in which that food fits into the overall diet. Food labels contain so much information that it's often difficult to know what you should be looking for and what it all means. But if you want to improve your diet and make healthy choices, it's important to get into the habit of checking the label.

FOOD LABELS IN THE USA

In many parts of the world, labels are not yet standardized, but in the USA, food labeling is standardized as specified by the Nutrition Labeling and Education Act of 1990. All packaged foods, except those produced by small businesses and those in packages too small to fit the labeling information, must be labeled. Food labeling laws regulate about 75% of all food consumed in the USA.

The information on food labels usually includes the name of the product; the name and contact details of the manufacturer, packager, or distributor; the net contents or weight of the package; and the date by which the product must be sold. The format of the nutrition facts label is identical on all products to make comparing foods easier and contains information about the typical serving size (indicated near the top of the label), ingredients in the food, expressed in amounts (g or mg) per typical serving size and also expressed as a percentage of the daily value (%DV). The %DV for protein is not required unless a protein claim is made for the product or the product is to be used by infants or children under four years of age.

As illustrated in figure 3.1, the nutrition facts label in the USA has a main top section that includes information that can vary with each product (serving size, energy content, and nutrition information). The lower part contains footnote information with daily values based on a 2,000-kcal diet.

The place to start when looking at the nutrition facts label is the serving size and number of servings per package. Serving sizes are expressed in familiar terms like cups and pieces followed by the weight in grams. The next line on the label indicates the energy content in calories, which are actually kilocalories (more on this in chapter 5). The label then informs the consumer about key nutrients and the percentage of daily value.

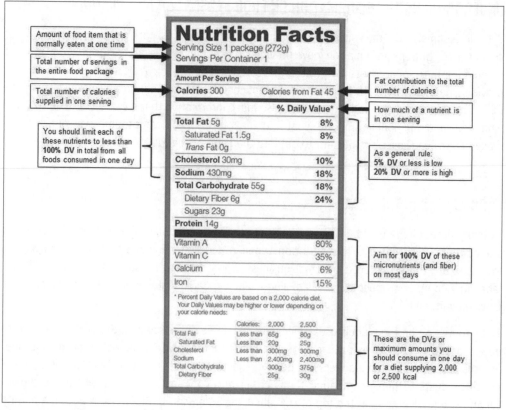

Figure 3.1: How to read a US food label. Adapted from US Food and Drug Administration,
https://www.accessdata.fda.gov/scripts/InteractiveNutritionFactsLabel/#whats-on-the-label

The nutrients are categorized by those whose intake should be limited, such as total grams of fat, saturated fats, *trans* fats, cholesterol, and sodium. Next are total carbohydrate (including the amount of added sugars) and protein, and below these are amounts of selected micronutrients.

Only since 2016 has the amount of added sugars been required to be on the label. This was introduced because it was recognized that it is difficult to meet nutrition needs while staying within calorie limits if more than 10% of total daily energy comes from added sugars. The carbohydrate entry is divided into fiber (which should be encouraged), and total sugars and added sugars (which should be limited). The nutrients are expressed in grams or milligrams per serving size but also as a percentage of daily value based on a 2,000-kcal diet. No %DV is given for total sugar because no such value has been established, but the %DV for added sugars is shown. Keep in mind that the total sugars on the label include the natural sugars in the product as well as the added sugars.

Labels often contain information that might be of interest to the consumer such as "low-fat," "reduced fat," "fat-free," "light," and "lean." The use of these and other terms is also regulated, and definitions of these terms have been established (see table 3.3). A consumer who buys a product with "low-fat" on the label can be sure that it meets the definition established by the FDA (which is less than 3 gof fat per serving).

Table 3.3: Definitions of nutrient content claims

Nutrient	Calories	Total fat	Sugars
Free (zero, no, without, trivial source of, negligible source of)	Calorie free: Less than 5 kcal per reference amount and per labeled serving	Fat-free: Less than 0.5 g per reference amount and per labeled serving (or for meals and main dishes, less than 0.5 g per labeled serving)	Sugar free: Less than 0.5 g sugars per reference amount and per labeled serving (or for meals and main dishes, less than 0.5 g per labeled serving)
Low (little, few for calories, contains a small amount of, low source of)	Few calories: 40 kcal or less per reference amount (and per 50 g if reference amount is small); meals and main dishes: 120 kcal or less per 100 g	Low-fat: 3 g or less per reference amount (and per 50 g if reference amount is small); meals and main dishes: 3 g or less per 100 g and not more than 30% of calories from fat	Not defined; no basis for recommended intake
Reduced or less (lower, fewer for calories)	Fewer calories: At least 25% fewer calories per reference amount than an appropriate reference food; reference food may not be low-calorie	Reduced fat: At least 25% less fat per reference amount than an appropriate reference food; reference food may not be low-fat	Reduced sugar: At least 25% less sugars per reference amount than an appropriate reference food
Comments	Light or lite: If 50% or more of the calories are from fat, fat must be reduced by at least 50% per reference amount; if less than 50% of calories are from fat, fat must be reduced by at least 50% or calories must be reduced by at least 1/3 per reference amount	__% fat-free: Allowed if food meets the requirements for low-fat. If 100% fat-free, food must be completely fat-free	No added sugars, or without added sugars: Allowed if no sugar or sugar-containing ingredient is added during processing; state whether food is not low-calorie or reduced-calorie

Reference amount = reference amount customarily consumed. Small reference amount = reference amount of 30 g or less or two tablespoons or less (for dehydrated foods that are typically consumed after being rehydrated with water).

FOOD LABELS IN THE UK AND EU

Nutrition labels are often displayed as a panel or grid on the back or side of packaging. For example, figure 3.2 shows the nutrition label on a loaf of white bread.

Nutrition Information				
Typical values	100 g contains	Each slice (typically 44 g) contains	% RI*	RI for an average adult
Energy	985 kJ 235 kcal	435 kJ 105 kcal	5%	8400 kJ 2000 kcal
Fat	1.5 g	0.7 g	1%	70 g
of which saturates	0.3 g	0.1 g	1%	20 g
Carbohydrate	45.5 g	20.0 g		
of which sugars	3.8 g	1.7 g	2%	90 g
Fibre	2.8 g	1.2 g		
Protein	7.7 g	3.4 g		
Salt	1.0 g	0.4 g	7%	6 g
This pack contains 16 servings *Reference intake of an average adult (8400 kJ/2000 kcal)				

Figure 3.2: Example of a UK/EU food label found on the side or back of packaged foods. In this example the food item is a loaf of sliced white bread.

This type of label includes information on energy in kilojoules (kJ) and kilocalories (kcal), fat, saturates (saturated fat), carbohydrate, sugars, protein and salt. Sometimes sodium is listed rather than salt. To convert sodium into salt, multiply the amount on the label by 2.5. The label may also provide additional information on certain nutrients, such as fiber (spelt as fibre in the UK). All nutrition information is provided per 100 grams (or 100 mL for beverages such as milk) and sometimes per portion of the food. The above will also be shown on the label usually as a percentage of an adult's **Reference Intake** (%RI) although some labels just show the absolute values for the daily RI for comparison with what is in the product. The RI has replaced the recommended daily amount (RDA) and is equivalent to the daily value (DV) shown on North American food packaging. Reference intakes are useful guidelines on the amount of energy and nutrients you need for a healthy balanced diet each day. The %RI tells you how much of your daily healthy maximum is in the portion of the product and is based on the following values: 2,000 kcal energy, 70 g fat, 20 g saturated fat, 90 g sugars, and 6 g salt (or 2.4 g sodium).

In order to know whether a food is high in fat, saturated fat, sugar, or salt, use the following guidelines:

Sugars

- High: more than 22.5 g of total sugars per 100 g

- Low: 5.0 g of total sugars or less per 100 g

Salt

- High: more than 1.5 g of salt per 100 g (or 0.6 g sodium)

- Low: 0.3 g of salt or less per 100 g (or 0.1 g sodium)

Total fat

- High: more than 17.5 g of fat per 100 g

- Low: 3.0 g of fat or less per 100 g

Saturated fat

- High: more than 5.0 g of saturated fat per 100 g

- Low: 1.5 g of saturated fat or less per 100 g

For example, if you are trying to cut down on saturated fat, limit your consumption of foods that have more than 5 g of saturated fat per 100 g.

Bear in mind that the serving or portion size indicated on the label is the manufacturer's recommendation for one portion of the product and that the %RI displayed on the label is worked out based on this portion size. Your idea of a portion size may be larger this, which means that even if a product looks healthy, if you have more than what the manufacturer recommended, you may end up consuming more energy, saturated fat, or salt than you realize.

Most of the big supermarkets and many food manufacturers also display nutritional information on the front of pre-packed and canned foods. This is very useful when you want to compare different food products at a glance. These labels provide information on the amount (in grams) of fat, saturated fat, sugars, and salt, and the amount of energy (in kJ and kcal) in a serving or portion of the food. But again, be aware that the manufacturer's idea of a portion may be different from yours, and check exactly what it is. In foods like cooking sauces, it may be that the portion size is one third of a jar or for a can of soup it might be half a can of soup. Never assume that the portion size on the label represents what the whole jar, can, or package contains, as usually it does not.

Some front-of-pack nutrition labels also provide information about reference intakes usually displayed as %RI or as percentage of daily guideline amounts (which is the same thing). Some front-of-pack nutrition labels use red, amber, and green color coding. Color-coded nutritional information, as shown for a spaghetti Bolognese ready meal in photo 3.1, tells you at a glance whether the food has high, medium or low amounts of fat, saturated fat, sugars, and salt.

- Red means high

- Amber means medium

- Green means low

Table 3.4 shows how low, medium and high levels of fat, saturated fats, total sugars and salt in foods are classified for front of pack labels in the UK. The amounts are per 100 g except for the "per portion" values in red which are used where portions are 50 g or more.

Table 3.4: Levels of fat, saturated fats, total sugars, and salt in foods used to classify foods for front of pack labels in the UK as green (low), amber (medium), or red (high).

RATING	LOW	MEDIUM	HIGH	
Color code	Green	Amber	Red	
Fat	< 3.0 g/100 g	> 3.0 to £ 17.5/100 g	> 17.5/100 g	> 21.0 g/portion
Saturated fat	< 1.5 g/100 g	> 1.5 to £ 5.0/100 g	> 5.0/100 g	> 6.0 g/portion
Total sugars	< 5.0 g/100 g	> 5.0 to £ 22.5/100 g	> 22.5/100 g	> 27.0 g/portion
Salt	< 0.3 g/100 g	> 0.3 to £ 1.5/100 g	> 1.5/100 g	> 1.8 g/portion

< equal to or less than; > more than

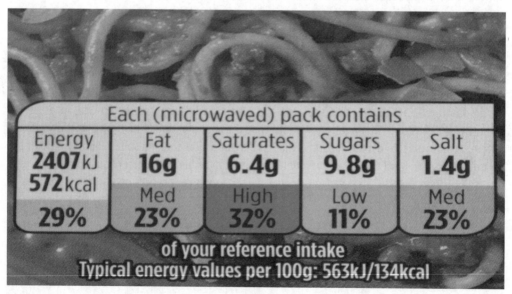

Photo 3.1: Example of a front-of-pack UK color-coded food label

In short, the greener the label, the healthier the choice. If you buy a food that has all or mostly green on the label, you know straight away that it's a healthier choice than one that contains any amber or red. As amber means neither high nor low, you can eat foods with all or mostly amber on the label most of the time. However, any red on the label means the food is high in fat, saturated fat, salt, or sugars, and these are the foods we should cut down on. Try to eat these foods less often and in small amounts (see the next chapter for details on exactly how to eat a healthy diet).

Most pre-packed food products also have a list of ingredients on the packaging or an attached label. The ingredients list can also help you work out how healthy the product is.

Ingredients are listed in order of weight, so the main ingredients in the packaged food always come first. That means that if the first few ingredients are high-fat ingredients, such as cream, butter, or oil, then the food is almost certainly a high-fat food. Many ingredient lists on food packages also highlight items that are potential allergens such as peanut and gluten containing cereals like wheat. The list may also include a statement that there are "no artificial colors, flavors, or hydrogenated fat" in the product.

HEALTH CLAIMS ON FOOD LABELS

Until relatively recently, many of the foods that we bought had statements on the label about their beneficial effects on the body, such as "Helps maintain a healthy heart" or "Aids digestion." These are examples of health claims. Previously, the rules on claims were extremely general, making it difficult for people to know what certain terms meant. In most countries, specific rules now help protect consumers from misleading claims, which means that any claims made about the nutritional and health benefits of a food will be allowed only if they are based on good science. In Europe, new rules came into effect on July 1, 2007, and the food industry was given some additional time to change its processes and comply with the new rules. The European Food Standards Agency (EFSA) has collated a list of claims that will need to be approved in Europe, and so far, only relatively few claims have been allowed in cases where sufficient scientific evidence was provided.

General claims about benefits to overall good health, such as "Healthy" or "Good for you," will be allowed only if accompanied by an appropriate and approved claim. This rule means that general claims must be backed up by an explanation about why the food is "healthy" or what makes it a **"superfood."** Labels cannot claim that a food can treat, prevent, or cure any disease or medical condition. These sorts of claims can only be made for licensed medicines. For instance, although calcium-rich products such as milk may reasonably claim to protect against osteoporosis, no such claims are allowed on food labels. Only the claims summarized in table 3.5 are legal (detailed information on health claims can be found on the FDA Web site). Health claims can be used only when a certain percentage of the DV is present in the food product, and the claims must be backed up by scientific evidence. In the USA, health claims must be accompanied by a disclaimer or be otherwise qualified.

Table 3.5: Health claims allowed on food labels

Health issue	Health Claim
Calcium and osteoporosis	Adequate calcium intake throughout life helps maintain bone health and reduce the risk of osteoporosis. A food must contain 20% or more of the DV for calcium.
Sodium and hypertension	Diets high in sodium may increase the risk of high blood pressure in some people; hence, a diet low in sodium may protect against hypertension.
Dietary fat and cancer	Diets high in fat increase the risk of some types of cancer; hence, low-fat diets may be protective.
Saturated fat and cholesterol and risk of coronary heart disease	Diets high in saturated fat and cholesterol increase blood cholesterol and thus the risk of heart disease. A diet low in saturated fat may therefore reduce this risk.
Foods high in fiber and cancer	Diets low in fat and rich in fiber-containing grain products, fruits, and vegetables may reduce the risk of some types of cancer.
Foods high in fiber and risk of coronary heart disease	Diets low in saturated fat and cholesterol and rich in fruits, vegetables, and grain products that contain fiber, particularly soluble fiber, may reduce the risk of coronary heart disease.
Folic acid and birth defects	Adequate folic acid intake by the mother reduces the risk of birth defects of the brain or spinal cord in her baby.
Dietary sugar and dental caries	Sugar-free foods that are sweetened with sugar alcohols do not promote tooth decay and may reduce the risk of dental caries.

A food carrying a health claim must be a naturally good source (10% or more of the daily value) for one of six nutrients (vitamin A, vitamin C, protein, calcium, iron, or fiber) and must not contain more than 20% of the daily value for fat, saturated fat, cholesterol, or sodium.

ARE THE CLAIMS ABOUT SUPERFOODS FOR REAL?

The term "superfood" is actually a marketing term for food with supposed health benefits as a means to sell more products. Scientists do not use the term, and nutritionally speaking, there is no such thing as a superfood. No single food item holds the key to good health or prevention of disease although it is true to say that certain food groups can contribute to some health benefits when eaten as part of a healthy balanced diet. Such foods include dark leafy green vegetables that are rich in fiber and phytonutrients, berries that have a high content of antioxidants, eggs that are rich in vitamins, protein and some unique antioxidants (e.g., lutein and zeaxanthin, which are known to protect vision and eye health), oily fish like salmon and mackerel that have a relatively high content of vitamin D and omega-3 fatty acids which have anti-inflammatory actions, herbs such as garlic, ginger, and turmeric which have some medicinal properties and vegetables that have a high **nitrate** content (e.g., beetroot and rhubarb) that are known help to lower blood pressure. The downside often is that you have to consume rather a lot of these foods to get the specific health benefits that are claimed. For example, to get 4 millimoles of nitrate (the effective dose to lower blood pressure by 5-10 mm Hg), you would need to consume about 200 g of beetroot which is rather a lot. However, there are some products now available that supply beetroot as a juice (you need about 400 mL to get the effective dose) or better still as a shot of concentrated juice (you only need about 70 mL for the required dose). Others like turmeric and garlic can be taken in capsule form. However, the bottom line is that achieving optimal health through food and nutrition is more than about just focusing on one or two of the latest food trends.

Good health is best supported by eating a variety of nutritious foods every day. There are also some hidden dangers in labelling foods as superfoods. For example, people may assume that because they are super healthy, they can eat them in unlimited quantities, but they still contain calories, and you can gain weight from eating too much healthy food. It may also encourage people to eat one kind of food over another and can lead to certain good foods being excluded from the diet just because they do not appear on a superfood list. Although superfoods might be a good introduction to healthy eating, and while understanding the influence that food can have on your health can be interesting and enlightening, it is your overall diet that is the most important factor in determining how good your health can be. Alongside getting enough exercise and sleep, practicing good hygiene, and avoiding bad habits like smoking and binge drinking, that is.

DO I NEED TO TAKE ANY SUPPLEMENTS?

Guidelines for a healthy balanced diet are given in the next chapter. If these guidelines are adhered to then there is no need to take supplements of vitamins, minerals, **essential fatty acids**, or protein as all will be supplied in adequate amounts by such a diet. One possible exception is vitamin D which unlike all the other essential vitamins, is synthesized in the skin when sunlight exposure is adequate. Most of the vitamin D in the body is produced internally this way, and only a small proportion normally comes from the diet. Therefore, in the winter months, when the strength of the sun is insufficient to produce vitamin D in the skin, a daily supplement of 1000 IU (25 micrograms) of vitamin D3 is desirable to maintain vitamin D status at its peak summer-time levels. Other situations where a supplement might be considered are as follows:

1. When a person is consuming a low energy diet in order to lose weight, then a daily multivitamin tablet can be taken to ensure that no deficiencies occur during the period of restricted food intake.

2. **Caffeine** in a dose of 1-3 mg per kg body weight can help to reduce perceived effort during exercise lasting an hour or more. This can be taken as a supplement using 50 mg tablets, but enough caffeine is contained in a cup of strong coffee to supply the required dose. This should be drunk about one hour before exercise for optimal effect.

3. **Probiotics** are "friendly" live bacteria which when ingested in sufficient amounts, modify the gut microbial population (called the **microbiota**) and can have some beneficial health effects. Probiotics are a particularly useful supplement to take after a course of antibiotic medication (usually prescribed to treat bacterial infections), as many antibiotics destroy a significant proportion of the microbiota. Taking probiotics at this time ensures that the microbiota is restored with good bacteria rather than bad ones. There is some scientific evidence that certain probiotics can also reduce the incidence of respiratory and gastrointestinal infections making them a potentially useful daily supplement for individuals who are particularly prone to infection (see chapter 11 for further details).

Key Points

- Essential nutrients cannot be synthesized in the body and are therefore required for some critical functions throughout life, and they are required in the diet for growth, health, and survival. Absence from the diet or inadequate intake results in characteristic signs of a deficiency, disease, and ultimately death.

- Humans have an essential requirement for over 40 nutrients. Nonessential nutrients can be synthesized in the body from their precursors.

- Some countries including the USA, UK, and Australia have developed a set of nutrient requirements and specific nutrient recommendations for individuals as well as groups. These were traditionally focused only on providing sufficient essential nutrients to prevent deficiency diseases such as scurvy or beriberi but now also provide guidelines for reducing the risk of diet-related chronic conditions such as heart disease, type 2 diabetes, hypertension, and osteoporosis while still providing sufficient essential nutrients.

- Guidelines have also become more specific and have been developed for various sex and age groups (and for pregnant and lactating women). Groups will have different reference values.

- Food labeling that includes information about amounts of the more important nutrients is now compulsory for many products in industrialized countries. Food labels help consumers make choices by providing detailed information about the nutrient content of food and the way in which that food fits into the overall diet. Any general claims about specific foods must be backed up by scientific evidence and an explanation about why the food is "healthy" which satisfies the relevant regulatory authority.

- Superfoods are particular food items that have supposed health benefits, but the term is actually something used in marketing to sell more products. Scientists do not use the term and nutritionally speaking, there is no such thing as a superfood.

- Supplements are generally unnecessary with the possible exception of vitamin D during the winter months.

Chapter 4

How to Eat a Healthy Balanced Diet

Objectives

After reading this chapter, you should be able to do the following:

- Understand why excessive intakes of some nutrients or certain subgroups and nonessential nutrients can have harmful effects on health

- Know why deficiencies of some nonessential nutrients can mean that our diets will not deliver what we need for optimal function and health

- Understand the current guidelines for a healthy diet

- Appreciate the differences in the dietary guidelines from different countries

- Understand the effects of food processing

In the previous two chapters, the functions and recommended intakes of the various nutrients were described. When people sit down for a meal, however, they eat food, not nutrients. Most people do not think about the individual nutrients or the combination of nutrients that they are consuming. Instead, they are concerned about the flavor, the texture, the palatability, and the smell of the food. Although many people recognize the importance and nutritional value of food and may be aware of some of the health implications of what they eat and drink, food choices are based on many factors, including previous experiences, personal preferences, availability, cost, and convenience. Advice is offered by numerous government departments (e.g., health, agriculture) and other agencies (e.g., World Health Organization) about foods or combinations of foods that will deliver certain amounts of nutrients. This chapter explores the recommendations given to people in various countries.

All of us should want to remain healthy – in both the short and long term – so it is important to understand the basis of a healthy diet. This chapter examines what a healthy diet means in relation to preserving long term health, avoiding weight gain, and reducing the risk of developing chronic cardiovascular and metabolic diseases. This obviously includes a discussion about how people can achieve a healthy diet through appropriate food choices and eating to maintain energy balance and avoiding excesses. The topic of energy requirements will be dealt with in more detail in the next chapter.

HEALTH EFFECTS OF CONSUMING INADEQUATE OR EXCESSIVE AMOUNTS OF NUTRIENTS

We all need certain amounts of energy and specific nutrients in order to survive and be healthy. We need energy from the food we eat to maintain our bodies and to be able to move. The main energy sources in our diet are carbohydrates and fats. We need protein to which enables our cells to divide, grow, develop, and function. And we need vitamins and minerals which play numerous vital roles in the body. They are needed for bone structure, nerve transmission, oxygen transport, wound healing, and immune function. They are also involved in metabolism and are needed for the function of many enzymes including those that convert food into energy, synthesize new molecules, and repair cellular damage. However, even if we consume adequate amounts of essential nutrients, this in itself does not guarantee the absence of potentially harmful effects on our health in relation to the food that we consume. Eating too much of some nutrients (e.g., carbohydrates, fats), or certain subgroups of nutrients (e.g., simple sugars, corn syrups, saturated fats, *trans* fatty acids), and other nonessential nutrients (e.g., alcohol, salt) can have harmful effects on our health. These effects may not always be obvious in the short term (i.e., days, weeks, or months), but in the long term (i.e., years), excess intakes increase our risk of developing chronic metabolic and cardiovascular diseases and cancer. Consuming sufficient vitamins and certain minerals is essential for good health, but consuming too much of high dose **(megadose)** supplements actually will have negative health effects. Also, deficiencies of some of the nonessential nutrients (e.g., fiber, phytonutrients) can mean that our diets will not deliver what we need for optimal function and health. Here some of the science and controversies regarding these important health issues are examined, and a summary of the current guidelines and recommendations is provided.

CARBOHYDRATE INTAKE AND HEALTH EFFECTS

Carbohydrate intake varies enormously in different parts of the world. For instance, in many parts of Africa, the diet typically consists of 80% carbohydrate (as a percentage of total daily energy intake), whereas in the Western world, carbohydrate intake averages 40% to 50%. In Caribbean countries, carbohydrate intake is about 65%. A carbohydrate intake of 40% to 50% is equivalent to approximately 300 g of carbohydrate per day in a relatively sedentary person. A more active person would likely consume more than this, and individuals who engage in regular sport, particularly endurance sports, tend to have more than 60% of their total energy intake as carbohydrate and may eat up to 900 g per day.

There is absolutely no doubt that both the quantity and quality of carbohydrate we regularly consume has important influences on the risk of developing obesity, cardiovascular disease, and type 2 diabetes. Sugar consumption is a proven cause of weight gain, and obesity is strongly associated with increased risk of cardiovascular and metabolic diseases. In the Western diet, about half of the daily carbohydrate intake is in the form of sugars, especially sucrose and high-fructose corn syrups. Numerous studies indicate that dietary fiber has an important influence on satiety (the feeling of fullness after a meal that inhibits our desire to eat more), and that relatively high intakes of dietary fiber can reduce weight gain and also protect against cardiovascular disease. Other studies have shown that some important sources of carbohydrate such as vegetables and fruits protect against coronary heart disease (CHD) and cancer, whereas whole grains provide protection against cardiovascular disease, type 2 diabetes, and weight gain.

The old adage "everything in moderation" seems to apply to the amount of carbohydrate we consume in our diet. Indeed, eating carbohydrates in moderation seems to be optimal for health and living longer as one important new research study published in 2018 has shown. The study involved over 15,400 US adults aged 45-64 years and investigated the association between the percentage of energy from carbohydrate intake and all-cause **mortality** and was extended to a **meta-analysis** (pulling together results from multiple studies to come up with a summary outcome or recommendation) from seven other multinational studies involving cohorts totaling over 432,000 participants from 20 different countries. A particular interest of the researchers was to determine whether the substitution of calories from animal or plant sources of fat and protein for carbohydrate affected mortality. In the US cohort study, there was a U-shaped association between the percentage of energy consumed from carbohydrate and mortality; the lowest risk of mortality appears to be when 50-55% of a person's energy needs were derived from carbohydrate. In the meta-analysis of all cohorts, both low-carbohydrate consumption (<40%) and high-carbohydrate consumption (>70%) conferred greater mortality risk than did moderate intake, consistent with the U-shaped association identified in the US cohort study. However, results varied by the source of macronutrients for participants who consumed relatively low-carbohydrate diets. Mortality rate increased by 18% when carbohydrates were exchanged for animal-derived fat or protein (e.g., from lamb, beef, pork, and chicken), but mortality decreased by 18% when the substitutions were made with plant-based protein (e.g., from vegetables, nuts, peanut butter, and whole-grain breads). The take home message is that both high and low-carbohydrate diets were associated with increased mortality, with minimal risk observed at 50-55% carbohydrate intake. That is reassuring as the Western diet actually contains about 50% carbohydrate, and this is the percentage currently recommended by health authorities in North America, the UK and Europe. Eating plant sources of fat and protein protected against the higher mortality risk when consuming low-carbohydrate diets, indicating that the source of food notably modifies the association between carbohydrate intake and mortality.

SUGAR INTAKE AND HEALTH EFFECTS

Over the past century, the intake of simple sugars has increased dramatically to approximately 50 kg per person per year—25 times more than 100 years ago. Most of this increase is due to increased consumption of soft drinks, but candy, cookies, cakes, pies and sauces have also contributed to the increase (figure 4.1).

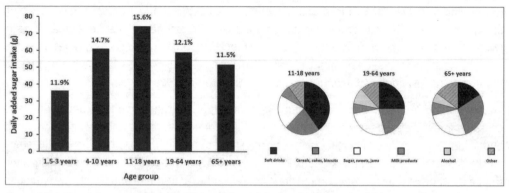

Figure 4.1: Sources of sugar intake in the Western diet: (a) Daily added sugar intake by age group and (b) where different age groups get their added sugar from. Data from UK National Diet and Nutrition Survey Rolling Programme (2008/2009-2011/12), published 2014. Available at https://www.gov.uk/government/collections/national-diet-and-nutrition-survey.

Evidence is accumulating that the intake of large amounts of simple sugars is linked to increased risk of obesity and cardiovascular disease. There is still considerable debate about this, however, because the results of studies to date are not conclusive, and the picture is often complicated by the fact that a higher sugar intake is often accompanied by higher saturated fat intake and higher energy intake as well. Therefore, sugar could just be a contributor and an indicator of an overall higher energy intake. A recent analysis of food availability data in the United States has confirmed that this is the case. It was found that between 1970 and 2014 the intake of all major **food groups** increased. Sugar intake increased, but so did the consumption of fats and oils; even fruit intake increased! Since the 1950s Americans have been eating more and more. In contrast participation in sports and levels of physical activity in general have declined among the majority, and many people now have sedentary lifestyle behaviors (e.g., occupations that involve minimal exercise, driving rather than walking or cycling, sitting watching television, playing computer games, spending lots of time texting and using social media platforms on tablets and mobile phones, etc.), so it is easy to understand how the obesity epidemic has developed. It may not be just increased intake of carbohydrate or sugar per se that is the problem, but this is very likely a contributor.

Generally, diets low in fiber and high in simple sugars are associated with weight gain and increased risk of **non-insulin-dependent diabetes mellitus (NIDDM)**, or type 2 diabetes, which is characterized by a lack of sensitivity to the hormone insulin. For more information on the characteristics of this disease – which affects millions of people worldwide – see the sidebar. If you have been diagnosed with prediabetes (a condition that precedes type 2 diabetes) or type 2 diabetes, then you should read my new book on beating type 2 diabetes (to be published by

Meyer & Meyer in 2020) which tells you everything you need to know about type 2 diabetes, including its diagnosis, causes, consequences, treatment, monitoring and management, and how to get yourself rid of it.

What Does It Mean to Be Diagnosed With Non-Insulin-Dependent Diabetes Mellitus (NIDDM), or Type 2 Diabetes?

An increasing number of people are being diagnosed as suffering from type 2 diabetes by their medical practitioner. The diagnosis is usually made after a blood test reveals a glycated hemoglobin A1c concentration of 48 mmol/mol (or 6.5%) or higher. Hemoglobin is the red pigment in your blood cells that carries oxygen, and it is said to be glycated when some sugar (glucose) molecules become attached to it, which only occurs when the blood sugar levels remain higher than normal for too long. The level of glycated hemoglobin reflects the average blood glucose concentration over the previous 2-3 months. A high level indicates that the body tissues are becoming less responsive to the hormone insulin which normally stimulates glucose uptake from the blood by muscle, liver and adipose tissue. The condition is caused by being overweight usually as a result of overeating (even if it is only a small excess of calories each day) and a lack of exercise. If uncontrolled blood glucose stays much higher for longer after feeding and even fasting, blood glucose concentrations can become extremely high. Fat breakdown and mobilization is normally inhibited by insulin, and reduced insulin action will therefore result in increased fatty acid concentrations in the blood. This reduced insulin sensitivity (which is also called increased insulin resistance) has far-reaching consequences and may result in many serious clinical complications including cardiovascular disease, kidney disease, blindness, nerve damage, more frequent infections, and poor wound healing. Type 2 diabetes also forms part of the metabolic syndrome, a term that is used to describe the common co-occurrence of several known cardiovascular disease risk factors, including insulin resistance, obesity, high blood cholesterol, and high blood pressure (hypertension).

Globally, the estimated diabetes prevalence for 2017 was 425 million and is expected to affect about 630 million people by 2045 if current trends continue. More than 110 million US adults are now living with diabetes or prediabetes, according to a 2017 report from the Centers for Disease Control and Prevention (CDC). Over 30 million Americans – almost 10% of the US population – have type 2 diabetes. Another 84 million have prediabetes, a condition that if not treated, often leads to type 2 diabetes within five years. In the UK about 9% of adults (aged over 16) have diabetes. This means that, including the number of undiagnosed people, there is estimated to be over 4 million people living with diabetes in the UK at present. The proportion of people who have diabetes increases with age: 9% of people aged 45 to 54 have diabetes, but for over 75s it is 24%. Diabetes at older ages has even bigger health implications as people are more likely to be suffering from other diseases, particularly cardiovascular diseases. Diabetes is more common in men (10% compared with 8% for women) and people from south Asia as well as; Hispanic and black ethnic groups are nearly twice as likely to have the disease compared with people from white, mixed, or other ethnic groups (15% compared with 9%).

If you have Type 2 diabetes you may be prescribed medication to help manage your blood sugar levels. The most common tablet form is metformin which decreases liver glucose production, decreases intestinal absorption of glucose, and improves insulin sensitivity by increasing tissue glucose uptake. There are numerous other types of medication as well, including sulfonylurea drugs, which stimulate the pancreas to produce more insulin. Insulin (by injection) is not usually given in the first five years after diagnosis. The best treatment is to get rid of the condition by going on a diet to lose weight and doing more physical activity. Research shows that the longer you have type 2 diabetes, the harder it is to reverse, so it obviously makes sense to take action as soon as possible after you have been diagnosed with the condition. Going on a very low energy diet (800 kcal/day) for 20 weeks has recently been shown to be effective in reversing type 2 diabetes, but it takes a lot of willpower to stick to such a diet for a long time. Losing the excess body fat and weight by a combination of less severe dieting and exercise could theoretically achieve the same goal and is easier to stick to. My new book on how to beat type 2 diabetes (to be published in 2020) explains exactly how you can do this. Chapter 13 describes how you can safely lose 7-10 kg of body weight in only 10 weeks using this combination approach. Exercise is known to improve insulin sensitivity independent of weight loss and comes with other health benefits that are described in chapter 9.

There are numerous large-scale population studies (that scientists call **epidemiological studies**) that link sugar intake to increases in obesity and type 2 diabetes. The WHO commissioned a number of reviews to assess the effects of increasing or decreasing intake of free sugars on excess weight gain and dental caries. It has been suggested that the consumption of a diet high in total carbohydrate adversely affects insulin sensitivity compared with consumption of a high-fat diet. Simple sugars, particularly fructose, appear to have adverse effects on insulin action although these findings apply to a population with extremely low levels of physical activity, and therefore the observations may not relate only to the carbohydrate intake. Endurance athletes, who generally consume diets with large amounts of carbohydrate, have higher than average insulin sensitivity confirming that regular exercise offers protection against type 2 diabetes (more about this in chapter 9).

Although a dose response relationship between sugar consumption and obesity cannot be definitively determined at this time, the evidence was of sufficient strength and consistency for the WHO to officially launch guidelines in 2015 for sugar intake in adults and children. In these, they recommend adults and children reduce their daily intake of free sugars to less than 10% of their total energy intake, and they suggest that a further reduction to below 5% or roughly 25 g (6 teaspoons) per day would provide additional health benefits. The UK has recently adopted the Scientific Advisory Committee on Nutrition's recommendation that no more than 5% of energy intake should be from free sugars. The term "free sugars" includes any sugar added by the manufacturer or during cooking plus natural free sugars in honey, syrups, and fruit juices but excludes any natural sugars in fresh fruit.

Another adverse effect of certain carbohydrates (primarily glucose, fructose, and sucrose, but also starches) is on **dental caries** (bacterial tooth decay) by providing a substrate for bacterial fermentation; bacteria in dental plaque metabolize dietary sugars to acids which then dissolve dental enamel and dentine. In many countries, the severity of dental caries increased in parallel with importation of sugar, reaching its zenith in the 1950s and 1960s. Since then, severity has declined in many countries, due to the widespread use of fluoride especially in toothpaste, but dental caries remains a disease of medical, social, and economic importance. Within the EU in 2011, the cost of dental treatment was estimated to be 79 billion euros. The evidence that dietary sugars are the main cause of dental caries is extensive; without sugar, caries would be negligible. Sucrose in particular increases the prevalence and progression of dental caries. Sugars are most detrimental if they are consumed between meals and in a form that is retained in the mouth for a long time. For example, sweets and candy often consist of sucrose and have a relatively long contact time with teeth. If sugar is consumed in acidic beverages (such as soft drinks or sports drinks), the risk of dental caries and teeth erosion is further increased. Risks can be decreased by drinking fluoridated water, brushing or flossing teeth (removing plaque), and reducing frequency and duration of contact with these carbohydrates by reducing sugar intake (see chapter 12 for further details).

SUGAR-SWEETENED BEVERAGE INTAKE AND HEALTH EFFECTS

Soft drink consumption in the Western world has increased considerably in the past two decades, particularly among children. On average, US adolescents and adults consume over 150 kcal/day from **sugar-sweetened beverages (SSBs)**. During 2011-2014 in the US, on average, about 7% of the total daily calories for children and adults were obtained from SSBs. Globally there has been a steady upward trend in consumption of SSBs from 2005 to 2011. This is why some states (and also some countries such as the UK) are experimenting with sugar taxes: adding tax to SSBs in an attempt to discourage sales. However, it is worth noting that data from the US Department of Agriculture indicates that between 1970 and 2010 in the USA average total daily energy intake increased by 474 kcal per person. Virtually all of this increase in energy intake (~94%) can be attributed to an increase in flour and cereal products and added fats, while added sugars only contributed 7% of the total increased calorie intake. Thus, data related to added sugar intake as a potential significant contributor to weight gain and obesity must be treated with caution; although it is likely to be a contributor to weight gain, it is only part of the problem. Moreover, public policy attempts to limit sugar consumption as a mechanism for helping individuals control weight seem unlikely to succeed; most people appear willing to pay a little more for their daily sugar fix!

Studies of SSB intake by children have shown regular consumption of these beverages results in larger weight gain compared with children who consume SSBs less often or rarely. This may relate to the lack of satiation (feeling of fullness) provided by these drinks as well as the calories they contain. Masking (i.e., hiding) replacement of SSBs with low or zero calorie beverages containing artificial sweeteners has been found to reduce weight gain in children. Several meta-analyses (large-scale statistical analyses based on data from numerous previously published studies) have suggested that SSBs are associated with weight gain and obesity in both children and adults and that the weight gain appears to be due to the increased energy consumption rather than any unique aspect of sugars themselves. Very high SSB consumption may increase risk of CHD, at least in those with a sedentary lifestyle where SSB intake contributes to a positive energy balance (i.e., where daily energy intake exceeds daily energy expenditure; you can find more detail on this in the next chapter).

HIGH FRUCTOSE INTAKE AND HEALTH EFFECTS

Some of the concerns about the health effects of excess carbohydrate intake have specifically focused on the monosaccharide fructose and corn syrup, which has high fructose content. Fructose was only present in our diet in very small quantities up to a few hundred years ago, but it has now become a major constituent of our diet. Our main dietary sources of fructose are sugar in the form of the disaccharide sucrose from beet or cane, high fructose corn syrup, fruits, fruit juices, and honey. Fructose, like glucose, is a 6-carbon sugar but its metabolism differs markedly from that of glucose due to its almost complete uptake by the liver where it is converted into glucose, glycogen, or fat. High fructose intake has been shown to cause increased blood cholesterol and to impair liver insulin sensitivity. In large amounts, dietary fructose leads to greater adverse metabolic changes than equivalent amounts of glucose, although the extent to which fructose itself is contributing to many of the metabolic changes found in the obese, as distinct from the calories it provides, is still a matter of debate.

FIBER INTAKE AND HEALTH EFFECTS

In the US and Canada, a fiber intake of at least 14 g per 1,000 kcal (4.2 MJ) of dietary energy intake is recommended. For most people, this intake would equal 25 to 30 g of fiber per day. The typical fiber intake in Western countries, however, is only about 15 g per day for females and 18 g per day for males. In African countries, the intake of fiber is much higher, in fact as much as 40 to 150 g per day. A low fiber intake is associated with increased risk of cardiovascular disease whereas higher than average intakes of fiber from cereal, fruit and vegetable sources are inversely associated with risk of both CHD and other cardiovascular diseases.

Fruit, vegetables, and plant fiber have also long been thought to protect against cancer. Indeed, high intake of fruits and vegetables is associated with reduced incidence of some cancers; however, this may be related not only to fiber intake but also to intake of folic acid and phytonutrients (see later in this chapter). The European Prospective Investigation into Cancer and Nutrition, a *prospective cohort study* (a study that follows over time a group of similar individuals, known as a cohort, to determine how certain factors affect rates of a certain outcome) that includes over half a million participants from 10 European countries, has examined associations between fruit, vegetable, or fiber consumption and the risk of cancer at 14 different sites. This large-scale study has thus far reported that the risk of cancers of the upper gastrointestinal tract was inversely associated with fruit intake but was not associated with vegetable intake. The risk of **colorectal cancer** (also known as bowel cancer) was inversely associated with intakes of total fruit and vegetables and total fiber, and the risk of liver cancer was also inversely associated with the intake of total fiber. The risk of cancer of the lung among smokers was inversely associated with fruit intake but was not associated with vegetable intake. There was a borderline inverse association of fiber intake with breast cancer risk. For the other nine cancer sites studied (stomach, biliary tract, **pancreas**, cervix, endometrium, prostate, kidney, bladder, and lymph nodes) there were no reported significant associations of risk with intakes of total fruit, vegetables, or fiber.

Potential mechanisms for reduced risk of some cancers with high fiber intake include reduced transit time of food (the time that food spends in the gut) which could reduce the uptake of **carcinogenic** substances. A second possible mechanism would be that the fiber itself absorbs some of these carcinogenic substances. In addition, a change in fiber intake may be the result of an alteration of nutritional habits that reduce the presence of carcinogenic substances (e.g., an increase in fiber intake is often accompanied by decreased meat and saturated fat intake). Higher fiber intake has also been associated with better weight maintenance. Therefore, increasing dietary fiber intake is often recommended because of its apparent protective effects against cancers, cardiovascular diseases, and type 2 diabetes.

FAT INTAKE AND HEALTH EFFECTS

According to a large nutrition survey in the US called National Health and Nutrition Examination Survey (NHANES), fat intake has declined from 36.9% to 33.5% of total energy intake for men and from 36.1% to 33.9% for women in the period 1971 through 2004. Although at first sight that seems like a good thing, the actual amount of fat intake (in grams) increased slightly because of an increase in total daily energy intake. In the period 2004 through 2010 there has been a slight reduction in both total energy and fat intake. However, few people in Western countries have a fat intake below 20%. Over 95% of the daily fat intake is in the form of triglycerides. The other fats such as phospholipids, fatty acids, cholesterol, and plant sterols make up the remainder. The daily triglyceride intake in the North American diet is about 100 to 150 g/day. The average person in the US consumes about a third of fat from plant origin (vegetables) and two-thirds from animal sources. Animal fat is higher in saturated fat than fat from plant sources and saturated fat typically represents about 11% of the total energy intake.

SATURATED FAT INTAKE AND HEALTH EFFECTS

Higher levels of blood cholesterol are associated with high intakes of saturated fats. More than half of the cholesterol in the body is actually synthesized by cells of the body with the liver and intestines each producing about 10-15% of the total daily amount, and only about 20% is directly obtained from the diet. Normal adults typically synthesize about 1 g of cholesterol per day, and the total body content is about 35 g. Typical daily additional dietary intake of cholesterol in the US and other Western countries is about 0.2 to 0.3 g. The body compensates for cholesterol intake by reducing the amount synthesized. Cholesterol is found in eggs, red meat, organ meat (heart, liver, and kidney), shellfish, and dairy products such as whole milk, butter, cheese, and cream. Foods of plant origin contain no cholesterol. But even if a cholesterol-free diet is consumed, the body synthesizes 0.5 to 0.9 g of cholesterol per day. In the blood stream, cholesterol is mostly transported in lipoprotein particles.

Research has shown that populations that consume diets high in saturated fats have relatively high levels of blood cholesterol and suffer a high prevalence of CHD. Particularly, **low density lipoprotein (LDL)** cholesterol promotes the development of arteriosclerosis and predisposes to cardiovascular disease. **High density lipoprotein (HDL)** cholesterol, on the other hand, seems to protect against cardiovascular disease. Reducing blood LDL cholesterol decreases the risk for CHD, thus providing evidence for a direct causal relationship. Various ways by which LDL cholesterol in the blood can be lowered seem effective in reducing the risk of cardiovascular disease, such as reducing the intake of saturated fat, increasing physical activity, and consuming cholesterol-lowering drugs such as statins which inhibit cholesterol synthesis. A reduction in cardiovascular events was seen in studies that primarily replaced saturated fat calories with polyunsaturated fat, whereas no effects were seen in studies replacing saturated fat with carbohydrate or protein.

The Seven Countries Study compared CHD mortality in 12,000 men aged 40 to 59 in seven countries and found positive correlations between CHD mortality and total fat intake in 1970, then in 1986 between CHD mortality and saturated fat intake. A migrant study of Japanese men living in different cultures confirmed in 1974 that men in California had the diet richest in saturated fat and cholesterol and the highest CHD rates, those in Hawaii had intermediate saturated fat and CHD rates, and those in Japan had a diet lowest in saturated fat and cholesterol and the least CHD.

Some studies have suggested a correlation between high dietary fat intake and obesity, but currently the evidence that high-fat intake contributes to obesity is insufficient to make definitive recommendations for a very low-fat diet. Therefore, the 2015 *Dietary Guidelines for Americans* state that fat intake should be moderate (rather than low). In fact, a very low-fat, high-carbohydrate intake may have adverse health effects. Reducing dietary fat to below 20% of energy intake while replacing the calories from fat with those from carbohydrate results in elevated plasma triglycerides, increased LDL cholesterol, and decreased HDL cholesterol. These metabolic changes increase the risk of cardiovascular disease and predispose to CHD, particularly for those with a sedentary lifestyle.

High-fat intake (along with low fiber intake) has been linked with increased incidence of colon and prostate cancer and with increased body weight. Epidemiological studies suggest that, as with cardiovascular diseases, the type of fat is important to cancer risk. The associations between high-fat intake and cancer may be due to the intake of animal fat (saturated fat), not vegetable fat (unsaturated fat), raising the possibility that fat per se is not the most important factor. In contrast, omega-3 fatty acids from fish seem to protect against cancer. For example, the native Inuit of Alaska and populations in Japan, who rely heavily on fish and thus have a relatively high intake of fish oil, have lower incidences of cancer.

TRANS FAT INTAKE AND HEALTH EFFECTS

Trans fatty acids are unsaturated fatty acids that contain at least one double bond in the *trans* instead of the *cis* configuration (see chapter 2 for details). Unlike other dietary fats, *trans* fats are neither essential nor desirable, and in fact, there is convincing evidence indicating that *trans* fatty acid intake raises blood LDL cholesterol levels and lowers HDL cholesterol levels, increasing the risk of cardiovascular disease. The two main sources of dietary *trans* fatty acids nowadays are meat and dairy products. Previously, partially hydrogenated fats from margarine were also a major source of *trans* fats, but because of a number of factors, including changes in federal labeling requirements for packaged foods, and local bans and grassroots pressure on the use of partially hydrogenated fat, *trans* fat intake has declined in recent years. Similar to saturated fatty acids, *trans* fatty acids increase plasma LDL-cholesterol concentrations. In contrast to saturated fatty acids, trans fatty acids do not increase HDL-cholesterol concentrations so their overall effect is to increase the LDL/HDL ratio, which is an important risk factor for cardiovascular disease. Thus, dietary recommendations from many countries are to limit *trans*-fat intake. The 2015-2020 *Dietary Guidelines for Americans* recommends keeping *trans*-fat intake as low as possible. Results from the most recent UK National Diet and Nutrition Survey (NDNS) rolling program (2012/13 – 2013/14) show that children and adults, including older adults, are eating 0.5-0.6% of food energy as *trans* fats. The UK Scientific Advisory Committee on Nutrition recommends that average intakes of *trans* fatty acids should not exceed 2% of food energy, so on average, the UK is well-within recommended maximum levels. But that doesn't mean we should be complacent about *trans* fats in foods, especially foods that may not have ingredients lists or labels, like takeaway and fast food items.

Is Margarine Healthier Than Butter?

There has been a long-simmering controversy over the health risks associated with regular consumption of butter compared with margarine. Although butter and margarine have the same (high) energy density and total fat content, their fatty acid composition is different. Margarine is manufactured from plant-derived polyunsaturated fatty acids that are partially hydrogenated (meaning the addition of hydrogen atoms) to prevent them from becoming rancid and to keep them solid at room temperature. Until the 1980s about 20% of the fatty acids in margarine were *trans* fatty acids compared with 7% in butter. Health concerns about these fats have more recently led to many manufacturers reducing the amounts of *trans* fats in foods such as margarines. Production methods for margarines and spreads have now altered due to concerns between *trans* fats and risk of cardiovascular disease. This has led to the reformulation of many margarines and spreads to make them much lower and, in some products, virtually free of *trans* fats. Margarine does not contain cholesterol, because it is manufactured from vegetable oil, whereas each gram of butter contains 10 to 15 mg of cholesterol, and butter contains much more saturated fat. Therefore, nowadays, margarines are probably healthier than butter. In some respects, today the butter-versus-margarine issue is really a false one. From the standpoint of heart disease, butter is on the list of foods to use sparingly mostly because it is high in saturated fat, which aggressively increases levels of LDL. Margarines, though, aren't so easy to classify as the older stick margarines that are still widely sold are high in *trans* fats, and are worse for you than butter, whereas some of the newer margarines that are low in saturated fat, high in unsaturated fat, and free of *trans* fats are fine as long as you don't use too much (as they are still rich in calories).

PROTEIN INTAKE AND HEALTH EFFECTS

In the developed world, where protein deficiency is uncommon, dietary protein intake is less critical and not related to disease. But in developing countries, protein deficiency is more common and can result in **kwashiorkor** (a pure protein deficiency, mainly in children, characterized by a bloated belly caused by edema as well as impaired immunity with increased susceptibility to infections) or **marasmus** (a protein deficiency resulting from a total dietary energy deficiency, characterized by extreme muscle wasting). Extreme protein deficiency is ultimately fatal due to vital organ breakdown or infection, and it is a sad reflection of today's society and global politics that such problems in poorly developed countries are still tolerated or ignored. This is my personal view, but I am sure it is shared by many others.

Although it has sometimes been suggested that long-term consumption of a high-protein diet may result in impaired kidney function, evidence for this is nonexistent. A meta-analysis by scientists at McMaster University in 2018 has confirmed that there is no need for concern on this issue.

The researchers examined 28 studies involving over 1,300 participants that had investigated the effects of high protein diets on glomerular filtration rate, an index of kidney function which generally falls when kidneys become damaged or diseased. The studies included in their meta-analysis involved participants who were healthy, obese, or had type 2 diabetes or high blood pressure, and the high protein diets contained 1.5 g of protein per kilogram of body weight per day, at least 20% of total caloric intake coming from protein or at least 100 g of protein per day. They found that there is simply no evidence linking a high protein diet to kidney disease in healthy individuals or those who are at risk of kidney disease due to conditions such as obesity, hypertension, or even type 2 diabetes. For people suffering from preexisting kidney problems, this circumstance may be different and an upper limit to protein intake of 1.6 g per kilogram body weight per day may be advised. In normal health, most of the excess amino acids are broken down, and the resulting (toxic) ammonia nitrogen is excreted mainly as urea by the kidneys, and there is no risk to health, at least with intakes up to about 2.5 g per kilogram body weight per day which are sometimes reached by bodybuilders. Another health concern related to a high dietary protein intake is that consuming large amounts of red meat and processed meat has been shown to increase the risk of colorectal cancer. For further details, see the following sidebar.

Is Red Meat Unsafe to Eat?

Evidence derived from numerous large-scale prospective epidemiological studies and their meta-analyses shows that red meat (beef, lamb, and pork) and processed meat (including bacon, ham, and salami) increases colorectal cancer risk by 20-30%. According to current dietary guidelines, the recommended amount of red meat for healthy people is 500 g/week or 70 g/day. It is also recommended to limit intake of processed meat. In contrast, white meat (fish and poultry) is thought to be safe to eat and is not associated with colorectal cancer risk. A likely cause of the carcinogenic effects of red and processed meat is the presence of heterocyclic amines which are produced when meat is cooked at high temperature. Processed meat also contains other carcinogens called nitrosoamines and nitrosoamides. The formation of heterocyclic amines can be diminished by not exposing meat surfaces to flames and using aluminum foil to wrap meat before oven roasting. To reduce the carcinogenic effects of heterocyclic amines, the diet should be high in dietary fiber sources such as wholegrain foods and vegetables. Red meat can be made safer to eat by trimming any visible fat before cooking. These health concerns about red meat do not mean we should all become vegetarians. Meat is an important source of nutrients including essential amino acids, iron, zinc, and vitamin B12. The take-home message is that meat should be consumed in moderation and balanced with other foods, particularly high-fiber vegetables.

ALCOHOL INTAKE AND HEALTH EFFECTS

Alcohol (also known as ethanol), is a nonessential nutrient that provides 7 kcal of energy per gram (28 kJ/g). Average alcohol intake in the USA is currently about 2 to 3% of daily energy intake. Alcohol is the most widely abused addictive drug and, in the short-term, causes intoxication which impairs mental function. In the longer term, regular drinking is known to cause damage to the liver and other organs. Death can result from both acute binge drinking and longer term alcoholism. Alcohol is responsible for approximately 6% of deaths worldwide. In the USA between 2006 and 2010, an estimated 88,000 people (approximately 62,000 men and 26,000 women) died from alcohol-related causes annually. By the way, these figures do not include alcohol-related homicides and alcohol-impaired driving fatalities which accounted for about an additional 10,000 deaths annually. However, alcohol may have health benefits when ingested in moderation. Moderate alcohol consumption reduces stress and raises levels of HDL cholesterol, which has a protective effect against cardiovascular diseases such as CHD and stroke.

Numerous studies have consistently shown that moderate drinkers (those that consume 14 **units of alcohol** per week or less, equivalent to one 175 mL glass of wine or one pint [568 mL in UK but 473 mL in US] of beer per day) tend to have fewer heart attacks and better life expectancy than those who drink a lot or not at all. In a recent study in the UK, researchers examined the health records of almost 2 million adults aged over 30 who were free from heart disease and provided their general practitioner with details of their drinking habits. Over a period of six subsequent years, moderate drinkers had the lowest rates of heart disease and lowest risk of overall death. A large intake of alcohol, however, increases blood pressure, which outweighs the positive effects of alcohol consumption.

Protection may also be provided by polyphenols in red wine, antioxidant compounds that reduce lipoprotein oxidation and thereby prevent or reduce the formation of atherosclerotic plaques (fatty deposits in blood vessels that impair or block blood flow). The polyphenols in red wine may also be responsible for protection against prostate cancer as a recent meta-analysis of 17 previous studies covering more than 600,000 men concluded that drinking one glass of red wine per day reduces the risk of prostate cancer by about 12%. In contrast, drinking white wine actually increased the risk of prostate cancer which correlates with other studies showing that consumption of alcohol in any amount has been shown to increase the risk of cancer of the oropharynx (throat), esophagus (gullet or food pipe connecting the mouth to the stomach), and breasts.

Despite these studies indicating the likely benefits of moderate alcohol consumption, a large global study published in the Lancet in 2018 strongly suggests that overall there is no safe level of alcohol consumption. Although moderate drinking may protect against heart disease and male prostate cancer, the worldwide study found that the risk of cancer and other diseases outweighs these protections. The Global Burden of Disease study looked at levels of alcohol use and its health effects in people aged 15 to 95 in 195 countries, including the USA and UK, between 1990 and 2016. Comparing people who did not drink at all with those who had one alcoholic drink a day, it was found that out of 100,000 non-drinkers, 914 would develop an alcohol-related health problem such as cancer or suffer an injury. For people who drank one alcoholic drink per day the number increased to 918 – an increased risk of 0.5%. For people who had two alcoholic drinks a day, the relative risk increased to 7% (977 people), for those who consumed five drinks every day, there was an increase of 37% (1,252 people), and for those who consumed ten drinks every day the increased risk was 125% (2,056 people) as illustrated in figure 4.2. Overall, the researchers concluded that although several previous studies have found a protective effect of alcohol on some conditions, the combined health risks (particularly for cancer, injuries, and infectious diseases) associated with alcohol increases with any amount of alcohol and offsets the protective effects for heart disease. Now many of us (including myself) may consider a 0.5% increase in health risk to be an acceptable one to take in return for carrying on drinking one nice glass of wine per day with our meals. It is all a matter of judgement when it comes to choices about what level of risk you want to take.

Globally, one in three people are thought to drink alcohol, and it is linked to nearly a tenth of all deaths in those aged 15 to 49. Drinkers around the world have three drinks per day and the biggest drinkers are from Eastern European countries with the men from Romania topping the list at an average of eight drinks per day. In several counties, the government recommended levels of alcohol consumption for men and women is no more than 14 units a week - equivalent to six pints of average strength beer or seven glasses of wine (figure 4.3).

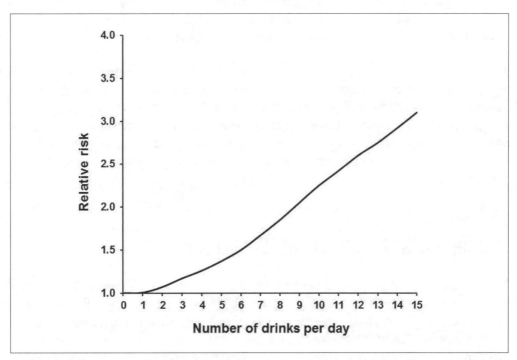

Figure 4.2: Alcoholic intake and the relative risk of all causes of death, illness, and disability. Alcohol intake is shown as the number of standard drinks (equivalent to 10 g alcohol) per day. Data from GBD 2016 Alcohol Collaborators (2018).

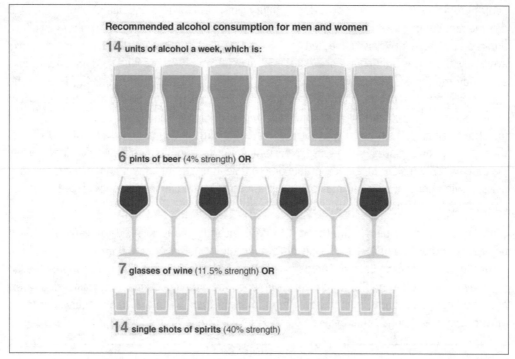

Figure 4.3: Current UK and US recommended upper limits of weekly alcohol intake

The energy content of alcohol can also be a significant contributor to the development of obesity. A 750 mL bottle of red wine contains about 600 kilocalories (2.5 MJ) which is equivalent to two hamburgers and a 500 mL bottle of beer contains around 220 kilocalories (900 kJ); despite this, the energy content of alcoholic beverages is rarely shown on the bottle. Therefore, in the interests of health, alcohol should only be consumed in moderation and at appropriate times (i.e., not before driving or participating in sport or work). Furthermore, alcohol should be avoided during pregnancy.

MICRONUTRIENT INTAKE AND HEALTH EFFECTS

The effects of inadequate intakes of the various vitamins and minerals (collectively known as the micronutrients) were covered in the previous two chapters. Deficiencies of any of the 13 vitamins or the essential minerals listed in the first sidebar of chapter 3 result in various forms of illness that can ultimately be fatal. However, excess intakes of both vitamins and minerals can be toxic and also result in ill health and death. For example, excess vitamin A causes nausea, headache, fatigue, liver damage, joint pain, skin peeling, and abnormal development of the fetus during pregnancy. Similarly, an excess of calcium can result in impaired absorption of essential trace elements, heart arrhythmia, constipation, and kidney stones. Many of us consume too much sodium in our diet, and this issue is covered in some detail in the next subsection.

SODIUM INTAKE AND HEALTH EFFECTS

Sodium is found in many foods, which is not surprising as it is the major mineral in the extracellular fluids of animals. It is also commonly added as salt (sodium chloride) to foods to enhance flavor and act as a preservative. Sodium deficiency is very rare, but when it does occur, it results in a fall in blood volume that subsequently leads to a drop in blood pressure, a serious health condition which may manifest itself in symptoms such as fatigue and lethargy. A temporary but debilitating low level of sodium in the blood (known as **hyponatremia**) can be caused by drinking far too much water, and this condition has sometimes been observed in people taking part in long duration endurance events such as a marathon. Symptoms may include changes to a person's mental state, headache, nausea, and vomiting, tiredness, muscle spasms, and seizures. Severe hyponatremia can lead to coma and can be fatal. Until fairly recently, the condition was often misdiagnosed as dehydration as the symptoms are remarkably similar. Unfortunately, this meant that the sufferers were treated by intravenous infusion of fluids which, of course, only made matters worse.

Excess sodium intake is related to the development of high blood pressure (known as hypertension). In most healthy young adults, the resting blood pressure is usually below 120 mmHg (**systolic**, when the heart contracts and ejects blood from the ventricles into the arteries) and below 80 mmHg (**diastolic**, when the heart is relaxed, and the ventricles are filling with blood). Blood pressure is largely determined by the degree of constriction of blood vessels and by sodium and water retention in the kidneys. When blood volume is increased due to sodium and water retention or constriction of the blood vessels, like when we are under stress, blood pressure rises. If resting blood pressure is chronically above a critical level of 140/90 mmHg (which is used to define the condition of hypertension), the risk of arteriosclerosis, heart attack, stroke, kidney disease, and early death increases. Blood pressure between 120 and 139 mmHg systolic and 80 and 89 mmHg diastolic is referred to as prehypertension and may indicate increased risk for the diseases mentioned earlier. Medication is often prescribed at this point to prevent blood pressure from rising further.

There is very strong evidence that a high dietary salt intake contributes to the development of high blood pressure, and this seems to arise because our kidneys are not capable of excreting large excesses of salt. In the past, most of our sodium intake would have come from eating meat and seafood, which may not have been frequently available, and our bodies are only adapted to ingest and excrete about one gram of salt per day, which is about eight times less than the average salt intake currently observed in many developed countries! As long-term consumption of high-salt diets appears to be a major factor involved in the frequent occurrence of hypertension and cardiovascular diseases in human populations, many governments and health or nutrition agencies recommend a low salt (or sodium) diet. The 2015-2020 *Dietary Guidelines for Americans* recommends an intake of no more than 2.3 g of sodium (equivalent to 5.8 g of salt) per day. People are advised to choose and prepare foods with less salt and restrict their intake of processed foods - which generally have a high salt content - and substitute salty snacks such as potato chips, pretzels, and salted peanuts with healthier alternatives like fresh fruit or raw vegetables (e.g., celery, carrot) which are low in sodium.

PHYTONUTRIENT INTAKE AND HEALTH EFFECTS

Phytonutrients are organic compounds found in plants (including many of the fruit and vegetables in our diet) that are thought to promote human health, but they differ from vitamins because they are not considered an essential nutrient. That means that without them, people will not develop a nutritional deficiency or disease, but these phytonutrients may well be needed for optimal health. Several mechanisms have been proposed by which phytonutrients such as carotenoids and polyphenols may protect human health. Among the possible mechanisms contributing to health benefits are that phytonutrients act as antioxidants, enhance immune responses, enhance cell-to-cell communication, alter estrogen metabolism, cause cancer cells to die, and help repair DNA damage caused by smoking and exposure to other toxic substances.

Evidence that fruit and vegetable consumption protects human health has come from a number of large-population studies, and at least some of these effects are thought to be caused by phytonutrients. The following are results of a few selected population studies and meta-analyses from the literature that link fruit and vegetable consumption to health. For example, fruit and vegetable consumption has been linked to decreased risk of stroke. In one study, each increment of three daily servings of fruits and vegetables equated to a 22% decrease in the risk of stroke. A recent meta-analysis of 20 prospective cohort studies, involving 16,981 stroke events among 760,629 participants, found that the relative risk of stroke decreased by 32% and 11% for every 200 g per day increment in fruit and vegetable consumption, respectively. Among older people, those with a high intake of dark green and deep yellow vegetables have half the risk of heart disease and cancer compared to those with low intakes. This difference in health outcomes arises from relatively small differences in vegetable intake (on average, 2.1 vs 0.7) servings of dark green or deep yellow vegetables per day. This evidence suggests that small, consistent changes in vegetable consumption can make important changes in health outcomes. In summary, it is reasonable to conclude that fruit and vegetable intakes are associated with reduced risk of cardiovascular disease, cancer, and all-cause mortality.

On average, Americans consume 3.3 servings of vegetables a day. But dark green vegetables and deep yellow vegetables currently each represent only 0.2 daily servings. On any given day, about half the population does not consume the minimum number of servings of vegetables recommended (three servings per day), and about 10% of the population consumes less than one serving of vegetables per day. On any given day, about 71% of the population does not consume the minimum number of servings of fruit recommended (two servings per day), and about half the population consumes less than one serving of fruit a day. This seems to be a worldwide trend; a study in 2009 showed that 78% of men and women from 52 mainly low- and middle-income countries consumed less than the minimum recommended five daily servings of fruits and vegetables.

Intake of one particular class of phytonutrients, the **flavonoids**, has been linked to lower risk of heart disease in many studies. Older Dutch men with the highest flavonoid intake had a risk of heart disease that was about 58% lower than that of counterparts with the lowest intake. Similarly, Finnish men with the highest flavonoid intake had a risk of mortality from heart disease that was about 40% lower than that of men with the lowest intake. In a 2017 meta-analysis of ten epidemiological studies, the risk of all-cause mortality for the highest versus lowest category of total flavonoids intake was 18% lower. Dose-response analysis showed that those consuming 200 mg/day of total flavonoids had the lowest risk of all-cause mortality.

PRACTICAL GUIDELINES FOR A BALANCED HEALTHY DIET

Although governments and other agencies provide recommendations and guidance on nutrient requirements to avoid deficiencies and excesses, they are not a practical way of informing people about the best food choices for optimal health. For example, even though there is a clear recommendation for adults to consume about 0.8 g/kg of body weight of protein per day and there are minimum recommended daily intakes for essential minerals like calcium and iron and vitamins like B12 and folic acid, how do people know whether they are meeting these recommended amounts from the food they are eating? A healthy diet is often referred to as a balanced diet that emphasizes the need for variety and moderation, so that the 46 essential nutrients can be supplied in sufficient amounts to support normal or optimal functioning. But how do we achieve a balanced diet? Well, the answer comes from some simple and comprehensive food guides that have been developed and progressively evolved by various expert groups of nutritionists during the past 100 years. For example, in the USA a food guide called **MyPyramid** was developed based on a previous version called the food guide pyramid. This was replaced in 2011 with **MyPlate** which distinguishes six main food groups:

- Dairy (e.g., milk, yogurt and cheese)
- Protein (e.g., meat, poultry, fish, eggs, dry beans and nuts)
- Grains (e.g., bread, cereal, rice and pasta)
- Vegetables
- Fruits
- Fats, oils and sweets

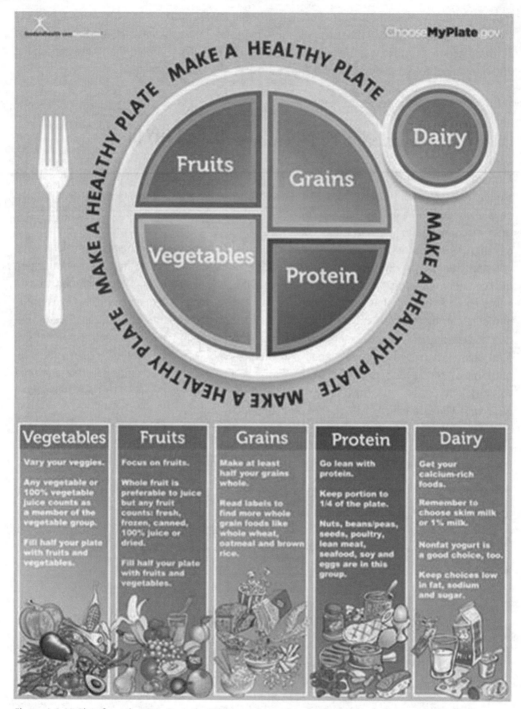

Figure 4.4: MyPlate from the USA. From the US Department of Agriculture's Center for Nutrition Policy and Promotion.

Only the first five groups are depicted on the MyPlate diagram (figure 4.4) as the fats, oils and sweets group is considered to be only a minor contributor to a healthy diet. The foods in each category make a similar nutrient contribution. MyPlate is an integral part of the latest 2015-2020 *Dietary Guidelines for Americans* produced by the US Department of Agriculture's Food and Nutrition Service. In previous versions of the guide, the only macronutrient with an RDA was protein. The latest version, however, includes recommendations for carbohydrate and fat to minimize the risk of chronic diseases. For adults the recommendation is that 45 to 65% of energy intake should be from carbohydrate, 20 to 35% from fat, and 10 to 35% from protein. Carbohydrates are found in the bread, cereal, rice, and pasta category as well as in the vegetable category and fruit category. But carbohydrates can also be found in the beans category and the sweets category. Proteins and fats are found mostly in the meat, poultry, fish, eggs, dry beans, and nuts category. Fats are a major component of the fats, oils, and sweets category.

Recommendations for healthy eating can be drawn up based on MyPlate, the 2015-2020 *Dietary Guidelines for Americans*, the 2016 *Eatwell Guide* from the UK and recommendations published by organizations and institutions in various other countries. These guidelines are based on the latest status of research and may be helpful in the prevention of obesity and associated chronic diseases, including cardiovascular disease, type 2 diabetes and cancer. The latest version of the UK's *Eatwell Guide* (2016) is shown in figure 4.5; it contains somewhat more information than MyPlate.

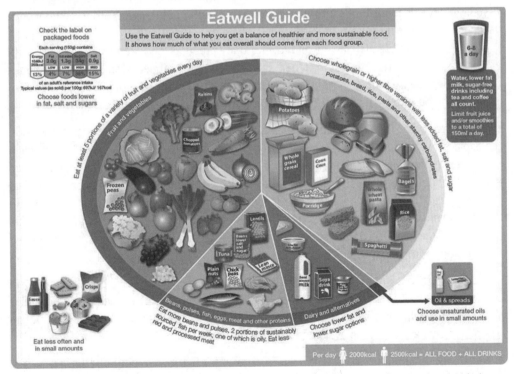

Figure 4.5: The Eatwell Guide from the United Kingdom. © Crown copyright material is reproduced with the permission of the Controller of HMSO and Queen's Printer for Scotland.

This list of guidelines shown below is quite detailed and comprehensive, so for a shortened summary version of the more important points, see the sidebar that follows. These guidelines also include some recommendations about amounts of exercise that people should do for the benefit of their health. In the following list, the recommendation is first stated, and then the reasons for this recommendation are briefly summarized.

- *Recommendation:* Follow a healthy eating pattern across the lifespan. *Why?:* Eating patterns are the combination of foods and drinks that a person eats over time. Healthy eating patterns include a variety of nutritious foods like vegetables, fruits, grains, low-fat and fat-free dairy, lean meats and other protein foods, and oils, while limiting saturated fats, *trans* fats, added sugars, and sodium. A healthy eating pattern is adaptable to a person's taste preferences, traditions, culture, and budget.

- *Recommendation:* Eat a wide variety of nutrient-rich or nutrient-dense foods. *Why?:* By eating a variety of foods from within each food group and between food groups, people will likely ingest adequate amounts of all essential nutrients. The term "nutrient-dense" indicates the nutrients and other beneficial substances in a food have not been "diluted" by the addition of calories from added solid fats, sugars, or refined starches, or by the solid fats naturally present in the food. Thus, nutrient-dense foods are those that provide vitamins, minerals, and other substances that contribute to adequate nutrient intakes or may have positive health effects but contain little or no solid fats, added sugars, refined starches, and sodium. Ideally, these foods also are in forms that retain naturally occurring components, such as dietary fiber. All vegetables, fruits, whole grains, seafood, eggs, beans, and peas, unsalted nuts and seeds, fat-free and low-fat dairy products, and lean meats and poultry— when prepared with little or no added solid fats, sugars, refined starches, and sodium— are nutrient-dense foods. These foods contribute to meeting food group recommendations within the desirable calorie and sodium limits.

- *Recommendation:* Eat a diet rich in vegetables, fruits, and whole-grain and high-fiber foods. People should eat at least five portions of fruit and vegetables daily. *Why?:* Consuming vegetables, fruits, and whole-grain and high-fiber foods will help to achieve the recommended carbohydrate intake and increase fiber intake which is good for digestive and cardiovascular health. In addition, these foods contain relatively large amounts of phytonutrients, which have some beneficial health effects. Epidemiological studies have generally shown that diets high in whole-grain products (bread and cereals), legumes (beans and peas), fruits, and vegetables have significant health benefits.

- *Recommendation:* Eat a variety of protein foods. *Why?:* Consuming a variety of high-protein food sources including seafood, lean meats and poultry, eggs, legumes (beans and peas), soy products, and nuts and seeds that provide 10-15% of daily calories should ensure that protein requirements are met while avoiding excessive fat intake.

- *Recommendation:* Choose a diet moderate in total fat but low in saturated fat, trans fats, and cholesterol. *Why?:* Apart from the essential fatty acids linoleic and α-linolenic acid, there is no specific requirement for fats. Too much saturated and *trans*-fat intake is linked to cardiovascular disease. But some fat is needed to help with the intake of fat-soluble vitamins.

Because most foods contain some fats, the intake of these vitamins is usually not a problem. To lower total fat intake, dairy products that are fat-free or low in fat are recommended. The standard recommendation is to have an intake of saturated fatty acids below 10% of total energy intake, limit cholesterol intake to 0.3 g or less per day, and keep *trans*-fat intake to a minimum.

- *Recommendation:* People should eat fewer commercially prepared processed foods, baked goods, and avoid fast foods. *Why?:* These foods are generally high in energy and fat and contain a significant amount of *trans* fatty acids which are harmful to cardiovascular health. Consumption of small amounts of oils is encouraged, including those from plants: canola, corn, olive, peanut, safflower, soybean, and sunflower. Oils also are naturally present in nuts, seeds, seafood, olives, and avocados.

- *Recommendation:* Cut back on beverages and foods high in calories and low in nutrition. *Why?:* Beverages such as soft drinks and foods with added sugar contribute significantly to energy intake while not adding useful nutrients. The US National Academy of Sciences advised that added sugars should make up no more than 25% of the total daily energy intake but that reducing this to 10% may be a healthier alternative. Indeed, the 2015-2020 *Dietary Guidelines for Americans* recommends that less than 10% of daily calorie intake should come from added sugars. As discussed earlier in this chapter, added sugar intake has been associated with high blood triglyceride concentrations, dental cavities, and obesity.

- *Recommendation:* Use less sodium and salt. *Why?:* Too much sodium raises blood pressure, a risk factor for cardiovascular disease. Healthy adults are generally advised to reduce sodium intake to 2.3 g of sodium (equivalent to 5.8 g salt) per day or less. Most people consume, on average, about 3.4 g of sodium (8.5 g salt) per day. One teaspoon or 5 g of salt contains 2.0 g of sodium. People should choose foods with little salt and prepare food with minimal amounts of salt. At the same time, they should consume potassium-rich foods, such as fruits and vegetables.

- *Recommendation:* Those who drink alcohol should drink in moderation. *Why?:* Alcohol is a non-nutrient but contains 7 kcal per gram (28 kJ/g). It can add significant energy to total daily intake without adding nutrients. Current evidence suggests that light to moderate alcohol intake (one drink per day) will cause no real risk for healthy adults. During pregnancy, alcohol should be avoided. Current guidelines recommend drinking no more than one drink per day for women and two drinks per day for men. A drink is defined as 360 mL (12 fl oz) of regular strength beer (5% alcohol), 150 mL (5 fl oz) of wine (12% alcohol), or 45 mL (1.5 fl oz) of spirits (40% alcohol).

- *Recommendation:* Avoid excessive intake of questionable food additives and nutrition supplements. *Why?:* Although most food additives used in processed foods are safe, it is often recommended to avoid these additives. In addition, nutritional supplements are often claimed to have various positive health effects or performance benefits, but negative effects may occur. Nutrition supplements are not under strict regulation, may contain substances that are not listed on the label, and therefore pose a greater risk to health.

- *Recommendation:* Practice food hygiene and safety. *Why?:* Food should be stored appropriately to avoid accumulation of bacteria. This practice often means refrigerating perishable foods and not storing foods for too long. Food should be cooked to a safe temperature to kill microorganisms, but people should be aware that excess grilling of meat can produce carcinogenic substances called heterocyclic amines. To avoid microbial food-borne illness, people should clean hands, food-contact surfaces, and fruits and vegetables. Meat and poultry should not be washed or rinsed. People should avoid raw (unpasteurized) milk or any products made from unpasteurized milk, raw or partially cooked eggs, or foods containing raw eggs, raw or undercooked meat and poultry, unpasteurized juices, and raw sprouts.

- *Recommendation:* Cook food in ways that preserve the integrity of nutrients and remove some of the fat. *Why?:* The way that we cook food influences its nutrient and energy content. Grilling or roasting meat, poultry, and fish and discarding the fat is better than pan frying or deep fat frying. Photo 4.1 illustrates the weight of fat (406 g) that drains from a whole 2.2 kg chicken after being cooked in a roasting bag in a hot oven for two hours. Losing the fat by this method of cooking makes the meat much healthier to eat, as it is now low in fat but still high in protein. Steaming rather than boiling vegetables will retain more of the vitamins and phytonutrients. Remember that some vegetables are good to eat raw such as grated carrot, diced onion, celery, cucumber, tomato, and salad leaves.

- *Recommendation:* Balance food intake with physical activity to maintain a healthy weight. *Why?:* Consuming moderate food portions and being physically active are important steps toward the prevention of obesity.

- *Recommendation:* Be physically active. *Why?:* People should aim to do at least 30 minutes of physical activity on most, if not all, days as this is the amount needed for the average healthy adult to maintain health and reduce the risk for chronic disease. The American College of Sports Medicine (ACSM) and the American Heart Association (AHA) recommend moderately intense **aerobic exercise** for 30 minutes a day, five days a week or vigorously intense aerobic exercise for 20 minutes a day, three days a week. Alternatively, people can undertake resistance exercise by performing 8 to 12 repetitions of each of 8 to 10 strength-training exercises twice a week. Moderate-intensity physical activity means working hard enough to raise the heart rate and break a sweat yet still being able to carry on a conversation. Note that to lose weight or maintain weight loss, 60 to 90 minutes of daily physical activity may be necessary.

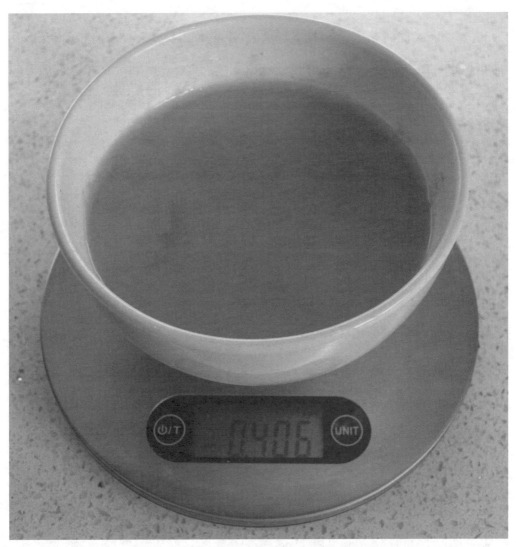

Photo 4.1: The amount of fat (406 g) that drains from a whole 2.2 kg chicken after being cooked in a roasting bag in a hot oven for two hours

10 Top Tips That Summarize How to Achieve a Healthy Balanced Diet

1. Eat meals at regular times of the day. Don't skip breakfast, and don't eat snacks between meals.

2. Eat at least five portions of a variety of fruit and vegetables every day.

3. Try to choose a variety of different foods from the six basic food groups. That means including ones from the milk group (e.g., milk, cheese, yogurt), the meat group (e.g., meat, fish, poultry and eggs, with dried legumes and nuts as alternatives), fruits, vegetables, and the breads and cereals group and limited amounts of oils and fats.

4. The main source of energy for meals should come from potatoes, bread, rice, pasta or other starchy carbohydrates. Have only small to medium portions of these, and choose wholegrain or higher-fiber produce where possible.

5. Choose lower-fat and lower-sugar options where available for things like dairy products, coleslaw, yogurts etc.

6. Eat some beans, pulses, fish, eggs, meat, and other high-protein foods. Aim for two portions of fish every week, one of which should be oily, such as salmon or mackerel.

7. Choose unsaturated oils and spreads, but only eat them in small amounts.

8. Drink plenty of fluids (six to eight cups or glasses per day are recommended), particularly water (plain, mineral or soda), low-calorie (diet) versions of popular beverages (e.g., cola, lemonade and tonic water), and fruit juices with no added sugar. Tea and coffee are also fine in moderation but if you like them to taste sweet use an artificial sweetener rather than sugar.

9. Limit your intake of alcohol by drinking no more than one 175 mL glass of wine or 350 mL beer with your main meal of the day and only on three days of the week.

10. Try to limit foods and drinks that are high in fat, salt and sugar by having these less often and in small amounts.

These guidelines for healthy eating apply to all adults who are above 18 years of age, and most of them are generally applicable to younger people from the age of four. In other words, although not the focus of this particular book, your children should be eating pretty much the same as the adult members of the family, but because the youngsters are smaller, they should be given smaller portions. For women who are pregnant, there are some differences in the recommendations of what should be eaten, how much should be eaten, and which foods should be avoided. These differences are summarized in the following sidebar.

Which Foods to Eat During Pregnancy and Which Foods to Avoid

A healthy diet is an important part of a healthy lifestyle at any time but is especially vital during pregnancy both for the health of the mother and to help the baby develop and grow. Most pregnant women find that they are hungrier than usual, and they have an increased requirement for protein and most vitamins, but it is not necessary to "eat for two" – even when expecting twins or triplets. Nor is there a need to go on a special diet, but it is important to eat a variety of different foods every day to get the right balance of nutrients that are needed. It's best to get vitamins and minerals from food, but most agencies recommend taking a daily folate (also known as folic acid or vitamin B9) supplement as well (this can be part of a daily multivitamin supplement) to minimize the risk of birth defects of the fetal brain and spine.

During pregnancy, women should follow the guidelines for healthy eating described in this chapter and try to have a healthy breakfast every day because this can help to avoid the temptation to snack on foods that are high in fat and sugar later in the day. For the health of the mother and the developing fetus, there are some foods to avoid and few additional recommendations to follow:

Additional recommendations during pregnancy

- Eat plenty of fruit and vegetables because these provide vitamins and minerals, as well as fiber which helps digestion and can help prevent constipation.

- Make sure poultry, burgers, sausages, and whole cuts of meat such as lamb, beef, and pork are cooked all the way through. Check that there is no pink meat, and that juices have no pink or red in them to minimize the risk of food poisoning.

- Try to eat two portions of fish a week, one of which should be oily fish such as salmon, sardines, or mackerel, but don't have more than two portions of oily fish a week because it can contain some pollutants (toxins) like dioxins and polychlorinated biphenyls.

- Dairy foods such as milk, cheese, fromage frais, and yogurt are important in pregnancy because they contain calcium and other nutrients that mother and baby need. Choose low-fat varieties wherever possible.

Foods to avoid in pregnancy

There are some foods to avoid or take care with during pregnancy, as there is a risk of illness or harm to the baby.

- Avoid eating raw or partially cooked eggs, as there is a risk of salmonella.

- Don't eat mold-ripened soft cheese (cheeses with a white rind) such as brie and camembert. This includes mold-ripened soft goats' cheese such as chèvre. These cheeses are only safe to eat in pregnancy if they've been cooked. The same goes for soft blue-veined cheeses such as Danish blue, gorgonzola, and Roquefort. Soft blue cheeses are only safe to eat in pregnancy if they've been cooked.

- It is safer to avoid some soft cheeses because they're less acidic than hard cheeses and contain more moisture, which means they can be a suitable environment for harmful bacteria, such as listeria, to grow in. Listeria infection, although rare, has been known to cause miscarriage, stillbirth, or severe illness in a newborn. All hard cheeses are safe in pregnancy and some soft cheeses are OK to eat, provided they're made from pasteurized milk (e.g., cottage cheese, mozzarella, feta, ricotta, halloumi, goats' cheese, and processed cheeses, such as cheese spreads).

- Avoid all types of pâté, including vegetable pâtés, as they can contain listeria.

- Avoid liver or products containing liver, such as liver pâté, liver sausage, or haggis, as they may contain a lot of vitamin A. Too much vitamin A can harm your baby.

- Avoid eating any shark, swordfish or marlin because of their relatively high mercury content. Mercury consumed during pregnancy has been linked to developmental delays and brain damage.

- Restrict the amount of tuna you eat to no more than two portions per week because tuna contains more mercury than most other types of fish.

- Avoid all raw shellfish including mussels, lobster, crab, prawns, scallops, and clams when you're pregnant, as they can contain harmful bacteria and viruses that can cause food poisoning.

- Do not take any high-dose multivitamin supplements, fish liver oil supplements, or any supplements containing vitamin A.

- Be cautious with cold cured meats in pregnancy as many including salami, prosciutto, chorizo, and pepperoni, are not cooked; they're just cured and fermented. This means there's a risk they contain parasites that can cause **toxoplasmosis**.

- The amount of caffeine consumed should be limited to no more than 200 mg per day, as high levels of caffeine can result in babies having a low birthweight, which can increase the risk of health problems in later life. Too much caffeine can also cause miscarriage. Remember that caffeine is naturally found in lots of foods, such as coffee, tea (including green tea), and chocolate (particularly dark chocolate). Caffeine is also added to some soft drinks, energy drinks, sports drinks, and some cold and flu remedies.

DIETS THAT ARE KNOWN TO BE VERY HEALTHY

There are several diets that are known to be good for health because they have been consumed by certain large populations for long periods of time, populations which have been shown to have relatively low risk of major chronic illnesses such as cardiovascular disease, type 2 diabetes, and cancer. Two stand-out examples are the Mediterranean diet and the Japanese diet. You might not want to adopt these particular diets on a full-time basis, but you could try adding some of their typical meals into your regular eating plan. Both these diets contain foods that combat chronic inflammation which is a major contributor to the development of chronic metabolic and cardiovascular diseases that plague Western societies. Therefore, one of the most powerful tools to combat inflammation comes not from the medicine cabinet but from your kitchen. Components of some foods or beverages have anti-inflammatory effects, so if you choose the right foods, you may be able to reduce your risk of illness. Consistently pick the wrong ones, and you could accelerate the inflammatory disease process. Anti-inflammatory foods include tomatoes, fresh fruit (e.g., strawberries, cherries, blueberries), nuts (e.g., almonds, pecan, walnuts), olive oil, and leafy greens (e.g., broccoli, kale, spinach), and oily fish (e.g., mackerel, salmon, tuna). The Mediterranean diet is particularly rich in these types of food while the Japanese diet includes lots of seafood, vegetables, and fruit but avoids most forms of refined and processed foods (e.g., bread, cake, fried foods, sugar, soft drinks, lard, and fatty or processed meat) which are the food types that promote inflammation.

THE MEDITERRANEAN DIET

The Mediterranean diet (see photo 4.2) is the traditional diet of many of the poorer people who lived in the Mediterranean region (particularly the southern parts of Spain, Italy, Sicily, Greece, and Crete) a generation ago. It does not include the pizzas and pasta favored by many in parts of southern Europe today. In a study published in 2013, Spanish researchers recruited over 7,400 Spanish overweight, middle-aged men and women and randomly allocated them to either a Mediterranean or a low-fat diet. Both groups were encouraged to eat lots of fresh fruit, vegetables, and legumes (such as beans, lentils, and peas). They were discouraged from consuming sugary drinks, cakes, sweets, or pastries and from eating too much processed meat such as bacon or salami. Furthermore, only those allocated to the Mediterranean diet were asked to eat plenty of eggs, nuts, and oily fish, use lots of olive oil, and encouraged to eat some dark chocolate, and enjoy the occasional glass of wine with their evening meal. In contrast, the low-fat diet group were told to eat low-fat dairy products and lots of starchy foods such as bread, potatoes, pasta, and rice. The researchers followed the volunteers for just under five years, getting them to fill in food diaries and keeping a check on their health via medical examinations, questionnaires, and blood and urine samples. All volunteers were given an 'M score', according to how closely they stuck to the Mediterranean diet. Within only three years, dramatic differences between the two groups appeared. Those who had a high M score were slimmer and much healthier, with their risk of heart attack or stroke reduced by 30%, type 2 diabetes reduced by 58%, and a reduced risk of cognitive decline. For women, there was also a 51% reduced risk of breast cancer. In order to achieve a high M score and enjoy the benefits of a Mediterranean diet, this is what you should be aiming to eat and avoid:

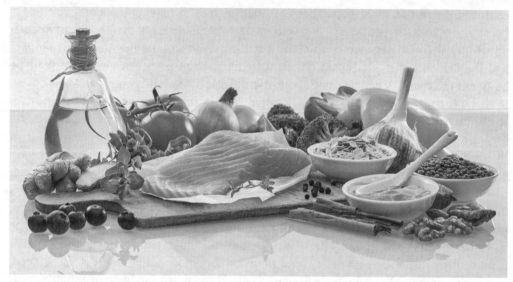

Photo 4.2: A selection of foods found in the Mediterranean diet

Eat the following:

- Fresh, lean meat such as pork, chicken, turkey, and lamb; oven roasted, grilled, or fried with a little olive oil.

- Fresh fish such as sardines, mackerel, and salmon; grilled or oven-baked.

- Eggs; poached or boiled, or as an omelet.

- Whole grain foods such as quinoa, whole rye, bulgar wheat, and pearl barley.

- Rice, preferably brown.

- Unsalted nuts such as walnuts, almonds, and cashews.

- Full-fat dairy such as yogurt, milk, and feta cheese.

- Legumes including beans, chickpeas, lentils, and peas.

- Olives, tomato, onion, and cucumber.

- Fruits such as orange, lemon, grapes, and water melon.

- One glass of wine (preferably red) per day.

- Wholegrain, wholemeal or rye bread.

- Raisins, grapes, or nuts make healthy snacks.

- Olive oil rather than vegetable oil or lard for frying.

- Herbs and garlic for added flavor.

Avoid the following:

- Potatoes on more than two days per week.

- Tropical fruit such as honeydew melon, pineapple, and bananas.

- Processed meats like ham, bacon, sausage, and salami.

- White bread, pasta, and pizza.

- Processed foods, cakes, pastries, milk chocolate, and sweets.

Some typical Mediterranean dishes include:

- Rice paella with peas, chicken, or seafood.

- Greek salad with tomato, cucumber, onion, feta cheese, olives, and lemon juice.

- Grilled sardines, tomato, and salad greens with wholegrain bread.

- Tuna salad dressed with lemon and olive oil.

- Omelet with mixed vegetables and olives.

- Grilled lamb, pork or chicken on a skewer with tomato, pepper, and onion.

- Lean lamb mince with diced aubergine and baked potato.

- Lean beef or lamb casserole with onions, tomato, aubergine, and figs.

- Fruit salad with yogurt and walnut.

THE JAPANESE DIET

The Japanese people are known to have a long life expectancy, which is higher than almost anywhere else in the world. So why is the Japanese diet so healthy, and what do they eat? The traditional Japanese diet (see photo 4.3) is largely fresh and unprocessed, uses fish, shellfish, and tofu as its major protein sources, with very few refined foods, bread, sugar, and dairy products. A recent study published in the British Medical Journal found that those who stuck closer to the Japanese dietary guidelines – a diet high in grains and vegetables, with moderate amounts of animal products, fruit and soy but minimal dairy – had a reduced risk of dying early and suffering from heart disease or stroke. As the Japanese diet is traditionally high in soy and fish this may also play a significant role in this reduced risk of cardiovascular disease.

The Japanese also have the lowest rates of obesity among men and women as well as long life expectancy. Okinawa, in southernmost Japan, has the highest number of centenarians in the world, as well as the lowest risk of age-related diseases such as type 2 diabetes, cancer, **arthritis**, and **Alzheimer's**. This has partly been attributed to their traditional Japanese diet, which is low in calories and saturated fat yet high in nutrients, especially phytonutrients such as antioxidants and flavonoids, found in different colored vegetables and seasonal fruits. This also includes phytoestrogens, or plant-based estrogens, that may help protect against hormone-dependent cancers, such as breast cancer. Fermented foods containing probiotic bacteria are also popular, and these can positively influence the gut bacterial population (known as the microbiota) which is now recognized to play an important role in health maintenance. The diet of the Okinawan people has been little influenced by the Western diet, which has been seen in more urban parts of Japan.

The traditional Japanese diet isn't that dissimilar to a traditional Chinese diet, with rice, noodles made from wheat flour, cooked and pickled vegetables, fish, meat, and soy products being staple choices. However, because Japan is actually a group of over 6,500 islands, its residents consume a lot more fish and shellfish compared to other Asian countries. They also eat raw fish in sushi and sashimi, plus a lot of pickled, fermented and smoked foods. The main sources of carbohydrate are rice and noodles made from rice or wheat. Bread, potatoes, and cookies are generally absent from the Japanese diet.

Soy beans, usually in the form of tofu or fresh edamame, are another key part of the Japanese diet, along with other beans such as aduki and various mushrooms. Increasingly, fermented foods have been shown to support a healthy digestive system. Fermented soy bean products such as miso and natto are staples of the Japanese diet. Miso pastes (a traditional Japanese seasoning produced by fermenting soybeans with salt and the fungus Aspergillus oryzae, known in Japanese as kōjikin, and sometimes rice, barley, or other ingredients) are a popular way of flavoring food and can be categorized into red (akamiso), white (shiromiso), or mixed (awase). Natto is traditionally consumed at breakfast and has a probiotic action that has been shown to help reduce **irritable bowel syndrome** (IBS) and may help blood clotting. The Japanese also consume a wide variety of vegetables, both land and sea vegetables such as seaweed, which is rich in minerals, and may help to reduce blood pressure. Fruit is often consumed with breakfast or as a dessert, especially Fuji apples, tangerines, and persimmons in preference to cakes, pastries, puddings, and sweets.

Alongside their diet, the Japanese like to drink green tea which is high in antioxidant compounds called **catechins**, which have been linked to fighting cancer, viruses, and heart disease. Furthermore, the Japanese tend to have a healthy attitude to food and eating. They have a saying, "hara hachi bu", which means to eat until you are 80% full, and it is not uncommon to teach it to children from a young age. The way the Japanese serve their food is also an important characteristic contributing to their general avoidance of high-calorie intake. Rather than having one large plate, they often eat from a small bowl and several different dishes, usually a bowl of rice, a bowl of miso, some fish or meat, and then two or three vegetables dishes, often served communally and eaten in rotation. The Japanese are also strong believers of 'flexible restraint' when it comes to treats and snacks, enjoying them from time to time but in smaller portions. Other than the occasional beer and sake rice wine, they are not great drinkers of alcoholic beverages.

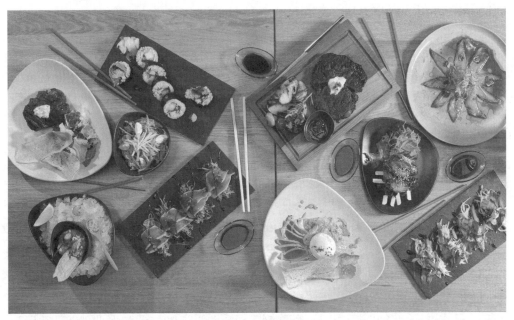

Photo 4.3: A selection of foods found in the Japanese diet, served as is usual in Japan, in small bowls or plates

Some typical Japanese dishes include:

- Miso chicken and rice soup.

- Japanese salmon and avocado rice.

- Teriyaki noodle broth.

- Soba noodle and edamame salad with grilled tofu.

- Japanese salad with ginger soy dressing.

- Miso marinated salmon.

- Miso brown rice and chicken salad.

- Japanese-style brown rice.

- Chicken or beef teriyaki with white rice.

VEGETARIAN AND VEGAN DIETS

Vegetarian and vegan diets are associated with lower health risks compared with diets containing meat. A vegetarian diet generally excludes meat and meat products with most food of vegetable or plant origin. Some versions of the diet allow the consumption of dairy products (e.g., milk, butter, cheese, yogurt) and eggs. A vegan diet is a very strict type of vegetarian diet in which no animal products are allowed. Research shows that a vegetarian diet can reduce a person's risk of heart disease, stroke, metabolic syndrome, and type 2 diabetes by about one third. This is probably because people who consume plant-based diets tend to have a lower body mass index (BMI) than meat eaters, their prevalence for obesity is lower, and they have higher intakes of phytonutrients and fiber. Overall cancer incidence is also 11% lower in vegetarians and 19% lower in vegans compared with meat eaters.

However, being vegetarian isn't always healthy; it depends on what types of plant foods are consumed and in what amounts. In fact, it has been reported that some plant-based diets can actually raise the risk of heart disease. For example, a US study found a vegetarian diet based on less healthy food options, such as refined grains, starchy vegetables like potatoes, and foods with high sugar content increased the risk of heart disease whereas those eating a healthy plant-based diet high in wholegrains, fruits, vegetables, and healthy fats were less likely to get heart disease. Essentially, the diet advice for vegetarians is the same as it is for nonvegetarians: eat a balanced diet with at least five portions of fruit and vegetables per day, choose wholegrain carbohydrates where possible, and limit intake of sugar, salt, and saturated fat. Eating too much starchy vegetables (e.g., potatoes) and dairy products (particularly cheese) and bread can also be fattening and so should be avoided.

An appropriate selection of foods is important for vegetarians and vegans to avoid deficiencies of protein, vitamin B12 (which is only found in animal products although nowadays some foods [e.g., breakfast cereals and milk] are fortified with vitamin B12, calcium [if dairy products are not consumed], and iron [heme iron is only found in foods containing animal meat, heart, liver, kidney, and blood and the nonheme iron present in plants is not as readily absorbed]). For vegans, in particular, a daily vitamin B12 supplement suppling 100% of the RDA is recommended. Because meat, poultry, and fish are the most common sources of protein, vegetarians and vegans could be at risk for marginal protein intake. Vegetarians and vegans often compensate by eating more grains and legumes, which both are excellent protein sources. But grains and legumes do not contain all essential amino acids. Grains (e.g., wheat, rice, oats, cornmeal, barley) lack the essential amino acid lysine, and legumes (e.g., peas, beans, chickpeas, lentils) lack methionine. An exception may be well-processed soybean protein, which is a high-quality protein comparable in quality to protein from animal sources. The potential problem for vegetarians of missing essential amino acids can be solved by not eating grains and legumes in isolation but combining both grains and legumes in their meals (together with other protein sources such as cheese or egg). Good sources of iron on a vegetarian diet include tofu, legumes (lentils, dried peas and beans), wholegrain cereals (in particular, iron-fortified breakfast cereals), green vegetables (broccoli, watercress, and kale), nuts, dairy products, and eggs. The intake of fat – particularly unhealthy saturated fat – will be considerably lower on a vegetarian diet. On such a diet, fat will be provided by margarine, salad dressing, vegetable oils, nuts, and some dairy products.

FOOD SHOPPING TIPS

Supermarkets and food manufacturers now highlight the energy, fat, saturated fat, sugar, and salt content on the front of the packaging, alongside the reference intake for each of these as described in detail the previous chapter. Other products will show nutrition information on the back or side of packaging. You can use nutrition labels to help you choose a more balanced diet. If you're standing in the supermarket aisle looking at two similar products such as a ready meal, trying to decide which is the healthier choice, check to see whether there's a nutrition label on the front of the package, and then see how your choices stack up when it comes to the amount of energy, fat, saturated fat, sugars, and salt. If the nutrition labels use color coding as introduced in the UK in 2013 and more recently in France, you will often find a mixture of traffic light colors: red, amber, and green. I suggest that you interpret these as follows: RED means STOP, and think whether you really want this product, as it contains high amounts of fat, saturated fat, sugars, or salt. If just one of these is RED, then maybe consider it, but more than two is a definite no-no if you want to eat healthily. AMBER means BE PREPARED to consider choosing this product, as it has medium amounts of fat, saturated fat, sugars, or salt. GREEN means GO AHEAD and buy the product as it has low amounts of fat, saturated fat, sugars or salt. So, when you're choosing between similar products, try to go for more greens and ambers, and fewer reds, if you want to make a healthier choice. But remember, even some of the healthier ready meals may be higher in energy, fat, sugar, and salt than the homemade equivalent. If you make the meal yourself, you have full control of the ingredients, and you could save money, too!

A PRIME EXAMPLE OF HEALTHY FOOD SELECTION: WHAT TO EAT FOR BREAKFAST

Often hailed as the 'most important meal of the day', a decent breakfast certainly has a range of health benefits. As well as providing nutrients, a regular healthy breakfast can help to maintain blood sugar, suppress hunger, and minimize unhealthy snacking later on. It also fuels your body to help you function better during a busy day. If you consume a good breakfast, then it is likely that you will not be particularly hungry in the middle of day and will only want a light lunch such as a salad or sandwich rather than a full meal.

When it comes to breakfast time, cereal remains a popular, convenient, and speedy choice. With the choice on supermarket shelves growing over the years, it can be tricky to choose the healthiest option. Breakfast cereals tend to be based on grains – some are wholegrains such as bran, oats, and wheat, and others are refined grains such as maize (corn), and rice. Many also have nuts, seeds, and dried fruit added to them. Wholegrain cereals release glucose more slowly as they are classed as a low **glycemic index** food (that means they cause less of a spike in blood glucose in the hours following their ingestion). Many cereals contain fiber which is important for gut health and can help lower cholesterol. Some cereals also contain vitamins and minerals such as iron, vitamin D, vitamin C, and B vitamins such as folic acid. However, some cereals that may appear healthy, including some that contain fruit and fiber, are not always as good for you as they seem because they can contain high amounts of free sugars and are lower in fiber than is recommended.

The calories and composition of some example cereals are shown in table 4.1 based on the usual serving size (40 g unless otherwise stated). To these you will need to add up to 100 mL of milk. If you add 100 mL of semi-skimmed milk, this will add an extra 47 kcal, 4.8 g carbohydrate, 1.8 g fat and 0.1 g salt). For other types of milk, see table 4.2 which compares the composition of whole, semi-skimmed, skimmed, and soya milks. Please note that the nutritional information provided does not include any sugar that you might add, and brand names are not disclosed.

Also shown for comparison is the calorie and composition of a full English breakfast (one egg, one slice of bacon, one sausage, all fried plus one cup of baked beans, and one slice of bread).

Table 4.1: Energy content (kcal) and composition (g) of breakfast cereals per usual serving size (40 g unless otherwise stated)

Name	kcal	Carbo-hydrate	Of which sugars	Fat	Of which saturated fat	Salt	Fiber
Oat and Fruit Granola	180	25.6	9.0	4.4	0.4	0.1	3.0
Shredded Wheat 2 pieces 45 g	144	30.1	0.4	1.0	0.2	0.1	5.4
All Bran	134	19.0	7.2	1.4	0.3	0.4	11.0
Bran Flakes 30 g	108	19.0	4.2	1.0	0.2	0.2	4.5
Weetabix 2 pieces 30 g	136	26.0	1.7	0.8	0.2	0.1	3.8
Ready Brek 30 g	112	17.0	4.8	3.0	0.0	0.1	2.4
Porridge Oats	150	24.0	0.4	3.2	0.6	0.1	3.6
Muesli	150	26.5	15.6	1.0	0.2	0.1	3.5
Fruit and Fiber	152	28.0	9.6	2.4	1.4	0.4	3.6
Full English Fry-Up	850	19.4	12.0	40.4	16.1	2.7	6.4

The cereal servings also contain 3-5 g protein and 100 mL added milk supplies 3-4 g protein.

Table 4.1 will help you make informed decisions about what you eat and drink by showing the levels of fat, sugar, and salt (light gray = low; medium gray = medium; dark gray = high). Two of the breakfast cereals – Shredded Wheat and Weetabix – are all light gray, meaning they're low in sugar, fat, saturated fat, and salt. These are good choices as long as you don't add sugar to them. Bran-based cereals are the highest in fiber but can have moderate sugar content.

Other cereals have moderate to high amounts of sugar and fat. The cereals that score high in fat but low in saturated fat are ones in which the fat mainly comes from unsaturated sources. Three of the cereals – the Oat and Fruit Granola, Muesli, and the Fruit and Fiber–score high for sugar. This sugar comes from sweetened dried fruit added to the cereal, along with added sugar. The full English breakfast provides a whopping 850 kcal with lots of fat, saturated fat, and salt; the sugar mostly comes from the baked beans and bread. The one plus for it is that it contains 48 g protein. A healthier alternative that will contain about half the calories is poached egg, steamed or grilled bacon and sausage, and the no added sugar version of baked beans.

Table 4.2: Energy content (kcal) and composition (g) of different milks (cow or soya) per 100 mL

Type of milk	kcal	Carbo-hydrate	Of which sugars	Fat	Of which saturated fat	Protein	Salt
Whole	68	4.7	4.7	3.7	2.4	3.5	0.1
Semi-skimmed	48	4.8	4.8	1.8	1.1	3.6	0.1
Skimmed	37	5.0	5.0	0.3	0.1	3.6	0.1
Sweetened soya	42	2.5	2.5	1.9	0.3	3.4	0.1
Unsweetened soya	39	0.4	0.4	1.6	0.3	3.0	0.1

Practical Tips When Choosing Your Breakfast Cereal

- Be aware of portion sizes - check whether the portion size suggested on the box is the same as the portion size you're consuming. Many people pour a larger bowl and therefore consume more calories than they expect. This is important if you're counting calories to control weight, or if you are diabetic, and carbohydrate count to adjust the correct dose of insulin.

- Weigh your cereal a couple of times to get an idea of the amount you usually consume, and then keep a note of this along with other foods you consume on a regular basis. Use this weight against the per 100 g values on the pack to calculate your intake.

- Another tip when calorie or carbohydrate counting - remember to allow for any extras you have added to your cereal such as milk, sugar, honey, fruit, or yogurt.

- The type of milk you choose to put on your cereal can also contribute to overall health – choosing semi-skimmed or skimmed instead of whole milk can reduce your overall fat and calorie intake for the day (e.g., whole milk contains 20 kcal and 2.2 g fat more per 100 mL than semi-skimmed).

- Check the label for fiber and try to choose a cereal with a higher fiber content.

- Try to choose cereals that are graded green for sugar, where possible.

PROCESSED FOODS

The term processed food refers to food that has been treated to extend its storage life or to improve its taste (by adding sugar, seasoning, or flavorings), nutrition (by adding certain micronutrients), color, or texture. Processing includes adding preservatives, colorings, or flavorings; fortifying, enriching, dehydrating, smoking, drying, or freezing; and a number of other treatments. Concern has been expressed that the nutritional quality of food has declined during recent years because the amount of processing has increased. Indeed, modern foods contain greater amounts of refined sugar, extracted oils, and white flour, products from which nutrients are lost in the refinement process. For example, in the bleaching of flour, over 20 known essential nutrients are lost.

Many processed products are completely artificial including synthetic fruit juices, numerous soft drinks, and nondairy creamers. Refined or artificial products may contain few or no nutrients but have the same energy content as their natural counterparts; in fact, the energy content of many processed foods and beverages is often higher due to added sugar. Thus, the **nutrient density** (the amount of essential nutrients per unit of energy) of refined or artificial products is usually extremely low unless they have been fortified with vitamins (e.g., B12, D3) or minerals (e.g., iron). However, although some nutrients are lost during processing, modern techniques used by most food manufacturers prevent major losses of nutrients in some products. Frozen and canned vegetables, for example, contain amounts of essential nutrients similar to those in fresh vegetables. The increased use of refined sugar, oils, unenriched white flour, salt, and questionable additives is a greater concern. Food labels can help consumers make decisions about the quality of processed foods, but in general, to ensure a healthy and nutritious diet, it is best to avoid processed foods as much as possible and make your own meals from natural products.

Care should be taken to avoid loss of nutrients during cooking at home. When vegetables are boiled, vitamins and minerals may end up in the water. This is less likely to happen with steaming, especially for foods where the cooking time can be relatively short (e.g., spinach, peas, asparagus, tenderstem broccoli). With other cooking methods (grilling, frying, baking), heat-sensitive vitamins may be lost if the food is overcooked.

Key Points

- Even if we consume adequate amounts of essential nutrients, this in itself does not guarantee the absence of potentially harmful effects on our health in relation to the food that we consume. Deficiencies of some of the nonessential nutrients (e.g., fiber, phytonutrients) can also mean that our diets will not deliver what we need for optimal function and health.

- Excessive intakes of some nutrients (e.g., carbohydrates, fats) or certain subgroups (e.g., simple sugars, corn syrups, saturated fats, *trans* fatty acids) and other nonessential nutrients (e.g., alcohol, salt) can have harmful effects on our health, particularly in the long term, increasing our risk of developing chronic metabolic and cardiovascular diseases and cancer.

- There is compelling evidence that carbohydrate quantity and quality have important influences on obesity, cardiovascular disease, the metabolic syndrome, and type 2 diabetes, particularly in those with a sedentary lifestyle. Dietary fiber is an important determinant of satiety and weight gain, and also protects against cardiovascular disease. Vegetables, fruits, and grains protect against cardiovascular diseases. Sugar consumption is a proven cause of weight gain, and obesity is strongly associated with increased risk of cardiovascular and metabolic diseases.

- Both the type and quantity of fat in the diet are important to the risk of cardiovascular diseases and some cancers.

- General guidelines for healthy eating include balancing food intake with physical activity to maintain a healthy body weight; being physically active; eating a wide variety of nutrient-rich and nutrient-dense foods; eating a diet rich in vegetables, fruits, whole-grain foods, and high-fiber foods; selecting a diet that is moderate in total fat but low in saturated fat, *trans* fat, and cholesterol; cutting back on beverages and foods that are high in energy but low in nutrients; consuming less sugar; using less sodium and salt; drinking alcohol in moderation; practicing food hygiene and safety; and avoiding excessive intake of food additives and supplements.

- Recently introduced updated dietary guidelines from several countries including the US, UK and Australia focus on advice about consuming recommended portions of various food groups and shifting food choices to healthier options. The overall aim is to achieve adequate intake of essential nutrients while meeting (but not exceeding) energy requirements. Most guidelines now also encourage increased physical activity.

- Two well established healthy diets are the Mediterranean diet and the Japanese diet. Both are healthy but for different reasons. Vegetarian diets can also be healthy provided that appropriate food choices are made to avoid deficiencies of protein, vitamin B12, calcium, and iron.

- The term processed food refers to food treated to extend storage life or to improve taste, nutrition, color, or texture. Processing includes adding preservatives, colorings, or flavorings; fortifying, enriching, dehydrating, smoking, drying, or freezing, as well as a number of other treatments. Concern has been expressed that the nutritional quality of food has declined during recent years because the amount of processing has increased.

Chapter 5

How to Achieve Energy Balance: Calories In and Calories Out

Objectives

After studying this chapter, you should:

- Know what energy is and how it is expressed

- Understand the various components of human energy expenditure and their respective contributions to daily energy expenditure in active and inactive persons

- Know how to estimate your own resting metabolic rate

- Know what diet-induced thermogenesis is and why it is not the same for protein, carbohydrates, and fats

- Understand the concept of energy balance and how it relates to body weight

- Know how you can achieve energy balance

The human body needs energy to survive and function. Every cell in the body needs energy to function, muscle fibers need energy to contract, nerves need energy to generate impulses, and energy is needed for the biosynthesis of large molecules. Heat energy is continuously generated from chemical reactions in the cells of the body, and this is used to maintain a normal body temperature of about 37 °C. Although the human body has some stored energy reserves, most of its energy must be obtained through nutrition. During exercise, energy requirements increase, and energy provision can become critical to exercise performance. In some forms of intensive exercise, the rate of energy expenditure can be 10-20 times more than at rest. Different types of exercise and sports have different energy requirements which depend on the mode, duration, and intensity of exercise performed.

FORMS OF ENERGY AND ENERGY TRANSFORMATIONS

Forms of energy range from light energy to chemical energy. Plants use light energy in the process of photosynthesis to produce carbohydrate, fat, or protein. The energy in food is stored in the chemical bonds of various molecules, and so it is called potential chemical energy. Breaking these bonds releases the energy, and it becomes available for conversion into other forms of energy. For instance, when glucose is broken down during a sequence of reactions called **glycolysis**, chemical energy is converted to another form of chemical energy in the form of **adenosine triphosphate (ATP)** and ultimately transformed into mechanical energy (muscle contraction) or used for transport of molecules across membranes, propagation of nerve impulses, or is used for the synthesis of large molecules such as proteins. None of these energy transfers or conversions is 100% efficient, and the "waste" energy appears as heat, which allows us to maintain a body temperature of 37°C (98.6 °F) and permits all the metabolic reactions in the body to occur at faster rates than they would at lower temperatures.

In physiology, energy represents the capacity to do work, which is often referred to as mechanical energy. Walking, running, throwing, and jumping require the production of mechanical energy. Work (energy) is the product of force times the vertical distance covered:

Work = Force x distance, or W = F x d

If work is expressed per unit of time, the term **power** (P) is used:

Power = Work/time, or P = W/t

The rate of **energy expenditure (EE)** refers to the amount of energy used (in kilocalories [kcal] or **kilojoules [kJ]**) per unit of time to produce power. During conversion of one form of energy into another, no energy is lost. This is usually referred to as the first law of thermodynamics, also known as law of conservation of energy, which states that energy cannot be created or destroyed in an isolated system. For example, during the oxidation of carbohydrate and fat, chemical energy is converted into mechanical energy (muscle contraction) to perform movement, and some heat energy is released due the inefficiency of the process. The sum of the mechanical energy and heat energy produced will be the same as the amount of chemical energy used up.

The human body is not efficient in its use of energy from the breakdown of carbohydrate and fat. During cycling exercise, for instance, only 20% of that energy is converted to power. The remainder of the energy becomes heat. This heat can be partly used to maintain body temperature at 37 °C (98.6 °F), but during exercise, heat production may be excessive, and body temperature usually rises by one or two degrees Celsius (°C). To prevent body temperature from rising too high, various heat-dissipating mechanisms such as increased skin blood flow and sweating must be activated.

UNITS OF ENERGY

Energy is often expressed in calories (the Imperial system) or joules (the metric system). One calorie expresses the quantity of energy (heat) needed to raise the temperature of 1 g (1 mL) of water by 1 °C (1.8 F) (from 14.5 °C to 15.5 °C [58.1 °F to 59.9 °F]). Thus, food containing 200 kcal (kilocalories) has enough energy potential to raise the temperature of 200 L of water by 1 °C (1.8 °F). In everyday language, kilocalories are often referred to as Calories (written with a capital C, although on many food items this is not done, and the energy is listed as calories). Because this may be a source of confusion, the term kilocalorie (abbreviated kcal) is used in this book.

The SI (International System of Units) unit for energy is the **joule**, named after the British scientist Sir Prescott Joule (1818–1889). One joule of energy moves a mass of 1 g at a velocity of 1 meter per second (m/s). A joule is not a large amount of energy; therefore, kilojoules are more often used; one kilojoule equals 1,000 joules. To convert calories to joules or kilocalories to kilojoules, the calorie value must be multiplied by 4.184.

When discussing energy expenditure or intake over 24 hours, megajoules (MJ) are often used to avoid large numbers; one megajoule equals 1,000 kilojoules or 1,000,000 joules. Because joules are not yet part of everyday language, both units are often mentioned on food labels, and in this book, kcal will be used, with the equivalent in kJ usually given in parentheses.

Converting Kilocalories to Kilojoules

1 calorie (cal) = 4.184 J
1 kcal = 4.184 kJ
1 kcal = 1,000 cal (or 1 Cal)
1 kJ = 1,000 J
1 MJ = 1,000 kJ

For example:

500 kcal = 500 x 4.184 = 2,092 kJ = 2.092 MJ (megajoules)
1 MJ = 1,000 kJ = 1,000/4.184 = 239 kcal

ENERGETIC EFFICIENCY

Efficiency is the effective work performed after muscle contraction, and it is expressed as the percentage of total work. As already mentioned, during physical activities such as cycling, only about 20% of the energy produced in the body is used to accomplish work (movement). Therefore, when exercising, humans are approximately 20% efficient. Other processes in the body that require energy such as the pumping of the heart, nerve impulse propagation, membrane transport mechanisms, and biosynthesis of large molecules are also rather inefficient and typically average an efficiency of no more than 40%. Many of these mechanisms are essential for survival and maintaining **homeostasis** (i.e., the ability or tendency to maintain internal stability in the body such as constant temperature, blood pressure, cellular and body fluid electrolyte concentrations etc.), but a major part of the energy used in these transformations is lost and wasted as heat. But in this sense, humans are not very different from other systems that transform chemical energy to do useful work. In fact, no system is 100% efficient. For example, a gasoline engine is 20% to 30% efficient, and a diesel engine is a little better, operating at an efficiency of 30% to 40%. Some people may be more efficient than others for various reasons. The efficiency of movement for humans depends on the type of activity (e.g., cycling is more efficient than running) and how accustomed a person is to the activity. For example, a novice cyclist will not be as efficient as an experienced cyclist, and their efficiencies could be around 16 and 22%, respectively.

WHAT YOU NEED TO KNOW ABOUT YOUR ENERGY METABOLISM

The energy we need comes from food, mostly in the form of carbohydrate, fat, and protein. Most of this is in the form of large molecules: plant starches for carbohydrate, triglyceride for fat and whole proteins. These are broken down into smaller molecules by enzymes in the gastrointestinal tract – sugars for carbohydrate, glycerol, fatty acids for fats, and amino acids for proteins – and are absorbed in the small intestine. Fats are reassembled into triglyceride in the intestinal cells and pass into the blood via lymph vessels as particles called chylomicrons. These are further processed in the liver to form lipoproteins and enter the circulation. Amino acids that pass into the blood from the gut are taken up by tissues and converted into tissue proteins and other compounds such as nucleic acids and neurotransmitters. Most excess amino acids are oxidized although some can be converted into glucose or fat. Glucose that passes into the blood from the gut is taken up by tissues to be used as fuel or is converted into the polysaccharide glycogen in liver and muscle. Excess glucose is taken up by adipose tissue where it is converted into fat. The triglyceride in chylomicrons and lipoproteins are also added to the fat stores in adipose tissue. The synthesis of glycogen and triglyceride is energetically cheap, but the synthesis of proteins is far costlier. Proteins serve useful functions in the body as structural components, enzymes, transporters, etc. and are only a minor fuel for both resting and exercising energy requirements.

When we need energy (e.g., for exercise), some of the stored glycogen and triglycerides are broken down in a process that requires oxygen and generates carbon dioxide (CO_2) and water (H_2O). Glucose is first converted to pyruvate in the cytoplasm of the cell in an anaerobic series of reactions that collectively are known as glycolysis. Anaerobic metabolism does not use oxygen. The oxidation of pyruvate, fatty acids, and some amino acids takes place in the intracellular organelles called mitochondria (figure 5.1). Oxidation is an oxygen-requiring **(aerobic)** process. Fatty acids and pyruvate can be completely oxidized to carbon dioxide (CO_2) and water (H_2O). The carbon and hydrogen atoms in amino acids can also be completely oxidized, but the nitrogen atoms cannot. For amino acids, the amino groups (NH_2) are first removed, then converted into ammonia (NH_3) and urea ($CO(NH_2)_2$), and subsequently excreted in urine that is formed in the kidneys. The energy released in the oxidation of pyruvate, fatty acids, and amino acids is used to convert adenosine diphosphate (ADP) to adenosine triphosphate (ATP) which is the energy currency of the cell.

Functions of the Mitochondria

The **mitochondria** are small organelles that are found in the cell. Their most important role is to oxidize fuel obtained from the breakdown of fat and carbohydrate and use the energy released in this process to produce (or more accurately, resynthesize) the energy currency of the cell, adenosine triphosphate (ATP, via the addition of a phosphate group to ADP).

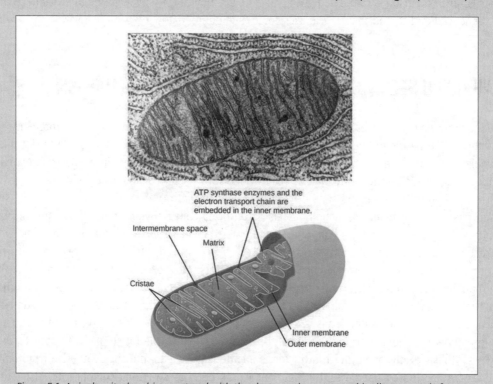

Figure 5.1: A single mitochondrion captured with the electron microscope and in diagrammatic form

All of the oxidation of fuels (carbohydrates, fats, and amino acids) takes place in the mitochondria. At rest they produce most of the ATP for energy requiring processes such as membrane transport, nerve conduction, and protein synthesis. During aerobic exercise, they produce most of the ATP that is used to fuel muscle contraction. The reactions that result in ATP production take place in the inner matrix of the mitochondrion and are collectively known as the **tricarboxylic acid (TCA) cycle**, citric acid cycle, or Krebs cycle after the German-born British biochemist Sir Hans Adolf Krebs who discovered it in the 1930s.

The breakdown of ATP to ADP releases energy which is used to perform all forms of biological work: muscle contraction, membrane transport, synthesis of biomolecules, etc. Without a sufficient supply of ATP, our cells would not be able to function or survive, and therefore without energy from food, we first use up our energy reserves then break down our tissues and organs and consequently die. We need food to survive, and we have evolved to be good at storing excess energy that we consume as fat, as this is our main storage form of energy and is needed in times of starvation. The problem with this is if we overindulge and eat too much food over a prolonged period, we become very fat, and this is bad for our health; being overweight or obese markedly increases or risk of developing chronic metabolic disease, cardiovascular diseases, and cancers and consequently reduces our life expectancy. While it is fine to have a certain amount of body fat, ideally, if we have a normal body weight (see chapter 7 for more about this), we should just eat enough to supply our daily needs, not too little and not too much, which brings us to the concept of energy balance.

ENERGY BALANCE

Energy balance refers to the balance between energy intake and energy expenditure. Simply put it is the difference between energy in and energy out. It can be measured on a day-to-day basis but probably makes more sense to measure it over a period of several days or weeks. When energy intake is greater than energy expenditure (i.e., when more calories come in than go out), the energy balance is said to be positive, and weight gain will occur, as most of the excess energy gets converted into body fat. When energy intake is below energy expenditure, the energy balance is negative, and weight loss will result. Therefore, to maintain energy balance and a stable body weight, energy expenditure must match energy intake. Over the long term, energy balance is maintained in weight-stable individuals even though this balance may be either positive or negative on a day-to-day basis. People who want to lose weight should increase energy expenditure relative to energy intake, which can be achieved either by increasing energy expenditure (by exercising more), reducing energy intake (by eating less), or a combination of both. There is no escaping this fact, and there are no quick-fix solutions to losing excess weight after it has been gained over a period of positive energy balance.

ENERGY INTAKE

Food contains energy in the form of carbohydrate, fat, and protein, which all have energy stored within their chemical bonds. To determine the gross energy content of food, a technique called direct calorimetry is used. The food is combusted (i.e., burned and completely oxidized), and the resulting heat is used as a measure of the energy content. The measurement takes place in a bomb calorimeter and has yielded the following information about macronutrient energy content:

- Carbohydrates have varying energy content, depending on the type of carbohydrate and the arrangements of atoms within the carbohydrate. The combustion of glucose, for instance, gives 3.7 kcal/g (15.7 kJ/g), whereas the combustion of glycogen and starch provides about 4.2 kcal/g (17.6 kJ/g). The latter figure is normally used as the energy value of carbohydrate.

- The energy content of fat also depends on the structure of the triglyceride or fatty acid. A medium-chain fatty acid, such as octanoic acid (eight-carbon fatty acid) may contain 8.6 kcal/g (36.0 kJ/g), whereas a long-chain fatty acid such as oleic acid (eighteen-carbon fatty acid) may contain up to 9.6 kcal/g (40.2 kJ/g). The energy content of fat in the average diet is 9.4 kcal/g (39.3 kJ/g).

- The energy content of protein depends on the type of protein and the nitrogen content. Nitrogen does not provide energy, and, therefore, proteins with higher nitrogen content contain less energy per gram. Nitrogen content in foods may vary from 15% (whole milk) to approximately 19% (nuts and seeds). The energy content of protein in the average diet is 5.7 kcal/g (23.7 kJ/g).

However, the gross energy value is not necessarily the same as the amount of energy that would be available if the food was eaten, particularly in the case of protein. Proteins are made up of amino acids all of which contain at least one nitrogen atom as an amino group (NH_2). In the body, the nitrogen in amino acids cannot be oxidized, so it is mostly excreted by the kidneys as urea, which has the chemical formula $CO(NH_2)_2$. Thus, some of the hydrogen atoms present in the amino acid are also excreted along with nitrogen in urea and therefore cannot provide energy. For this reason, about 20% of the potential chemical energy of the amino acid will be lost. If a bomb calorimeter shows that protein contains 5.7 kcal/g (23.7 kJ/g) of potential chemical energy, only 4.6 kcal/g (19.3 kJ/g) is actually available in the human body. This value is the net energy of protein in food.

Another thing that has to be taken into consideration is that food is sometimes not completely absorbed. Incomplete digestion and absorption will, of course, result in decreased availability of energy as some will appear in the feces. Wilbur Olin Atwater (1844–1907), one of the pioneers in studying human energy balance, determined this fact. After measuring many different kinds of foods with varying macronutrient content, Atwater came up with energy values for foods that accounted for differences in their digestibility. Conveniently, these energy values were rounded to whole numbers. The energy contents of carbohydrate, fat, and protein were found to be 4 kcal/g, 9 kcal/g and 4 kcal/g, respectively (17 kJ/g, 37 kJ/g and 17 kJ/g). These correction factors are often referred to as the **Atwater factors** or Atwater energy values and represent what is called the metabolizable energy value of food.

Nowadays, for many of the foods that are part of our regular diet, we know the percentage of food energy that is completely digested and absorbed. This percentage value averages 97% for carbohydrate, 95% for fat, and 92% for protein (see table 5.1) and is known as the **coefficient of digestibility**. Adding food items that are high in fiber to a meal generally reduces the coefficient of digestibility because fiber makes the food move faster through the gastrointestinal system, leaving less time for absorption processes to take place. Thus, a smaller amount of energy is available to the body from a food item high in fiber than from a food item with identical energy content but low in fiber. In several plant foods, some of the macronutrient content is encased in indigestible cell walls made of cellulose and other forms of fiber and so cannot be broken down and absorbed. Such foods have a much lower coefficient of digestibility. For example, for wheat bran protein it is only 40%, and its energy contribution is just 1.8 kcal/g (7.6 kJ/g), significantly less than the 4 kcal/g (17kJ/g) for protein estimated by Atwater. Furthermore, the coefficient of digestibility of wheat bran carbohydrate is 56%, and its energy contribution is only 2.4 kcal/g (9.8 kJ/g), again, far below the 4 kcal/g (17 kJ/g) for carbohydrate used by Atwater.

Table 5.1: Energy content of nutrients and the availability of energy in the body

	Energy content by combustion in kcal (kJ) per gram	Energy available in body in kcal (kJ) per gram	Coefficient of digestibility (%)
Protein			
Animal food	5.65 (23.7)	4.27 (17.9)	97
Meats, fish, and poultry	5.65 (23.7)	4.27 (17.9)	97
Eggs	5.75 (24.1)	4.37 (18.3)	97
Dairy products	5.65 (23.7)	4.27 (17.9)	97
Plant food	5.65 (23.7)	4.27 (17.9)	85
Cereals	5.80 (24.3)	3.87 (16.2)	85
Legumes	5.70 (23.9)	3.47 (14.5)	78
Vegetables	5.00 (20.9)	3.11 (13.0)	83
Fruits	5.20 (21.8)	3.36 (14.1)	83
Average protein	5.65 (23.7)	4.05 (17.0)	92
Fat			
Animal food	9.40 (39.3)	8.93 (37.4)	95
Meat and eggs	9.50 (39.8)	9.03 (37.8)	95
Dairy products	9.25 (38.7)	8.79 (36.8)	95
Vegetable food	9.30 (38.9)	8.37 (35.0)	90
Average fat	9.40 (39.3)	8.93 (37.4)	95
Carbohydrate			
Animal food	3.90 (16.3)	3.82 (16.0)	98
Vegetable food	4.15 (17.4)	4.03 (16.9)	97
Cereals	4.20 (17.6)	4.11 (17.2)	98
Legumes	4.20 (17.6)	4.07 (17.0)	97
Vegetables	4.20 (17.6)	3.99 (16.7)	95
Fruits	4.00 (16.7)	3.60 (15.1)	90
Sugars	3.95 (16.5)	3.87 (16.2)	98
Average carbohydrate	4.15 (17.4)	4.03 (16.9)	97

The coefficient of digestibility reflects the percentage of energy in a nutrient that is actually available after digestion and absorption in the gut has taken place.

Nowadays many extensive databases are available that list the composition and available energy content of a vast array of food items. One of the largest and most comprehensive databases is the USDA National Nutrient Database. There is a section for Standard Reference that is freely available (https://www.ndb.nal.usda.gov/ndb/) and can be downloaded in several different formats for use on your computer. An online search tool is also provided so you can look up the nutrient content of over 7,700 different foods directly from the home page. It is the major source of food composition data in the United States and provides the foundation for most food composition databases in the public and private sectors. There is also a USDA Branded Food Products Database **(https://www.ndb.nal.usda.gov/ndb/)** which is also freely accessible.

The UK **(https://www.gov.uk/government/publications/composition-of-foods-integrated-dataset-cofid)** has its own data base with its own specific products as do many other countries such as Australia **(https://www.foodstandards.gov.au/science/monitoringnutrients/ausnut/foodnutrient/)**. Some professional software programs combine all these international databases to provide a very comprehensive collection of foods.

Many apps on mobile devices can be used to record food intake and estimate the intake of energy, macronutrients, and micronutrients. Often these apps use the same databases, but many apps allow users to enter their own foods and values and share these items publicly. This means that not all values in these apps have been verified, and some nutrition information is inaccurate or incomplete. It is important to be aware of such limitations when using them for diet planning.

ENERGY EXPENDITURE

Energy is needed for various processes in the body, including basal functions, digestion, absorption, metabolism, and storage of food. In addition, active people expend energy during exercise. The three components of energy expenditure: resting metabolic rate, diet-induced thermogenesis, and exercise-related energy expenditure, are explained in this section.

RESTING METABOLIC RATE

The largest component (60% to 85%) of daily energy expenditure in a relatively inactive person is the **resting metabolic rate (RMR)**, the energy required for the maintenance of normal body functions and homeostasis in resting conditions. Factors such as maintaining body temperature at 37 °C, sympathetic nervous system activity, thyroid hormone activity, cell membrane transport activity, biosynthesis of large molecules, pumping of the heart, contraction of the muscles involved in breathing and maintaining posture contribute to the RMR. Another measure is the **basal metabolic rate (BMR)** which was originally developed for use in a clinical setting to measure the lowest oxygen uptake in resting thermoneutral conditions for patients with thyroid problems. Measurements were often performed in the morning after a 12-hour to 18-hour fast, but this is inconvenient for most people, and the RMR has become the far more popular measure. The RMR is primarily related to the lean body (fat-free) mass and is influenced mainly by age, gender, body composition (particularly degree of muscularity and adiposity), as well as genetic factors (some people naturally have slower metabolism than others).

Different body tissues and organs have very different resting energy requirements. Organs that have large metabolic demands, such as the liver, gut, brain, and kidney, and the tissues that need to intermittently contract like the heart (to pump blood around the circulation), and the respiratory muscles like the diaphragm (to inflate the lungs during breathing), have the highest energy requirements per gram of tissue. In a lean adult, these organs account for about 75% of RMR, although they constitute only around 10% of total body weight. Apart from the continuously working respiratory muscles, other skeletal muscles account for only 20% of RMR, although they make up about 40% of total body weight. Adipose tissue uses very little energy and accounts for less than 5% of RMR even though it usually represents at least 20% of body weight. The RMR decreases with age (2% to 3% per decade), and males generally have a higher RMR than females (because of their larger body size and higher proportion of lean mass). Part of the drop in RMR with age is due to **sarcopenia** which is the name used by clinicians to describe the gradual loss of muscle mass as we get older

Resting energy expenditure (REE) correlates closely with the amount of lean mass which is often referred to as **fat-free mass**. Although the energy expenditure of metabolically active organs is responsible for the largest component of RMR and REE, the fat-free mass, which is mostly composed of skeletal muscle, accounts for most of the variability in energy expenditure between individuals in the resting state. The REE includes the RMR plus the small (10-30%) transient increases in energy expenditure that occur following feeding. This phenomenon is referred to as the thermic effect of food or diet-induced thermogenesis.

How to Calculate Your Own Resting Metabolic Rate (RMR)

To most accurately calculate the RMR, a scientist would take measurements of oxygen uptake and carbon dioxide production after a subject has fasted for 12 hours and has had eight hours of sleep. However, a rough estimation of this data is possible using the Mifflin-St. Jeor equation which was introduced in 1990. This equation is currently considered to be the best for estimating RMR.

Mifflin St. Jeor Equation:

For men: RMR (kcal/day) = 10 x weight (kg) + 6.25 x height (cm) − 5 x age (years) + 5

For women: RMR (kcal/day) = 10 x weight (kg) + 6.25 x height (cm) − 5 x age (years) − 161

The RMR will be about 5-10% higher for a man than a woman of the same age and body weight since body composition (ratios of lean muscle, bone and fat) differ between men and women. The heavier you are, the more energy you need to sustain the larger muscle mass and larger organs, which is why heavier and taller individuals have a higher RMR. The other important factor is age, as your RMR decreases as you get older because muscle mass declines by 5-10% each decade after the age of 30, unless that is, you participate in regular resistance training to prevent this (and believe me it is preventable). Nowadays many apps on mobile devices can be used to calculate RMR.

DIET-INDUCED THERMOGENESIS

The **diet-induced thermogenesis (DIT)**, or **thermic effect of food (TEF)**, is the increase in energy expenditure above RMR that occurs for several hours after ingestion of a meal. DIT is the result of digestion, absorption, and the subsequent storage or metabolism of food and normally represents about 10% of the total daily resting energy expenditure. The magnitude of DIT mostly depends on the size of the meal and its macronutrient composition, which in turn determines the energy cost of its storage. The cost of storing fat in adipose tissue is approximately 3% of the energy of the ingested meal, whereas if carbohydrate is stored as glycogen in the liver and muscles, about 7% of the energy is lost. The energy cost for the synthesis of new body protein is around 20-25% of the available energy. Energy expenditure can be increased up to eight hours following a large meal. The largest DIT occurs after eating a large meal high in protein which can result in a 30% increase in the RMR. Meals that are predominantly composed of carbohydrate and/or fat generally raise the RMR by less than 10%. The **sympathetic nervous system** seems to play an important role in DIT. We know this because when the effects of the sympathetic nervous system are reduced by administering a β-blocker drug (e.g., propanolol), DIT is also reduced.

THERMIC EFFECT OF EXERCISE

The third component of daily energy expenditure is the **thermic effect of exercise (TEE)**, or energy expended in physical activity, including all daily tasks that involve movement (e.g., walking, climbing stairs, gardening, household chores, and even minor activities like typing or playing a musical instrument), as well as participation in any sport or exercise, is by far the most variable component of daily energy expenditure. It includes all energy expended above the RMR and DIT. The TEE has both an intentional voluntary component (exercise) and an involuntary component (shivering, fidgeting, or postural control) which both require muscle contraction and therefore some use of energy over and above the REE. In completely sedentary people, or individuals who are confined to bed due to illness, the TEE may be no more than 100 kcal/day (400 kJ/day). In recreationally active people, the TEE will often be several hundred kilocalories per day, and in extremely active people such as those involved in professional sport, the TEE may be a few thousand kilocalories per day. The highest TEE in humans is probably found among elite endurance athletes when they compete in prolonged endurance events such as road race cycling with extremes of up to 6,000 kcal/day (25 MJ/day) having been reported for cyclists on some race days in the Tour de France. Thus, the TEE can vary from an average of 5% of the daily energy expenditure up to 80% in extreme conditions during heavy endurance training or competition. The amount of exercise we do is therefore extremely important for the maintenance of our daily energy balance. It is not only the most variable component of 24-hour energy expenditure but also the main component that can we can control voluntarily. Since all forms of exercise count towards an individual's TEE, it is useful to have an idea of how much energy is expended in various activities. Regular exercise also improves our fitness and brings many health benefits; these are explained in detail in chapter 9.

ENERGY COST OF DIFFERENT ACTIVITIES

Some physical activities obviously expend more energy than others, as shown in tables 5.2 and 5.3. The amount of energy expended per minute is related to the intensity of the exercise, but the total amount of energy expended is more closely related to the duration of the activity or the total distance covered. But even in the same activity, there can be considerable differences in the energy expenditure, depending on the level at which it is performed. Tennis, for example, has relatively low energy expenditure if played recreationally, and because each player has to move less when playing doubles, the energy cost is lower than for singles. At this level of play, it could be classified as a light-to-moderate activity, although at occasionally during a game, the activity can sometimes be extremely intense, requiring high rates of energy expenditure but only in short bursts lasting no more than a few seconds. However, the majority of the time, recreational tennis and even moderate level club play involve longer periods of low-intensity activity like moving side to side, walking, standing, and even some sitting (at change of ends). This is why the average energy expenditure for tennis is relatively low. The advantage, of course, is that this game can be enjoyed by many people right into old age. In contrast, tennis played at a high level has shorter periods of rest, and the average exercise intensity is much higher. The players are fitter and more skillful, meaning that rallies can be prolonged, and a lot more energy is expended. A five-set match in men's grand slam events can often last over four hours and total energy expenditure may exceed 2,500 kcal (10.5 MJ). Games like soccer, rugby, and American football also involve intermittent activity but match duration is fixed by the rules of the sport, so the average amount of energy expended (e.g., typically 1,600 kcal or 6.7 MJ for professional soccer) does not vary much from game to game. Continuous sports such as cycling and running, which usually include little or no recovery during the activity, will generally have the highest energy expenditures.

Table 5.2: The energy cost of various activities

Activity	(kcal/min)	(kJ/min)	Examples
Resting	1	4	Sleeping, reclining, sitting in relaxed pose
Very light activities	2-5	8-21	Standing activities including most household chores, and some active sitting activities such as driving, card playing, typing
Light activities	5-7	21-29	Walking (3 to 5 km/h), baseball, bowling, horseback riding, golf, gardening
Moderate activities	7-9	29-38	Cycling at 10-15 km/h, hiking, jogging, badminton, basketball, soccer, swimming, tennis, volleyball
Strenuous activities	9-13	38-54	Cycling at 20 km/h, running at 10-13 km/h, cross-country skiing (8 to 10 km/h)
Very strenuous activities	>13	>54	Cycling at 35 km/h, running at >14 km/h, cross-country skiing at >12 km/h

Table 5.3: The estimated energy cost of various sporting activities in kcal/min (kJ/min) according to body weight in kg (lbs.)

Activity	Body weight				
	50 kg (110 lbs.)	60 kg (132 lbs.)	70 kg (154 lbs.)	80 kg (176 lbs.)	90 kg (198 lbs.)
Aerobics	7.0 (29)	8.3 (35)	10.0 (42)	11.3 (47)	12.8 (54)
Badminton	5.0 (21)	5.7 (24)	6.7 (28)	8.3 (35)	9.3 (39)
Ballroom dancing	2.8 (12)	3.3 (14)	3.8 (16)	4.3 (18)	4.8 (20)
Basketball	7.2 (30)	8.8 (36)	10.0 (42)	11.5 (48)	13.0 (54)
Boxing	11.5 (48)	14.0 (58)	16.3 (68)	18.5 (77)	21.0 (88)
Sparring in ring	7.2 (30)	8.8 (37)	10.0 (42)	11.5 (48)	13.0 (54)
Canoeing Easy	2.3 (10)	2.8 (12)	3.3 (14)	3.8 (16)	4.3 (18)
Hard	5.5 (23)	6.5 (27)	7.5 (31)	8.5 (35)	9.8 (41)
Circuit training	5.5 (23)	6.5 (27)	7.5 (31)	8.5 (35)	10.0 (42)
Baseball/ Cricket (batting)	4.3 (18)	5.3 (22)	6.0 (25)	7.0 (29)	8.0 (33)
Cycling 10 km/h	3.3 (14)	4.0 (17)	4.5 (19)	5.3 (22)	6.0 (25)
15 km/h	5.3 (22)	5.7 (24)	6.7 (28)	8.3 (35)	9.5 (40)
25 km/h	8.8 (35)	10.5 (42)	12.3 (49)	14.0 (56)	15.8 (63)
Football/Soccer	7.0 (29)	8.3 (35)	9.8 (41)	11.0 (46)	12.5 (52)
Golf	4.5 (19)	5.5 (23)	6.3 (26)	7.0 (29)	8.0 (33)
Gymnastics	3.5 (15)	4.0 (17)	4.8 (20)	5.5 (23)	6.3 (26)
Hockey	4.5 (19)	5.0 (21)	6.0 (25)	7.3 (30)	8.3 (34)
Judo	10.3 (43)	12.3 (51)	14.3 (60)	16.3 (68)	18.3 (76)
Running 11 km/h	10.0 (43)	12.3 (51)	14.3 (60)	16.3 (68)	18.3 (76)
12 km/h	11.0 (46)	13.0 (54)	15.3 (64)	17.5 (73)	19.5 (82)
13.5 km/h	12.0 (50)	13.8 (57)	16.3 (68)	18.8 (78)	21.3 (89)
15 km/h	13.5 (56)	16.3 (67)	19.0 (79)	21.8 (91)	24.5 (102)
Skiing Cross-country	8.8 (35)	10.5 (43)	12.3 (49)	14.0 (58)	15.8 (66)
Downhill (easy)	4.5 (18)	5.5 (21)	6.3 (25)	7.3 (29)	8.3 (33)
Downhill (hard)	7.3 (29)	8.8 (35)	10.0 (40)	12.3 (49)	13.8 (55)
Squash	11.0 (44)	13.3 (53)	15.5 (62)	17.8 (71)	19.8 (79)
Swimming					
Freestyle	8.3 (35)	10.0 (42)	11.5 (48)	13.0 (54)	14.8 (61)
Backstroke	9.0 (37)	10.8 (45)	12.3 (51)	14.0 (58)	15.8 (66)
Breaststroke	8.5 (35)	10.3 (43)	11.8 (49)	13.5 (55)	15.3 (61)
Table tennis	3.5 (15)	4.3 (18)	4.8 (20)	5.8 (24)	6.5 (27)
Tennis Social	3.8 (16)	4.3 (18)	5.0 (21)	5.8 (24)	6.5 (27)
Competitive	9.3 (39)	11.0 (46)	12.5 (52)	14.5 (60)	16.3 (68)
Volleyball	2.5 (10)	3.0 (13)	3.6 (16)	4.3 (18)	4.8 (20)
Walking 4 km/h	3.9 (16)	4.7 (20)	6.0 (25)	6.9 (29)	7.5 (31)
6 km/h	5.3 (22)	6.5 (27)	7.5 (31)	8.8 (37)	9.8 (41)

HOW TO ACHIEVE ENERGY BALANCE

As explained earlier in this chapter, in order to remain weight-stable, we need to achieve energy balance, and that means that over a period of time (say one week), our energy expenditure has to match our energy intake as illustrated in figure 5.2.

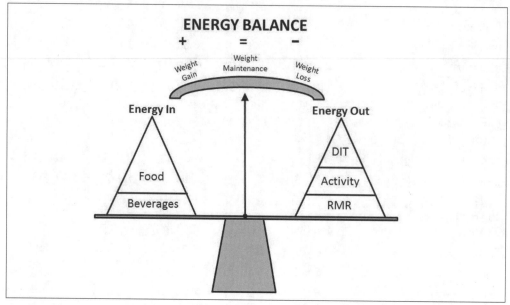

Figure 5.2: The concept of energy balance: DIT, diet-induced thermogenesis; RMR, resting metabolic rate

So, in practical terms it makes sense to estimate your own weekly total energy expenditure and use this as a guide to the average amount of food energy you should aim to consume on a daily basis. You can do this as follows:

First, estimate your RMR using the Mifflin-St. Jeor equation. Let's take as an example a 30-year-old male, who is 180 cm tall and weighs 80 kg. The appropriate equation is:

For men: RMR (kcal/day) = 10 x weight (kg) + 6.25 x height (cm) − 5 x age (years) + 5

Inputting weight, height, and age gives:

RMR (kcal/day) = 10 x 80 (kg) + 6.25 x 180 (cm) − 5 x 30 (years) + 5

= 800 + 1,125 − 150 + 5

= 1,780

To this value, add 10% to account for the DIT component of daily energy expenditure, so that means your daily resting energy expenditure is 1,780 + 178 = 1,958 kcal/day.

Now we need to add any energy expended in physical activities; for just moving around the house, daily chores, going up and down stairs, etc., we can add about 100 kcal, making your daily energy expenditure 2,058 kcal/day. Multiply this by 7 to give the amount of energy you expend in one week, which in this case would be 14,406 kcal.

Now add the energy you have expended on each day of the week doing any of the activities listed in tables 5.2 and/or 5.3. As these values are shown in kcal/min, multiply that value for the particular activity you did by the number of minutes you spent doing it. For example, if on one day you went for a 40-minute brisk walk and covered about 4 km your additional energy expenditure was 8.8 kcal/min x 40 min = 352 kcal.

Do this for what you did for each day of the week, add them all up (this is the amount of energy you expended in physical activity in one 7-day week), and add this to the weekly resting energy expenditure. To simplify the example we have used, let's say you did a 40-minute walk every day but nothing else. Then we add 7 days x 352 kcal/day = 2,464 kcal to 14,406 kcal to give the weekly average energy expenditure which is 16,870 kcal. Divide this by 7 to get the average daily energy expenditure which is 2,410 kcal. This is the amount of food energy you should consume each day (on average) to achieve energy balance and maintain your current weight.

Second, you should calculate your typical daily dietary energy intake. As this will vary on a day-to-day basis, it is best to average this over a period of one week. It involves recording every item of food you consume, noting the weight or portion size, and determining its calorie content to determine your daily energy intake. This used to be a laborious process as all the information had to be looked up in food composition tables. Nowadays such data bases are available online, and there are several computer programs and apps for mobile devices that can be downloaded for free (or at least for a 7-day trial) that enable you to select from thousands of commercial food items such as breakfast cereals, breads, and sauces as well as loose items such as fresh meats, vegetables, and fruits, and beverages including tea, wine, and beer. You can also use Google to find out how many calories there are in specific food items (this information is usually given as calories per 100 g and calories per typical portion size).

Now compare your average daily energy intake with your average daily energy expenditure. If they are exactly the same, then you are in energy balance and likely to remain weight stable. If your energy intake is less than expenditure, then you are in negative energy balance and likely to lose weight if this is sustained over time. If your energy intake is more than expenditure, then you are in positive energy balance and likely to gain weight if this is sustained over time. Let's say you find that this is the case, and your daily energy intake is 100 calories (kcal) greater than your energy expenditure. It might not sound like a lot, but if maintained, that is 700 kcal excess in one week, 2,800 kcal excess in one month or 33,600 kcal excess in one year. That equates to 4.4 kg (9.8 lbs.) of fat gain in one year! So, it pays to know if you are in energy balance. Some of the apps that have recently become available will do both food calorie counting and estimate your daily energy expenditure and even let you know whether you are in positive or negative energy balance, so why not download one now and try it out.

THE LOWEST LIMIT OF ENERGY EXPENDITURE

The lowest limit of energy expenditure is determined by the sum of RMR, DIT, and a minimum level of physical activity needed to carry out daily living, even if that is only walking from one room to another in your home! DIT is directly affected by the amount of food consumed. Reducing food intake results in decreased DIT, and it may also indirectly influence the RMR. This is because after a few weeks of reduced dietary energy availability, the body adapts by slowing the metabolic rate by up to 10%, meaning that it becomes harder to lose weight when dieting (see chapter 7 for further details). One of the problems associated with reducing energy intake to very low levels is the possibility of marginal nutrition or even malnutrition, particularly of essential nutrients, such as fat-soluble vitamins, calcium, iron, and essential fatty acids.

Key Points

- All biological functions require energy, and although the human body has some stored energy reserves, most of the energy must be obtained through nutrition.

- Energy is the capacity to do work. The various forms of energy include light energy, chemical energy, heat energy, and electrical energy.

- Energy is often expressed in calories (English system) or joules (metric system); 1 calorie equals 4.184 joules.

- Efficiency describes the effective work performed after muscle contraction and is usually expressed as the percentage of total work. Humans are approximately 20% efficient.

- The energy content of 1 g of carbohydrate is 4.2 kcal (17.6 kJ). Fat contains between 8.6 kcal/g (36.0 kJ/g) and 9.6 kcal/g (40.2 kJ/g) (on average, about 9.4 kcal/g [39.3 kJ/g]), and protein contains about 5.65 kcal/g (23.7 kJ/g). The coefficient of digestibility represents the proportion of consumed food actually digested and absorbed by the body.

- Coefficients of digestibility average about 97% for carbohydrates, 95% for fats, and 92% for proteins. The net energy values of carbohydrate, fat, and protein are therefore 4 kcal (17 kJ), 9 kcal (37 kJ), and 4 kcal (17 kJ), respectively, and these are referred to as the Atwater energy values or Atwater factors.

- Human energy expenditure can be divided into several components: resting metabolic rate, thermic effect of food, and exercise-related energy expenditure. The resting metabolic rate is the largest component (60% to 85%) of the daily energy expenditure in relatively sedentary people, the thermic effect of food represents about 10%, and the remainder is 5% to 30% for exercise-related energy expenditure. The latter can be considerably higher in more active people, and for endurance athletes, it could be as high as 80%.

- Different activities and sports have different energy requirements, which are based on the muscle mass involved, and the mode, duration, and relative intensity of the exercise. Some sports, including road race cycling, triathlon, and ultra-endurance running are sports that may require total energy expenditures as high as 8,000 kcal/day (33 MJ/day) on competition days.

- Energy balance is usually calculated over long periods (days or weeks) and represents the difference between energy intake and energy expenditure. Energy balance is achieved when energy intake equals energy expenditure when measured over about a week. When energy intake exceeds energy expenditure, a positive energy balance occurs, which results in weight gain. When energy intake is lower than energy expenditure, energy balance is negative and results in weight loss.

Chapter 6

What Controls Your Appetite and How Hunger Can Be Abated When Dieting

Objectives

After studying this chapter, you should:

- Understand the factors that control appetite

- Appreciate the difference between appetite and satiety

- Know which gastrointestinal hormone stimulates feelings of hunger

- Understand the factors that influence satiety

- Know which macronutrient has the biggest impact on satiety

- Know what can help to make us feel full without ingesting excess calories

- Know how hunger can be abated when dieting by appropriate food choices

- Be aware of the problem of food addiction

We generally eat when we are feeling hungry, and most people will consume at least two or three meals during the day and may also eat a few snacks in between meals. You will probably already know that some meals can be more filling than others and will abate our hunger for longer; it is not just about the amount of food or calories in a meal. Several factors influence how satisfying a meal is to an individual, and these include the smell, texture, and flavor of the food, the macronutrient composition, the energy content, and the volume (bulk) of the meal. Sensory information about these influences from the nose, mouth, and gut are sent to the appetite center in the brain and affect when we stop eating (because we feel full), and the time that elapses before we feel that we want the next meal (because we feel hungry again). Although both physiological and environmental factors contribute to our **appetite** and eating behavior, it is widely accepted that strong social and environmental influences can easily overcome our normal physiology. This chapter will explain how our appetite is controlled and provides some ideas as to how hunger can be abated, at least to some degree, when dieting, by appropriate food choices.

HOW OUR APPETITE IS CONTROLLED

An important processing region in the brain called the **hypothalamus** plays a key role in controlling eating behavior in humans (figure 6.1). The hypothalamus, in particular the part of it known as the arcuate nucleus, constantly receives and processes various signals from the periphery. These signals are transferred to the hypothalamus by nerves and hormones, and the hypothalamus can also detect the concentration of certain nutrients (e.g., glucose) in the blood. These continuous sensory inputs enable it to maintain energy homoeostasis by adjusting dietary energy intake. But that is not all, as the information processed by the hypothalamus also influences our energy expenditure by promoting the desire for rest or increased physical activity. Other than the nose and mouth, sensory signals are generated mainly by the gastrointestinal tract but also by other organs and tissues such as the liver, pancreas, and adipose tissue. The human gut is lined with more than 100 million nerve cells that link to the vagus nerves and spinal cord, meaning that the gut actually talks to the brain directly via a neural circuit that allows it to transmit signals in a matter of seconds. Following the ingestion of a meal, the gastrointestinal tract detects the presence of nutrients, signals this to the brain via the aforementioned neural connections, and also produces several appetite regulating hormones such as **cholecystokinin (CCK)**, glucagon-like peptide-1 (GLP-1), and peptide YY. Most of these hormones provide signals that influence **satiety** (feeling of fullness and satisfaction during and after a meal) but **ghrelin**, produced mostly by the stomach, plays an important role by stimulating appetite or hunger. When the stomach is empty, ghrelin secretion increases and elevated blood ghrelin concentration stimulates the conscious sensation of hunger that makes us want to eat food. After eating meals, ghrelin returns to baseline concentrations. Meal size and composition influence the secretion of these hormones and contribute to the sensation of satiety, as the foods consumed are digested and absorbed.

Our body also generates signals that are related to the size of our body fat stores. These adiposity signals such as insulin and **leptin** act in the arcuate nucleus of the brain to provide a background tone, which in turn determines the sensitivity of the brain to signals that influence satiety, and therefore how much food is eaten at any one time. This background tone, however, has only a relatively minor and subtle influence on our food intake during any given meal. Numerous other influences including social factors (e.g., religion, wealth, and peer pressure to eat everything that the cook puts on our plate), **palatability** (how agreeable the food tastes), habits (e.g., what we normally eat for breakfast), stress (e.g., from our relationships and job as well as hard physical activity) are always at work, influencing not only when meals occur but also how much food is consumed. In fact, only when these external influences are tightly controlled in laboratory experiments, or when ingestion is precisely monitored and quantified over periods of days or weeks in free-feeding humans, do the effects of these adiposity signals become apparent.

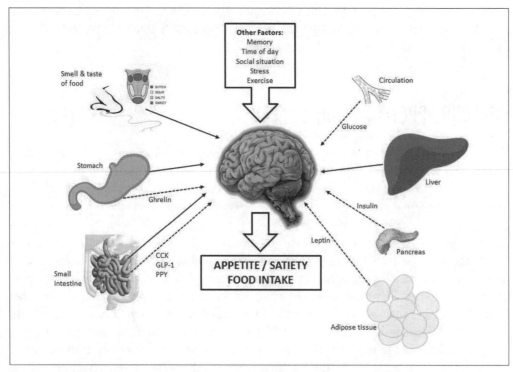

Figure 6.1: Appetite is sensed in the brain. The brain constantly receives and processes nervous, metabolic, and hormonal signals from the periphery. In addition, many other factors influence the eventual outcome: our food intake. Solid arrows indicate nervous signals, and dashed arrows indicate blood-borne signals.

CONTROL OF FEEDING BEHAVIOR

Over the past thousands of years, humans have regularly experienced periods of feast and famine. To protect the human species from extinction through periods when food is scarce, mechanisms have evolved to help us be resistant to fat loss and maintain body weight. The hypothalamus and brainstem regulate feeding behavior by promoting food intake or suppressing appetite in response to peripheral hormonal and nervous signals. Feeding behavior is also influenced by the brain's reward systems. The hypothalamus plays a key role in monitoring, processing, and responding to the incoming sensory signals. The hunger hormone, ghrelin, or the sight and smell of appealing, high-calorie foods, and the usual mealtime habits prompt people to eat. Satiety hormones, particularly the various **brain-gut peptides**, act to inhibit feeding behavior. These short-term effects are modulated by the longer-term effects of the circulating levels of insulin and leptin. In addition, parts of the brain concerned with cognition are also involved in this process, which means that our feelings and emotions can also influence our eating behavior.

The hypothalamus comprises several different regions which include the arcuate nucleus, the dorsomedial nucleus, the paraventricular nucleus, the ventromedial nucleus, and the lateral hypothalamic area, and all of them are involved in the control of energy balance. Sensory nerve endings in the gut and digestive organs provide information to the brain about incoming nutrients, and this information is transmitted as nerve impulses in the vagal nerves and the ascending spinal cord. Gut peptide hormones secreted from the gastrointestinal tract in response to the appearance of various nutrients communicate information via blood circulation and binding to receptors in the hypothalamus. Receptors in the hypothalamus also detected levels of some nutrients in the blood (e.g., glucose) that are elevated after feeding. The arcuate nucleus is adjacent to the third ventricle and the median eminence, where there is a thin blood-brain barrier allowing hormones and nutrients to directly cross into the cerebrospinal fluid. Thus, both nervous signals and blood-borne hormones and nutrients influence the arcuate nucleus to give it a major role in the control of feeding behavior.

Receptors in the gut sense the presence of nutrients and transfer this information via the vagal nerves to the brain. Most of the vagal sensory (afferent) nerve fibers that innervate the gastrointestinal tract and digestive organs project to brain regions that influence food intake through actions that activate motivation and reward-related areas. The reward system of the brain, which is located in a number of limbic and cortical areas that communicate with each other, together with the hypothalamus determine the pleasantness of food in concert with the emotional and cognitive aspects of eating behavior. What we refer to as "comfort foods", which are almost always highly flavored, energy-dense food items, can override normal eating control mechanisms and generate paradoxically high but ineffective levels of appetite-suppressing hormones because of their strong influence on the reward system of the brain. In other words, a part of our brain is actually tricking us into consuming unhealthy foods just because eating them is pleasurable. You need to forego the immediate pleasure and make the conscious decision not to eat comfort foods because you know they are not good for your long-term health. Or learn to enjoy healthy foods more than the unhealthy ones.

THE ROLE OF BRAIN–GUT PEPTIDE HORMONES

The gastrointestinal tract is the largest **endocrine** (hormone secreting) organ in the body, and the gastrointestinal peptide hormones it produces influence feeding behavior by acting as appetite promotors or appetite suppressants. Collectively they are called brain-gut peptides. There are two types of brain-gut peptides:

1. short-term signals, which are kept in step with each episode of eating; these include amylin, CCK, gastric inhibitory polypeptide (GIP), ghrelin, GLP-1, glucagon, nesfatin-1, neuropeptide Y, oxyntomodulin, pancreatic polypeptide, and peptide YY, to name a few; and

2. long-term signals, which reflect the metabolic state of adipose tissue, such as insulin and leptin. Both the short- and long-term signals interact with each other to determine eating behavior.

Ghrelin is mostly secreted into the bloodstream by the stomach and increases food intake by promoting appetite via the receptors located in the hypothalamic ventromedial nucleus and arcuate nucleus. Ghrelin is secreted when the stomach is empty, so that during fasting, the plasma concentration of ghrelin increases to stimulate hunger. After food is ingested and the stomach fills and distends, the secretion of ghrelin is inhibited, and its plasma concentration falls. Currently, ghrelin is the only known gut peptide hormone to stimulate appetite and promote food intake, and therefore its actions may facilitate weight gain. Following a meal, the reduction in ghrelin secretion and the subsequent drop in plasma ghrelin levels is influenced by the relative proportion of macronutrients in a meal, with a greater decrease after protein and carbohydrate ingestion than after fat ingestion. Ghrelin is also produced in the hypothalamus, where it acts as a neurotransmitter to adjust appetite and also influence the reward system in the brain, in which the emotional wanting or reward value for those highly desirable "comfort foods" is increased. In summary, ghrelin can be thought of as the enemy of someone on a weight-loss diet. Low-calorie and particularly low volume diets as well as poor sleep are known to increase ghrelin levels, so it is advisable to ensure good sleep quality (as explained in chapter 10), add low-calorie but bulky foods to your diet, drink plenty of fluid to increase and prolong stomach distension (remember that inhibits ghrelin secretion), and eat a high-protein diet because protein increases feelings of fullness and reduces hunger via a reduction in plasma ghrelin concentration.

CCK was the first gut hormone discovered to affect feeding and appetite. CCK is secreted mostly from cells located in the wall of the first part of the small intestine (which is called the **duodenum**), mainly in response to the presence of fatty acids. Plasma CCK levels increase within 15 minutes following a meal, but it is short acting and is only present in the circulation for a few minutes. Both the vagus nerve and hypothalamus possess CCK receptors that can detect elevated levels of CCK in the blood and lead to early meal termination and reduced food intake.

In addition to CCK, several gut peptides including neuropeptide Y, pancreatic polypeptide, and peptide YY are secreted following feeding and act to inhibit appetite and eating. Pancreatic polypeptide is released from the pancreas in proportion to the amount of ingested calories, and its actions via the brainstem and hypothalamus result in the suppression of appetite. Peptide YY is secreted in proportion to the amount of nutrients (particularly fat) ingested, and it also acts as an appetite suppressant. GLP-1 is produced by cells in the wall of the small intestine and also by parts of the hindbrain. GLP-1 is released in proportion to the amount of calories ingested, predominantly from carbohydrate and fat. The actions of GLP-1 in the hypothalamus lead to satiety and reduced hunger.

Some drugs used to promote weight loss in obese people act as appetite suppressants by stimulating brain chemicals to induce a feeling of fullness. One such drug called lorcaserin works by specifically activating brain receptors for **serotonin**, a neurotransmitter that affects appetite by triggering feelings of satiety and satisfaction. Lorcaserin is sold as Belviq in the US and is the first weight loss medicine to successfully pass a long-term safety study now required by regulators to stay on the market. Researchers hope that passing this milestone will encourage more widespread use of this oral medication and pave the way for approval in other countries, including the UK. At the present time, there are no appetite suppressants available on the National Health Service, and experts say there is a need for treatments that plug the gap between lifestyle modification and surgery. Other weight loss pills that are used to treat obesity, such as those that increase resting metabolic rate or promote fat burning, have a history of serious complications, and none are currently recommended for general use.

THE ROLE OF LEPTIN AND INSULIN IN LONG-TERM FEEDING CONTROL

The brain-gut peptides described previously all play a role as short-term signals in the control of feeding behavior. Two other hormones – leptin and insulin – act as long-term signals of feeding behavior. Leptin is produced by adipose tissue, and the amount of leptin released into the circulation is proportional to body fat content. Leptin acts directly on the feeding control centers in the brain to both reduce food intake and increase energy expenditure. It therefore plays a role in preventing obesity by inhibiting appetite. Genetic defects that result in an absence of leptin or cause a leptin receptor dysfunction may lead to overeating and obesity. Insulin, which is secreted from the pancreatic islets into the circulation in response to an increase in the blood glucose concentration, also acts to inhibit appetite via its actions on the hypothalamus.

Nutrients and Satiety

Humans eat in intervals; that is, they eat meals. Before a meal begins, the sensation of hunger rises, and this motivates food-seeking behavior. After eating starts, hunger declines, and people report that they start to feel full. The term satiation describes the processes that bring a meal to an end. An interval of time then elapses before eating begins again. Satiety refers to the inhibition of eating following a meal, and it is measured both by the length of the interval between meals and by the amount of food consumed when it is next offered. Different macronutrients have different effects on satiety. It has been demonstrated that protein has a much stronger effect on satiety than fat and carbohydrate do.

NUTRIENTS AS SIGNALS IN FEEDING CONTROL

Nutrients can also transfer satiating signals to the hypothalamus. Specific receptors or transporters sense the signals from nutrients like carbohydrate, fat, and protein. These receptors are mostly located in specialized cells in the lining of the small intestine and can trigger the release of gastro-intestinal regulatory peptides such as CCK, ghrelin, peptide YY, and GLP-1 among others. Levels of blood glucose can also be detected by the hypothalamus in the brain, and when blood glucose is higher than normal, it reduces the sensation of hunger. Receptors in the small intestine can sense the presence of fatty acids which are produced during the digestion of dietary fat, and this information is sent to the brain by the vagal nerves. After digestion, proteins are degraded to amino acids and small peptides which are detected by receptors in the nerve cells located in the wall of the portal vein (which transfers blood from the gut to the liver), and these signals are sent via both vagal and ascending spinal cord nerves. Certain proteins such as whey protein (from milk) are more rapidly digested than others and cause a relatively larger increase in the plasma amino acid concentrations following ingestion. This generates signals that have a greater stimulatory effect on the secretion of gastrointestinal hormones such as CCK and GLP-1, and these effects probably account for the greater satiety after ingesting protein compared with carbohydrate and fat. How slowly or quickly we eat our food when we sit down for a large meal (maybe with two or three courses) also influences the development of the satiety signals. It is better to eat food slowly and chew it well before swallowing, as this not only aids digestion but also allows more time for nutrients to be digested and absorbed and the satiety signals to kick in. That means that you start to feel full and satisfied earlier – well before you have finished eating everything on your plate – so you may end up eating smaller portions or no longer want a dessert after your main meal.

Our perspectives on the roles of the macronutrients (carbohydrate, fat, and protein) in appetite and energy intake have changed over the past few decades. Their digestion products and/or circulating metabolites have been viewed as

1. signals to stimulate and initiate eating, thus determining eating frequency;

2. signals to stop eating thereby controlling meal size; and

3. signals that activate brain reward systems that may, to some degree, dysregulate healthy eating.

In the past few decades, various diets have been proposed, accentuating or minimizing each macronutrient to achieve a desired effect on appetite and/or energy intake; however, none has been widely successful. This is likely due to their failure to adequately address effects on eating frequency and meal size concurrently, as well as the fact that eating behavior is strongly influenced by many cognitive and environmental factors in addition to sensory appeal, appetite and the various metabolic, hormonal, and nervous signals arising from food intake, digestion, and subsequent metabolism. There may be health or sport performance reasons to emphasize one macronutrient over another in a diet, but from the perspective of energy balance, total energy intake, rather than its source, is the most important factor to address. An important take home message is that meals high in good quality protein and bulky but with low energy density (achieved by having a high water and/or fiber content and low in fat, starch and sugars) are more likely to satisfy our appetite without promoting weight gain. If you are aiming to lose body fat, then take note of your gut feelings while you are eating meals. That means stop eating when you feel full (or better still when you feel 80% full) rather than routinely eating everything that is on your plate, even at the risk of offending the cook!

So What Makes Us Feel Full Without Consuming Excess Calories?

There are several things you can do to make you feel fuller and more satisfied when eating a meal without eating more calories. These are useful things to know when you are dieting. The strategies listed below will help to abate your hunger when dieting to lose weight, making it more likely you will stick to your diet for longer.

Drinking water before eating: Drinking a glass or two of water or low-calorie beverage before eating a meal is a good idea, as it makes the stomach feel fuller quicker.

Foods and beverages that increase the volume in the stomach but with low energy density: Eating foods with a high water and/or fiber content but low-fat and sugar content (e.g., beansprouts, tomato, melon, salad leaves, celery, zucchini (courgette), green beans, broccoli, asparagus, pickled vegetables) also add to the bulk volume of a meal which is one of the things that signals satiety.

Eating meals with high-protein content: Because protein has a much stronger effect on satiety than fat and carbohydrate do, meals with high-protein content (e.g., from meat, fish, and beans) are satisfying even when relatively low in calories.

Eating the high-protein and lower energy food items on your plate first: Because you may start to feel full before you start consuming the higher energy food items containing carbohydrate and/or fat.

Eating your food slowly: Because this will allow more time for nutrients to be digested and absorbed and the satiety signals to kick in, meaning that you may eat smaller portions or no longer want a dessert after your main meal.

Sprinkling dried mixed herbs and a little salt over your food: Because this adds to the flavor and satisfies your desire for salted tasty foods without adding much salt at all. Two or three shakes of the salt cellar over your food will only add about 0.2 g salt.

THE PROBLEM OF FOOD ADDICTION

Everyone knows that it is possible to become addicted to drugs, and that the dangers to health of high intakes are very real and in some cases potentially fatal. Addictive drugs include not only illegal substances such as heroin, cocaine, and amphetamines but also the legal and socially accepted drugs nicotine (in tobacco products and e-cigarettes), alcohol (in beer, wine, and spirits) and caffeine (in coffee, chocolate, and energy drinks). But is it possible to become addicted to some food items that do not contain any drugs? Many scientists are becoming increasingly convinced that the answer is yes. The evidence comes from brain imaging and other studies of the effects of compulsive overeating on pleasure centers in the brain. Experiments in animals and humans show that, for some people, the same reward and pleasure centers of the brain that are stimulated by addictive drugs like cocaine and heroin are also activated by food, especially highly palatable foods that are rich in sugar, fat, and salt.

Like addictive drugs, very tasty and enjoyable foods trigger feel-good brain chemicals such as **dopamine**. Once people experience pleasure associated with increased dopamine transmission in the brain's reward pathway from eating a particular type of food or a specific food item, the desire to eat another quickly arises again. As mentioned earlier in this chapter, reward signals from highly palatable foods may override other signals of fullness and satisfaction as well as overriding our common sense because, in truth, we really know that we should not be eating more. As a result, people keep on eating, simply for the pleasure it gives, even when they're not hungry. Taken to the extreme, this effect is called compulsive overeating. It is a type of behavioral addiction meaning that someone can become preoccupied with a behavior (such as eating, or gambling, or shopping) that triggers intense pleasure and becomes a pressing need to have on a regular basis. Psychological dependence has also been observed with this condition such that withdrawal symptoms occur when consumption of these favorite foods stops or is replaced by foods low in sugar and fat. People with food addictions have essentially lost control over their eating behavior and find themselves spending excessive amounts of time involved with food and overeating or anticipating the emotional rewards of compulsive overeating. Just like with most addictive drugs, people who show signs of food addiction may also develop a kind of tolerance (to food). They eat more and more, only to find that food satisfies them less and less, and their response is to eat even more! Overeating results in a daily positive energy balance (in some recorded cases daily energy intakes have exceeded 5,000 calories) that can soon make a person become obese with all the associated health problems that come with excess adiposity.

Many compulsive overeaters engage in frequent episodes of uncontrolled eating that could be called binge eating. The term binge eating means eating an excessive and unhealthy amount of food while feeling that one's sense of control has been lost. People who engage in binge eating may feel frenzied and consume a large number of calories before stopping. Food binges are often followed by feelings of guilt and depression, but unlike the condition known as **bulimia nervosa**, binge eating episodes are not compensated for by so-called "purging behavior" to lose the extra calories such as vomiting, using laxatives, fasting for a prolonged period, or doing lots of exercise. When compulsive overeaters overeat through binge eating and experience feelings of guilt after their binges, they can be said to have **binge eating disorder**. In addition to binge eating, compulsive overeaters may also engage in "grazing" behavior, during which they continuously eat snacks (e.g., chips, cookies, cake, chocolate, and candy) throughout the day in addition to their regular meals. These actions result in an excessive overall number of calories consumed, even if the quantities eaten at any one time may not be particularly large.

It is thought that up to 20% of people may suffer from food addiction or addictive-like eating behavior, and this number is even higher among people with obesity (no doubt because it has already contributed to their excess fat accumulation). The take home message is that food addiction involves being addicted to food in the same way as drug addicts are addicted to drugs. It is really not that different from the alcoholic who is addicted to alcohol or the smoker who is addicted to nicotine. People who have food addiction have effectively lost the ability to control their intake of certain foods. This does not apply to all foods because people don't just get addicted to any food. The addiction is usually for one or more specific food items or particular food types. As explained in the sidebar that follows, some foods are much more likely to cause symptoms of addiction than others.

What Are the Most Addictive Food Items?

Researchers from the University of Michigan studied addictive-like eating in 518 participants. They used the Yale Food Addiction Scale as a tool to assess food addiction. All participants got a list of 35 foods, which included both processed and unprocessed food items. They rated how likely they were to experience problems with each of the 35 foods, on a scale from 1 (not at all addictive) to 7 (extremely addictive). In this study, about 10% of participants were diagnosed with full-blown food addiction but shockingly, nine out of ten participants had addictive-like eating behavior towards some foods. Although they repeatedly had the desire to quit eating them, they felt they were unable to. Here is a list of the top 12 foods that were found to be the most addictive (the number following each food is the average score given in the study):

- Pizza (4.0)
- Chocolate (3.7)
- Chips (known as crisps in the UK and EU) (3.7)
- Cookies (known as biscuits in the UK and EU) (3.7)
- Ice cream (3.7)
- French fries (3.6)
- Cheeseburger (3.5)
- Sugary soft drinks (3.3)
- Cake (3.3)
- Cheese (3.2)
- Bacon (3.0)
- Fried chicken (3.0)

Scientists at Yale University's Rudd Center for Food Science and Policy have developed a questionnaire to identify people with food addictions. Some of the questions used are listed below and you can answer these to determine if you have a food addiction. Simply answer yes or no.

Do you:

- End up eating more than planned when you start eating certain foods?

- Keep eating certain foods even if you're no longer hungry?

- Eat to the point of feeling ill?

- Worry about not eating certain types of foods or worry about cutting down on certain types of foods?

- Go out of your way to obtain certain foods when they aren't available when you want them?

- Eat certain foods so often or in such large amounts that you start eating food instead of working, spending time with the family, or doing recreational activities?

- Avoid professional or social situations where certain foods are available because of a fear of overeating?

- Have problems functioning effectively at your job or college because of food and eating?

- Have problems such as depression, anxiety, self-loathing, or guilt after eating food?

- Need to eat more and more food to reduce negative emotions or increase pleasure?

- Not gain the same amount of pleasure by eating food in the way you used to?

- Have symptoms such as anxiety or agitation when you cut down on certain foods (excluding caffeinated and alcoholic beverages)?

If you answered yes to five or more of the above questions, you are likely to have a food addiction. A copy of the full 25-item questionnaire can be found at **https://www.midss.org/sites/default/files/yale_food_addiction_scale.pdf**, and the instructions how to score it are available at **https://www.midss.org/sites/default/files/yfas_instruction_sheet.pdf**

If you think you are addicted to a certain type of food or even only one specific food item, the only real way to end the addiction is to cut out the food item from your diet completely for at least three weeks and then reintroduce it sparingly, as a treat, perhaps only once or twice per week and stick to a reasonable amount that you have decided upon in advance. Of course, recovery from a food addiction may be more complicated than recovery from other kinds of addictions. Alcoholics, for example, can ultimately abstain from drinking alcohol altogether, but people who are addicted to food still need to eat. In extreme cases of addiction to multiple foods or compulsive overeating, a nutritionist, psychologist, or doctor who is educated about food addiction may be able to help you break the cycle of compulsive overeating.

Key Points

- Appetite is sensed in the brain, which constantly receives and processes nervous, metabolic, and hormonal signals from the periphery. In addition, a large number of external factors influence eventual food intake.

- Feeding behavior is controlled in the hypothalamus of the brain which is influenced by various gut peptide hormones whose secretion is determined by the presence or absence of food digestion products in the gastrointestinal tract.

- Ghrelin is produced when the stomach is empty and is the only gut peptide hormone that stimulates appetite and promotes food intake.

- All the other known gut peptide hormones (e.g., CCK, neuropeptide Y, peptide YY) are secreted when food is ingested, digested, and absorbed following a meal. Their actions are to suppress appetite and promote satiety.

- The term satiation describes the processes that bring a meal to an end. An interval of time then elapses before eating begins again. Satiety refers to the inhibition of eating following a meal, and it is measured both by the length of the interval between meals and by the amount of food consumed when it is next offered.

- Different macronutrients have different effects on satiety with protein having a much stronger effect on satiety than fat and carbohydrate do.

- Calories from different food sources can have markedly different effects on hunger, hormones, energy expenditure, and the brain regions that control food intake. Meals that are high in good quality protein and bulky but with low energy density are more likely to satisfy our appetite without promoting weight gain.

- Some people can become addicted to eating certain foods that are usually energy dense and rich in fat, sugar, or salt. This food addiction can lead to compulsive overeating which can be a major contributor to the development of obesity.

Chapter 7

How to Lose Weight by Dieting

Objectives

After studying this chapter, you should:

- Be aware of the possible risks and pitfalls of dieting

- Understand how to tell whether you are overweight

- Understand how to tell whether you are overfat

- Know some reasons why calories from different foods are not the same when it comes to their influence on body weight

- Know how your body's metabolism adapts to restriction of food intake

- Know at least five different diets that have proven to be effective in achieving moderate weight loss

- Understand how a diet with a low energy density can be achieved

Weight loss is desirable for the health reasons explained in chapter 4 but only for people who are overweight because of an excess of body fat. In other circumstances, weight loss is not always a good idea, and if not done correctly (e.g., eating insufficient protein or cutting out major macronutrients or food groups from your diet) can often be accompanied by a reduction in muscle mass, and it may reduce liver and muscle glycogen stores as well, which will make doing any exercise feel harder and make you feel more tired. Excessive weight loss has also been associated with chronic fatigue, irritability, and increased risk of injuries. Too much emphasis on losing weight can lead to the development of micronutrient deficiencies and **eating disorders** such as **anorexia nervosa** and bulimia nervosa, which are harmful to health. The elderly and illness-prone individuals may actually benefit from being slightly overweight rather than underweight in order to have an energy reserve when they become ill and are unable to eat properly. These are good reasons to avoid extreme dieting.

For those who are determined to lose some weight, the first step in determining a healthy body weight goal is weighing in a normally hydrated state and measuring body composition. These measures can be used to determine how much body fat individuals should lose to put them within an optimal range for health. An energy deficit of 500 to 1,000 kcal below estimated daily energy needs is generally recommended for weight loss. However, individuals with lower energy needs (women, elderly adults, and children) should minimize their total energy deficit to ensure they are getting enough nutrients for good health, growth, development, and reproductive functioning. As with any weight loss plan, always seek medical advice before you start if you:

- Have a history of eating disorders.

- Are taking prescribed medication.

- Are pregnant or breastfeeding (unless you have been advised to lose weight for health reasons by your physician).

- Have a significant medical or mental health condition.

Don't go on a diet if you are under 18 (unless it is done under medical supervision), if you are very lean or underweight (BMI below 21 kg/m^2), or are recovering from illness or surgery or are generally frail.

NORMAL LEVELS OF BODY FAT

Body fat consists of essential body fat and storage fat. Essential body fat is present in all cell membranes, nerve tissues, bone marrow, and organs, and we cannot lose this fat without compromising physiological function. Storage fat, on the other hand, represents an energy reserve that accumulates when excess energy is ingested and decreases when more energy is expended than consumed. Essential body fat is approximately 3% of body mass for men and 12% of body mass for women. Women are believed to have more essential body fat than men do because of childbearing and hormonal functions. In general, the total healthy body-fat percentage (essential plus storage fat) is between 12% and 20% for young men and between 25% and 30% for young women (see table 7.1). As approximately 3% of body mass of males and 12% of body mass of females is essential body fat, no diet should ever aim to get rid of all fat from the body. For those aged over 40, the acceptable body fat percentages are a bit higher (table 7.2) because as we get older we tend to lose some lean muscle mass and – particularly in postmenopausal women – some bone mass.

Table 7.1: Body-fat percentages for men and women aged 18-40 and their classification

Men	Women	Classification
5-10%	8-15%	Athletic
11-14%	16-23%	Good
15-20%	24-30%	Acceptable
21-24%	31-36%	Overweight
Over 24%	Over 36%	Obese

Note that these are rough estimates. The term athletic in this context refers to sports in which low body fat is an advantage.

Table 7.2: Body-fat percentages for men and women aged 41-70 and their classification

Men	Women	Classification
8-13%	12-20%	Athletic
14-18%	20-27%	Good
19-22%	28-34%	Acceptable
23-28%	35-39%	Overweight
Over 28%	Over 40%	Obese

Note that these are rough estimates. The "athletic" values are those found in very fit people who participate regularly in sports or other strenuous physical activities.

HOW CAN I TELL WHETHER I AM OVERWEIGHT OR OVERFAT?

In order to determine whether you are overweight or overfat, a variety of measurements can be made, but bear in mind they all have some limitations. Body composition can be measured reasonably accurately by some methods but only by those that will normally found in a science lab or hospital (e.g., Dual Energy X-Ray Absorptiometry, Computed Tomography, Magnetic Resonance Imaging, Air Displacement Plethysmography) or which require expertise (e.g., using skinfold calipers, underwater weighing). Here I will only describe some methods that the general public could do for themselves. These can provide a rough estimate rather than a very accurate measure of body composition.

HEIGHT–WEIGHT RELATIONSHIP

Height–weight tables, such as the one shown in figure 7.1, provide a normal range of body weights for any given height. Such figures and tables have limitations, especially when applied to people who have a large muscle mass. For instance, a muscular man who is 180 cm tall and weighs 100 kg may have low body fat but could be classified as overweight, but in his case the "extra" weight is muscle, not body fat, which would lead to erroneous classification and possibly mistaken advice.

BODY MASS INDEX

A rough but better measure than the height–weight tables is the body mass index (BMI), also known as Quetelet index. Also derived from body mass and height, BMI in units of kg/m^2 is calculated by dividing the body mass in kg by the height in meters and then dividing again by the height in meters:

BMI = (body mass in kilograms/height in meters)/height in meters

A person who is 1.75 m (5 ft 9 in) tall and weighs 75.0 kg (165 lbs.) has a BMI of $(75.0)/(1.75)^2 = 75.0/3.06 = 24.5$ kg/m^2 (figure 7.2). The normal range is between 18.5 kg/m^2 and 25.0 kg/m^2. People with a BMI of 25-29 kg/m^2 are classified as overweight, people with a BMI of 30 kg/m^2 or higher are classified as obese, and people with a BMI of 40 kg/m^2 or higher are classified as morbidly obese. People with a BMI below 18.5 kg/m^2 are classified as underweight.

Even when using BMI rather than just body weight, our muscular man weighing 100 kg and 1.80 m tall would be classified as overweight or even obese because the equation does not take into account body composition (his BMI = $(100/1.80)/1.80 = 30.9$ kg/m^2). It is quite possible that two individuals could have the same BMI but completely different body compositions. One could achieve his or her body weight with mainly muscle mass as a result of hard training, whereas the other could achieve his or her body weight by fat deposition as a result of a sedentary lifestyle or overeating. Without information about body composition, they both might be classified as obese. In children and older people, the BMI is difficult to interpret because muscle and bone weights change in relationship to height.

The BMI, however, does provide useful information about risks for various diseases and is used in many epidemiological and clinical studies. For example, BMI correlates with the incidence of cardiovascular complications (hypertension and stroke), certain cancers, type 2 diabetes, kidney disease, and dementia. The BMI, however, is best used for populations rather than individuals. When used for individual assessment, BMI needs to be used in coordination with other measurements such as waist circumference or body composition because it is possible to be within normal weight or BMI yet have unhealthily high levels of visceral fat.

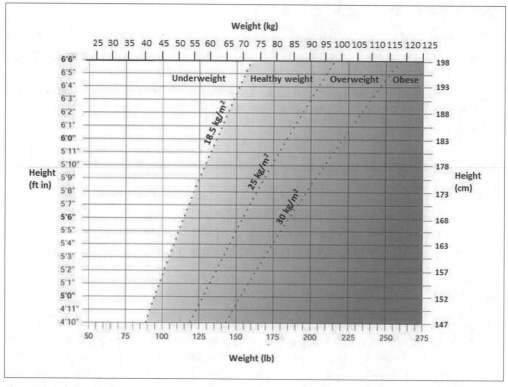

Figure 7.1: Relationship between height, weight, and body mass index (BMI), and criteria for underweight, normal (healthy), overweight, and obesity. BMI measures weight in relation to height (kg/m2). The BMI ranges shown are for adults and should not be applied to children. They are not exact ranges of healthy and unhealthy weights, but health risk increases at higher levels of overweight and obesity. Even within the healthy BMI range, weight gains can carry health risks for adults. Directions: Find your weight (unclothed) on the bottom (lbs.) or top (kg) scale of the graph. Go straight up or down from that point until you come to the line that matches your height (without shoes). Then look to find your weight group. Adapted from Dietary Guidelines for Americans (2000), https://www.health.gov/dietaryguidelines/dga2000/document/frontcover.htm.

WAIST CIRCUMFERENCE AND WAIST-TO-HIP RATIO

The waist-to-hip ratio (WHR) measurement gives an index of body-fat distribution (figure 7.2). Because it gives an indication of the body fat distributed around the torso, it can be used to help determine the degree of obesity. Excess fat around the waist is associated with increased risk of chronic disease. The distribution of fat is evaluated by dividing waist size by hip size. A person with a 34-inch (86.5 cm) waist and 42-inch (106.7 cm) hips would have a ratio of 0.81 (figure 7.2); one with a 40-inch (101.6 cm) waist and 41-inch (104.2 cm) hips would have a ratio of 0.98. The higher the ratio, the higher the risk of heart disease and other obesity-related **morbidity**. The WHR reflects increased visceral fat better than BMI. Females with a WHR greater than 0.80 and males with a WHR greater than 0.91 have a higher risk of developing cardiovascular disease, diabetes, hypertension, and certain cancers. A WHR smaller than 0.73 for women and 0.85 for men indicates a low risk of developing chronic disease. WHR is also a better predictor of mortality in older people than waist circumference or BMI although some studies have found waist circumference alone to be a good indicator of cardiovascular risk factors, body fat distribution and hypertension in type 2 diabetes.

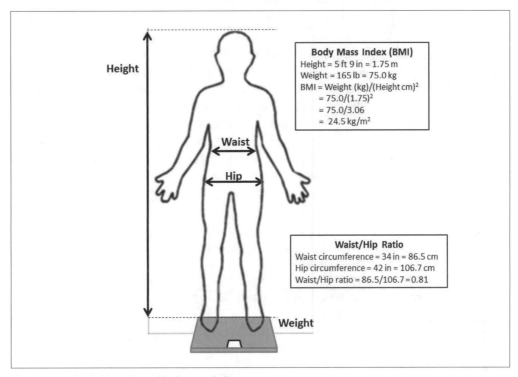

Figure 7.2: Waist-to-hip ratio and body mass index measurement

BIOELECTRICAL IMPEDANCE ANALYSIS

In scientific studies, body fat percentage is usually estimated using dual energy X-ray absorptiometry (DEXA), air displacement plethysmography (commonly known as Bodpod), or is derived from skin fold caliper measurements made by a skilled technician at three or more body sites. However, the simplest way to measure body fat for most people who do not have access to a science lab is to use an electronic scale that incorporates a bioelectrical impedance device. **Bioelectrical impedance analysis** (BIA) is based on the principle that different tissues and substances have different impedance (resistance) to an electrical current. For example, impedance or conductivity is quite different for fat tissue and water. Adipose tissue —of which only 5% is water—has high resistance, or impedance, whereas muscle—of which up to 77% is water—has low resistance. A BIA device sends a small, safe electrical current through the body to measure impedance and so can be used to estimate percentage body fat.

WAYS OF LOSING BODY FAT AND WEIGHT

The various ways to lose body fat and weight include pharmacological and surgical procedures (see the sidebar), but here the focus is on the weight loss strategies that involve altering the diet. Numerous different diets designed to promote weight loss exist, some of which have been commercialized. Some diets have proved to be effective, whereas others (probably the majority) are not and may be based on a list of erroneous assumptions and unjustified claims. For the individual wanting to lose some weight while remaining healthy, distinguishing between the facts and the fallacies is often difficult. Weight loss with dieting is mostly dependent on the size of the weekly energy deficit; that is, by how many calories you have reduced your energy intake, compared to when you are weight stable and in energy balance. Research indicates that an energy deficit of 3,500 kcal (14.7 MJ) – which could be achieved by a daily energy deficit of 500 kcal/day (2.1 MJ/day) for seven days – will normally result in a loss of 1 lb. (0.46 kg) of body fat and a similar or slightly greater reduction in body weight. This chapter reviews some of the most common dietary regimens and weight loss methods. The use of different types of exercise to lose weight by increasing energy expenditure is dealt with in the next chapter. Further general tips on dieting and a personalized combination weight loss plan incorporating multiple diets and your preferred choice of exercise can be found in chapter 13.

Methods That Can Be Used to Achieve Weight Loss

Dietary methods:

- Energy restriction (moderate or severe)
- Fasting
- Very low energy diet
- Intermittent fasting diet (e.g., the 5:2 Fast diet)
- Low-fat diet
- Food-combining diet
- Low Glycemic Index (GI) diet
- High-protein diet
- Zone diet
- Paleo diet
- Low-carbohydrate ketogenic diet (e.g., Atkins diet, Sugarbusters)
- Low-energy density diet
- Calcium and dairy product diet
- Mediterranean and Japanese diets (described in chapter 4)

Exercise:

- Increased physical activity of any kind

- Regular exercise (e.g., daily walking)

- Endurance exercise (e.g., jogging, cycling, swimming for 30 minutes or more)

- High intensity interval exercise (repeated sprints with short recovery periods)

- Resistance exercise (e.g., weight lifting)

- Participation in sport

Pharmacological methods:

- Drugs that stimulate metabolism or fat burning

- Drugs that suppress appetite

- Drugs that promote satiety

- Drugs that make the stomach feel fuller

- Drugs that reduce fat absorption

Surgical procedures:

- Stomach (gastric) band – a band is placed around the stomach, so you don't need to eat as much to feel full

- Stomach (gastric) bypass – the top part of the stomach is joined to the small intestine, so you feel fuller sooner and don't absorb as many calories from food

- Sleeve gastrectomy – some of the stomach is removed, so you can't eat as much as you could before, and you'll feel full sooner

- Intra-gastric balloon – A soft balloon filled with air or salt water that's placed into your stomach so that you won't need or be able to eat as much before you feel full

- Removal of a section of the small intestine so that you are unable to digest and absorb food as effectively

- Liposuction – Sucking out small areas of fat that from areas of the body where deposits of fat tend to collect, such as the abdomen, buttocks, hips, and thighs

ABOUT FOOD CALORIES AND THE EFFECTS OF ENERGY RESTRICTION

First, it is important to appreciate that some food calories are not the same as others. Different food sources are metabolized differently in the body, and the energy cost of this metabolism is higher for some than others. In addition, ingested calories from different food sources can have very different effects on satiety, hormones, and the brain regions that control food intake. In this sense, not all calories from food are equal (see the sidebar that follows for further details).

In response to reduced energy intake, metabolic adaptation or adaptive thermogenesis occurs which results in a decrease in resting metabolic rate (RMR), makes weight loss even harder. Additionally, any lean body (muscle) mass that is lost over time will lower resting energy expenditure further and make exercise more efficient (so a little less energy will be expended during weight-bearing activities such as walking and running), which again makes losing weight harder to achieve. The adaptations explain why it is harder to lose more weight the longer you're on a diet and why people regain weight after stopping a diet (known as weight cycling or the yo-yo effect). However, it remains controversial as to whether the magnitude of the reduced resting energy expenditure is actually greater than predicted by changes in the thermic effect of food (see chapter 5 for details) and body composition so that it exceeds the original calorie deficit prescribed for weight loss.

In a study, three groups of moderately overweight people were subjected to energy restriction for six months. One group was energy restricted by reducing food intake by 25%, one group was subjected to energy restriction (12.5%) and an increase in physical activity by structured exercise (12.5%), and the third group served as the control group with unchanged food intake. Weight loss was similar in the two energy-restricted groups (both lost 10% of their initial body weight). RMR decreased beyond values expected from changes in weight and body composition as a result of the energy deficit that was achieved through a food-based diet after three months and a food-based diet plus structured exercise after six months. The control group did not experience a decrease in RMR. At month six, the combined data from the dieting groups demonstrated that RMR was lower than expected, resulting in 91 kcal less energy expenditure per day compared with control participants, even after differences in **lean body mass** were taken into consideration. This decrease in resting metabolism is an **autoregulatory feedback** mechanism by which the body tries to preserve energy. This **"food efficiency"** may occur independently of a person's body mass or dieting history. It usually causes a reduction or even a plateau in weight loss and is a common source of frustration for dieters.

Essentially, this means that during periods of prolonged (more than a few weeks) dietary energy restriction, the previously mentioned equivalency of a loss of 1 lb. (0.46 kg) of body fat from an accumulated 3,500 kcal (14.7 MJ) dietary energy deficit no longer holds, because of the interrelationships between energy intake, energy expenditure, and body weight as outlined above. In this situation, it may take an energy deficit of over 4,200 kcal (17.3 MJ) to lose 1 lb. (0.46 kg) of body fat.

Why All Calories Aren't the Same

While it is true that in absolute terms all calories have the same amount of energy, when it comes to your body, things are not that simple. Of course, no matter what the food source, one dietary Calorie (kilocalorie) contains 4,184 joules of energy and represents the amount of energy needed to raise the temperature of one liter of water by one degree Celsius. In that respect, a calorie IS a calorie. But in the body, different foods go through different biochemical pathways, starting with digestion and absorption followed by metabolism, and including the biosynthesis of macromolecules (e.g., glycogen from glucose, protein from amino acids, triglycerides from fatty acids), all of which have different energy costs. Some of these metabolic pathways are more inefficient than others and cause more of the energy from the food that was ingested to be lost as heat. This means that the energy available is somewhat less than the original gross chemical energy of the foodstuff as determined in a bomb calorimeter.

Furthermore, different macronutrients and food items have varying effects on the hormones and brain centers that control our hunger and eating behavior. Indeed, the foods that we eat can have a big impact on the physiological and psychological processes that have a controlling influence on when, what, and how much we eat. The following are six evidence-based examples of why a calorie is not simply a calorie:

- *The metabolic pathways for protein are less efficient than the metabolic pathways for carbohydrates and fat.* Protein contains 5.3 kcal/g, but some of this is not available, as the nitrogen component cannot be oxidized and gets excreted from the body as urea. That reduces the energy available to 4 kcal/g. In addition, a significant portion of protein calories are lost as heat when they are metabolized by the body. The thermic effect of food (see chapter 5) is a measure of how much a particular macronutrient or food item increases the resting metabolic rate (i.e., the resting energy expenditure) following its ingestion. The thermic effect of fat is 1-3%, for carbohydrates it is 5-10%, but for protein it is considerably higher at 20-30%, so clearly protein requires much more energy to metabolize than fat and carbohydrate. What this means is that 100 kcal of dietary protein would end up as 70-80 kcal of stored energy, while a 100 kcal of fat would end up as 97-99 kcal of stored energy. Therefore, calories from protein are considerably less fattening than calories from carbohydrates and fat, because protein takes more energy to metabolize. Whole foods also require more energy to digest than processed foods.

- *Protein reduces appetite more effectively and so makes you eat fewer calories.* Protein is known to be the most fulfilling macronutrient by far. If people increase their dietary protein intake as a percentage of their total daily energy intake (in other words they substitute some fat and carbohydrate for extra protein), they can start losing weight without counting calories.

- *Different simple sugars are metabolized differently and have different effects on appetite.* The two main simple sugars in the diet are glucose and fructose, and although they have the same chemical formula ($C_6H_{12}O_6$), glucose can be metabolized by all of the body's tissues, but fructose can only be metabolized by the liver in any significant amount. Following feeding, fructose does not reduce levels of the appetite-stimulating hormone ghrelin (see chapter 6) as much as glucose, meaning that we will tend to want to eat more calories with fructose. Furthermore, fructose does not stimulate the satiety centers in the brain as strongly as glucose, which makes us want to eat for longer until we feel full.

- *Studies show that refined carbohydrates lead to faster and bigger spikes in blood sugar, which leads to cravings and increased food intake.* Refined carbohydrates tend to be very low in fiber, and they get digested and absorbed quickly. This results in more rapid and larger spikes in the blood glucose concentration, meaning that they have a high glycemic index (GI), which is a measure of how quickly foods raise blood sugar. However, within one to two hours of eating a food that causes a rapid spike in blood sugar, the blood sugar levels fall below normal (known as the insulin rebound effect). When blood sugar levels drop, it stimulates the appetite center in the brain, and we get cravings for another high-carbohydrate snack. Indeed, studies show that people eat up to 80% more calories when given ad libitum access to a high GI meal compared to a low GI meal.

- *Different foods have different effects on satiety.* Because some foods affect satiety more than others, it affects how many calories we end up consuming in subsequent meals. This is measured on a scale called the Satiety Index. The satiety index is a measure of the ability of foods to reduce hunger, increase feelings of fullness, and reduce energy intake in the hours following a meal. If you eat foods that are low on the satiety index, then you are going to be hungrier and want to eat more to reach the same level of satisfaction that you would get from eating foods higher on the satiety index. Conversely, if you choose foods that are high on the satiety index, you will probably end up eating less and increase your chances of losing weight. Some examples of foods with a high satiety index are meat, eggs, boiled potatoes, beans, and fruits, while foods that are low on the satiety index include doughnuts, cookies, and cake.

- *Low-carbohydrate diets lead to reduced dietary energy intake.* Studies that have compared weight loss on low-carbohydrate versus low-fat diets consistently show that more weight is lost (often two to three times as much) on the low-carbohydrate diets. One of the main reasons for this is that low-carbohydrate diets markedly reduce appetite, and so energy intake tends to be less than on a low-fat diet. Also, low-carbohydrate diets cause significant water loss in the first week or two and low-carbohydrate diets tend to include more protein (with its higher thermic effect) than low-fat diets.

The take home message is that calories from different food sources can have markedly different effects on hunger, hormones, energy expenditure, and the brain regions that control food intake. Even though calories are important, in many cases, altering food selection to change the macronutrient composition can lead to the same (or slightly better) results for weight loss than just limited calorie restriction on a mixed diet. However, there is no escaping the fact that significant weight loss (i.e., more than a few kilograms) can only be achieved by more substantial reductions in energy intake and improved further with increased energy expenditure with exercise.

FAD DIETS AND WHY YOU SHOULD AVOID THEM

Every year there seems to be at least one new diet that gets promoted by the media and endorsed by some television, film, music, or fashion celebrities. These are mostly what can be called fad diets and only seem to reign in popularity for a few months until the next new fad diet comes along. I will not bore you with a long list of those that have come and gone over the years. Many such diets are based on pseudoscience, myths, and ignorance but often receive much media attention. The simple fact is that many of these diets are complicated, not based on scientific evidence, and when tested in an appropriate controlled manner, do not lead to sustained long-term weight loss. Quite frankly, most of them do not actually do what they claim to do. There are several good reasons to avoid fad diets including:

- Some diets, especially those that require crash dieting, can make you feel tired and lethargic, and some can actually make you ill.

- Diets that require you to cut out certain foods altogether (e.g., meat, fish, cereal, or dairy products) could prevent you from getting enough of the essential vitamins, minerals, and other essential nutrients that your body needs to function properly.

- Some diets may be low in sugar and other carbohydrates, but instead they are high in fat which can cause its own problems such as bad breath, tiredness, headaches, and constipation.

- Some diets claim to "detoxify" your body and that a build-up of toxins can be removed by eating certain foods and avoiding others. This is complete nonsense. They only work because your calorie intake is reduced as a result of the restrictions the diet plan places on what you can actually eat. Toxins do not normally build up in the body. Any potentially toxic substances like ammonia and urea are excreted in the urine well before they can accumulate to high enough levels to cause problems.

- The problem with many fad diets is that they are extreme in one form or another, and while weight loss might be achieved in the short term, they are very difficult to stick to for more than a few weeks. Furthermore, diets that are unbalanced are more likely to be bad for your health, even if you do manage to stick with them!

COMMON DIETS

Some diets have been designed specifically for weight loss while others have been designed with some other useful purpose in mind such as to lower and stabilize blood sugar, lower blood pressure, treat irritable bowel syndrome, etc. although they may also help to facilitate some weight loss. In this chapter I will focus on the diets that are intended to make you lose body fat and body weight. A number of these diets have stood the test of time and are still popular because people have found that they work, and science has proved that they have some degree of success in achieving weight and/or fat loss. Some, however, are better than others either in terms of their effectiveness for weight and/or fat loss or by virtue of not having side effects or unwanted health problems associated with their use. The ones that have proven to have some degree of success are described in the pages that follow, together with my comments on their efficacy.

FASTING

Fasting literally means going without any food and only drinking water. Although this is the most effective form of dieting in the short-term, there are significant dangers to health if it is maintained for more than even a few days due to the deficiencies of protein and micronutrients. There will also be a significant loss of lean tissue (muscle) as well as fat, and you will constantly be feeling hungry, tired and irritable, so forget it.

VERY LOW-ENERGY DIETS

Very low-energy diets (VLEDs) or very low-calorie diets (VLCDs) are used as therapy to achieve rapid weight loss in obese people. These diets are usually in the form of liquid meals that contain the recommended daily intakes of micronutrients but only 400 to 800 kcal/day (1.6 to 3.2 MJ/day). These liquid meals contain a relatively large amount of protein to reduce muscle wasting and a relatively small amount of carbohydrate (less than 100 g/day). Such diets are extremely effective in reducing body weight rapidly. In the first week, the weight loss is predominantly glycogen and water. Fat and protein are lost as well during the initial phase, but those losses are a relatively small proportion of the total weight loss. After the initial rapid weight loss, the weight reduction is mainly from adipose tissue, although some loss of body protein occurs. The restricted carbohydrate availability and increased fat oxidation results in ketosis (formation of ketone bodies, mostly in the form of acetoacetate and β-hydroxybutyrate). Ketone bodies have a specific odor that is easily detectable on the breath and does not smell nice! After ketosis begins, hunger feelings may decrease somewhat as the ketone bodies can be used as a fuel by the brain compensating for the reduced availability of blood glucose.

Because carbohydrate intake is low, blood glucose concentration is prevented from falling too low by synthesizing glucose from various non-carbohydrate precursors (glycerol from fat and amino acids from protein). Because of the associated chronic glycogen depletion, exercise capacity is severely impaired. For this reason, such diets are not advised for athletes, who would likely be unable to complete their normal training sessions and because the loss of body protein can be significant. Side effects of such diets include nausea, halitosis (bad breath), hunger (which may decrease after the initiation of ketosis), light-headedness, and low blood pressure. Dehydration is also common with such diets and electrolyte imbalances may occur. Although effective and have been shown to reverse type 2 diabetes if maintained for long enough (see following sidebar), such diets are hard to stick to unless you are highly motivated and determined to lose weight quickly (i.e., within weeks rather than months).

Reversal of Type 2 Diabetes With a VLED

Importantly, for people diagnosed with type 2 diabetes, a recent study in the UK has shown that losing weight and body fat by sticking with a VLED can reverse the condition. Until relatively recently, the medical profession generally described type 2 diabetes as progressive and incurable with a need for more and more medication over time to keep symptoms under control. But the medication doesn't actually prevent a doubling of the risk of having a heart attack, a stroke, or developing dementia compared with someone of the same age who is not diabetic. However, a new study has demonstrated that type 2 diabetes can be reversed and essentially cured by going on a VLED for 20 weeks. In the UK study, about 300 people diagnosed with type 2 diabetes were put on a VLED or remained on conventional care and were followed with for up to one year. On average, those on the VLED lost 10 kg (22 lbs.), and 50% of them had put their diabetes into remission. Those getting conventional care lost 1 kg (2 lbs.) and only 6% went into remission.

INTERMITTENT FASTING DIETS

Intermittent fasting diets (IFD), of which there are several, have become popular in recent years, in part because of a lot of media coverage and backing from television and film celebrities. However, there is reasonable evidence that they can be effective, as all of them will reduce weekly energy intake to some degree. They may not be quite as beneficial for women as men and may also be a poor choice for people who are prone to eating disorders. It is also important to bear in mind that you should aim to eat healthily as well (see chapter 4) during the normal eating phase of the diets.

The alternate-day fasting diet means fasting every other day. This can be a complete fast, or some versions of this diet allow you to consume up to 500 kcal on the fasting days. A full fast every other day seems rather extreme and could lead to insufficient protein intake with negative consequences for muscle mass, so it is not recommended for athletes and other highly physically active people. The version where you eat normally on four days of the week and consume only about 500 kcal on alternate days is sometimes referred to as the 4:3 diet. A less extreme version of this IFD diet is the 5:2 diet (also commonly known as the "Fast Diet"), popularized by the British television medic Dr. Michael Mosley, which involves eating normally on five days of the week, while restricting intake to 500 kcal (for women) or 600 kcal (for men) on two days of the week (usually these are separated by two to three days such as fasting on Mondays and Thursdays). On the fasting days (note this is not strictly fasting, rather just eating much less than normal on two days of the week), you could eat two small meals (250 kcal per meal for women, and 300 kcal for men). These should be high-protein meals for better satiety (as mentioned in chapter 6) and to maintain muscle mass. A slightly less drastic version with a lower risk of consuming inadequate amounts of protein is to allow up to 800 kcal on the fasting days. Dr. Mosley has more recently promoted a modified version of the 5:2 diet in which he recommends a healthy Mediterranean diet (see chapter 4 for details) on the non-fasting days. This is a very sensible recommendation in my opinion, especially if it incorporates some high-protein and low energy density meals on the non-fasting days (see later in this chapter for the reasons why). Alternatively, for a change of foods and flavors, you could try adopting the Japanese diet on the non-fasting days.

Another IFD involves fasting from evening dinner one day to dinner the next (i.e., skipping both breakfast and lunch for a day), amounting to a 24-hour fast, and doing this on two days of the week. You should eat a normal meal at dinner on these days and not compensate for your hunger by eating more than usual; eating slowly and having a high-protein meal will again help with satiety. Another simple IFD is to skip one meal (usually lunch) during the day. The Warrior Diet was popularized by ex-army fitness expert Ori Hofmekler and involves eating small amounts of raw fruits and vegetables during the day, then eating one large meal in the evening. The diet also emphasizes food choices (whole, unprocessed foods) that are quite similar to a **Paleo diet** (described later in this chapter) in which you are encouraged to eat anything we could hunt or gather way back in the Paleolithic era (also known as the Stone Age), including foods like meats, fish, nuts, leafy greens, regional vegetables, and seeds but avoiding processed foods, ready meals, pasta, bread, cereal and candy. Another type of IFD is what is known as **time-restricted feeding**. This is a daily eating pattern in which all your food is eaten within an 8-12-hour timeframe every day, with no deliberate attempt to alter nutrient quality or quantity. This usually involves abstaining from breakfast, thus extending the duration of your normal overnight fast (the time when you are asleep and not eating), which gives your body more time to burn fat and do essential repairs. Outside of this time-restricted eating period, a person consumes no food items apart from drinking water or low-calorie beverages to stay well hydrated. Such beverages could also include black unsweetened coffee or green tea (without milk). Time-restricted eating is a type of intermittent fasting because it involves skipping breakfast or both breakfast and lunch. It is a pattern of eating that probably is similar to what our ancient ancestors adopted: most of the daytime would be spent hunting and gathering food, and most of the eating would take place after dark.

Although time-restricted eating will not work for everyone, some may find it beneficial. Some recent studies have shown that it can aid weight loss, improve sleep quality, and may lower the risk of metabolic diseases, such as type 2 diabetes. Modern humans, due to societal pressures, work schedules, and with the availability of night-time indoor illumination and entertainment, stay awake longer, which enables food consumption for longer durations of time. This extended duration itself, in addition to the caloric surplus, can be detrimental to health by reducing sleep time. A recent study using a smartphone app to monitor eating time has revealed more than 50% of adults spread their daily food and beverage intake over 15 hours or longer. Such extended eating of high fat or high or high glycemic index diets is known to predispose laboratory animals to metabolic diseases.

It is probably best to start a time-restricted eating plan gradually. Try starting with a shorter fasting period and then gradually increasing it over time. For example, start with a fasting period of 10:00 pm to 6:30 am. Then increase this by one hour every two days to reach the desired fasting period (usually around 8:00 pm to 1:00 pm the next day – leaving a time-restricted eating period of seven hours). Studies have suggested that restricting feeding periods to less than six hours is unlikely to offer additional advantages over more extended feeding periods.

The largest evidence base for the efficacy of IFDs derives from studies that have used some of the more extreme forms, such as alternate day fasting, which, according to several studies, can lead to significant body weight loss amounting to 3-8% over a period of 3-24 weeks. With alternate-day fasting the rate of weight loss averages about 0.7 kg/week (1.5 lbs./week); with other IFDs the rate of weight loss is less at about 0.25 kg/week (0.5 lbs./week). Studies comparing intermittent fasting and continuous calorie restriction show no difference in weight loss if calories are matched between groups.

LOW-FAT DIETS

Because fat is the most energy dense nutrient (each gram of fat contains 9 kcal compared with only 4 kcal for carbohydrate and protein) reducing the dietary fat intake can be a very effective way to reduce total daily energy intake and promote weight loss. Fat is also less satiating than either protein or carbohydrate, so we tend to eat more calories when consuming mostly fatty foods. Furthermore, fat is stored efficiently and requires little energy for digestion, and the thermic effect of food ingestion is lowest for fat compared with protein and carbohydrate, so consuming fat results in only a very small increase in energy expenditure and fat oxidation.

Reducing dietary fat is best achieved by eliminating foods with high-fat content from the diet. That means cutting out fatty meats, sauces, cheese, creams, pizza, cakes, and cookies and substituting some foods or beverages with lower fat alternatives (e.g., skimmed milk, low-fat yogurt, and reduced fat coleslaw). Scientific evidence from large scale population studies suggests that reducing the percentage of fat in the diet is more effective in reducing body weight than is reducing the absolute amount of fat. However, the most important factor is always the reduction in energy intake. An important advantage of reduced fat intake is that relatively high-carbohydrate content can be maintained, resulting in reasonable glycogen stores and better recovery from exercise for those who also want to include exercise as part of their weight loss program. Indeed, many athletes who want to lose some body fat also adopt a diet that is low in fat with a small reduction in energy intake, so that they can still replenish their carbohydrate stores to maintain their high training loads. This type of diet seems to be a sensible way of reducing weight, although weight reduction will occur relatively slowly. The magnitude of body weight and body fat losses on a low-fat diet will largely depend on by how much daily energy intake is reduced. See the section on low-carbohydrate diets for a comparison of the efficacy of these with low-fat diets for weight loss.

FOOD-COMBINING DIETS

Food-combining diets are based on a philosophy that certain foods should not be combined. Although many types of food-combining diets exist, most advise against combining protein and carbohydrate foods in a meal. It is often claimed that such combinations cause a "buildup of toxins" (which, quite frankly, is utter nonsense) with "negative side effects such as weight gain." These diets are often tempting to overweight people because they promise an easy way to rapid weight loss, and they are claimed to work for some people. However, when these diets are strictly followed, energy and fat intake are likely to be reduced compared with the normal diet, and it is this reduction in energy and fat that is the main reason for the success of the diet rather than the fact that certain foods were not combined. This is one dietary strategy I definitely do not recommend.

LOW GLYCEMIC INDEX DIETS

A low **glycemic index (GI)** diet is helpful for people who have type 2 diabetes or are at risk of developing it, as it can help to control body weight by minimizing spikes in blood sugar and insulin levels. Low GI diets have also been linked to reduced risks for cancer, heart disease, and other conditions. A low GI diet is an eating plan based on how the foods you eat (in particular the items that are your main sources of carbohydrate) affect your blood sugar level. The GI is a system of assigning a number to carbohydrate-containing foods according to how much each food increases your blood sugar. The GI values are based on experimental studies that have examined the impact of individual food items on the blood sugar level and how much it is increased over the two hours following a portion of the food item that contains 50 g carbohydrate compared with ingesting 50 g of pure glucose (which has the highest possible GI of 100). For example, boiled white potato has an average GI of 82 relative to glucose, which means that the blood glucose response to the carbohydrate in a potato containing 50 g carbohydrate (which will be in the form of starch) is 82% of the blood glucose response to the same amount of carbohydrate in pure glucose. In contrast, cooked brown rice has an average GI of 50 relative to glucose. The GI itself is not a diet plan but a useful tool to guide food choices. The GI principle was first developed as a strategy for guiding food choices for people with diabetes. An international GI database is maintained by Sydney University Glycemic Index Research Services in Sydney, Australia (available at https://www.researchdata.ands.org.au/international-glycemic-index-gi-database/11115). The database contains the results of studies conducted there and at other research facilities around the world and provides an extensive list of foods and their GI values.

In general, the GI value is based on how much a food item raises blood glucose levels compared with how much pure glucose raises blood glucose. GI values are generally divided into three categories:

- Low GI: 1 to 55
- Medium GI: 56 to 69
- High GI: 70 and higher up to a maximum of 100

Obviously, foods that contain very little or no carbohydrate like meat, fish, poultry, nuts, oils etc. have a zero GI value.

A GI diet prescribes meals primarily of foods that have low values and can include some foods with medium values. All high GI foods are studiously avoided. Examples of foods with low, middle, and high GI values include the following:

- Low GI: Green vegetables, most fruits, tomato, raw carrots, kidney beans, chickpeas, lentils, pizza, sweetcorn, milk, muesli, brown rice, spaghetti, and bran breakfast cereals
- Medium GI: Couscous, muffin, fruit loaf, bananas, raw pineapple, raisins, cookies, oat breakfast cereals, and multigrain, oat bran, or rye bread
- High GI: White rice, white bread, potatoes, pancakes, scones, cornflakes, watermelon, jelly beans, and candy

The low GI diet is a specific diet plan that uses the index as the primary or only guide for meal planning. Unlike some other plans, a GI diet doesn't necessarily specify portion sizes or the optimal number of calories, carbohydrates, or fats for weight loss or weight maintenance. Therefore, it can only be effective for weight loss if overall daily calorie intake is reduced below normal. Several of the popular commercial diets, including the Zone Diet, Sugar Busters, and the Slow-Carb Diet are based on the low GI principle. Most scientific studies of the low GI diet suggest that a GI diet can help achieve some loss of body fat and body weight. However, you might be able to achieve the same or even greater weight loss by eating the other diets described in this chapter and/or doing more exercise.

Comparing GI values, therefore, can help guide healthier food choices. For example, an English muffin made with white wheat flour has a GI value of 77. A whole-wheat English muffin has a GI value of 45. However, there are several limitations of GI values, and probably the most important one is that they do not reflect the likely quantity you would eat of a particular food. For example, watermelon has a GI value of 80, which would put it in the category of food to avoid. But watermelon has relatively few digestible carbohydrates in a typical serving. In other words, you have to eat a lot of watermelon to significantly raise your blood glucose level.

To address this problem, researchers have developed the idea of **glycemic load (GL)**, a numerical value that indicates the change in blood glucose levels when you eat a typical serving of the food. Glycemic load is calculated by multiplying the grams of available carbohydrate in the food (for a typical serving size) by the food's GI and then dividing by 100. For example, a 120 g serving of watermelon has a GL value of 5, which would identify it as a healthy food choice. Sydney University's table of GI values also includes GL values. The values are generally grouped in the following manner:

- Low GL: 1 to 10

- Medium GL: 11 to 19

- High GL: 20 or more

Examples of foods with low, middle and high GL values include the following:

- Low GL: Green vegetables, most fruits, raw carrots, kidney beans, chickpeas, lentils, pizza, milk, muesli, brown rice, fruit loaf, scones, watermelon, tomato, and bran breakfast cereals,

- Medium GL: White bread, boiled potato, sweet corn, couscous, muffin, fruit loaf, doughnut, bananas, raw pineapple, raisins, cookies, oat breakfast cereals, and multigrain, oat bran, or rye bread

- High GL: White rice, baked potato, pancakes, raisins, cornflakes, spaghetti, jelly beans, and candy

However, even when using the GL rather than the GI there are still several other important limitations:

- The GI or GL value tells us nothing about other nutritional information. For example, whole milk has a GI value of 31 and a GL value of 4 for a 250 mL serving. But because of its high-fat content, whole milk is not the best choice for weight loss or weight control; semi-skimmed or skimmed milk are better.

- The published GI database is not an exhaustive list of foods but a list of those foods that have been studied. Many healthy foods with low GI values are not in the database.

- The GI value of any food item is affected by several factors, including how the food is prepared, how it is processed and what other foods are eaten at the same time.

- Also, there can be a range in GI values for the same foods, and some nutritionists argue it makes it an unreliable guide to determine food choices.

Selecting foods based on their GI or GL value may help you manage your weight because many foods that should be included in a well-balanced, low-fat, healthy diet with minimally processed foods — whole-grain products, fruits, vegetables, and low-fat dairy products — have low-GI values. Avoiding high GI foods generally means eliminating candy, chocolate, sugar sweetened beverages, most sauces, many processed foods, and starchy vegetables like potato as well as rice, bread, and pasta from your diet. However, when trying to decide which diet is best for you, never forget the most important principle of energy balance: In order for you to maintain your current weight, you need to burn as many calories as you consume. To lose weight, you need to burn more calories than you consume. Weight loss is best achieved by a combination of reducing the number of calories you consume each day and increasing your weekly amount of physical activity. For these reasons a low GI diet is not one I would recommend if your main goal is effective weight loss.

HIGH-PROTEIN DIETS

For most diets, protein will provide 10 to 15% of the calories; with high-protein diets, this is increased to about 30%. Many of the most popular or fad diets recommend increased consumption of protein usually to replace calories from fat or carbohydrate. One main reason that is often given is that high-protein diets suppress the appetite, which might be a mechanism that could help to promote weight loss. Protein also has a larger thermic effect and a relatively low coefficient of digestibility compared with a mixed meal of equal total calorie content. Several studies have demonstrated that increased protein content of the diet, particularly in combination with regular exercise, may improve weight loss and reduce the loss of lean body mass in overweight and obese individuals who are consuming a low-energy diet. It is also known that less weight regain occurs after the energy-restricted period ends when protein intake is high compared with more normal dietary compositions.

On a high-protein (30% protein, 50% carbohydrate, 20% fat) diet, satiety is increased compared with a normal weight-maintaining diet (15% protein, 50% carbohydrate, 35% fat) of equal calorie content. In one study, when subjects were on an ad libitum (eat as desired) high-protein diet for 12 weeks, their mean spontaneous daily energy intake decreased by 441 kcal, and they lost an average of 4.9 kg (11 lbs.) of body weight and had a mean decrease in fat mass of 3.7 kg (8 lbs.). As protein has a greater effect on satiety than both carbohydrate and fat, it can be helpful in weight-maintenance or weight loss situations. Of course, increasing the proportion of protein in the diet also permits a simultaneous reduction in the proportion of fat which is good because extra calories from fat (and carbohydrate) are more fattening than calories in the form of protein.

Another effect of protein that can facilitate weight loss is its thermogenic effect as described in chapter 5. The net metabolizable energy (that is the energy available from a nutrient after it has been digested and absorbed) of dietary protein is 4 kcal/g (17 kJ/g). Protein, however, is particularly thermogenic, and the net metabolizable energy is actually only 3.1 kcal/g (13 kJ/g) (that is the available energy after taking into account the energy lost as heat in its metabolism), making it lower than either carbohydrate or fat (4 kcal/g [16 kJ/g] and 8.1 kcal/g [34 kJ/g], respectively). Reported values for diet-induced thermogenesis for separate nutrients are 0 to 3% for fat, 5 to 10% for carbohydrate, and 20 to 30% for protein. Thus, a high-protein diet induces a greater thermic response in healthy subjects compared with a high-fat diet. This conclusion implies even higher fat oxidation, thus a negative fat balance and a positive protein balance. The relatively strong thermic effect of protein may be mediated by the high energy costs of protein synthesis following the absorption of amino acids from digested protein after a meal. In one study, increasing the amount of dietary protein from 10 to 20% of total energy intake resulted in a 63 to 95% increase in protein oxidation, depending on the protein source. Protein from meats (e.g., pork, beef) generally produces higher diet-induced thermogenesis than protein derived from plants (e.g., soy).

A third possible mechanism by which a high-protein intake may aid weight loss is by maintaining muscle mass during periods of dietary energy-restriction. A high-protein intake helps to prevent some of the muscle mass loss that is otherwise inevitable with energy restriction. This means that a larger muscle mass can be maintained, and because muscle is the most active tissue metabolically, the resting metabolic rate can be better maintained, thus helping weight loss. In one study, 31 overweight or obese postmenopausal women were put on a reduced-calorie diet of 1,400 kcal/day (with 15%, 65%, and 30% calories from protein, carbohydrate, and fat, respectively) and randomized to receive either 25 g of a whey protein or carbohydrate (maltodextrin) supplement twice a day for the 6-month study period. The group receiving the additional protein lost 4% percent more body weight than the carbohydrate group and preserved more muscle mass. In another intervention study, young, overweight, recreationally active men were placed on an intense 4-week diet and exercise program that included circuit training and sprints to help build muscle. Their diet contained 40% less energy each day than necessary for weight maintenance. Half of the men were randomly selected to receive a higher protein diet (2.4 g/kg body weight, 35% protein, 50% carbohydrate, and 15% fat), and the others were placed on a lower-protein diet (1.2 g/kg body weight, 15% protein, 50% carbohydrate and 35% fat). Both groups lost body weight, with no significant difference between groups. However, men in the higher-protein group gained 1.2 kg (2.6 lbs.) of muscle and lost 4.8 kg (10.6 lbs.) of body fat, while men in the lower-protein group gained only 0.1 kg (0.2 lbs.) of muscle and lost 27% less fat. Both groups similarly improved measures of strength and power in addition to aerobic and anaerobic capacity.

Some of the more important reasons for selecting a high-protein diet are summarized in the following sidebar.

Dietary Protein in Weight Loss and Maintenance

Protein may be an effective and healthy means of supporting weight loss and maintenance for several reasons:

- Eating protein makes you feel fuller for longer as protein has a greater effect on satiety than carbohydrate or fat does.

- Ingested protein has less **metabolizable energy** available than carbohydrate or fat does, as its nitrogen component cannot be oxidized, and it has a higher thermogenic effect.

- A high-protein intake helps to maintain muscle mass during periods of dietary energy restriction thereby preserving metabolically active tissue.

- High-protein diets are associated with less severe hunger pangs because the levels of ghrelin, the hormone that stimulates appetite are lower.

- The amino acids obtained from the digestion of ingested protein can be used to support glucose synthesis in situations of low-carbohydrate availability.

- High-protein diets are associated with lower plasma triglyceride concentrations.

For these reasons, a high-protein diet is one that I highly recommend for safe and effective weight loss.

ZONE DIET

The Zone diet was proposed in 1995 by Barry Sears in his book The Zone: A Dietary Road Map. The diet is essentially a high-protein but relatively low-carbohydrate diet. By reducing carbohydrate intake, plasma insulin responses following meals are lower. The benefits are increased fat breakdown and improved regulation of **eicosanoids**, hormone-like derivatives of fatty acids in the body that act as cell-to-cell signaling molecules. The diet is claimed to increase the "good" eicosanoids and decrease the "bad" eicosanoids which will promote blood flow and oxygen delivery to muscle tissue and stimulate fat oxidation. The diet is also claimed to reduce "diet-induced inflammation". To "enter the zone," the diet should consist of 40% carbohydrate, 30% fat and 30% protein divided into a regimen of three meals and two snacks per day. The diet is also referred to as the 40:30:30 diet. On the Zone diet, you need to stick to a rather strict and restrictive regimen. You're supposed to eat a meal within an hour of waking, never let more than five hours go by without eating, and have a snack before bedtime. Worst of all, you need to stick to the 40% carbohydrate, 30% fat and 30% protein formula at every meal and snack. You can't eat mostly carbohydrate for lunch and eat lots of protein for dinner.

Although some arguments by Sears are scientifically sound, several previous diet manipulation studies have been unsuccessful in stimulating the synthesis of good eicosanoids relative to bad eicosanoids. The book contains some errors in assumptions, some contradictory information, and the scientific studies referenced in support of the Zone diet are just a limited few that show positive outcomes for hormonal influences on eicosanoid metabolism, while any opposing evidence is conveniently left out.

Following the consumption of a meal containing some carbohydrate, only very small rises in insulin concentration are needed to reduce fat breakdown and oxidation significantly, and these effects persist for up to six hours after a meal. To avoid reductions in fat breakdown after a meal, the carbohydrate intake must be extremely small; much less, in fact, than the amount of carbohydrate in the Zone diet. Furthermore, from a practical standpoint, meals with the 40:30:30 carbohydrate:fat:protein ratio are quite difficult to compose, unless, of course, the dieter buys the 40:30:30 energy bars specially formulated and marketed by Sears.

Although the Zone diet seems has been shown to achieve some degree of weight loss when applied to overweight people, such success really should be expected because the Zone diet is essentially a lower than normal energy diet supplying 1,000 to 2,000 kcal/day (4 to 8 MJ/day). Although the theory of opening muscle blood vessels by altering eicosanoid production is correct in theory, there is very little evidence available from human studies to support any significant contribution of eicosanoids to this proposed effect. In fact, the key eicosanoid reportedly produced in the Zone diet and responsible for improved muscle oxygenation is not found in human skeletal muscle. Therefore, there is little reason to recommend this diet.

PALEO DIET

The Paleo (short for Paleolithic) diet is based on eating just like our ancient ancestors did. The aim is to eat as naturally as possible, opting for grass-fed lean meats, an abundance of fruit and vegetables and other wholefoods like nuts and seeds. Some less strict versions of the diet allow some foods (e.g., low-fat dairy products and root vegetables like potatoes, carrots and turnips) that were not necessarily available during the Paleolithic era – also known as the early Stone Age – which began around 2.5 million years ago and lasted until around 10,000 BC. The diet encourages the consumption of lean proteins, fruit, vegetables, and healthy fats from whole foods such as nuts, seeds, olive oil, and grass-fed meat. A consequence of this, of course, is that the diet results in a low intake of sugar, salt, saturated fat and zero processed foods. The diet is relatively low in carbohydrate but rich in lean protein and plant foods. These plant foods contribute the important fiber, unsaturated fats, vitamins, minerals, and phytonutrients. The diet is not low-fat but instead promotes the inclusion of natural fats from pasture-fed livestock, fish, and seafood as well as nuts, seeds and their oils. Although people who adopt this diet are generally more concerned with healthy eating or have a digestive problem with cereals, grain or dairy products rather than a strong desire for weight loss, the absence of such a wide range of foods like grains, dairy, processed foods, fatty foods, and sugar means the diet is more than likely to lead to some weight loss. In fact, a number of small studies have suggested that those following a Paleo diet report positive health outcomes, including weight loss, improved blood sugar control, and a reduction in the risk factors for heart disease.

However, there are some drawbacks as the Paleo diet ignores the health benefits of consuming whole-grains as well as beans, legumes, and starchy vegetables. Numerous studies have reported a reduced incidence of heart disease in those who regularly consume three or more servings of whole-grains per day. The low glycemic index properties of beans and legumes make them especially useful for those with blood sugar issues and starchy vegetables are an excellent source of nutrient-dense energy. All of these foods supply essential B vitamins, which among other things help us unlock the energy in our food by acting as cofactors of enzymes involved in energy metabolism. Finally, omitting dairy may limit the intake of minerals like calcium, which is essential for development and maintenance of the skeleton as well as nerve and muscle function. The diet also has the problem that it is difficult to stick to especially when socializing and eating out because of the restriction on grains, dairy, starchy vegetables, and all processed foods. Very few cafes or restaurants have menus that allow the restrictions of the Paleo diet to be satisfied. For these reasons, although it is a healthy diet, it is not one I recommend for weight loss.

LOW-CARBOHYDRATE DIETS

Some of the best-known low-carbohydrate (ketogenic) diets are the **Atkins diet** and Sugarbusters that were introduced in the 1990s. These diets are based on the premise that reducing carbohydrate intake results in increased fat oxidation. When carbohydrate is severely restricted to less than 20 g per day, the production of ketone bodies (acetone, acetoacetate, and β-hydroxybutyrate) will increase, which may suppress appetite. Ketone bodies may also be present in urine, which could result in loss of some "calories" through urination. Although all of the preceding may be true, the loss of calories achieved via the excretion of ketone bodies in urine is small at no more than 100 to 150 kcal/day (400 to 600 kJ/day). Such diets can be effective for weight loss, but they are no more effective than a well-balanced, energy-restricted diet. Although these diets may provide better satiety than high-carbohydrate diets, most of the effect can be attributed to the relatively high-protein content. For active individuals, these very low-carbohydrate or ketogenic diets are detrimental because of reduced glycogen stores which limit the ability to perform prolonged aerobic exercise due to an earlier onset of fatigue.

The main idea behind the Atkins diet is that severely limiting carbohydrate intake confers a so-called "metabolic advantage" allowing large amounts of fat to be consumed without significant weight gain. With a very low-carbohydrate intake, circulating insulin levels are substantially and continuously reduced, and this promotes fat breakdown and oxidation. This, in turn, increases energy expenditure by 400-600 kcal/day and should therefore result in body fat loss over time. These ideas have collectively become known as the "carbohydrate-insulin hypothesis". However, some recent studies that have rigorously investigated it have reported that although low levels of plasma insulin and increased fat oxidation do indeed occur, the desired outcomes of increases in energy expenditure and body fat loss do not. In fact, the studies reported less body fat loss with low-carbohydrate diets than with low-fat diets when protein and energy intake were matched.

The Atkins Diet had been tested in large number of clinical trials and overall the evidence supports its efficacy in achieving meaningful long-term body weight loss. However, body weight loss was the only outcome measure in most of these studies, and the effects of the diet on body composition (i.e., percentage body fat) were not considered. A recent comprehensive meta-analysis that considered the results of 32 controlled feeding studies involving over 500 subjects did not support the use of low-carbohydrate diets for body fat loss. In all these studies the participants had some of their dietary carbohydrate calories replaced by an equal number of calories from fat, but dietary protein content remained the same. As the proportion of dietary carbohydrate to fat changed, daily energy expenditure and body fat changes were recorded, which allowed a direct comparison of the efficacy of low-fat and low-carbohydrate diets across a wide range of study conditions. The main findings were that the average rate of body fat loss was 16 g/day (or 0.5 kg/month) greater with lower fat diets. In fact, only three out of the 32 studies examined showed a greater body fat loss with the low-carbohydrate diet, whereas the overwhelming majority showed greater body fat loss with the low-fat diet. These results do not support the carbohydrate-insulin hypothesis and fail to confirm any so-called "metabolic advantage" of consuming low-carbohydrate diets. Despite these reservations, as the Atkins diet works for some people, it is a diet you can consider for weight loss, although it is not my number one choice.

LOW ENERGY DENSITY DIETS

The **energy density** of the diet can play an important role in weight maintenance. A small quantity of food rich in fat has very high energy content. Visual cues that may prevent a large intake of energy on a high-carbohydrate diet, which is commonly of high bulk and volume, may be absent in a high-fat diet. Several studies have shown that subjects tend to eat a similar weight of food regardless of the macronutrient composition. Because a 500 g meal consisting mainly of carbohydrate will contain significantly less energy than a 500 g high-fat meal, lower energy intake will automatically result.

Studies in the 1990s showed that when subjects received a diet that contained 20%, 40%, or 60% fat and could eat ad libitum (i.e., they were free to choose as much as desired), the weight of the food that they consumed was the same (see figure 7.3). Because of differences in energy density, however, the total amount of energy consumed with the higher-fat diets was greater, and therefore weight gain was greater. This result happened in both controlled laboratory conditions and free-living conditions. When the fat content of the diet was altered, but the energy density was kept the same, the subjects still consumed the same weight of food, indicating that the energy density of the meals is a major determinant of energy intake.

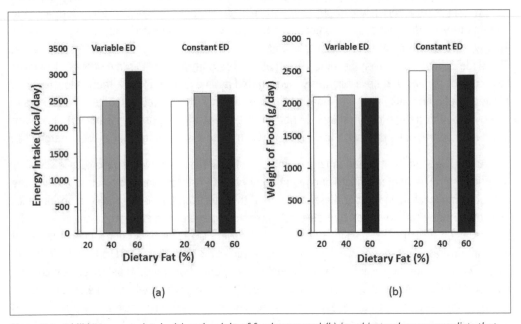

Figure 7.3: Ad libitum energy intake (a) and weight of food consumed (b) in subjects who consume diets that have 20, 40, and 60% of their energy as fat. In one of these projects the energy density (ED) between diets was different (variable ED). In the other study, the energy density was the same despite differences in composition (constant ED). Data from Stubbs et al. (1995) and Stubbs et al. (1996).

Several large scale longitudinal and cross-sectional studies involving thousands of participants have clearly shown that an increase in energy density results in an increase in energy intake, whereas a decrease in the energy density of the diet results in a decrease in intake as illustrated in figure 7.4. These studies clearly demonstrate the important role of the energy density of the diet and suggest that manipulation of energy density is a good tool in weight management. What these studies also indicate is that normal-weight people consume diets with a lower energy density than obese people and that people who have a high fruit and vegetable intake have the lowest dietary energy density values and the lowest prevalence of obesity. This is not surprising as fruits and vegetables generally have high water and fiber content which provides bulk but less energy than most other food sources. Only subtle changes to the diet are needed to alter its energy density. For example, the energy density of many popular foods such as pies, pizzas, sandwiches, and stews can be decreased by reducing the fat content and through the addition of vegetables and/or fruits without noticeably affecting palatability or portion size. In fact, the portion size will generally be larger for a low energy density meal and the changes to food selection can lead to healthier eating patterns consistent with the 2015-2020 *Dietary Guidelines for Americans* as explained in chapter 4.

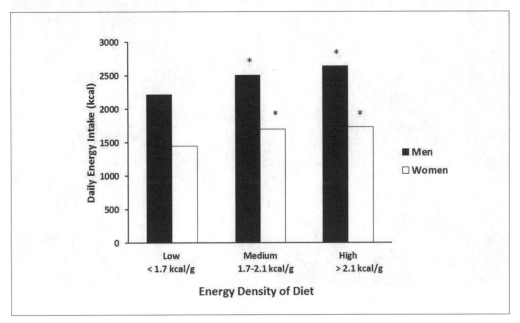

Figure 7.4: Energy intakes of men (closed columns) and women (open columns) consuming a low-, medium-, or high-energy-dense diet. Data are from a cross-sectional study involving 7,356 participants by Ledikwe et al. (2006).

The low energy density diet provides a total of 1,300 to 1,500 kcal/day with an energy density of less than 1.5 kcal/g. The diet typically contains 25-30% protein with low-fat (less than 30 g/day) and limited carbohydrate (less than 130 g /day). The main principle of a low energy density diet is to avoid fatty foods (or use reduced fat versions of foods like cheese and milk), use only lean meat (trim off any visible fat and remove skin from poultry), and fish, and include lots of fruit and non-starchy vegetables such as spinach, broccoli, cauliflower, green beans, or salad leaves with tomatoes, onion, celery, etc. Gourds (a fleshy, typically large fruit with a hard skin – a selection is illustrated in photo 7.1) including eggplant (aubergine), squash, marrow, melon, and zucchini (courgette) are a particularly good choice, as all have an energy density less than 0.5 kcal/g. In fact, most vegetables have an energy density less than 1.0 kcal/g (e.g., salad leaves and spinach are only 0.2 kcal/g, carrots are 0.4 kcal/g, and beans are about 0.9 kcal/g). The energy density of some common foods is illustrated in figure 7.5. Using the principles of energy density, it is possible to achieve a lower calorie intake which will help towards weight loss, whilst allowing generous, voluminous portions of food and get an overall balanced diet that is high in protein, fiber, micronutrients, and phytonutrients. Another significant advantage of consuming a low energy density diet is that because the majority of the ingredients contain relatively few calories per gram, you can eat more of it. This helps to avoid the hunger pangs that are many a diet's downfall. For these reasons, a low energy density diet with high-protein is my number one choice for safe and effective weight loss.

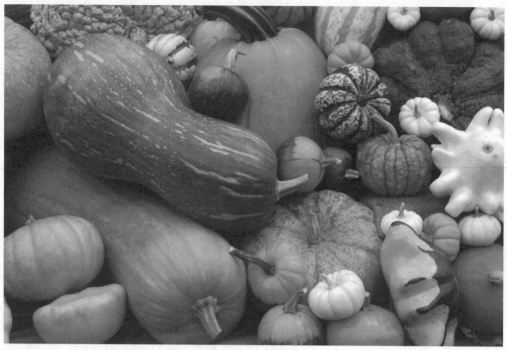

Photo 7.1: A selection of gourd vegetables, all of which have a low-energy density

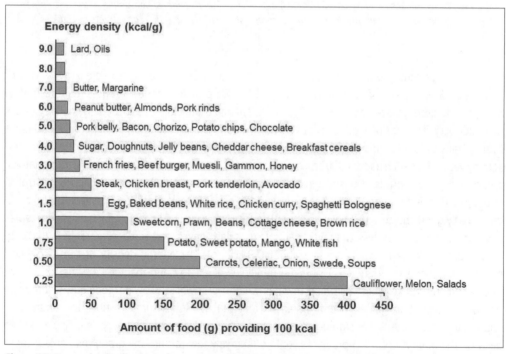

Figure 7.5: Energy density (kcal/g) of some common foods, and the amount of food (in grams) that provides 100 kcal

DIETS HIGH IN CALCIUM AND DAIRY PRODUCTS

The discovery that dietary calcium and dairy intake can contribute to weight loss was made by accident. It had been known for some time that a relatively high calcium intake through high consumption of dairy products was associated with reduced blood pressure in hypertensive individuals. In one study, a higher dairy intake that provided 1,000 mg of calcium per day reduced hypertension compared with a control diet that provided 400 mg of calcium per day. But the authors also reported the surprising finding that the participants in the dairy supplemented group lost 4.9 kg (11 lbs.) of body fat whereas the control group subjects were, on average, relatively weight stable. In several subsequent large population-based studies, similar trends were observed.

A possible mechanism by which increased dairy and calcium consumption could work is via a negative influence of dietary calcium on levels of the hormone calcitriol or $1,25\text{-}(OH)_2$-vitamin D. This hormone regulates calcium absorption, uptake, and the intracellular calcium concentration which plays a crucial role in fat metabolism in adipocytes. It has been suggested that reducing calcitriol by increasing dietary calcium intake results in increased fat breakdown and a gradual reduction of body fat even in the absence of dietary energy restriction. In combination with energy restriction it may result in increased losses of body fat and body weight. Dairy calcium appears to be more effective than just calcium, because the protein and amino acids in dairy products may have additional benefits such as increased satiety.

However, despite some reports of improved fat loss with higher dairy and calcium intake, the most recent meta-analysis reviews, in which the outcomes of multiple studies were considered, have concluded that neither calcium supplementation nor increased dairy food intake significantly affects body weight or body fat compared with control or placebo treatments. However, sub-analyses of studies in which calcium supplementation or increased dairy food intake took place in combination with lower than normal energy intake revealed an important positive outcome. Although, in the presence of dietary energy restriction, dairy supplementation resulted in no change in body weight, it did result in about a 1 kilogram greater reduction in body fat over a mean of four months compared with control. Therefore, this meta-analysis strongly suggests that increasing dietary calcium intake by supplements or increasing dairy intake in isolation is not itself an effective weight reduction strategy for overweight adults, but that approximately three servings of dairy per day may facilitate fat loss on weight reduction diets at least in the short term. It would be sensible for these dairy products to be of the low-fat variety (e.g., skimmed milk, cottage cheese, low-fat yogurt). In my opinion, there are far superior diets than this if your primary goal is body weight loss.

COMPARISONS OF THE DIFFERENT DIETS FOR WEIGHT LOSS

Many scientists still support the view that weight changes are not primarily determined by varying proportions of carbohydrate and fat in the diet but instead by the number of calories ingested. I certainly agree that overall daily calorie intake in comparison with daily energy expenditure is the most important factor when it comes to weight and fat loss. Diet-induced changes in energy expenditure, which metabolic pathways are used, and other considerations are quite modest when compared with the importance of actual calorie intake. Table 7.3 provides a summary of expected body fat losses on different diets.

Table 7.3: A summary of the efficacy of different diets for body fat loss in slightly overweight adults

Diet	What it involves	Weekly energy deficit	Weekly body fat loss
Very low energy	800 kcal/day (3.4 MJ/day) liquid meals high in protein	8,400 kcal (35.2 MJ)	1.0 kg (2.2 lbs.)
Alternate day fast	Fast completely every other day	7,000 kcal (29.3 MJ)	0.8 kg (1.8 lbs.)
4:3	Only 500 kcal (2.1 MJ) on 3 days/week	4,500 kcal (18.8 MJ)	0.5 kg (1.1 lbs.)
5:2	Only 500 kcal (2.1 MJ) on 2 days/week	3,000 kcal (12.6 MJ)	0.35 kg (0.8 lbs.)
Skip lunch	No 500 kcal (2.1 MJ) lunch 3 days/week	1,500 kcal (6.3 MJ)	0.17 kg (0.4 lbs.)
Low-carbohydrate (Atkins)	1,500 kcal/day (6.3 MJ/day) with <20 g carbohydrate daily in first 2 weeks, up to 50 g/day thereafter	3,500 kcal (14.7 MJ)	0.4 kg (0.9 lbs.)
Zone	1,500 kcal/day (6.3 MJ/day) with 40% CHO, 30% fat, and 30% protein	3,500 kcal (29.3 MJ)	0.4 kg (0.9 lbs.)
Low-fat	1,500 kcal/day (6.3 MJ/day) with <10% fat	3,500 kcal (14.7 MJ)	0.4 kg (0.9 lbs.)
High-protein	1,500 kcal/day (6.3 MJ/day) with 30% protein	4,200 kcal (17.6 MJ)	0.5 kg (1.1 lbs.)
Low energy density	1,400 kcal/day (5.8 MJ/day) with 25% protein	4,900 kcal (20.5 MJ)	0.6 kg (1.3 lbs.)

Assumes (1) normal energy intake is 2,000 kcal/day with 15% coming from protein, (2) some diets will reduce appetite compared with normal due to higher protein or lower energy density, (3) body fat losses are average weekly loss over a 10-week period on each diet, and (4) approximately 0.46 kg of body fat is lost for each 3,500 kcal energy intake deficit in the first five weeks and 0.34 kg is lost for each 3,500 kcal energy intake deficit thereafter (accounting for metabolic adaptation to energy restriction). Note that body weight losses with be higher than the losses of body fat shown here as some diets will also cause some loss of body water, glycogen, and lean tissue (see main text for details).

When it comes to choosing which is the best diet for yourself, you need to take into account not only the efficacy of the diet for body weight and fat loss but also how likely you are going to be able to stick to the diet for 10 weeks or more, how healthy (or unhealthy) the diet is, and how safe it is. Table 7.4 below shows my own personal ratings and overall rankings for the 10 diets that were listed in the previous table.

Table 7.4: My own personal star ratings and overall rankings of the different diets after considering how effective they are for body fat loss together with taking into account how easy they are to stick to, their health effects, and their safety

Diet	Efficacy for body fat loss	How easy to stick to	Health and safety	Overall rating (and rank)
Very low energy	*****	*	*	** (8=)
Alternate day fast	****	**	**	** (6=)
4:3	***	***	***	*** (4=)
5:2	**	****	****	**** (3)
Skip lunch	*	****	****	*** (4=)
Low-carbohydrate	**	***	**	** (8=)
Zone	**	*	***	* (10)
Low-fat	**	***	***	** (6=)
High-protein	***	****	****	***** (2)
Low energy density	***	****	*****	***** (1)

* = lowest rating; ***** = highest rating

USING NONNUTRITIVE SWEETENERS IN THE DIET

Nonnutritive sweeteners or **artificial sweeteners** are substances that are used instead of sugars (i.e., sucrose, corn syrup, honey) to sweeten foods, beverages, and other products, such as toothpastes and some medicines. Some come from natural sources and are known as natural sugar substitutes (see sidebar). Some, like fructose, have similar energy content per gram as cane sugar (sucrose) but are sweeter so that less is needed. Some, like maltitol, have a similar sweetness to sucrose but contain less energy per gram (maltitol has only 2.1 kcal/g compared with 4 kcal/g for sucrose). Maltitol is one of a number of sugar alcohols that are incompletely absorbed and metabolized by the body, and consequently contribute fewer calories than most sugars. Other commonly used sugar alcohols include sorbitol, mannitol, xylitol, lactitol, and erythritol. Other natural sugar substitutes are extremely sweet proteins like mabinlin which are extracted from plant seeds. Other potent sweeteners are chemically synthesized compounds. Five of these artificial nonnutritive sweeteners with intense sweetening power have FDA approval (acesulfame-K, aspartame, neotame, **saccharin**, and sucralose). The advantage of these artificial sweeteners is that they contain very little energy and you only need very small amounts to achieve the equivalent sweetness of a spoonful of cane sugar. Therefore, they can assist in lowering daily sugar and energy intake while maintaining diet palatability. In theory this should contribute to weight loss for dieters with little or no influence on appetite; however, evidence of long-term efficacy for their use in weight management is not currently available. Of course, the addition of nonnutritive sweeteners to the diet will provide no benefit for weight loss unless there is overall restriction of daily energy intake.

Nonnutritive Sweeteners Showing Their Sweetness Relative to Sucrose by Weight or by Food Energy

Natural sugar substitutes:

- Brazzein–protein 800 x sweetness of sucrose (by weight)
- Curculin–protein 550 x sweetness (by weight)
- Erythritol 0.7 x sweetness (by weight), 14 x sweetness of sucrose (by food energy)
- Fructose 1.7 x sweetness (by weight and food energy)
- Glycyrrhizin 50 x sweetness (by weight)
- Isomalt 0.45–0.65 x sweetness (by weight), 0.9–1.3 x sweetness (by food energy)
- Lactitol 0.4 x sweetness (by weight), 0.8 x sweetness (by food energy)
- Lo Han Guo 300 x sweetness (by weight)
- Mabinlin–protein 100 x sweetness (by weight)
- Maltitol 0.9 x sweetness (by weight), 1.7 x sweetness (by food energy), E965
- Mannitol 0.5 x sweetness (by weight), 1.2 x sweetness (by food energy), E421
- Monellin–protein 3,000 x sweetness (by weight)
- Pentadin–protein 500 x sweetness (by weight)
- Sorbitol 0.6 x sweetness (by weight), 0.9 x sweetness (by food energy), E420
- Stevia 250 x sweetness (by weight)
- Tagatose 0.92 x sweetness (by weight), 2.4 x sweetness (by food energy)
- Thaumatin–protein 2,000 x sweetness (by weight), E957
- Xylitol 1.0 x sweetness (by weight), 1.7 x sweetness (by food energy), E967

Artificial sugar substitutes (with examples of brand names and E numbers):

- Acesulfame potassium 200 x sweetness (by weight), Nutrinova, E950
- Aspartame 160–200 x sweetness (by weight), NutraSweet, Equal, Sugar Twin, E951
- Neotame 8,000 x sweetness (by weight), Newtame, E961
- Saccharin 300 x sweetness (by weight), E954
- Sucralose 600 x sweetness (by weight), Splenda, E955

Key Points

- Negative energy balance is required to lose weight. In addition, negative fat balance will help to promote fat loss.

- Calories from different macronutrients or food items can have markedly different effects on hunger, hormones, resting energy expenditure, and the brain regions that control food intake. Even though calories are important, in many cases, simple changes in food selection can lead to the same (or slightly better) results for weight loss than limited (i.e., cutting back by less than 300 kcal/day) calorie restriction.

- Substantial weight loss (i.e., more than a few kilograms) can only be achieved by more substantial reductions in energy intake (i.e., eating at least 500 kcal/day less than normal) and improved further with increased energy expenditure through doing more exercise.

- The resting metabolic rate decreases in response to weight loss. This effect, referred to as food efficiency, makes losing weight more difficult.

- Another effect that contributes to a lower resting metabolic rate with dieting is the loss of lean muscle mass that occurs when dietary protein intake as well as total energy intake is reduced.

- Eating a high-protein diet helps to maintain muscle mass and resting metabolic rate during periods of dietary energy restriction.

- A common problem is the yo-yo effect, or weight cycling. After weight loss is achieved, the lost weight is often regained in a relatively short period when a normal diet is resumed.

- Studies clearly demonstrate the important role of energy density of the diet for voluntary food intake and suggest that manipulation of energy density is a useful tool in weight management.

- Common diet strategies to lose weight include very low-energy diets, intermittent fasting diets, low-carbohydrate diets, low-fat diets, food combination diets, high-protein diets, and low energy density diets. For individuals seeking to lose weight, energy restriction and reduced fat intake while maintaining or even increasing dietary protein are recommended. This strategy allows a reasonable carbohydrate intake (needed for those who want to exercise) without major reductions in lean body mass.

- Perhaps the most effective yet safe and healthy diet for weight loss is one that incorporates the principles of eating mostly low energy density meals in combination with a high intake of lean protein. Another safe, healthy and effective diet is the 5:2 or 4:3 intermittent fasting diet in combination with the Mediterranean or Japanese diet on the non-fasting days.

- The use of non-nutritive sweeteners can help dieters reduce their intake of free sugars in food and beverages.

Chapter 8

How to Lose Weight by Exercising

Objectives

After studying this chapter, you should:

- Understand why fat burning is most effective at a moderate exercise intensity

- Know why resistance exercise and high intensity interval training (HIIT) are not effective ways of increasing energy expenditure to lose weight

- Appreciate the number of calories burned when performing different activities or sports for one hour

- Be aware of the influence of exercise on appetite

- Understand the influence of exercise on resting metabolic rate

As an alternative to dieting, exercise is another way to create a negative energy balance. In obese people (BMI of 30 kg/m² or more), the effectiveness of exercise programs to achieve weight loss has been questioned because of problems related to a lack of motivation to do physical activity, non-compliance with exercise programs lasting more than a few weeks, and impaired ability (e.g., poor fitness, flexibility or stamina) to perform some forms of exercise, particularly weight-bearing activities like jogging. In moderately overweight people (BMI of 25-29 kg/m²) with a real desire to lose weight, these factors are less likely to be a problem. Most people can include exercise sessions with the specific aim of increasing energy expenditure, and they can exercise at an intensity high enough or for a duration long enough to cause a significant increase in the amount of energy expended. Working people may have difficulty finding time to exercise, so for them higher intensity with relatively short duration would be the exercise of choice, at least on working days. For those lucky enough to have time on their hands such as retired folk like myself, long walks (e.g., 5 miles or 8 km taking about two hours) are a great way to exercise while enjoying the local scenery and still being able to engage in conversation.

Generally, adding exercise to a weight loss program results in weight loss that is fat loss (rather than lean tissue loss), and a combination of dieting and exercise is the most effective way to lower body weight and to maintain it at a lower level after weight reduction; it is nearly always more successful for weight loss than dieting or exercise alone (see the sidebar). The exercise, especially if it includes some resistance exercise and is followed by a high-protein post workout meal, will also help to maintain muscle mass and resting metabolic rate. Some forms of exercise can also increase the resting metabolic rate for several hours after exercise although this is not a significant factor in weight loss, despite some claims to the contrary by so-called fitness experts. In this chapter, the efficacy of different forms of exercise for weight loss will be explained. Let's begin by examining the impact of exercise intensity for aerobic exercise.

Is Dieting Better Than Exercise for Weight Loss?

It is often said that dieting is more effective for weight loss than doing more exercise. Indeed, the scientific evidence suggests that this is the case in most circumstances, even after taking into account the adaptive reduction in metabolic rate that occurs after a few weeks of reduced dietary energy intake. Of course, many authors of diet books hammer this point home and often one can be left thinking is it worth doing any more exercise at all? There are several reasons why dieting is more effective than exercise for losing weight, and the main ones are probably as follows:

- People who are not used to doing exercise are concerned that they will find the experience painful and unpleasant; some do and so they don't keep up the exercise regimen for long.

- They don't want to have to strip off or go to a gym where they may be surrounded by other people who are much slimmer than them as it is likely to make them feel embarrassed about their body.

- Doing exercise requires a significant time investment. For example, to incur a 500 kcal energy deficit by walking, you would have to cover about 5 miles (8 km) which would take the average person around two hours. In reality it is much easier to lose weight by cutting back on what we eat, and it can also save some time that is normally spent in preparing and eating food.

- It is simply much easier to skip a meal like lunch to achieve a 500 kcal energy deficit that it is to burn it off through exercise.

What the diet books generally don't tell you is that combining both dieting and exercising more is actually the best strategy for weight loss and for your health. This is backed up by the results of numerous scientific studies that indicate for a given daily calorie deficit, people will lose more body weight by a combination of dieting and exercise than with dieting alone. Not only is more weight lost but virtually all of it is achieved by a reduction in body fat. With dieting alone, some muscle mass is usually also lost which is undesirable, especially for people over 50 years of age when age-related loss of muscle (sarcopenia) becomes a significant concern. If the energy deficit achieved via reduced energy intake through dieting is supplemented by the energy burned with exercise, then the dieting can be less severe which reduces the impact on metabolic rate and makes it less likely that protein or micronutrient intakes will be insufficient to support optimal health. Exercise itself has its own health benefits by maintaining muscle and bone mass, improving fitness, flexibility, cardiovascular function, and immune function as well as increasing insulin sensitivity, a particular bonus for diabetics. Furthermore, exercise reduces the risk of health complications such as coronary heart disease, stroke, kidney disease, dementia, and some cancers in overweight and type 2 diabetic people.

EXERCISE INTENSITY

Aerobic exercise (also known as cardio) is physical exercise of low to high intensity that depends primarily on the aerobic (oxygen requiring) energy-generating process. During aerobic exercise, oxygen is used to oxidize stored fat or carbohydrate to provide energy in the form of ATP for muscle contraction. Generally, light-to-moderate intensity activities that are sufficiently supported by aerobic metabolism can be performed for extended periods of time and will predominantly use fat as the main fuel. High exercise intensities that approach the **aerobic capacity** (or maximal oxygen uptake) of the individual also activate anaerobic ATP production and cause **lactic acid** accumulation which contributes to fatigue. High intensity exercise (that is exercise at more than 70% of aerobic capacity) will predominantly use carbohydrate as the main fuel. Exercise at an intensity of 90-100% of a person's aerobic capacity can only be sustained for a matter of minutes. So what intensity of exercise is best for weight loss?

Some scientists argue that the optimal exercise intensity for weight and fat loss is related to fat oxidation and should be the intensity with the highest fat oxidation rate. Fat oxidation increases as exercise increases from low to moderate intensity, even though the percentage contribution of fat may decrease (see figure 8.1). Increased fat oxidation is a direct result of increased energy expenditure when going from light-intensity to moderate-intensity exercise. Compared with rest, light-intensity activities may increase the metabolic rate (i.e., energy expenditure) three to five-fold. At moderate exercise intensities, the metabolic rate may be six to nine times the value at rest. High intensity activities generally increase the metabolic rate more than 10 times the resting value (and up to about 20 times in elite endurance athletes). However, at high exercise intensities, fat oxidation is inhibited, and both the relative rate and the absolute rate of fat oxidation decrease to negligible values. In other words, high intensity exercise is really no good for fat burning.

The maximal rate of fat oxidation (typically around 0.4-1.0 g/min or 25-60 g/hour depending on an individual's aerobic capacity) generally occurs between 55% and 65% of aerobic capacity (maximum oxygen uptake) and has been referred to as the **"Fatmax"** intensity. In endurance trained people, Fatmax tends to occur at higher (62-65% of aerobic capacity or maximal oxygen uptake) than in less fit individuals (50-55% of aerobic capacity) because adaptations to exercise training result in an increased ability to burn fat as a fuel for exercise. If you are unfit or perform exercise occasionally, it is likely that your maximum rate of fat oxidation is around 0.5 g/min or 30 g/hour and will occur at about 55% of your aerobic capacity. At this intensity in a middle-aged relatively sedentary or recreationally active person, the heart rate will be about 140-150 beats/min and wearing a heart rate monitor will therefore enable you to know that you are exercising at the desired intensity. Whether regular exercise at the Fatmax intensity is more effective than exercise at other intensities for body weight and fat loss remains to be determined. However, one of the advantages of moderate intensity exercise is that it can be sustained for a long time (hours) and will feel easier when it is performed regularly.

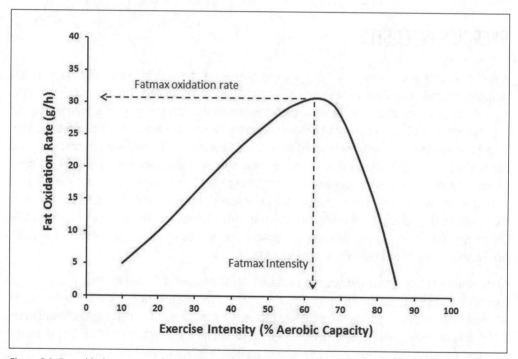

Figure 8.1: Fat oxidation rate as a function of exercise intensity. In this example the maximum rate of fat oxidation is about 31 g/hour and occurs at a relative exercise intensity of about 62% of aerobic capacity (maximum oxygen uptake).

How Can I Determine My Personal Fatmax Intensity?

For maximum fat burning during exercise, you should exercise aerobically at an intensity close to that which elicits your maximal fat oxidation rate. For a person of average fitness this will be about 60% of your aerobic capacity. In fact, measuring your aerobic capacity (or maximum oxygen uptake) requires specialist laboratory equipment and performing an incremental exercise test to exhaustion, so an alternative is to use a method that only requires the measurement of your heart rate using a simple and inexpensive heart rate monitor. Firstly, you can easily calculate your maximum heart rate which can be estimated as 220 minus your age in years. So, for a 30-year-old person, this would be 220 − 30 = 190 beats/min. Secondly, by wearing a monitor or counting your pulse at the wrist, measure your resting heart rate. Start the measurement after lying down and relaxing for 10 minutes. For a person of average fitness (and a non-smoker), this will be about 70 beats/min. Thirdly, calculate your heart rate reserve which is simply your maximum heart rate minus your resting heart rate. In our example, this would be 190 − 70 = 120 beats/min. Your Fatmax intensity (i.e., 60% of your aerobic capacity) will be achieved when exercising at a heart rate equal to your resting heart rate plus 60% of your heart rate reserve. In our example this would be 70 + (60/100 x 120) = 70 + 72 = 142 beats/min. So, when you go out for a run or cycle while wearing your heart rate monitor, start off slowly and gradually increase your pace until your heart rate reaches your personal target value and try to keep it at this value ±5 beats/min for the duration of your workout.

EXERCISE DURATION

The rate of fat oxidation during moderate intensity aerobic exercise increases as exercise duration increases (see figure 8.2), as it takes some time for fatty acids to accumulate in the blood (from the breakdown of fat stores in adipose tissue), so that the working muscles have a ready supply of fat fuel to burn. Thus, the longer you exercise, the more fat you burn.

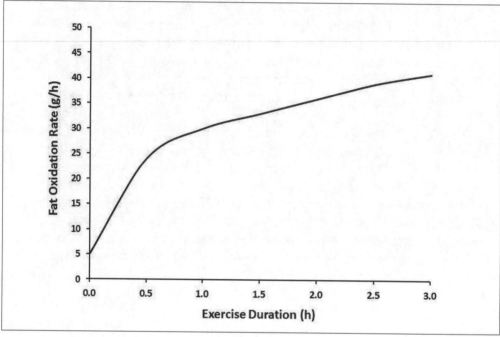

Figure 8.2: Fat oxidation rate as a function of exercise duration. In this example the exercise intensity is fixed at 55% of aerobic capacity (maximum oxygen uptake).

EXERCISE MODE

The mode of exercise also affects maximal rates of fat oxidation. As previously indicated, aerobic exercise is best for burning fat and losing weight, but there are several different modes of aerobic exercise, including walking, running, aerobics, cycling, and swimming. Fat oxidation has been shown to be significantly higher during uphill walking and running compared with cycling at the same relative exercise intensity or heart rate. Although no long-term studies have been conducted to compare different types of exercise and their effectiveness in achieving or maintaining weight loss, there have been numerous studies that have examined the volume of exercise or weekly amounts of energy expended in relation to weight loss. More on this later in the chapter, but before that, let's consider the case for two other popular forms of exercise, namely **resistance exercise** and **high intensity interval exercise**.

RESISTANCE EXERCISE

Comparisons of resistance training with endurance training have demonstrated some favorable effects on body composition but resistance training is not so effective in facilitating body-fat loss. However, resistance training certainly seems more effective in preserving or increasing lean muscle mass. In turn, the amount of metabolically active tissue also increases, and the increase is suggested as one of the mechanisms by which exercise helps to maintain lower body weight after weight loss that has been achieved mostly through dietary energy restriction. Resistance exercise preserves (or even increases) muscle mass, resulting in a smaller reduction (or even an increase) in the resting metabolic rate. The disadvantage of resistance exercise, however, is that it cannot be sustained for long periods and is intermittent rather than continuous as the muscles are worked hard and need time for recovery between sets of contraction repetitions. Thus, actual fat loss with resistance exercise is likely to be considerably less than with continuous, moderate intensity aerobic activities such as brisk walking, jogging, and cycling.

Few studies have compared the effectiveness of various types of exercise. Current evidence, however, indicates that resistance training is at least as effective as aerobic exercise in reducing body fat for the same (but relatively short) duration of actual exercise. The duration of the exercise is, of course, an important factor which largely determines the total amount of energy expended. People who can spend more time exercising at relatively high exercise intensities have a greater opportunity to achieve a negative energy balance and thus lose body fat and body weight. However, this is limited by fatigue, and in reality, it is easier to expend more energy in aerobic activities (e.g., walking, running, cycling, or swimming) that can be sustained for an hour or more.

Combining resistance training with aerobic training has been shown to be superior for body weight and fat loss and to result in greater lean body mass when compared with aerobic exercise alone in several randomized controlled trials. When resistance training is added to a reduced energy intake intervention, the energy restriction seems to overshadow the resistance training. None of the recently performed randomized controlled trials have observed a greater body weight loss for interventions lasting from 4 to 16 weeks. Most studies did not detect greater body fat loss with resistance training over dietary energy restriction alone, although one study examined body fat at various sites using magnetic resonance imaging and reported a superior loss of subcutaneous body fat with the combination of resistance training with diet compared to diet modification alone. On the other hand, most studies combining resistance training with dietary energy restriction report better maintenance or even increased lean body mass compared to dieting alone. The take home message is that resistance exercise helps to preserve muscle mass during periods of dieting but does not, in itself, assist much with fat loss. Combined resistance and aerobic exercise training can also provide some additional benefits for health and this issue is discussed in the following chapter.

HIGH-INTENSITY INTERVAL EXERCISE

Most exercise protocols designed to induce fat loss have focused on regular participation in relatively prolonged aerobic exercise such as walking and jogging at a low to moderate intensity. For most people, in the absence of dietary energy restriction, these kinds of protocols have led to rather slow and small losses of body fat and/or weight. This should not be surprising, as even exercising at the intensity that elicits maximal fat oxidation (i.e., 55-60% of aerobic capacity for a moderately fit individual) only results in a rate of fat oxidation of about 0.5 g/min, or 30 g/hour (i.e., one ounce per hour). Some scientists and fitness gurus have claimed that **high-intensity interval exercise (HIIE)** has the potential to be an economical and effective exercise protocol for reducing body fat in overweight individuals. But can it really be as effective as some are claiming? Let's stop to consider what HIIE actually involves.

HIIE protocols typically involve repeated bouts of brief sprinting at an all-out intensity (or at least at exercise intensities that exceed 90% of aerobic capacity) immediately followed by low intensity exercise or rest. The length of both the sprint and recovery periods has varied from six seconds to four minutes. A commonly used protocol has been the Wingate test, which consists of 30 seconds of all-out sprint cycling on a cycle ergometer with a hard resistance that is performed four to six times with each bout separated by two to four minutes of recovery. This protocol amounts to three to four minutes of actual exercise per session with each session being typically performed three to seven times a week. This form of training is commonly called **high-intensity interval training** (HIIT). Other less demanding HIIE protocols have also been utilized with either shorter sprints or exercise intensities of 90-150% of aerobic capacity but with shorter recovery periods. Thus, one of the characteristics of HIIT is that it involves markedly lower training volume, making it a time-efficient strategy for accruing training adaptations and possible health benefits (see the next chapter for further details) compared with traditional aerobic exercise programs. These benefits have been shown to include increased aerobic and anaerobic fitness, lowering of insulin resistance, and increased muscle capacity for fat oxidation. While this is good from the fitness and health perspective, there is limited evidence that HIIT results in significant body fat and weight loss even when performed for weeks or months.

Studies that have carried out relatively short HIIT interventions (e.g., three to six weeks) in young adults with normal body mass and BMI have reported negligible weight loss. Research examining the effects of longer term HIIT on body weight and fat loss in slightly overweight people has produced evidence to suggest that it can result in only rather modest reductions in body fat. Unfortunately, this type of exercise is usually distressing for those who are not used to it (photo 8.1). Heart rate and blood pressure are elevated and the hyperventilation it causes makes people who are unaccustomed to this form of exercise feel faint and sick which does not provide much motivation to stick with it. People who have existing hypertension and women who are pregnant should avoid any form of HIIE.

The mechanisms underlying the small degree of body fat reduction induced by HIIT appear to include elevated fat oxidation in the post-exercise period and suppressed appetite. However, the actual energy cost of HIIE is rather low; despite the intensity of the exercise being high, the duration is so short that actual amount of energy expended in each HIIE session usually does not exceed 100 kcal (420 kJ). Even taking into account a prolonged post-exercise elevation of resting metabolic rate (which could be as much as a 10% increase over the first 12 hours after the HIIE session) this only adds another 100 kcal at most, making the overall daily energy cost of a HIIE session to be no more than 200 kcal (840 kJ). If performed five times per week, this amounts to a 1,000 kcal (4.2 MJ) energy deficit. To put this into perspective, this amount of energy loss could be achieved with a single 10-mile (16-km) walk or run. Therefore, as previously mentioned, the moderately overweight person who seriously wants to lose body weight relatively quickly (i.e., in a matter of weeks or months) would be best advised to

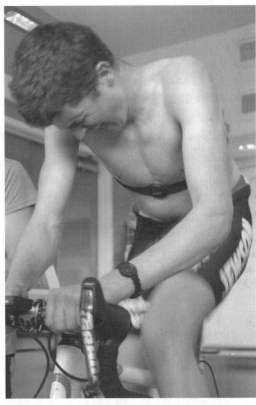

Photo 8.1: Performing a HIIE session can be distressing, even for individuals who are used to exercising.

exercise at relatively high but submaximal intensities for longer durations together with at least some degree of dietary energy restriction as will be further discussed in chapter 13.

HOW MUCH EXERCISE IS NEEDED TO ACHIEVE SIGNIFICANT BODY WEIGHT AND FAT LOSS?

A negative energy balance generated by regular exercise will result in weight loss and the larger the negative energy balance, the greater the weight loss. Extreme amounts of physical activity performed by military personnel, endurance athletes and mountaineers offer the potential for substantial weight loss; however, it is difficult for most individuals to achieve and sustain these high levels of physical activity.

A limited number of studies that have examined moderate levels of physical activity as the only intervention in sedentary overweight or obese individuals have reported about 2-3 kg decreases in body weight after 12 weeks. Therefore, most individuals who require substantial weight loss may need additional interventions (i.e., dietary energy restriction) to meet their weight loss needs. Better controlled studies that supervised and verified the volumes of exercise performed have generally found larger losses of body mass in overweight individuals, but as expected, the magnitude of the weight loss depended on the weekly volume (duration) of physical activity. Several studies that targeted 90-150 min/week of physical activity for 12 weeks found only small changes in body weight (0.5-1.5 kg), but increasing this to 150-225 min/week increased weight loss to 2-3 kg, and further increasing the exercise dose to 225-350 min/week (incurring a 500-700 kcal/day energy deficit) has generally resulted in body weight losses of 5.0-7.5 kg. Thus, as expected, a dose response effect is apparent for the impact of physical activity on weight loss.

As the energy expenditure of various activities has been measured in laboratory studies, it is possible to estimate the amount of body fat loss when regularly performing such activities for one hour per day, five days per week as illustrated in table 8.1.

Table 8.1: Weekly amounts of energy and body fat lost for a 70 kg person with different exercise protocols when exercising for one hour per day, five days per week

Activity	Daily energy deficit kcal (MJ)	Weekly energy deficit kcal (MJ)	Weekly fat loss kg (lbs.)
Aerobics	522 (2.2)	2,610 (10.9)	0.35 (0.8)
Badminton	480 (2.0)	2,400 (10.0)	0.32 (0.7)
Circuit training	450 (1.9)	2,250 (9.4)	0.30 (0.65)
Cycling 15 km/h	400 (1.7)	2,000 (8.4)	0.26 (0.6)
Running 11 km/h	860 (3.6)	4,300 (18.0)	0.57 (1.25)
Walking 4 km/h	275 (1.2)	1,375 (5.8)	0.18 (0.4)
Swimming	720 (3.0)	3,600 (15.0)	0.47 (1.0)

Table 8.2 shows the amount of exercise needed to incur a 500-kcal daily energy deficit and the amount of exercise needed to lose 0.46 kg (1 lb.) of fat (equivalent to 3,500 kcal) per week when exercising five days per week.

Table 8.2: Daily duration of exercise needed to (A) expend 500 kcal and (B) lose 0.46 kg (1 lb.) of fat (equivalent to 3,500 kcal) per week when exercising five days per week for a 70 kg person

Activity	(A) minutes	(B) minutes
Aerobics	56	79
Badminton	61	86
Circuit training	66	92
Cycling 15 km/h	76	106
Running 11 km/h	34	48
Walking 4 km/h	109	153
Swimming	42	59

Remember that doing exercise, especially with family or friends can be fun. Some examples of enjoyable physical activities are shown in photos 8.2 to 8.5. You can tell from these pictures that the participants are not overexerting themselves as they all look happy!

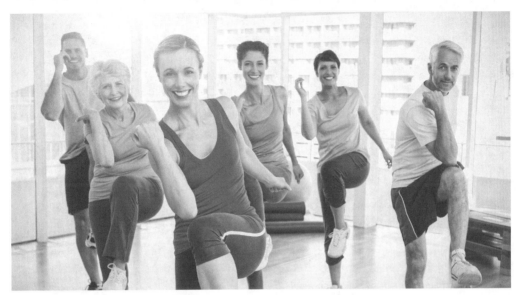

Photo 8.2: A simple aerobics class is good for cardiorespiratory fitness, flexibility, and fun.

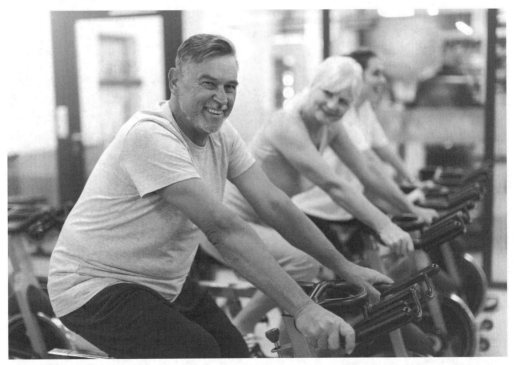

Photo 8.3: A stationary cycling (spinning) class is a non-weight-bearing aerobic exercise which is great for overweight people.

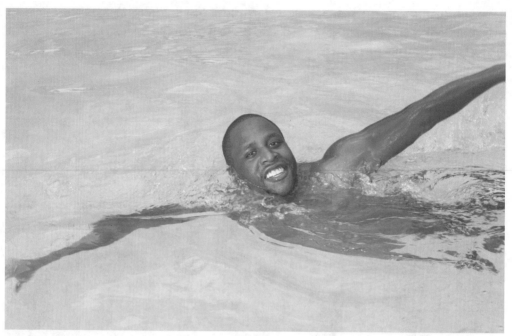

Photo 8.4: Swimming is another form of non-weight-bearing aerobic exercise which is great for overweight people and will improve cardiorespiratory fitness and flexibility.

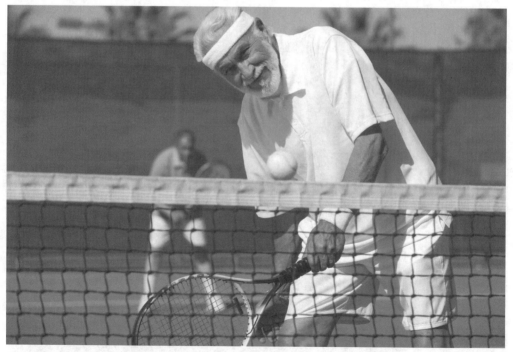

Photo 8.5: Games like doubles tennis involve intermittent physical activity but can burn significant amounts of fat when played for a couple of hours.

How to Estimate Your Energy Expenditure for Walking or Running Using a Pedometer

Simple inexpensive pedometers that record steps taken and distance covered for walking are available and usually just require the user to input their normal stride length which can be determined by measuring the distance covered when walking a given number (e.g., 20) of strides. The device can then reasonably estimate the distance covered over a long walk (say 6 miles or 10 km). For running, the stride length will, of course, be longer than it is for walking, so you will have to measure this as you did for walking but while running at your usual pace. If you have one of the more expensive devices that incorporates a Global Positioning System (GPS) function (just like the satnav in your car) the distance covered on a walk or run can be even more accurately determined without having to know your stride length. There is a relatively simple relationship between the distance covered (either walking or running) and the amount of energy expended. A person expends 1 kcal (4.184 kJ) per km distance covered per kg body mass, so the following equation can be used to estimate the energy expended when completing any known distance on foot:

- Amount of energy expended (kcal) = Distance covered (km) x body mass (kg) or

- Amount of energy expended (kJ) = Distance covered (km) x body mass (kg) x 4.184

Thus, a person weighing 70 kg (154 lbs. or 11 stone) would expend 700 kcal (2.93 MJ) if they covered a distance of 10 km (6 miles). As a rough approximation you can say about 100 kcal per mile (or 70 kcal per km). This is for covering distance over relatively flat terrain. The amount of energy expended would be ~10-20% higher if walking mostly uphill (photo 8.6).

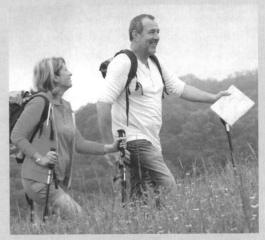

Note though that it is the distance covered, not the pace at which it is covered, nor the time taken to complete the distance that determines the amount of energy expended.

Photo 8.6: Walking is great for fat burning at about 100 kilocalories per mile on the flat and about 10-20% more when walking uphill.

For a 70 kg runner, the amount of energy expended when completing a marathon race (26.2 miles or 42.2 km) is 42.2 x 70 kcal which is 2,954 kcal or 12.4 MJ.

EFFECT OF EXERCISE ON APPETITE

Performing exercise has an effect on our appetite. Appetite and post-exercise energy intake depend on many factors including the intensity, duration, and mode of exercise. High-intensity exercise suppresses appetite for a short period but does not influence food intake when measured over several days. Hunger is suppressed only when the exercise is long enough (60 minutes or more) and intense enough (more than 70% of aerobic capacity). The mode of exercise (e.g., running versus cycling) does not seem to be important. Although anecdotal evidence indicates that swimming increases appetite more than other activities do, no scientific evidence backs this up. One study compared cycling submerged in cold (20 °C) water to cycling in neutral temperature (33 °C) water and observed an increased appetite in the cold conditions, suggesting an effect of water temperature rather than the exercise mode.

Evidence suggests that in the short to medium term (up to three weeks), exercise is able to produce a negative energy balance, with no substantial compensatory responses in energy intake. In the long term (more than three weeks), however, an increase in energy intake is likely to be observed. This compensation is usually partial and incomplete, generally accounting for only 30% of the energy cost associated with exercise, therefore still allowing the attainment of a negative energy balance and some degree of weight loss. In the short term, exercise may in fact be more effective than dieting in producing a negative energy balance. This notion is supported by the finding that acute energy deficits of about 500-700 kcal created by dietary restriction induce a significant increase in subjective hunger, subsequent energy intake, and food cravings during the day. On the other hand, a similar energy deficit created by exercise does not induce any significant change in these variables, thereby allowing the attainment of a short-term negative energy balance.

A study in 2016 investigated the effect of fasting compared with eating breakfast prior to a one hour bout of moderate intensity exercise (that expended 920 kcal) on 24-hour energy intake. It found that total 24-hour energy intake was 20% lower in the no-breakfast (fasting) treatment even though the subjects reported feeling hungrier before exercise, after exercise, and before lunch (see figure 8.3). Also, the rate of fat oxidation during exercise was higher in the no-breakfast treatment. Therefore, fasting before morning exercise may be a useful means of boosting fat burning and creating a larger daily energy deficit to promote weight loss.

Although appetite is controlled in the short term by the episodic secretion of gut peptides including ghrelin, CCK, GLP-1, as well as other hormones such as insulin (see chapter 6 for further details), there are also important long-term influences of other hormones such as leptin (secreted from adipose tissue) and other factors including fat mass, lean body mass and resting metabolic rate. It is also clear that exercise can influence all of these factors, which influences the drive to eat and the selection of particular foods through the modulation of hunger and post-meal satiety. The effect of exercise on each of the aforementioned factors will vary in strength from person to person and with the intensity and duration of exercise. Therefore, individual appetite responses to exercise will be highly variable and rather difficult to predict. Even so, it is safe to say that compared with moderate energy deficits resulting from exercise alone, acute dietary energy restriction results in rapid changes in appetite that result in compensatory eating, which may initially limit potential success in weight loss efforts.

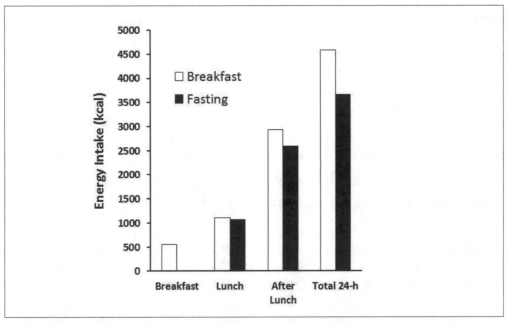

Figure 8.3: Dietary energy intake for breakfast, lunch, evening meal, and the total 24-hour period when performing 60 minutes of moderate intensity running in the morning with or without breakfast beforehand. Data from Bachman et al. (2016).

EFFECT OF EXERCISE ON RESTING METABOLIC RATE

Resting metabolic rate (RMR) is an important component of daily energy expenditure. It has been suggested that exercise can increase RMR and thereby increase energy expenditure during the rest of the day. The increase in RMR post-exercise is often measured as the **elevated post-exercise oxygen consumption** (EPOC). It is well established that immediately after exercise, oxygen uptake and RMR will be elevated, although this may only occur if the exercise is long enough and vigorous enough. Even so, the post-exercise increase in RMR seems only temporary and relatively small. After several hours RMR will return to baseline values. Suggestions that RMR is chronically increased have been refuted, and although some studies have reported an increased RMR, several other studies have even observed a decrease in RMR after a period of exercise training.

Another effect of exercise training could be an increase in muscle mass and thereby an increase in metabolically active tissue, though this will occur only with resistance exercise. So, exercise may have a small, short-term effect on RMR. The longer-term effects are unclear but are unlikely to be important in relation to total daily energy expenditure as previously explained for HIIE.

However, some other benefits arise from doing regular exercise. For instance, exercise training, especially aerobic exercise, results in a shift from carbohydrate to fat metabolism, and the oxidative capacity of the muscle is improved due to the production of more mitochondria and blood capillaries (see chapter 9 for further details). These effects allow an increase in the supply of blood-borne fuels and oxygen to the muscle as well as an increase in the capacity to take up oxygen and oxidize fat. Studies have consistently observed a decreased reliance on carbohydrate as a fuel and an increased capacity to oxidize fat in response to as little as four weeks of exercise training. This increased ability to oxidize fat may help to reduce fat mass even more in a situation of energy restriction.

The take home message is that combining some additional but regular exercise with dietary energy restriction is likely to be the most effective strategy for body fat and weight loss.

So What Sort of Exercise Is Best for Body Fat Loss?

Taken as a whole, the evidence suggests that for maximum fat burning during exercise itself, you should exercise aerobically at an intensity close to that which elicits your maximal fat oxidation rate. Depending on your fitness, this will be around 55-65% of your aerobic capacity (or 60-80% of your maximum heart rate which can be estimated as 220 minus your age in years). As for the duration and frequency of exercise sessions, the most important factor is your total energy expenditure over any given time period. So, for example, six dynamic exercise (e.g., cycling or running) training sessions per week of one-hour duration at 75% of your maximal heart rate would be equivalent to three sessions of two hours duration at the same relative exercise intensity. The goal is to increase your total volume of exercise (within reasonable limits), so that you will burn more fat. Fewer but longer sessions may be more advantageous as fat oxidation becomes an increasingly important fuel as the duration of exercise increases. An additional benefit of structuring sessions this way is that it allows longer periods of recovery in between each bout of exercise and/or some of that recovery time could be used to do HIIE sessions which should increase your aerobic capacity, further increasing your muscles' ability to burn fat. If you are undecided about whether to run or cycle, it is worth knowing that rates of fat oxidation have been shown to be slightly higher for a given rate of oxygen uptake during running compared with cycling.

Furthermore, any fat loss program should ideally include some resistance training because this increases muscle mass and lean body mass, which is desirable as lean tissue is metabolically far more active than adipose tissue. Increasing your muscle mass by including some resistance training means that your resting metabolic rate can be increased to a small degree, helping you to achieve your negative energy balance more easily. Two short (~30-minute) sessions of resistance training per week comprising of 8-12 exercises designed to work all the major muscle groups (one to two sets of 10-15 repetitions per exercise with enough weight set so that the repetitions can only just be completed) should produce good results in those who are not experienced resistance trainers.

GENDER DIFFERENCES IN WEIGHT LOSS

Numerous studies of weight loss after aerobic exercise training have shown that weight loss, although modest, was generally greater for males. These findings confirm earlier research in males concerning exercise-training effects on body mass and body composition and extend them both to females and to a broader range of exercise types including running, cycling, circuit training, and aerobics. These gender differences have been related to differences in body-fat distribution. Women store more fat in the buttocks and thighs, whereas men store more fat in the visceral (abdominal) area. Fat located in the upper body and abdominal regions (central fat) is more metabolically active and therefore has higher rates of fat breakdown in response to sympathetic nervous stimulation which occurs during exercise. This means that during exercise, fat is preferentially mobilized from these regions. In addition, fat storage after feeding may be higher in subcutaneous adipose tissue in women than in men. All these differences may play a role in the variation in net regional fat storage between men and women and women's greater resistance to weight loss with exercise.

Key Points

- Exercise can help to create a negative energy balance, maintain muscle mass, and compensate for the reductions in RMR seen after weight loss.

- Resistance exercise and high intensity interval exercise are not as effective for fat burning and weight loss as continuous aerobic exercise which can be sustained for much longer duration.

- For maximum fat burning during exercise itself, you should exercise aerobically at an intensity close to that which elicits your maximal fat oxidation rate. Depending on your fitness, this will be around 55-65% of your aerobic capacity (or 60-80% of your maximum heart rate).

- The mode, duration, and intensity of exercise influence the amount of energy expended and the amount of fat that is burnt. The most effective way to create a 500-kcal energy deficit is to exercise aerobically at low to moderate intensity for a continuous period of one to two hours.

- Compared with moderate energy deficits resulting from exercise alone, acute dietary energy restriction results in rapid changes in appetite that result in compensatory eating, which may initially limit potential success in weight loss efforts.

Chapter 9

How to Get the Health Benefits of Exercise

Objectives

After studying this chapter, you should:

- Understand how the body adapts to aerobic exercise training

- Understand how the body adapts to resistance exercise training

- Know how to improve your strength and endurance through appropriate training and nutrition

- Appreciate how regular exercise reduces the risk of chronic metabolic and cardio-respiratory diseases due to its metabolic, cardiovascular, and anti-inflammatory effects

- Be aware of these anti-inflammatory mechanisms

- Be able to list most of the major potential health benefits of exercise

- Appreciate that regular exercise is good for your mental health as well as your physical health

- Understand how exercise affects immune function and susceptibility to infection

Regular physical activity results in adaptations that eventually result in improved physiological function. Exercise training makes use of this principle by planning and systematically applying exercise activities with the goal of optimizing those adaptations and thus improve both health and performance. For ordinary people, improvements in stamina and strength may prove extremely useful in later life because as we get older, we tend to get less fit and lose muscle mass, which may compromise our ability to carry out everyday tasks such as walking to the shops, climbing a flight of stairs, or even getting off the toilet! Furthermore, exercise helps with weight loss and management, and some of the adaptations provide health benefits such as improving the blood lipid profile, lowering blood pressure, increasing the capacity to oxidize fat, and improving insulin sensitivity. These effects reduce the risk of developing chronic metabolic diseases such as type 2 diabetes and cardiovascular diseases such as arteriosclerosis, hypertension, peripheral vascular disease, and coronary heart disease. Regular exercise has also been shown to reduce the risk of some cancers. Being regularly active also reduces the risk of falling and breaking bones in old age and helps people remain independent.

Even with only moderate exercise training, a multitude of adaptations occurs at all levels and in different organs in the body, including increased capillarization of heart and muscle, fast-to-slow muscle fiber type conversion, increased heart size, increased muscle mitochondrial content, increased muscle mass, and so on. As well as training the limb muscles, exercise also trains the respiratory muscles and the heart. Table 9.1 lists a number of adaptations to exercise that can be gained with the regular performance of either resistance exercise or aerobic endurance exercise. A combination of both these major types of exercise may be best for health in the long term.

TRAINING ADAPTATIONS

Adaptations to exercise or exercise **training** are specific to the exercise performed. High-intensity (predominantly anaerobic) exercise will result in adaptations different from those resulting from moderate-intensity, longer-duration (aerobic) exercise.

Table 9.1: Training adaptations to endurance or strength training

	Endurance training	Strength training
Muscle blood capillary numbers	++	=
Muscle mitochondria number and size	++	+
Aerobic capacity	++	+/=
Muscle myoglobin	+	=
Muscle oxidative enzymes	++	-/=
Fat oxidation	++	+/=
Anaerobic capacity	-	+
Resting heart rate	-	=/-
Maximum heart rate	-	-
Maximum cardiac output	++	+/=
Blood volume	++	=
Muscle fiber number	=	=
Muscle fiber size	=	++
Muscle mass	=	++
Endurance	++	=
Strength	=	++
Power	=	++
Sprint speed	=	+

++ large increase; + increase; = no change; – decrease

Anaerobic exercise literally means "without the use or need for oxygen" and usually refers to short all-out efforts of dynamic exercise such as sprinting or more static forms of exercise such as muscle contractions against a strong resistance as in weight training. Resistance exercise typically results in effects that are different to those produced by aerobic endurance training. With resistance exercise, muscle hypertrophy is one of the main adaptations which increases strength and power whereas endurance training will not increase muscle mass but may improve muscle tone. Endurance training, however, will result in greater capacity to deliver and use oxygen, increasing the fatigue resistance of the muscles, and enhancing our stamina and endurance.

Resistance training results in a number of adaptations in the muscle, including an increase in the muscle cross-sectional area **(hypertrophy)** and altered neural recruitment patterns. For hypertrophy to occur, the rate of muscle protein synthesis must exceed the rate of muscle protein breakdown over a certain period of time, and an adequate supply of protein in the diet is essential for this to occur. Generally, resistance training does not increase the oxidative capacity of the muscle much, although some studies have observed small improvements in oxidative enzyme activity. The frequency, type, and intensity of resistance training, and the length of the recovery intervals will determine the degree to which such adaptations take place.

Endurance exercise training is characterized by the development of improved fatigue resistance partly because of increased numbers of skeletal muscle mitochondria (referred to as **mitochondrial biogenesis**) and the improved capacity for oxidative metabolism that this confers. Intramuscular glycogen stores as well as triglyceride stores increase after endurance training, although the amounts of both these fuel stores depend on the time since the last exercise session and the adequacy of nutrition in the post-exercise period. With endurance training, reliance on carbohydrate (glycogen) as a fuel for exercise decreases and the ability to oxidize fat increases. These changes result in sparing of muscle glycogen during exercise and delay the onset of fatigue. Endurance training does not greatly alter muscle fiber size, although an increase in the cross-sectional area of type 1 (slow, oxidative) fibers of around 20% has been observed in some studies. Endurance training can increase the mitochondrial protein content of the muscle by 50-100% within six weeks. The training adaptation is only temporary, and if the regular exercise stimulus is not maintained, mitochondrial proteins will be broken down again. Therefore, when the training stops, the hard-won adaptations will begin to be lost within a matter of weeks. This is why *regular* exercise rather than occasional bouts, no matter how strenuous, is so important.

Another important adaptation to training is the improvement in blood supply to the muscles involved in the exercise. This is caused by increased numbers of capillaries in the muscle, and this process is referred to as **angiogenesis**. These increases are greatest in type 1 and type 2A oxidative muscle fibers. It turns out that angiogenesis is tightly coupled with the mitochondrial content of the muscle fibers. If one increases, the other seems to increase in parallel. It is believed that shear stress on endothelial cells lining the **capillary** walls resulting from an increased blood flow and stretch of the muscle are the main triggers of angiogenesis. Small biopsy samples (approximately 100 mg) of leg muscles taken from endurance-trained athletes show that each muscle fiber is surrounded by a greater number of capillaries than are present in the muscles of untrained or sedentary individuals. Longitudinal training studies have also shown increases in the number of capillaries after training, even after only a few weeks of training. The major advantage of an increased capillary supply is an increased capacity for the delivery of oxygen to the active muscles. The distance that oxygen has to diffuse from the capillary to reach the deeper regions of the muscle fibers is reduced. There is also an increased capacity for the delivery of fuel—in the form of blood-borne glucose and fatty acids—to the muscle.

Myoglobin is an oxygen-binding protein similar in structure to one of the four subunits that make up the structure of hemoglobin. It has a reddish color and accounts at least for part of the deeper red color of muscle fibers that have a high oxidative capacity. Myoglobin can act as an oxygen store, releasing bound oxygen at times of high demand, but the total amount of oxygen made available in this way is fairly small. A more important function of myoglobin in highly oxidative fibers may be to assist the **diffusion** of oxygen through the cell. In response to endurance training, there is an increase in the amount of myoglobin in the muscles.

There is no doubt that training adaptations in muscle affect the mixture of fuels that are oxidized. Endurance training increases intramuscular content of glycogen and triglyceride and increases the capacity to use fat as an energy source during submaximal (i.e., moderate intensity) exercise. Trained subjects also appear to demonstrate an increased reliance on intramuscular triglyceride as an energy source during exercise. These effects and the aforementioned physiological effects of training, including increased maximum cardiac output and maximum oxygen uptake, improved oxygen delivery to working muscle, and diminished hormonal responses to exercise, decrease the rate of utilization of muscle glycogen and blood glucose and decrease the rate of accumulation of lactic acid during submaximal exercise. These adaptations contribute to the marked improvement in endurance capacity following training.

As moderate aerobic exercise causes the heart rate to more than double and the strength of cardiac contractions to increase, the heart itself undergoes training adaptations. Over a period of several months, this causes the heart to enlarge, and angiogenesis results in a higher numbers of capillaries in the cardiac muscle. With an enlarged heart, the stroke volume (the volume of blood pumped with each heart beat) increases, allowing a higher maximum cardiac output which is the main limiting factor determining the aerobic capacity of an individual. At rest, cardiac output is the same in the trained and untrained state at about 6 L/min. However, the higher stroke volume in the trained state means that the resting heart rate is 10-20 beats/min lower than the 70-80 beats/min in a sedentary individual. In elite endurance athletes, this difference can be even greater. For example, the 2018 winner of the Tour de France, Geraint Thomas, has a resting heart rate of only 45 beats/min.

Exercise will increase net muscle protein synthesis after both resistance and endurance exercise, provided that dietary protein and energy intakes are adequate. With resistance exercise, there is increased synthesis predominantly of proteins of the contractile machinery, namely actin and myosin, whereas endurance exercise results mostly in mitochondrial biogenesis and increased synthesis of oxidative enzymes with little or no change in the synthesis of proteins involved in muscle contraction. The increase in protein synthesis after resistance or endurance exercise may last for up to two to three days after the last training session.

Ultimately, all adaptations, whether an increase in muscle mass or an increase in mitochondrial mass, result from increases in certain proteins. The complex process of exercise-induced adaptation in skeletal muscle starts with a blend of stresses that trigger specific molecular events leading to the stimulation of muscle protein synthesis and altered gene expression. These stresses are different for endurance and for strength training; with strength training, stresses are mostly mechanical, while during endurance exercise, stresses are mainly metabolic.

The signaling events and the resulting increases in the synthesis of proteins, depend on the intensity and duration of exercise, the type of exercise performed, and the intake of specific nutrients. All individuals, including the elderly, can improve their performance by training. Furthermore, the more exercise you do, the easier it becomes.

TRAINING STRATEGIES AND THE ASSOCIATED ADAPTATIONS

The principles of overload, specificity, and reversibility govern the nature and extent of physiological and metabolic adaptations to training. Both physiological and biochemical adaptations occur as a result of the performance of repeated bouts of exercise over several days, weeks, or months. These adaptations improve performance in specific tasks. The nature and magnitude of the adaptive response is dependent on the intensity and duration of exercise bouts, the mode of training, and the frequency of repetition of the activity, genetic limitations in the ability to respond and adapt, and the level of prior activity of the individual.

In order to bring about effective adaptation a specific and repeated exercise overload must be applied. A general principle is that adaptation to training will only occur if the individual exercises at a level above the normal habitual level of activity for a sufficient time (e.g., at least 20-30 minutes per day) on a fairly frequent basis (e.g., on at least three days per week). By manipulating combinations of training intensity, duration, frequency, and mode, an appropriate overload can be achieved for any given individual. Another important principle is that physiological and metabolic adaptations to training are generally specific to the nature of the exercise overload. As previously mentioned, training for speed and strength induces adaptations that are different to those elicited by endurance training. The major effects of endurance training on skeletal muscle are on its oxidative capacity and its capillary supply. Strength or resistance training, however, mainly influences the size (cross-sectional area) of a muscle and thus its force-generating capacity. The specific exercise mode is also important; for example, the development of endurance capacity for running, cycling, swimming, or rowing is most effectively achieved when training involves the specific muscles to be used in the desired activity. This is because regular exercise induces adaptations that are both central (e.g., improvements in heart performance) and peripheral (e.g., improvements in local muscular performance).

Adaptations to training are essentially transient and reversible: after only a few days of detraining, significant reductions in both metabolic and work capacity are demonstrable, and many of the training improvements are lost altogether within several months of stopping regular exercise. Excessive training loads may cause breakdown and loss of performance, a condition referred to as 'overtraining syndrome', but this is only a real issue for elite endurance athletes. Sufficient time for regenerative recovery is required within a training program to allow the adaptations to occur. Muscle is an extremely plastic tissue and will adapt to training with functional benefits, but disuse (and particularly immobilization) results in protein breakdown and **atrophy** causing marked reductions in strength. This can be an important issue after a leg bone fracture or following a prolonged period of bed rest due to illness. However, any loss of muscle sustained by enforced inactivity due to injury or illness can be reversed by a suitable exercise training program and increased dietary protein intake. Even the loss of muscle mass that occurs with aging (sarcopenia) can be reversed by regular resistance training. Therefore, although genetic factors are the major determinant of the quantity and quality of muscle present in untrained people, considerable changes in the functional characteristics, size, and metabolic capacity can be induced by training in most people.

TRAINING FOR STRENGTH: INCREASING MUSCLE MASS

Training with weights can increase the force-generating capacity of the individual muscle fibers and cause them to increase in size and become stronger. Strength training is used by many athletes, not only in sports where peak force generation is important, but also where high power must be generated. The work done is the product of force and the distance through which it acts, and power is the rate at which work is done. Few sports call for the application of force without movement, but there are situations, as for example in a rugby scrum, where very high forces are generated without any external work being done (i.e., the distance moved is zero).

To some degree, all these characteristics—strength, power, and muscle mass—can be developed selectively by a suitable choice of training program. The specificity is not absolute, and some overlap will occur. Actin and myosin are the proteins in muscle that interact to generate force, so strength-training programs are aimed at increasing the muscle content of these proteins rather than simply increasing total muscle mass.

As with all training programs, the intensity and duration of training sessions will largely determine the training response. Intensity is critical, as this will dictate the extent to which the different muscle fibers are recruited and therefore subjected to a training stimulus. If the force that a muscle is asked to produce is low, this can be achieved without the need to activate all of the muscle fibers. Because of the way the neural control of contraction is organized within the central nervous system, the same fibers are always activated first. These are the slow-twitch **type 1 fibers**, which have a high oxidative capacity, a low anaerobic capacity and a high resistance to fatigue. The nerves that control the fast-twitch **type 2 fibers** are activated only if:

- The load exceeds that which can be lifted by the other (type 1) fibers, or

- The velocity of movement is very high, or

- Other fibers have been fatigued or damaged by prior exercise.

Just as training induces changes only in those muscles that are trained, so any muscle fiber that is not involved in force production will not experience a training stimulus. If the aim is to train the whole muscle, training must involve either high loads that will fully activate all of the muscle fibers or lighter forces that are repeated until fatigue of the slow-twitch fibers requires recruitment of the fast-twitch fibers to occur. If hypertrophy is to occur, the rate of protein synthesis must exceed the rate of protein breakdown. This can be achieved by an increase in the rate of synthesis, a reduction in the rate of breakdown or a combination of both.

The number of muscle fibers is fixed very early in life and even the most intense weight-training program does not seem to be able to induce growth of new muscle fibers. There has been some speculation as to whether increases in muscle size are the result of increases in the cross-sectional area of fibers alone (the process of muscle hypertrophy), or whether there is the possibility of an increase in the number of fibers (hyperplasia) as a result of the splitting of existing fibers. It has been suggested that once a fiber has increased in size (i.e., diameter) beyond a certain point, the internal stresses that result when that fiber is active will cause it to spit into two smaller fibers. The evidence for this is not strong, however, and results from animal models that involved the separation and counting of all the fibers in muscles from trained and untrained limbs have not provided evidence of a detectable increase in fiber number.

Responses begin within a few training sessions, and there are clearly adaptations occurring within the central nervous system that allow increased force production before there is any significant change in muscle fiber size. However, there are also changes to the contractile proteins within only a few training sessions, and measurable increases in muscle size are seen after about 15 training sessions. Some suitable resistance exercises for the arms include lifting hand-held weights (two to five kilograms) with the arms which can be done as part of other activities such as an aerobics class (photo 9.1) or even in the swimming pool. Alternatively, pushups in which your arms have to raise the weight of the upper body, are good for building arm strength (photo 9.2).

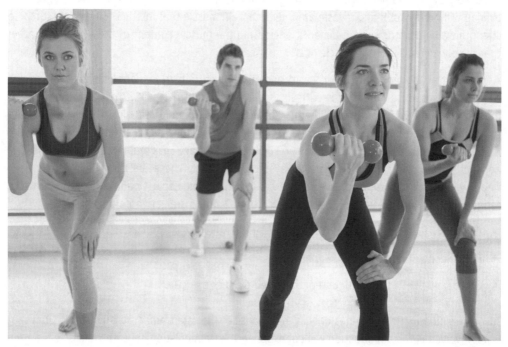

Photo 9.1: Doing some bicep curls as part of an aerobics class is a way of combining resistance and aerobic exercise.

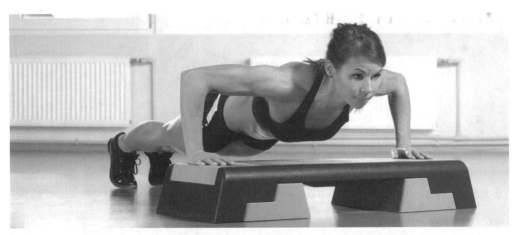

Photo 9.2: Push-ups are a good way of increasing the strength of your biceps. If this is too hard to begin with, try supporting your lower body with your knees rather than the toes until you have built up your strength sufficiently.

Some suitable resistance exercises for the legs include using a bench press to raise a cushioned weighted bar while in a seated position as shown in photo 9.3, or, if you prefer not to have to go to a gym, you can get your partner to provide resistance by using their arms as shown in photo 9.4. After performing several actions with both legs, you can swop around, so that you both get some arm and leg resistance exercise. For all resistance exercises, you should aim to do about 10-15 minutes per day, allowing about 30 seconds rest between successive efforts. You need to do these exercises on at least three days per week in order for effective adaptations to occur. In a few weeks you will start to notice that your limb muscles are getting a bit bigger and stronger, provided that your dietary protein intake is adequate (1.2 to 1.6 g protein per kg body mass per day is recommended for muscle building). Read on to learn more about the importance of nutrition for muscle building exercise.

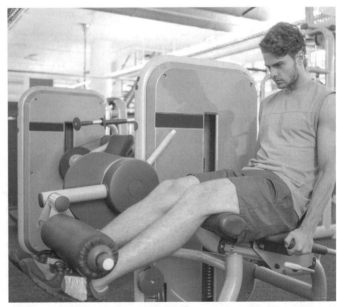

Photo 9.3: Performing a seated bench press leg raise of a cushioned weight to strengthen the thigh muscles

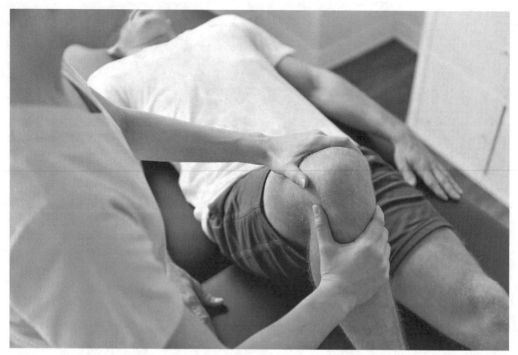

Photo 9.4: Performing a leg raise while lying on your back with your partner providing resistance with their arms to oppose your direction of movement. This exercise can also be performed in the reverse direction as you attempt to straighten your leg while your partner opposes the action.

Recent research indicates that muscle protein gain in response to resistance exercise training is influenced not only by the training load but also the amount, timing, and type of protein ingested in the following 24-48 hour period. Optimal adaptation to the training occurs when meals containing about 0.35 g protein per kg body weight (about 25 g protein for a person weighing 70 kg) are consumed shortly after a training session and up to three other meals distributed throughout the day with the aim of achieving a total dietary protein intake of about 1.4 g protein per kg body weight (about 100 g protein for a person weighing 70 kg) per day. Eating fewer meals with more protein is not as good as eating this optimal amount. The protein content of the post-exercise meal should be predominantly in the form of rapidly digested high-quality proteins with high leucine content. Such proteins include whey, skimmed milk, and eggs. This is because the essential amino acid leucine has a direct stimulatory effect on muscle protein synthesis (it is the only amino acid that has this special effect). The addition of carbohydrate to the post-exercise meal will only increase rates of protein synthesis when the amount of protein ingested is less than optimal.

The increase in muscle size and strength with resistance training can also be viewed as a health benefit, as it opposes the age-related decline in muscle mass (sarcopenia) that can result in weakness and incapacity in our later years of life. Although (as described in the previous chapter) the effects of resistance training on body weight and composition may be modest, resistance training has been associated with improvements in cardiovascular disease risk factors in the absence of significant weight loss. Resistance training has been shown to improve the blood lipid profile by increasing the concentration of the protective HDL while decreasing the concentrations of plasma triglycerides and LDL particles. Improvements in insulin sensitivity and reductions in glucose-stimulated plasma insulin concentrations have been reported after resistance training, effects which should reduce the risk of developing type 2 diabetes. Reductions in both resting systolic and diastolic blood pressure have also been reported after resistance training although it is important to be aware that resistance training will cause systolic blood pressure to increase considerably during the exercise itself. For this reason, resistance training should not be undertaken by people suffering from existing hypertension as there will be an increased risk of stroke.

TRAINING FOR ENDURANCE: INCREASING AEROBIC CAPACITY

Endurance training requires the performance of exercise at submaximal (i.e., moderate) intensities for at least 30 minutes per day three times per week. Greater adaptation will occur at exercise intensities that cause an elevation in blood lactic acid concentration and with more prolonged training sessions. Further improvements in aerobic capacity will occur with the addition of some interval training, which involves repeated higher intensity sessions (close to the intensity at which current aerobic capacity is reached), lasting one to two minutes with each session separated by only a few minutes recovery. Cardiovascular and metabolic adaptations to endurance training increase the capacity for fuel oxidation. The primary aim of an endurance-training program is to enhance the capacity for oxidative metabolism and in particular to increase the oxygen supply to the muscles and to increase the capacity for oxidation of fat.

Recent research indicates that training with low muscle glycogen might be a useful strategy to promote endurance-training adaptations. Low muscle glycogen levels can be attained by first doing an exercise session and then restricting carbohydrate intake, so that the next session will take place in a glycogen depleted state. For example, do a morning exercise session and then another in the afternoon with no carbohydrate intake in between. The same effect would be seen if training was performed during a period on a high-fat, low-carbohydrate diet. Studies show that under such conditions some metabolic adaptations in the muscles are enhanced, in particular mitochondrial biogenesis, increased oxidative enzymes, and an increased capacity to oxidize fat.

The physiological adaptations that accompany endurance training are well recognized, and the main ones are listed in table 9.1. An increased cardiac output resulting from an increased stroke volume (the volume of blood pumped into the arteries with each beat of the heart) and an increased perfusion of the muscle resulting from an increase in the density of the capillary network within the trained muscles are perhaps the two most important adaptations. Because there is a close coupling between the ability of the cardiovascular system to deliver oxygen and the ability of the muscles to use the oxygen that is supplied, it is hardly surprising that both cardiovascular function and muscle oxidative capacity are closely linked to performance in endurance events.

THE LINKS BETWEEN SEDENTARY BEHAVIOR, CHRONIC INFLAMMATION, AND CHRONIC DISEASE

The prevalence of obesity continues to rise worldwide and is being accompanied by proportional increases in a host of other medical conditions associated with derangements of metabolism such as insulin resistance, type 2 diabetes, cardiovascular diseases, **chronic obstructive pulmonary disease**, dementia, depression, and cancer. Inflammation appears to be an important causal factor in the appearance of all these conditions, and the development of a chronic low-grade inflammatory state as indicated by elevated levels of circulating inflammation markers such as C-Reactive Protein (CRP) and tumor necrosis factor-alpha (TNF-α) has been established as a predictor of risk for several of them. Importantly, physical inactivity and sedentary behavior in addition to overeating increase the risk of all these conditions.

An inactive lifestyle and a positive energy balance lead to the accumulation of abdominal (visceral) fat and consequently the activation of a network of inflammatory pathways that results in inflammation in adipose tissue, increased release of **adipokines** (peptides and proteins including some cytokines that are secreted from white adipose tissue), and the development of a low-grade systemic inflammatory state. The production of pro-inflammatory adipokines is increased with adipose tissue expansion, whereas the amounts of anti-inflammatory cytokines produced are reduced. This leads to the development of a state of persistent system low-grade inflammation which encourages the development of insulin resistance, atherosclerosis, neurodegeneration, and tumor growth, and subsequently the development of several diseases associated with physical inactivity such as atherosclerosis, coronary heart disease, and type 2 diabetes (figure 9.1). Atherosclerosis is further promoted by the deleterious changes in the blood lipid profile (namely a decreased HDL/LDL ratio and elevated blood triglycerides) associated with a lack of physical activity. Increased levels of fatty acids activate toll-like receptors (TLRs) on **macrophages** which also encourage inflammation. Such changes also increase the risk of developing dementia and several cancers.

A 2017 study of more than 1.3 million people from the UK, Europe, and USA found that those with a high body mass index (BMI) in their 50s were more likely to develop dementia two decades later. High BMI, an indicator of middle-aged spread, increased the risk of this neurological condition by up to a third. This may be due to the higher prevalence of type 2 diabetes in overweight people which is associated with numerous metabolic and circulatory defects that cause damage to blood vessels, potentially leading to reduced blood flow to the brain. Another study published in 2016 found that being overweight in middle-age makes the brain age by 10 years. The study, which scanned 473 brains, found changes in the brain structure of overweight people which are normally seen in those far older. The volume of white matter - the tissue that connects areas of the brain and allows information to be communicated between regions - shrunk far more in those with a BMI above 25 kg/m^2. Human brains naturally shrink with age, but scientists are increasingly recognizing that obesity - already linked to conditions such as diabetes, cancer, and heart disease - may also affect the onset and progression of brain aging.

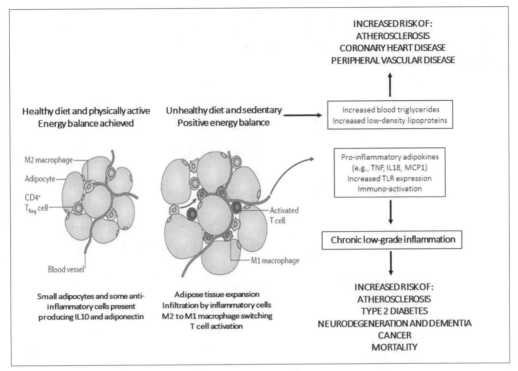

*Figure 9.1. In people who are not overweight, the amount of adipose tissue is relatively small and contains small adipocytes and some anti-inflammatory cells such as T-regulatory **lymphocytes** and M2 macrophages. Physical inactivity and positive energy balance lead to an accumulation of adipose tissue (particularly visceral fat stores) with expanded adipocytes which become infiltrated by pro-inflammatory immune cells called M1 macrophages and activated T lymphocytes. Adipose tissue then becomes inflamed and releases pro-inflammatory cytokines or adipokines that lead to a state of persistent low-grade systemic inflammation. This promotes the development of insulin resistance, tumor growth, neurodegeneration, and atherosclerosis. The latter is exacerbated by the deleterious changes in the blood lipid profile associated with a lack of physical activity. Increased levels of fatty acids activate toll-like receptors (TLRs) on macrophages which further promote inflammation. These effects increase the risk of developing several chronic and life-threatening diseases. Adapted from Gleeson et al. (2011).*

Exercise has anti-inflammatory effects and therefore, in the long-term, regular physical activity can protect against the development of these chronic diseases as well as having other benefits for health, functional capacity, and quality of life which are summarized in table 9.2. Furthermore, exercise can be used as a treatment for (or to ameliorate the symptoms of) many of these conditions, an insight which is increasingly being promoted as "exercise is medicine".

Obviously exercise increases energy expenditure and burns off some of the body fat that would otherwise accumulate when individuals eat more dietary energy than they need. In that simple sense, exercise reduces the risk of becoming overweight or obese. Regular exercise also imbues cardiovascular health benefits by improving the blood lipid profile, by decreasing the concentration of plasma triglycerides and LDL particles, and by increasing the concentration of protective HDL particles. These beneficial alterations in plasma lipids are presumed to limit the development of atherosclerosis. However, the protective effect of a physically active lifestyle against chronic inflammation associated diseases may, to some extent, be ascribed to an anti-inflammatory effect of exercise. This may be mediated not only via increased fat burning and a reduction in visceral fat mass (with a subsequent decreased production and release of adipokines) but also by induction of an anti-inflammatory environment with each bout of exercise. These benefits of exercise are depicted in figure 9.2.

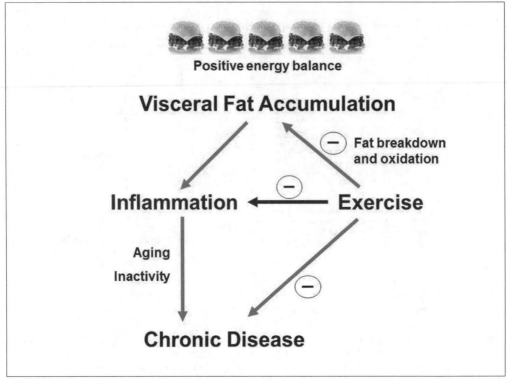

Figure 9.2: How exercise helps to prevent chronic diseases. Exercise promotes fat breakdown and oxidation which reduces visceral fat mass. Exercise also inhibits inflammation and via these mechanisms helps to prevent the development of chronic diseases.

WHAT ARE THE ANTI-INFLAMMATORY MECHANISMS OF EXERCISE?

The anti-inflammatory effects of exercise have mostly been ascribed to two possible mechanisms:

1. increased production and release of anti-inflammatory cytokines and in particular **interleukin** 6 (IL-6) from contracting skeletal muscle and

2. reduced expression of toll-like receptors (TLRs) on the cell surface of monocytes and macrophages, which are important in the initiation of inflammation.

However, the anti-inflammatory effects of exercise arise not only from these two mechanisms but also other effects of exercise that recently have been established, such as the inhibition of monocyte/macrophage infiltration into adipose tissue, switching of macrophages within adipose tissue from a pro-inflammatory subtype (the M1 macrophage) to a less inflammatory subtype (the

M2 macrophage), a reduction in the numbers of pro-inflammatory monocytes in the blood, and an increase the circulating numbers of interleukin-10 (IL-10) secreting regulatory T lymphocytes which play a role in dampening inflammation. These mechanisms are summarized in figure 9.3.

During exercise, the active skeletal muscle increases cellular and circulating levels of IL-6, which appears to be responsible for the subsequent rise in circulating levels of the anti-inflammatory cytokines IL-10 and interleukin-1 receptor antagonist (IL-1ra) and also stimulates the release of the anti-inflammatory hormone **cortisol** from the adrenal glands.

IL-1ra is secreted mainly by monocytes and macrophages and inhibits the pro-inflammatory actions of IL-1, whereas IL-10 is produced primarily by regulatory T lymphocytes and monocytes and has potent anti-inflammatory effects. Circulating levels of IL-10 are lower in obese subjects and acute treatment with IL-10 has been shown to prevent high-fat diet induced insulin resistance. IL-10 increases insulin sensitivity and protects skeletal muscle from obesity-associated macrophage infiltration; it also reduces the production of pro-inflammatory cytokines and their deleterious effects on insulin signaling and glucose metabolism.

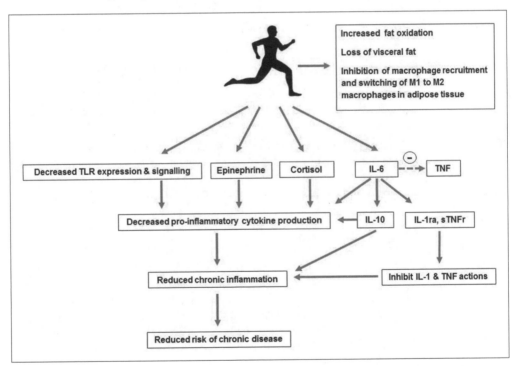

Figure 9.3 Potential mechanisms contributing to the anti-inflammatory effects of exercise. See the main text for details. Abbreviations as follows: TNF tumor necrosis factor, IL-1ra interleukin-1 receptor antagonist, IL-6 interleukin-6, IL-10 interleukin-10, M1 pro-inflammatory macrophage subtype, M2 anti-inflammatory macrophage subtype, Treg regulatory T lymphocytes (a major source of IL-10 a potent anti-inflammatory cytokine).

EXERCISE IS MEDICINE

In view of the anti-inflammatory effects of exercise described previously and the role of inflammation in the pathogenesis of disease, it is not surprising that exercise is now considered a prophylactic for preventing several major diseases as well as an effective therapy for many conditions/diseases (table 9.2).

Table 9.2: Summary of the effects of physical activity (PA) or physical fitness (PF) on disease risk and/or therapeutic value in treating diseases such as coronary heart disease (CHD)

Disease	Effects of physical activity (PA) or physical fitness (PF) on disease risk and/or therapeutic value in treating disease
Coronary heart disease	High levels of PA and PF are associated with a lower risk of developing CHD. Regular PA can favorably modify CHD risk factors including HDL/LDL ratio, hypertension, and obesity. PA improves survival in CHD patients.
Stroke	High levels of PA and PF reduce the risk of stroke.
Hypertension	PA can lower but not necessarily normalize blood pressure in hypertensive individuals.
Type 2 diabetes mellitus	High levels of PA/PF reduce risk of developing type 2 diabetes. Lifestyle interventions (diet and PA) can lower body mass, improve glucose tolerance, and reduce the risk of developing type 2 diabetes in high risk patients. In patients with type 2 diabetes, high levels of PA and PF are associated with a reduced risk of CHD and all-cause mortality.
Cancer	High levels of PA are associated with lower risk of colon and breast cancer. There is a therapeutic role for PA in preserving mobility and function in cancer patients.
Dementia	High levels of PA are associated with a lower risk of cognitive decline and dementia in older adults. PA induces modest improvements in cognition in people who are at increased risk of dementia and Alzheimer's disease.
Infections	Regular moderate PA improves some aspects of immune function and is associated with reduced incidence of respiratory infection such as the common cold. PA also improves vaccination responses in the elderly.
Other	PA enhances physical function and improves quality of life in those suffering from chronic heart failure, chronic obstructive pulmonary disease, depression, intermittent claudication (narrowing or blockage in the main arteries taking blood to the legs), osteoarthritis, and osteoporosis.

Table adapted from Gleeson et al. (2011).

Perhaps the strongest evidence for the role of exercise in disease prevention comes from randomized controlled trials evaluating the effectiveness of lifestyle intervention in preventing type 2 diabetes. These studies have demonstrated conclusively that lifestyle intervention – involving a combination of dieting and increased physical activity – is effective in preventing type 2 diabetes in groups of individuals who are at high risk of the disease because they have elevated blood glucose and/or impaired glucose tolerance as well as being overweight or obese.

A limitation of these studies is that they did not isolate the independent effects of exercise and diet in preventing type 2 diabetes but the effectiveness of exercise is supported by the finding in the 2001 Finnish Diabetes Prevention Study that among those in the intervention group who did not reach the goal of losing 5% of their initial body mass, but who achieved the goal of exercising for more than four hours per week, the risk of developing type 2 diabetes was 80% lower than in intervention participants who remained sedentary. Thus, although more needs to be learned about the role of exercise in preventing type 2 diabetes, it is clear that exercise makes a valuable contribution to an overall lifestyle package for preventing this disease.

The importance of exercise and physical fitness in reducing chronic disease risk is illustrated in figures 9.4 and 9.5. Increasing weekly exercise energy expenditure from less than 500 kcal to between 500 and 1,000 kcal decreases the risk of all-cause mortality by 23%, and there is a dose-related decrease in risk for exercise energy expenditures up to 3,500 kcal/week (figure 9.4). That is only 500 kcal per day which can be achieved by low-moderate intensity exercise such as walking, jogging, or cycling for one to two hours per day (see chapter 13 for further practical details). Figure 9.5 demonstrates that the biggest drop in all-cause mortality risk in terms of physical fitness comes from changing from being very unfit to a low-moderate level of fitness. This relatively small change, achievable through regular moderate exercise, halves the risk of all-cause mortality. In other words, it is far, far better to do some exercise than almost none at all.

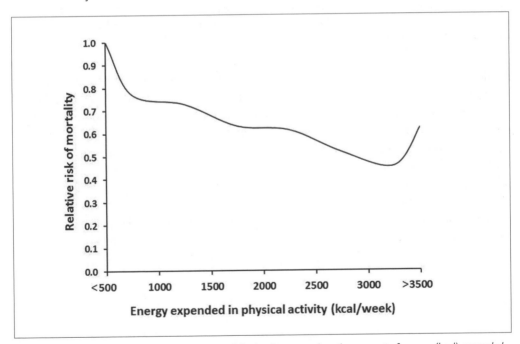

Figure 9.4: The relationship between physical activity level expressed as the amount of energy (kcal) expended in physical activity per week and the relative risk of all-cause mortality (mainly cardiovascular diseases, metabolic diseases, and cancer). Data from Paffenbarger et al. (1986).

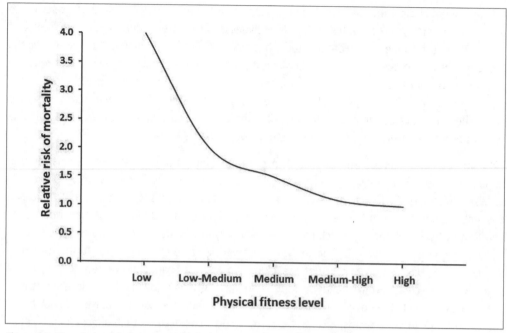

Figure 9.5: The relationship between physical fitness level (based on exercise test estimates of aerobic capacity) and the relative risk of all-cause mortality (mainly cardiovascular diseases, metabolic diseases and cancer). Data from Blair et al. (1989).

In addition, exercise appears to have major benefits for the treatment of type 2 diabetes. The findings of one non-randomized study (The 1991 Malmö Feasibility Study) showed that 54% of participants with early stage type 2 diabetes were in remission by the end of a 5-year diet and exercise intervention. Aside from its role in preventing and treating type 2 diabetes, there is good evidence that exercise is effective in preventing several other major diseases particularly cardiovascular disease, breast cancer, and colon cancer, and there is some evidence to support a role of exercise in preventing dementia. Moreover, while exercise should not be considered a panacea, there is evidence to support a role for exercise as a therapy for many diseases/ conditions beyond those mentioned previously including chronic obstructive pulmonary disease, chronic kidney disease, asthma, and osteoporosis.

EXERCISE AND BONE HEALTH

Our bones are living tissue and are constantly being remodeled. For the first 20-25 years of our lives, our bones continue to develop and strengthen. Our bones are most dense, and peak bone mass is attained in our late 20s – called peak bone mass. Every day some of our bone cells begin to dissolve bone matrix (resorption), while new bone cells deposit osteoid (formation); this process is known as remodeling. After the age of 30, our bones gradually lose mass and become less dense. In women this process accelerates after menopause as estrogen – a sex steroid hormone secreted by the ovaries that promotes bone formation – stops being produced. Bone mass and density are higher in men and are better maintained with aging because the production of testosterone – the male sex steroid hormone that promotes bone formation as well as sperm production – declines only slightly with aging. Osteoporosis, which literally means porous bone, is a disease in which the density and quality of bone are reduced and is far more common in elderly women. In this condition, the rate of bone loss outpaces the growth of new bone, so the bones become more porous and fragile, and the risk of fracture is greatly increased. The loss of bone generally occurs gradually with no obvious symptoms and may only be identified when the first fracture occurs and an X-ray or bone density scan (called a **DEXA** scan) is carried out. Worldwide, one in three women and one in five men are at risk of an osteoporotic fracture. The most common fractures associated with osteoporosis occur at the hip, spine, and wrist, and the risk of these fractures occurring increases with age in both women and men.

Of particular concern are vertebral (spinal) and hip fractures. Vertebral fractures can result in serious consequences, including intense back pain, limited mobility, and deformity. A hip fracture often requires surgery and may result in several months of limited mobility. Among the frail elderly, such events can result in loss of independence or premature death. Genetic factors play a significant role in determining whether an individual is at heightened risk of osteoporosis. However, lifestyle factors such as diet (particularly protein, calcium, and vitamin D intakes) and physical activity also influence bone development in youth and the rate of bone loss later in life.

After the age of about 30, the gradual thinning of bone is a natural process and cannot be completely stopped. However, the thicker your bones, the less likely they are to become thin enough to break as you reach your 60s or 70s. Young women in particular need to be aware of their osteoporosis risk and take steps to slow its progress and prevent fractures. Building strong bones starts during early childhood and essentially the prevention of osteoporosis begins with optimal bone growth and development in childhood and adolescence. It is estimated that a 10% increase of peak bone mass in children reduces the risk of an osteoporotic fracture during adult life by 50%. The sidebar explains how we can maximize bone mass during our childhood and teenage years.

How to Maximize Bone Mass During Youth

- Ensure a nutritious diet with adequate calcium intake.

- Avoid protein malnutrition and under-nutrition in general.

- Ensure an adequate supply of vitamin D through sufficient sun exposure and diet.

- Participate in regular physical activity, particularly weight-bearing activity such as walking, running, and jumping.

- Do not smoke and try to avoid the effects of second-hand smoking.

Adults should do the same but in addition should:

- Avoid under-nutrition, particularly the effects of severe weight loss diets and eating disorders.

- Maintain an adequate supply of vitamin D, and take a daily 1,000 IU vitamin D3 supplement in the winter months.

- Participate in weight-bearing activity at least 30 minutes per day and three days per week.

- Avoid heavy drinking of alcoholic beverages.

One safe way to prevent fractures is to positively affect bone mass and strength through mechanical stimuli. Lack of physical activity means a lack of mechanical stimuli which causes a rapid and substantial loss of bone mass. This may be particularly pronounced during periods of limb immobilization due to an injury or prolonged bed rest due to illness. Weight-bearing physical activity such as walking, running, and jumping, on the other hand, results in increased bone mineral content and density (these are known to be about 20% higher in the loaded bone regions of athletes). In general, high magnitude mechanical loads (as with jumping or skipping), as well as loads applied at high frequency (like running) are known to increase bone mass, while lower impact activities (like walking and cycling) have less effect on bone, even when applied for a longer duration. Unfortunately, exercise at a high intensity might be difficult for elderly people at risk of fractures, and the key may lie in building a sufficient "reserve" of bone mass at a young age. Indeed, bone mass at the age of 70 largely depends on peak bone mass reached before the age of 30. During growth, both high impact activity and low impact activity contribute to bone health. High impact physical activity in childhood, especially when initiated before puberty, results in increased bone width and increased bone mineral content in young girls and adolescent females. The mechanical loading of bones through exercise benefits bone mass at a later age as well as in our youth.

Besides daily physical activity, a healthy diet is among the most commonly advocated lifestyle measures to improve (skeletal) health. Guidance for the management of osteoporosis in postmenopausal women recommends a daily intake of at least 1000 mg/day for calcium, 800 IU/day for vitamin D, and one gram of protein per kilogram body weight for all women aged over 50.

EXERCISE AND MENTAL HEALTH

Regular exercise is known to be associated with benefits to mental health including a reduced incidence of depression, improved cognitive function in the elderly, and a reduced risk of developing dementia. Recent research has shown that regular moderate exercise improves mental health, but overdoing it does more harm than good. In 2018, a study of 1.2 million people in the US found those who exercised were stressed and depressed on fewer days than those who did not. Participants were asked about their physical activity habits and were also asked to estimate how many days in the past 30 they would rate their mental health as "not good" based on stress, depression, and emotional problems. The study findings revealed that exercising for 45 minutes three to five times a week was associated with the biggest benefits, and even doing household chores or some gardening cut the time spent depressed by 10%. Regular moderate exercise was associated with a lower mental health burden across people no matter what their age, race, gender, household income, and education level. The scientists found that team sports reduced the time spent in poor mental health by 22%, cycling by 21%, and going to the gym by 20%. Jogging resulted in a 19% reduction and walking 18%.

However, there was a threshold beyond which the benefits began to be reversed. Those who did the most exercise – more than five times a week or more than three hours a day – actually had worse mental health than those who did nothing at all. The researchers ascribed this effect to a problem of being 'addicted' to exercise to the extent where it starts to impact other aspects of life – like foregoing family and social activities because of the time needed to devote to exercise using up too much of people's spare time outside of work. In contrast, the mental health benefits of moderate participation in sport, and particularly team sports or exercising with others, could indicate that social activities promote resilience and reduce depression by reducing social withdrawal and isolation.

HOW MUCH EXERCISE DO I NEED TO GET HEALTH BENEFITS?

As explained previously, regular exercise reduces the risk of chronic metabolic and cardio-respiratory diseases, in part because exercise exerts anti-inflammatory effects. But how much exercise is needed to get these health benefits? Well, the good news is that the biggest reduction in chronic disease risk is between those who do no exercise whatsoever and those who do some exercise amounting to about 30 minutes of light-moderate intensity on a minimum of three days per week. Further improvements in health markers and reduced disease risk will come by doing more exercise than this, and a good target to aim for is about 60 minutes of moderate intensity exercise at least five days per week. Beyond that, the benefits become increasingly smaller and doing too much exercise can result in fatigue with an increased risk of injury and illness as well as potentially interfering with other social activities. If moderate intensity exercise such as jogging or aerobics is too hard for you, then you can achieve the same amount of work by exercising at a lower intensity (e.g., walking) for longer. If using a pedometer, you can aim for a target of 10,000 steps per day which is equivalent to about 4.5 miles (7 km) and will expend about 500 kcal (2.1 MJ) per day. The health benefits and improvements to your fitness will be better if you exercise at moderate rather than low intensity and brisk walking is better than a gentle stroll (see the sidebar), but always remember that doing some physical activity is far, far better than doing nothing at all. Besides, the more exercise you do, the fitter you become, and the exercise then feels easier than before. So, it's a win-win situation!

How Do I Know If I Am Walking at a "Brisk Pace"?

It is often mentioned that walking at a "brisk pace" is very good for getting the health benefits of exercise and is better than walking at a slow pace. While this is certainly true, what does a "brisk pace" actually mean? Obviously, the actual distance covered in a certain amount of time (say one hour) depends on a person's stride length and the stride rate or cadence (steps per minute), so the actual speed for brisk walking will be different for a tall person with long strides than for a shorter person with smaller strides when their stride rate is the same. The Centers for Disease Control and Prevention advice indicates that brisk walking is movement that calls for heavy breathing, so although you may be able to roughly approximate a brisk pace by asking "Am I getting a little breathless?" or "Am I moving faster than a leisurely stroll?", how do you really know if you're walking at what's considered a "brisk pace" without the use of scientific equipment to measure something like your rate of oxygen uptake? Well, a new review of research published in 2018 in the British Journal of Sports Medicine found that a cadence of about 100 steps per minute indicated a moderately intense brisk walk for most adults. Of course, you don't need to be at exactly 100 — some people might be at 95, others 105 — but close to 100 steps per minute constitutes a brisk walk, the research suggests, regardless of age, fitness or athletic ability. So, if this is what you want to achieve, the next time you're on a walk, take 20 seconds to mentally count how many steps you take, and then multiply that number by three to get your step count per minute. Obviously to be walking at 100 steps per minute you need to be completing about 33 steps every 20 seconds.

Pregnant women are often concerned about the sort of exercise they can do during the nine months that they are carrying a baby. The good news is that there are many forms of exercise that can still be undertaken with minimal risk to the health of the mother and her developing baby. For example, it is fine to take walks, participate in low impact aerobics, and dance or swim. But some exercises are not a good idea when you're pregnant. Knowing the difference can help keep you and your growing baby safe. See the sidebar for further details.

How Much Exercise Should I Get During Pregnancy?

You've probably heard about the benefits of exercising during pregnancy: your sleep quality and mood are usually better, and you will improve or at least maintain your strength and endurance. Regular exercise can also reduce back pain, ease constipation, and may decrease your risk of **pre-eclampsia**. The official advice of the American College of Obstetricians and Gynecologists is to aim for at least 20 to 30 minutes of some sort of physical activity every day of the week, right up until delivery. If that sounds somewhat daunting, bear in mind that all forms of physical activity count, including housework and walking. And those 30 minutes don't need to be done all at once; you can spread your exercise into five or six short sessions over the course of the day.

What exercises should I avoid when I'm pregnant?

There are plenty of exercises that are great for pregnant women. In fact, most physical activity is perfectly safe during pregnancy provided that you are healthy, and you have no complications during your pregnancy. But you have to make a few changes, be sensible, and realize that you should not exercise as hard or long as you might normally do. An hour of moderate intensity exercise per day is a reasonable upper limit to aim for. There are also a few exercises you should avoid:

- Sports that carry a higher risk of falling or abdominal injury, like gymnastics, downhill skiing, snowboarding, ice-skating, vigorous racket sports (squash or singles tennis), horseback riding, off-road cycling, contact sports (such as judo, boxing, ice hockey, soccer, or basketball), bungee jumping, and rollerblading.

- Exercising at high altitude. Unless you're living at high altitude already (and therefore well adapted to the conditions), avoid any activity that takes you up more than 2,000 meters. Sky diving is an obvious no-no.

- Scuba diving, which poses a risk of decompression sickness for your baby.

- Exercises that involve lying flat on your back for long periods of time after the first trimester, since the weight of your enlarging uterus could compress major blood vessels and restrict circulation to you and your baby.

- Exercise involving abdominal moves, like full sit-ups or double leg lifts, can pull on the abdomen, so they're best avoided altogether.

- Jumping, bouncing, and sudden, jerky motions are best avoided because your joints get looser during pregnancy, which can increase your risk of injury. So, cut out any high-impact aerobics or trampolining.

- Excessive or bouncy stretching as your ligaments are already looser than normal which increases the risk of injury. If something hurts, stop.

- Back bends or other contortions, as well as movements that involve deep flexion or extension of joints (like deep knee bends), can increase your risk of injury.

- Any activity that requires you to hold your breath (such as diving or swimming underwater) should be avoided, as both you and your baby need an uninterrupted flow of oxygen.

- Any exercise or environment that raises your body temperature more than 1°C (1.5°F) should be avoided, since it causes blood to be shunted away from your uterus and is redirected to your skin as your body attempts to increase heat loss. That means avoiding high intensity exercise, exercise in hot weather, and staying out of saunas and hot tubs.

Other considerations

- Avoid overexertion that makes you feel exhausted or dehydrated because dehydration is a risk factor for preterm birth, and there is a risk of not enough oxygen getting to your baby if you end up short of breath for long periods. That's why it's more important than ever to learn to listen to your body during pregnancy. Many experts recommend using what's known as the "Rating of Perceived Exertion" scale. Think of a scale that goes up from 1 to 10, where at 3 you're walking slowly and at 10 you're working out as hard as you can. Your goal is to keep your exertion rate between 5 and 6 on that scale, or at a somewhat hard rate but not so hard that you get out of breath or sweat profusely.

- Certain conditions can make exercise during pregnancy riskier. These conditions include anemia (which reduces the capacity of your blood to carry oxygen), chronic bronchitis (which causes difficulty breathing), poorly controlled diabetes (which causes wide variations in blood sugar), hypertension (because most forms of exercise will acutely raise your systolic blood pressure even higher), and being either obese (BMI of 30 kg/m² or more), or extremely underweight (BMI under 15 kg/m²). If you suffer from these or any other medical conditions, you may have to restrict your exercise during pregnancy. Check with your doctor before starting any exercise program.

- Most women feel tired in the third trimester, so it's not surprising if you feel your body is telling you to stop exercising and get some rest. Certainly, if you experience excessive fatigue, irritability, joint or muscle pain, or trouble sleeping, take these symptoms as a sign that you should be cutting back on your exercise routine. However, do try to remember that the right kind of prenatal exercise can actually give you a much-needed physical and mental health boost. You can also consider doing some kinder, gentler forms of exercise in the third trimester such as a yoga class, tai chi, a leisurely swim in the pool, or just practicing the breathing techniques you'll soon need.

INFLUENCE OF EXERCISE ON RISK OF INFECTIONS

We all suffer from colds at some time, but research indicates that a person's level of physical activity influences their risk of respiratory tract infections, most likely by affecting immune function. Moderate levels of regular exercise appear to reduce our susceptibility to illness compared with a sedentary lifestyle, but long hard bouts of exercise and periods of intensified training put endurance athletes and exercise addicts at increased risk of colds and flu.

Infections of the nose, throat, windpipe (trachea), or the two airways that branch from the trachea as it reaches the lungs (bronchi) are the most common infections that people get. These upper respiratory tract infections **(URTIs)** include the common cold, bronchitis, sinusitis, and tonsillitis, and most are due to an infection with a virus. The average adult has two to three URTIs each year, and young children have twice as many. We are constantly exposed to the viruses that cause these infections, but some people seem more susceptible to catching URTIs than others. Every day our immune system protects us from an army of pathogenic microbes that bombard the body. Immune function is influenced by an individual's genetic make-up as well other external factors such as stress, poor nutrition, lack of sleep, the normal aging process, lack of exercise, or excessive amounts of exercise. These factors can suppress the immune system making a person more vulnerable to infection.

The good news is that researchers have found a link between moderate regular exercise and reduced frequency of URTIs compared with a sedentary lifestyle. A study carried out over one year in over 500 adults found that participating in one to two hours of moderate exercise per day was associated with a one third reduction in the risk of getting a URTI compared with individuals that had a sedentary lifestyle. It appears that when about 40 minutes of moderate exercise is repeated on an almost daily basis, there is a cumulative effect that leads to a long-term improvement in immune response. In another study which examined the number of illness days reported by over 1,000 US adult participants during a 12-week period in the fall and winter months, the researchers reported that people who exercise two or more days per week have half as many sick days due to colds or flu as those who don't exercise. Other factors that were found to reduce infection risk included a high intake of fruit, being married, having a moderate or high level of fitness, and having a low level of mental stress. Interestingly, females reported 30% more sick days than men.

It seems though that more is not always better in terms of exercise volume, as other studies have reported a two- to six-fold increase in risk of developing an URTI in the weeks following marathon (42.2 km) and ultra-marathon (90 km) races. This is due in part to the anti-inflammatory effect of exercise and increased levels of stress hormones like **epinephrine** and cortisol which suppress white blood cell functions.

Key Points

- Exercise leads to adaptations that eventually result in improved physiological function. Exercise training makes use of this principle by planning and systematically applying exercise activities with the goal of optimizing these adaptations and thus improving fitness and performance.

- Adaptations to exercise or exercise training are specific to the exercise performed. Resistance exercise training results in muscle hypertrophy, making the muscle stronger, and endurance training results in increased oxidative capacity, making the muscle more fatigue resistant.

- Training adaptations in skeletal muscle may be generated by the cumulative effects of transient increases in gene transcription and altered protein synthesis during recovery from repeated bouts of exercise.

- The complex process of exercise-induced adaptation in skeletal muscle starts with specific molecular events that trigger an increase in protein synthesis. Signaling mechanisms triggered by exercise stress initiate replication of **deoxyribonucleic acid (DNA)** genetic sequences that enable subsequent translation of the genetic code into a series of amino acids to synthesize new proteins.

- Exercise results in an increase in the circulating and tissue levels of numerous cytokines; the production and/or release of some cytokines (notably IL-6) are increased when muscle glycogen content is depleted.

- IL-6 appears to act in a hormone-like manner and is involved in increasing substrate mobilization (release of glucose from the liver and fatty acids from adipose tissue) during prolonged exercise. IL-6 also induces secretion of cortisol, IL-1ra, and IL-10 and so has generally anti-inflammatory effects.

- Regular exercise reduces the risk of chronic metabolic and cardio-respiratory diseases, in part because exercise exerts anti-inflammatory effects.

- The health benefits of regular exercise may be mediated via a reduction in visceral fat mass (with a subsequent decreased release of pro-inflammatory adipokines) as well as the induction of an anti-inflammatory environment with each bout of exercise. Regular exercise also results in an improved blood lipid profile (lower plasma triglyceride and an increased HDL/LDL ratio).

- Various mechanisms may contribute to the anti-inflammatory effects of exercise, including increased release of IL-6 from working skeletal muscle, increased release of cortisol and epinephrine from the adrenal glands, reduced expression of TLRs on monocytes/macrophages, inhibition of monocyte/macrophage infiltration into adipose tissue, switching of macrophages to a less inflammatory subtype within adipose tissue, a reduction in the circulating numbers of pro-inflammatory monocytes, and an increase the circulating numbers of regulatory T lymphocytes.

- The minimum recommended amount of exercise to get significant health benefits is about 30 minutes of light-moderate intensity on a minimum of three days per week. Further improvements in health markers and reduced disease risk will come by doing more exercise than this, and a good target is about 45-60 minutes of moderate intensity exercise on four or five days per week. Beyond that, the benefits become increasingly smaller, and with some, aspects of mental health may be reversed. Doing too much exercise can also result in fatigue with an increased risk of injury and illness.

- Weight-bearing exercise together with adequate nutrition (particularly calcium, vitamin D, and protein) promote bone development and increase bone density, which helps to prevent osteoporosis in later life, a particular risk for postmenopausal women.

- Regular exercise is known to be associated with benefits to mental health including a reduced incidence of depression, improved cognitive function in the elderly, and a reduced risk of developing dementia.

- The anti-inflammatory effects of exercise are also likely to be responsible for depressed immunity that makes the elite endurance athlete more susceptible to common infections when training volumes are extremely high. This should not be a concern for recreationally active people, as regular moderate exercise actually improves immune function and reduces the risks of infectious illnesses such as the common cold and influenza.

Chapter 10

The Importance of Sleep and How to Sleep Well

Objectives

After studying this chapter, you should:

- Understand the causes and consequences of insomnia

- Know how much sleep we need

- Understand how our diet can influence how we sleep

- Understand how sleep quality can influence what we eat and our risk of chronic disease

- Appreciate that sleep quality can influence our susceptibility to the common cold

- Know how you can improve your sleep quality

Everyone knows that diet and exercise have important influences on our health, but sleep is often ignored. We spend more hours in bed than we do eating or exercising, so it should not come as a big surprise that the amount and quality of sleep we get can influence our quality of life, mood, mental state, and general heath (photo 10.1). Sleeping well means sleeping long enough (at least seven hours is the general recommendation) and sleeping soundly with few awakenings during the night, so that you feel refreshed on waking in the morning.

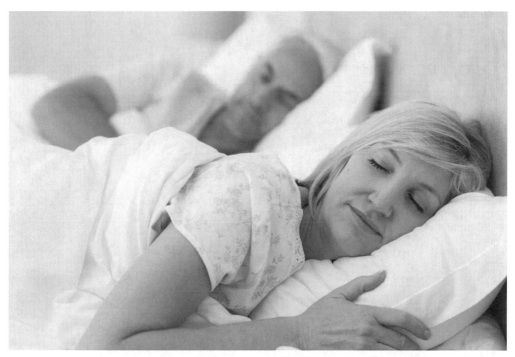

Photo 10.1: It is now recognized that getting enough good quality sleep is an important factor that helps to maintain our quality of life, mood, mental state, and general heath.

THE PROBLEM OF INSOMNIA

Habitual lack of sleep or poor sleep quality (e.g., frequently waking up during the night) is called **insomnia** and is linked to poor mood, increased use of health care resources, decreased quality of life, and increased risk of both infectious illness and chronic disease. Not getting enough sleep means that we do not feel refreshed in the morning, and consequently we feel more tired and listless throughout the day. It is a common problem thought to regularly affect around one in every four people in the USA and Europe and is particularly common in adolescents and the elderly. Studies have also shown that poor sleep results in increases in circulating stress hormone (cortisol and epinephrine) levels, decreased immunity, and increased markers of sympathetic nervous activity in both sleep-deprived healthy subjects and those with chronic insomnia. The medical literature shows that people who complain of chronic insomnia and shortened sleep have an increased incidence of type 2 diabetes, hypertension, and cardiovascular disease. They are also more susceptible to infectious illnesses such as the common cold.

If you have insomnia, you may:

- Find it difficult to fall asleep.

- Lie awake for long periods at night.

- Wake up several times during the night.

- Wake up too early in the morning and not be able to get back to sleep.

- Not feel refreshed when you get up.

- Find it hard to nap during the day, despite feeling tired.

- Feel tired and irritable during the day and have difficulty concentrating.

- Be prone to picking up upper respiratory tract infections.

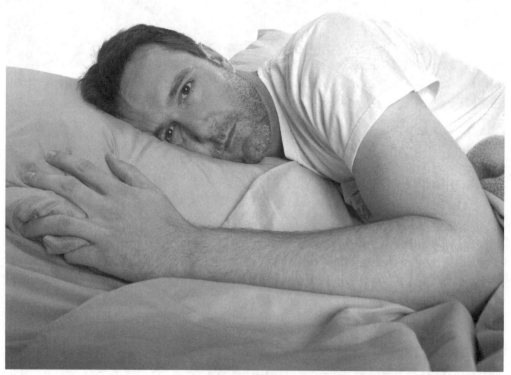

Photo 10.2: Habitual lack of sleep or poor sleep quality (insomnia) is linked to poor mood, decreased quality of life, and increased risk of both infectious illness and chronic disease.

How Much Sleep Do I Actually Need?

There are no official guidelines about how much sleep you should get each night because everyone is different. How much sleep we need and want is influenced by our genetics which explains why some people are "night owls" and some are "early birds". Some people seem to be able to cope well with as little as five hours of sleep per night but on average, a "normal" amount of sleep for an adult is considered to be between seven and nine hours per night. Babies and young children may sleep for much longer than this, whereas older adults may sleep somewhat less. What's important is whether you feel you get enough sleep such that you don't feel tired or lethargic during the daytime, and whether your sleep is good quality and you feel refreshed after waking in the morning. You're probably not getting enough good-quality sleep if you constantly feel tired throughout the day, and it's affecting your mood and ability to carry out the tasks of everyday life.

WHAT CAUSES INSOMNIA?

It's not always clear what triggers insomnia, but in otherwise healthy people it is often associated with:

- Stress and anxiety.

- A poor sleeping environment – such as an uncomfortable bed, or a bedroom that's too light, noisy, damp, hot, or cold.

- Lifestyle factors – such as jet lag, exercising hard, or working rather than relaxing in the evening.

- Watching television, looking at your phone or tablet, or playing computer games before bedtime.

- Sleeping during the day.

- Drinking alcohol or caffeine, smoking, or eating a heavy meal just before going to bed.

- A poor diet and/or micronutrient deficiencies.

Of course, there can be other reasons for not sleeping well during certain periods of your life. One of the major reasons can be who you sleep with! For example, you may start living with a partner who snores loudly or suffers themselves from insomnia. You might have a baby that cries a lot during the night, or you might have a partner who has some activities in mind other than sleep when you go to bed! You need to talk through these sorts of issues with your partner. For example, there are some suggested remedies to help people to stop snoring such as those described on the HelpGuide website **(https://www.helpguide.org/articles/sleep/snoring-tips-to-help-you-and-your-partner-sleep-better.htm)**. And bear in mind that while sexual intercourse may extend the time before you get to sleep, you should feel more relaxed afterwards and so may actually sleep better!

DIET AND SLEEP

A simple truth is what we eat can affect our sleep, and how we sleep can affect our food intake. The quality of the diet and the consumption of certain foods and nutrients can influence regulatory hormonal pathways that can alter both the quantity and quality of sleep. In turn, the amount of sleep we get and its quality influence the intake of total energy, as well as of specific foods and nutrients, through both physiological and behavioral mechanisms. Research in this field has examined the effects of both short and long sleep duration on patterns of food intake and nutritional quality. The latest evidence suggests that extremes of sleep duration (too little or too much) alter circulating hormone levels and circadian rhythms, which contribute to weight gain and other risk factors for the development of chronic disease such as type 2 diabetes and cardiovascular disease. These influences may begin in childhood and have impacts throughout the course of our lives.

HOW WHAT WE EAT CAN INFLUENCE OUR SLEEP

The composition of the diet influences our sleep duration, quality and behaviors. For example, diets that are low in fiber content, high in saturated fat, or high in sugar are all associated with lighter, less restorative sleep, over an ad libitum (eat what you like) diet. A high-carbohydrate/low-fat diet has been associated with poorer sleep quality compared with a normal balanced diet or a low-carbohydrate/high-fat diet. Deficiencies of total energy, protein, and carbohydrate have also been shown to be associated with shorter sleep duration. In contrast, one study reported that consuming high-glycemic index carbohydrate meals (that is meals that cause a rapid spike in the blood sugar concentration) about four hours before bedtime decreased the time it took to fall asleep after going to bed. This effect was attributed to a decreased plasma fatty acid concentration and a consequent increase in circulating free tryptophan after carbohydrate consumption. Tryptophan is an essential amino acid that is the precursor of the sleep-regulating hormone serotonin and is thought to be important in the proposed relationships between diet and sleep. Increases in tryptophan intake via protein ingestion in the evening have been shown to improve sleep in adults with sleep disturbances and result in enhanced alertness in the morning, most likely as a result of improved sleep quality.

Deficiencies of certain micronutrients have also been suggested to affect sleep duration and quality. For example, deficiencies of the vitamins folate and thiamin, as well as the minerals iron, magnesium, phosphorus, selenium, and zinc are associated with shorter sleep duration. Furthermore, lack of selenium and calcium make it more difficult to fall asleep and low intakes of vitamin D and lycopene (an antioxidant phytonutrient found in fruits and vegetables) impair our ability to stay soundly asleep. In contrast, the ingestion of certain micronutrients in non-deficient individuals appears to improve sleep quality. For, example, nightly intake of a magnesium or zinc supplement improved sleep quality in long-term care facility residents with insomnia, and in healthy subjects, zinc-rich foods improved sleep onset latency (i.e., shortened the time it takes to fall asleep after going to bed and turning off the lights) and increased **sleep efficiency** (i.e., fewer awakenings) compared with placebo. One study found that people who reported the healthiest sleep patterns also had the most varied diets, and based on this, the phrase "eat crappy, sleep crappy" has arisen!

Intake of beverages or foods containing chemical stimulants has negative effects on sleep quality. Caffeine (in coffee and some soft drinks) and theobromine (in tea) interfere with the actions of adenosine, a hormone that regulates sleep–wake cycles. The ingestion of caffeine or theobromine before bedtime alters sleep patterns for many hours, including making it harder to go to sleep, reducing total sleep time, and worsening perceived sleep quality. In addition, alcohol, although often regarded as a sedative, actually has a mixed impact on sleep. Imbibing alcoholic drinks tends to make falling asleep easier but may disrupt sleep later in the night due to its ability to influence levels of brain neurotransmitters including serotonin and norepinephrine.

It should be fairly obvious that we should avoid drinking large volumes of fluid (including plain water) in the hour before bedtime, otherwise we will feel the need to urinate during the night which will interrupt our sleep. Urine production is usually at its highest about one hour after consuming a large volume of water, so it is best to have your last drink a few hours before bedtime and visit the toilet just before going to bed. A cup (about 200 mL) of water or milk just before bedtime should be OK, but larger volumes than this should be avoided.

The consumption of certain whole foods in the hours before bedtime can also affect sleep quantity and quality. For example, consumption of cherries, kiwi fruits, milk, and oily fish have each been associated with beneficial effects on sleep quality. Some of these foods have a relatively high content of tryptophan, and this may be responsible for their sleep promoting effects. The intake of bread, pulses, fish, and shellfish appear to extend sleep duration. So, what we eat and drink, particularly in the last meal before bedtime can influence our sleep quantity and quality.

HOW SLEEP CAN INFLUENCE WHAT WE EAT AND OUR RISK OF CHRONIC DISEASE

Research suggests that both short (less than seven hours) and long (more than nine hours) sleep duration can influence the risk of several chronic diseases as illustrated in figure 10.1 for type 2 diabetes, and figure 10.2 for cardiovascular disease, and all-cause mortality. Short sleep duration has received more attention and has been shown to be associated with an increased risk of obesity, type 2 diabetes, and cardiovascular disease, particularly among women. It has been suggested that this is due to interference with the body's restorative processes that occur during sleep, leading to biological and behavioral (including food choice) factors that increase our risk for chronic disease development.

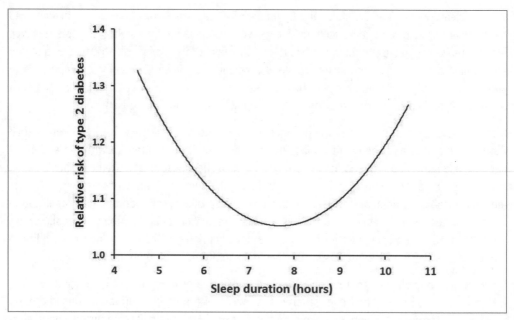

Figure 10.1: Association between sleep duration and relative risk of type 2 diabetes. Data from Shan et al. (2015).

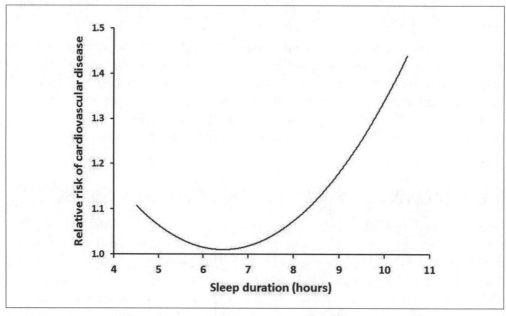

Figure 10.2: Relationship of sleep duration between all-cause mortality and cardiovascular events. Data from Yin et al. (2017).

Sleep influences the circulating levels of the appetite controlling hormones ghrelin and leptin. As explained in chapter 6, ghrelin stimulates hunger, and leptin signals satiety. Sleep deprivation or insomnia causes relatively high levels of ghrelin and low levels of leptin which would be predicted to increase appetite and induce overeating behaviors. Furthermore, circulating levels of adiponectin (an anti-inflammatory chemical secreted from adipose tissue that is found in lower levels in the plasma of individuals with obesity) were found to decrease following sleep restriction in Caucasian women and may be another mechanism by which reduced sleep duration promotes cardiovascular risk in this population. As explained in chapter 9, the development of chronic low-grade inflammation is a major risk factor for chronic metabolic and cardiovascular diseases.

Sleep loss, short sleep duration, and complaints of sleep disturbance are associated with increases in inflammation, which are thought to be due to the effects of sleep disruption on sympathetic nervous system activity that promotes inflammatory gene expression. This may be one of the mechanisms by which poor sleep quality and quantity put us at increased risk for cardiovascular disease and cancer.

Sleep deprivation is also associated with increased appetite and a higher motivation to consume energy-dense foods that are high in fat and sugar, leading to increased energy intakes and potential weight gain. But that is not all. Having only a short sleep time increases the opportunities for eating, and can induce psychological distress, greater sensitivity to food reward, and disinhibited eating. We tend to eat more for these reasons and because we need more energy to sustain extended wakefulness. Indeed, people who complain of short sleep duration are more prone to having irregular eating patterns, including more frequent consumption of energy-dense snacks outside of regular mealtimes, and higher total energy and fat intake. Other studies suggest that weight loss and weight maintenance through diet and lifestyle interventions can contribute to improvements in sleep quality.

It will come as no surprise to many parents that adolescents are at particularly high risk for short sleep duration, and the highest prevalence of insufficient sleep (69%) is reported for this age group. Their high use of electronic devices (television, computers, game stations, phones, tablets, etc.) as well as a tendency for unhealthy eating are among the behavioral risk factors that may account for this. In a recent large-scale survey in the USA, one in four adolescents reported using an electronic device "constantly", and 72% reported taking their mobile phones into their bedrooms and using them while trying to fall asleep!

In addition, another study showed that adolescents with short sleep duration eat significantly fewer servings of fruits and vegetables and are more likely to consume fast food items, compared with adolescents who sleep for eight hours per night. The combination of short sleep duration and poor-quality food consumption among adolescents may contribute to an increased chronic disease later in life. In fact, lack of sleep in adolescents is now known to be associated with a higher risk for obesity, decreased insulin sensitivity (predisposing to type 2 diabetes), and high blood pressure.

In recent years, evidence has emerged indicating that overlong sleep duration, usually defined as more than nine hours of sleep, is also associated with higher risk of type 2 diabetes, obesity, cardiovascular disease, chronic kidney disease, and depression although at present the mechanisms for these relationships are not clear. It may be that long sleep duration is actually associated with more sleep disruptions and indeed, the coexistence of poor sleep quality and longer sleep duration were shown to be associated with a higher incidence of coronary heart disease in one study. In summary, current evidence suggests that particularly short or long sleep durations are predictors of increased risk for unhealthy eating and the subsequent development of several chronic metabolic and cardiovascular diseases.

HOW SLEEP CAN INFLUENCE OUR RISK OF INFECTIONS

Sleep duration and quality also influence our risk of picking up infections such as the common cold because sleep affects immunity. Sleep deprivation and disturbance of sleep impair adaptive immunity, and this impairment is associated with reduced response to vaccines and increased susceptibility to infectious disease. Poor quality sleep and prolonged sleep deprivation induce a stress response that results in increases of cortisol and sympathetic nervous activity and decreased growth hormone secretion which are likely responsible for the link between sleep disturbance and reduced antiviral immune responses. Both an inadequate amount of nightly sleep and poor sleep quality have been shown to increase the risk of developing common cold symptoms when subjects are experimentally exposed to a dose of human rhinovirus in a nasal spray as illustrated in figure 10.3.

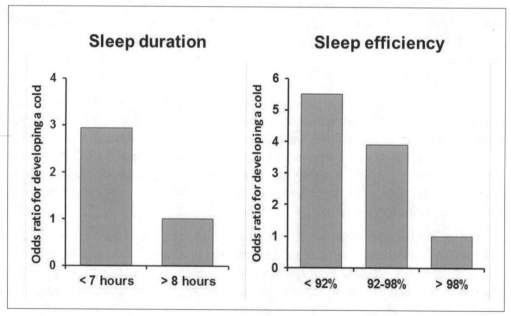

Figure 10.3: Lower sleep duration and efficiency (% time in bed asleep) are associated with increased risk of developing a cold following rhinovirus exposure via a nasal spray (< less than; > more than). Data from Cohen et al. (2009).

HOW TO BEAT INSOMNIA AND IMPROVE YOUR SLEEP QUALITY

The influence of poor sleep quality on various aspects of our health is summarized in figure 10.4.

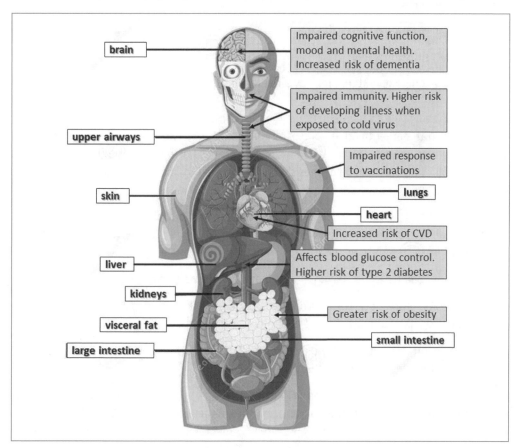

Figure 10.4: The impact of poor sleep quality on various aspects of our health

Although it is becoming increasingly clear that poor sleep quality has negative impacts on eating behavior and long-term health, there are very few official sleep recommendations available to guide health professionals and the general population. Although the *Dietary Guidelines for Americans* (2015-2020) include recommendations about physical activity and other aspects of a healthy lifestyle, they currently do not include recommendations on how to ensure sufficient sleep, and do not mention the relationship between sleep and diet. However, in the USA, the National Sleep Foundation has now published age-specific, evidence-based recommendations for sleep duration to lower the risk of chronic disease. The American Academy of Sleep Medicine has also recently provided recommendations on appropriate norms for sleep duration for children and adults.

By examining these sources and other relevant literature, I have identified a number of things you can try to help yourself get a good night's sleep if you have insomnia. Bear in mind that when you sleep, there are three main things that happen:

1. your muscles become relaxed,

2. your heart rate slows, and

3. your body core temperature drops by a degree or so.

Therefore, anything you do before bedtime to delay these effects may impair your ability to get off to sleep. On the other hand, if you spend the last hour or two before bedtime in a relaxed state, not getting excited, and in a comfortably warm but not hot room you can get to sleep easier. The following practical guidelines should be followed to improve your sleep quality if it is not already good:

- Set regular times for going to bed and waking up. Use an alarm clock so that you do not have to worry about waking up on time in the morning for work, etc. Avoid oversleeping or having a long lie in at weekends, as this disrupts your normal sleep schedule.

- Relax before bed time – try taking a warm bath or listening to calming music.

- In the bedroom use thick curtains or blinds, an eye mask, and earplugs to stop you being woken up by light and noise if these are potential problems.

- Have a comfortable, warm bed and pillows. Good quality cotton is best for sheets and pillows, and a duvet is cosier and lighter than blankets.

- Have a selection of duvets at hand (e.g., 5, 10 and 13 tog), and use them according to the night-time bedroom temperature. In hot countries, an air conditioning system that does not create much noise is a must.

- A bedroom temperature of 15-19°C is generally best for sleeping well.

- Avoid caffeine, nicotine, alcohol, heavy meals, and large volumes (over 200 mL) of fluid for at least a few hours before going to bed. Caffeine and nicotine are stimulants that will keep you awake. Alcohol in moderation may make you feel relaxed and tired, but it can disrupt sleep patterns by reducing the cycle of restorative rapid eye movement sleep. Furthermore, alcohol is a diuretic (a drug that increases urine production) which means that frequent trips to the bathroom are more likely and will disrupt your sleep.

- Don't do any exercise for at least a few hours before going to bed.

- A cup of hot or cold milk or chocolate milk before bedtime may help you sleep.

- Don't watch television or use phones, tablets, or laptop computers in bed shortly before trying to go to sleep. The blue light emitted from electronic devices suppresses the secretion of melatonin, the hormone that controls our body clock. Reduced levels of melatonin make it harder to fall asleep and stay asleep during the night.

- Avoid napping during the day.

- Think of pleasant things when you are trying to get off to sleep. Try to ignore your worries and ideas about how to solve them before going to bed to help you forget about them until the morning.

- If your partner is keeping you awake by snoring, do something to help them stop it, or sleep in the spare room.

- If you are overweight or obese, losing 5% of your body weight will help you sleep better. When you put on excess weight, the fat not only goes in your belly region, but also around your neck. Having a fat neck means you are more likely to snore (which will keep your partner awake), and you are more likely to develop obstructive sleep apnea, a disorder which causes people to stop breathing while sleeping and results in disrupted sleep with frequent awakenings.

- Some people find over-the-counter sleeping tablets helpful, but they don't address the underlying problem and can have troublesome side effects.

Key Points

- Sleep has a critical role in promoting health. Research has documented that sleep disturbance has a powerful influence on the risk of infectious disease, as well as the occurrence and progression of several major chronic diseases, including type 2 diabetes, cardiovascular disease, and the incidence of depression.

- About seven to eight hours of sleep is the norm.

- Insomnia complaints are highly prevalent, occurring in nearly 25% of the US population and adversely influence disease, illness, and mortality risk.

- Insomnia in otherwise healthy people is often associated with stress and anxiety, a poor sleeping environment, inappropriate lifestyle habits (e.g., late evening work or exercise), use of electronic visual devices before bedtime, sleeping during the day, drinking alcohol or caffeine, smoking, eating a heavy meal just before going to bed, a poor diet, and micronutrient deficiencies.

- Sleep deprivation and disturbance impair immunity; this impairment is associated with reduced response to vaccines and increased susceptibility to infectious illnesses such as the common cold.

- The quality of the diet and the consumption of certain nutrients can affect the regulatory hormonal pathways that influence sleep quantity and quality. Sleep, in turn, affects the intake of total energy, as well as of specific foods and nutrients, through a variety of physiological and behavioral mechanisms.

- There are a number of things you can try to help yourself get a good night's sleep if you have insomnia, including having regular times for going to bed and waking up, relaxing before bed time, having a dark, quiet, warm sleeping environment, and a comfortable bed, avoiding caffeine, nicotine, alcohol, heavy meals, large volumes of fluid, and exercise for a few hours before going to bed, and ignoring your worries.

Chapter 11

How to Avoid Common Illnesses

Objectives

After studying this chapter, you should:

- Know why extreme physical or mental stress can impair immunity

- Understand the role of nutrition in maintaining an effective immune system

- Appreciate that some supplements, including probiotics, plant polyphenols, vitamin D3, and bovine colostrum may benefit immunity and reduce risks of infection if taken regularly in sufficient doses

- Understand how to limit your exposure to the microorganisms that cause common infections

- Know the principles of good food hygiene that can reduce your risk of getting tummy bugs

- Understand how to maintain robust immunity and reduce your risk of picking up infections

- Understand the differences between infection, allergy, and intolerance

The previous chapters have mostly been concerned with our health in the long-term and particularly how we can minimize our risk of developing chronic diseases such as type 2 diabetes, hypertension, and coronary heart disease. Another more immediate concern is our risk of picking up infections like the common cold, influenza, tonsillitis, measles, and tummy bugs. Our immune system protects us against the viruses and bacteria that cause these infections, but because there is a genetic influence on the efficacy of our immune systems, some people are more prone to infections than others. However, just as with the risk of chronic disease, our susceptibility to common infectious diseases is also influenced by what we eat, how much exercise we do, and how well we sleep. In addition, other lifestyle behaviors such as good personal and food hygiene practices can help to reduce our risk of picking up infections. This chapter explains the various nutritional, behavioral, and lifestyle strategies that we can easily implement to help minimize our risk of infections. The chapter also explains the differences between infections and allergies, which together with food intolerances are forms of non-infectious illness.

COMMON INFECTIOUS ILLNESSES

The most common illnesses in the general population are viral infections of the upper respiratory tract (i.e., the common cold and influenza), which are more common in the winter months. Adults typically experience between two and four episodes of respiratory illness per year. The incidence is higher in young children who typically suffer about six illness episodes per year because their immune systems are not fully developed. Among the elderly, the incidence is lowest at about one to three episodes annually, but the impact of infection for older people can be more debilitating, and they have an increased risk of developing more serious complications such as chest (lung) infections, including bronchitis and pneumonia. Illness symptoms similar to the common cold (e.g., sore throat, runny nose, dry cough) can also be due to an allergy or inflammation affecting the mucosal lining of the upper respiratory tract caused by the inhalation of cold, dry, or polluted air. Other common illnesses are those affecting the skin, digestive tract, and genitourinary system. In some situations, poor food hygiene can be a problem with increased risk of gastrointestinal infections (i.e., what are commonly called tummy bugs) that cause symptoms such as bloating, vomiting, and diarrhea.

There are also some forms of non-infectious illness, including allergies that involve the respiratory tract, skin, or digestive system and are caused by a hypersensitivity of the immune system to certain molecules (often proteins) that are inhaled (e.g., pollen), come into contact with the skin (e.g., latex), or are eaten (e.g., wheat gluten). All of these involve the inappropriate activation of the immune system against a compound that is normally tolerated well by the majority of people. The inflammation caused by this hypersensitivity is the major cause of the illness symptoms. Similar symptoms may arise with intolerance to certain food items, although this does not directly involve immune system activation.

STRESS AND IMMUNITY

Excessive stress – both psychological and physical – impairs our immunity. Very prolonged bouts of strenuous exercise or intensified training and competition in elite athletes have been shown to result in transient depression of white blood cell functions, and it is suggested that such changes create an "open window" of decreased host protection, during which viruses and bacteria can gain a foothold, increasing the risk of developing an infection. In recreationally active people participating in endurance events like marathons, the incidence of respiratory infections is increased in the first one or two weeks that follow the event. Chronic psychological stress caused by problems in the workplace or family, caring for a loved one, bereavement, divorce, moving house, or worrying about exams can also cause depressed immunity. These effects are brought about by increases in stress hormones, particularly cortisol and epinephrine which depress immunity, weakening our defenses against pathogenic (disease causing) microorganisms. Other factors such as nutrient deficiencies (e.g., insufficient protein, iron, or vitamin D) and lack of sleep can also depress immunity and lead to increased risk of infection (figure 11.1). There are also some situations in which our exposure to infectious agents may be increased, which is the other important determinant of infection risk. Examples include coming into contact with sick people suffering from infections, working with children, exposure to large crowds (e.g., at music or sports events, airports, and shops), foreign travel (particularly long haul flights), unclean environments, and poor personal hygiene.

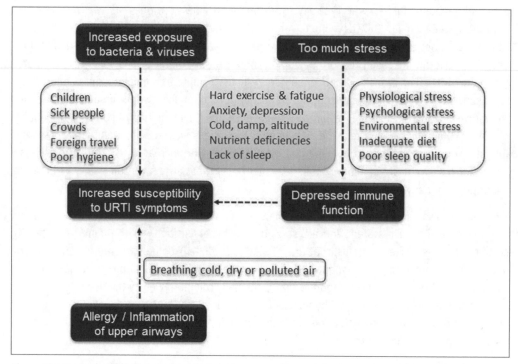

Figure 11.1: Factors contributing to the risk of picking up respiratory infections. Adapted from Gleeson (2015).

MAINTAINING AN EFFECTIVE IMMUNE SYSTEM

Adequate nutrition and in particular appropriate intakes of energy, protein, vitamins, and minerals are essential to maintain the body's natural defenses against disease causing viruses and bacteria. People are best advised to consume a sound diet that meets their energy needs and contains a variety of foods, as the key to maintaining an effective immune system is to avoid deficiencies of the nutrients that play an essential role in immune cell functions. Inadequate intake of dietary protein and energy or deficiencies of certain micronutrients (e.g., iron, zinc, magnesium, manganese, selenium, copper, vitamins A, C, D, E, B6, B12, and folic acid) decrease immune defenses against invading **pathogens** and make the individual more susceptible to infection. Even short-term dieting that results in a loss of a few kilograms body weight over the course of a few weeks can result in significant drops in several aspects of immune function. Thus, care should be taken to ensure adequate protein (and micronutrient) intakes during periods of intentional weight loss, and it should be recognized that individuals undergoing weight reduction are likely to be more prone to infection. In general, a broad-range multivitamin/mineral supplement is the best choice to support a restricted food intake, and this may also be suitable when travelling abroad in situations where food choices and quality may be limited.

It has only recently been recognized that Vitamin D plays an important role in bolstering immunity, and this is a concern as Vitamin D insufficiency is common in the general population, especially if exposure to natural sunlight is limited (e.g., in the winter months or when living or working mostly indoors). An increasing number of studies have provided evidence that sufficient vitamin D status optimizes immune function and helps defend against the common cold. Hence, individuals who think they could be deficient in vitamin D are likely to benefit from vitamin D3 supplementation.

GUIDELINES FOR MAINTENANCE OF IMMUNE HEALTH AND LIMITING THE RISK OF INFECTION

Although it is usually easy to treat infections like the common cold using over-the counter remedies, it would, of course, be preferable to prevent the infection from happening in the first place. Remember the old adage that "prevention is better than cure"? Although there is no single method that completely eliminates the risk of contracting an infection, there are several effective behavioral, nutritional, and lifestyle strategies that can limit the extent of stress-induced immunodepression and lower exposure to pathogenic microorganisms and so reduce the risk of infection. Unfortunately, vaccination – which can be very effective against certain infectious illnesses such as influenza (see the sidebar), cholera, and typhoid – is no good at preventing the common cold, as there are more than a hundred different varieties of viruses that can cause colds which means that no single vaccine is effective.

Is It Worth Having an Annual Vaccination Against Influenza?

Influenza or flu is a debilitating illness that can last a week or two and can be life threatening particularly for the elderly and very young. Being vaccinated is our best defense against flu. This has to be done every year (usually in the autumn as the vaccine takes 5-7 weeks to work) because different strains of flu virus become prevalent during winter from year to year. Having the flu vaccine protects you against the flu, and it also helps to protect your own family and the wider community. Typically, the flu vaccine will offer protection to 30-60% of the people who have it (in adults it is usually administered by injection). Occasionally its efficacy can drop to 10-15%, as the vaccine is produced six to nine months before it is needed based on expert predictions of which strain or strains are likely to be the most prevalent in the coming winter. Sometimes the experts get it wrong, or the flu virus mutates making the vaccine less effective. All vaccines contain an inactive harmless version of the virus that expresses several proteins (antigens) that allow the body's immune system to learn what it looks like and become prepared to mount a rapid and effective killing response when we come into contact with the real flu virus. Some vaccines may also contain an adjuvant which boosts the body's immune reaction and makes the vaccine more effective. In some countries such as the UK, the flu vaccine is available for free to certain parts of the population (e.g., those aged over 65, schoolchildren, and those with long term conditions such as diabetes that make flu complications more likely). Even if you have to pay for it my advice is to have the vaccination.

Certain supplements may boost immune function and reduce infection risk in individuals who are subjected to stress. While there are many nutritional supplements on the market that are claimed to boost immunity, such claims are often based on selective evidence of efficacy in animals, in vitro (test tube) experiments, children, the elderly, or severely ill clinical patients, and direct evidence for their efficacy in preventing stress-induced immune depression or improving immune system status in otherwise healthy adults is usually lacking. However, there are a limited number of nutritional strategies and supplements whose efficacy is supported by some scientific evidence and which work to reduce immune perturbations caused by stress and/or decrease the incidence of infection. These include fruits, probiotics, plant polyphenols such as flavonoids, vitamin D3 (in the winter months), bovine colostrum, vitamin C (in those exposed to stress or cold environments), and vitamin E (in the elderly).

LIMITING THE TRANSMISSION OF INFECTIONS

Some practical guidelines for limiting transmission of infections among people are shown in the sidebar. The most important of these are good hand hygiene and avoiding contact with persons that are infected. Hand washing (using the correct technique to ensure all parts of hands are cleaned effectively) with soap and water is effective against most pathogens but does not provide continuous protection. Hand gels containing a minimum of 60% alcohol disinfect effectively, but the protection they provide does not last more than a few minutes, so they need to be applied frequently, and this can cause dry skin and irritation. Other sanitization methods include the use of non-alcohol based antimicrobial hand foams that contain cationic biocides and hydrophobic polymers which are claimed to disinfect hands for up to six hours. However, individuals need to be aware that these products are removed by hand washing and excessive sweating, therefore they also need to be reapplied every few hours.

Behavioral and Lifestyle Strategies to Limit Transmission of Infections

- Minimize contact with infected people, young children, animals, and contagious objects.

- Avoid crowded areas and shaking hands.

- Keep your distance from people who are coughing, sneezing, or have a 'runny nose', and when appropriate, wear (or ask them to wear) a disposable mask.

- Use a face mask to protect airways from being directly exposed to very cold (below 0°C) and dry air during outdoor exercise.

- Wash hands regularly and effectively with soap and water, especially before meals, and after direct contact with potentially contagious people, animals, blood, secretions, public places, and bathrooms.

- Use disposable paper towels and limit hand to mouth/nose contact when suffering from symptoms of the common cold or gastrointestinal illness (putting hands to eyes and nose is a major route of viral self-inoculation).

- Carry anti-microbial foam/cream or alcohol-based hand-washing gel with you.

- Do not share drinking bottles, cups, cutlery, towels, etc. with other people.

- When abroad, choose cold beverages from sealed bottles, avoid raw vegetables and undercooked meat. Wash and peel fruit before eating.

- Ensure good hygiene in food preparation areas to reduce the risk of gastrointestinal infections caused by bacterial contamination.

- Wear flip-flops or similar footwear when going to the showers, swimming pool, and locker rooms in order to avoid dermatological diseases.

- Individuals should be updated on all vaccines needed at home and for foreign travel. Influenza vaccines take 5-7 weeks to take effect. But don't get vaccinated if you are currently suffering from any symptoms of illness.

Another important issue with regard to hygiene is taking care in how you store, prepare, and cook your food. Gastrointestinal infections can be very nasty and may cause bloating, abdominal discomfort, vomiting, and diarrhea that can last for days. These infections are caused primarily by eating food that has become contaminated with bacteria. This can be avoided by practicing good hygiene in the kitchen or other food preparation and storage areas. There are four main things to consider: cross-contamination, cleaning, chilling, and cooking. These are known as the 4 Cs, and further details, including useful guidance documents and hygiene training videos, can be found on the UK Food Standards Agency website (https://www.food.gov.uk/business-industry/food-hygiene). A summary of the more important guidelines is provided in the sidebar that follows:

Guidelines on Good Food Hygiene Practice

Follow these recommendations about cross-contamination, cleaning, chilling, and cooking (known as the 4 Cs) to reduce the risk of bacterial contamination of your food and avoid gastrointestinal infections.

Cross-contamination

Cross-contamination is when bacteria are spread between food, surfaces, or equipment. It is most likely to happen when raw food touches (or drips onto) ready-to-eat food, equipment, or surfaces. Cross-contamination is one of the most common causes of food poisoning. Here is what needs to be done to avoid it:

- Clean and disinfect work surfaces, chopping boards, and equipment thoroughly before you start preparing food and after you have used them to prepare raw food.

- Use different equipment (including chopping boards and knives) for raw meat/poultry and ready-to-eat food unless they can be heat disinfected in, for example, a commercial dishwasher.

- Wash your hands thoroughly before preparing food.

- Wash your hands after touching raw food.

- Keep raw and ready-to-eat food apart at all times, including packaging material for ready-to-eat food.

- Store raw food below ready-to-eat food in the fridge. If possible, use separate fridges for raw and ready-to-eat food.

- Separate cleaning materials, including cloths, sponges, and mops, should be used in areas where ready-to-eat foods are stored, handled and prepared.

Cleaning

- Effective cleaning gets rid of bacteria on hands, equipment, and surfaces. So, it helps to stop harmful bacteria from spreading onto food. You should do the following things:

- Wash and dry your hands thoroughly before handling food.

- Clean and disinfect food areas and equipment between different tasks, especially after handling raw food.

- Clear and clean as you go. Clear away used equipment, spilt food etc. as you work, and clean work surfaces thoroughly.

- Use cleaning and disinfection products that are suitable for the job, and follow the manufacturer's instructions.

- Do not let food waste build up.

Chilling

Chilling food properly helps to stop harmful bacteria from growing. Some food needs to be kept chilled to keep it safe; for example, food with a 'use by' date, cooked dishes and other ready-to-eat food such as prepared salads and desserts. It is very important not to leave these types of food standing around at room temperature. So, make sure you do the following things:

- Keep chilled food cold enough when returning from the supermarket; don't leave it in the trunk for longer than necessary. In hot weather, use an insulated cool box or bag to transport chilled food in.

- Check any chilled food that you have delivered to make sure it is cold enough.

- Put food that needs to be kept chilled in the fridge straight away.

- Cool cooked food as quickly as possible, and then put it in the fridge.

- Keep chilled food out of the fridge for the shortest time possible during preparation.

- Check regularly that your fridge and display units are cold enough (less than 8°C).

- For frozen food, ensure that food packages are stored at below 18°C, and ensure food is completely defrosted before cooking.

Cooking

Thorough cooking kills harmful bacteria in food. So, it is extremely important to make sure that food is cooked properly by following these guidelines:

- Cooking food at a temperature of 75°C or more will kill virtually all bacteria.

- When cooking or reheating food, always check that it is steaming hot all the way through. It is especially important to make sure that you thoroughly cook poultry, pork, rolled joints, and products made from minced meat, such as burgers and sausages. This is because there could be bacteria in the middle of these types of products. They should not be served pink or rare and should be steaming hot all the way through.

- Whole cuts of beef and lamb, such as steaks, cutlets, and whole joints, can be served pink/rare as long as they are fully sealed on the outside.

- Hot food that is not served immediately should be kept at a minimum of 63°C.

Adapted from Food Hygiene: A Guide For Businesses, Food Standards Agency© Crown Copyright 2013. This information is licensed under the Open Government Licence v3.0. To view this licence, visit **https://www.nationalarchives.gov.uk/doc/open-government-licence/OGL.**

MAINTAINING ROBUST IMMUNITY AND LIMITING STRESS

The other things that people can do to limit their risk of infection are to adhere to some practical guidelines to maintain robust immunity and limit the impact stress. These guidelines are listed in the next sidebar and relate mostly to nutritional, behavioral, and lifestyle strategies and are based on the findings of numerous research studies. The most effective nutritional strategies to maintain robust immune function are to avoid deficiencies of essential micronutrients, ingest *Lactobacillus* probiotics on a daily basis, and eat plenty of fruit and vegetables. Probiotics are live bacteria which when ingested in adequate amounts, modify the bacterial population (known as the microbiota) that inhabits our gut and modulate immune function by their interaction with the gut-associated lymphoid tissue, leading to positive effects on the systemic immune system. Some well-controlled studies in children, adults, endurance athletes, and the elderly have indicated that daily probiotic ingestion results in fewer days of respiratory illness and lower severity of infection symptoms, and a recent meta-analysis using data from multiple studies involving 3,451 subjects concluded that there is likely a benefit in reducing respiratory infection incidence. Another potential benefit of probiotics could be a reduced risk of gastrointestinal infections – a particular concern when travelling abroad.

Some studies suggest that regular consumption of fruits and plant polyphenol supplements (e.g., quercetin) or beverages that contain high amounts of polyphenols (e.g., non-alcoholic beer and green tea) can also reduce common cold incidence. Ensuring that the individual has adequate vitamin D may also be helpful, and supplementation with vitamin D3 (1,000-4,000 IU/day or 25-100 micrograms (µg)/day) may be warranted for some people, especially in the winter months for those living at latitudes of 48°North (equivalent to Paris, France and the USA-Canada border) and above since the skin is unable to form vitamin D between the months of October through to March because the sunlight is not strong enough. Bovine colostrum is the first collection of a thick creamy-yellow liquid produced by the mammary gland of a lactating cow shortly after birth of her calf, usually within the first 36 hours. Colostrum contains antibodies, growth factors, enzymes, gangliosides (acid glycosphingolipids), vitamins, and minerals and is commercially available in both liquid and powder forms. Numerous health claims have been made for colostrum ranging from athletic performance enhancement to preventing infections, but well-controlled studies are rare. The **gangliosides** in colostrum may modify the gut microbial population and act as decoy targets for bacterial adhesion as well as having some direct immune-stimulatory properties. A recent study in young children prone to URTI and gastrointestinal infections suggested that a daily bovine colostrum supplement reduced their incidence of both types of infection and some studies in adult athletes have indicated similar benefits.

Many other nutrition supplements, including β-glucan, echinacea, glutamine, and others, are on sale with claims that they can boost the immune system, but the scientific evidence that any of these are effective in preventing infections is not compelling.

When cold symptoms begin, there is some evidence that taking zinc lozenges (>75 mg zinc/day; high ionic zinc content) or certain herbal supplements (e.g., echinacea, ginseng, kaloba) can reduce the number of days that illness symptoms last for. However, these may not be any more effective than treating illness symptoms with over-the-counter cold remedies.

Nutritional and Behavioral Strategies
to Help Maintain Robust Immunity

- If you participate in regular exercise, avoid very prolonged training sessions (longer than two hours) and excessive periods of intensified training as this can depress your immunity.

- Wear appropriate outdoor clothing in inclement weather and avoid getting cold and wet after exercise.

- Get adequate sleep (at least seven hours per night is recommended). Missing a single night of sleep has little effect on immune function at rest or after exercise, but respiratory illness episodes are more prevalent in those who regularly experience low sleep quantity (less than seven hours per night) and poor sleep quality (frequent awakenings).

- Keep other life stresses to a minimum.

- Ensure adequate dietary energy, protein, and essential micronutrient intake.

- Vitamin D plays an important role in promoting immunity, and this is a concern as vitamin D insufficiency is common in people especially in situations where exposure to natural sunlight is limited (e.g., during the winter months or when living or working mostly indoors). A vitamin D3 supplement (1,000 IU/day or 25 µg/day) may be beneficial to optimize immune function from October to April in Northern hemisphere countries.

- Avoid crash dieting and rapid weight loss. Care should be taken to ensure adequate protein (and micronutrient) intakes during periods of intentional weight loss, as individuals undergoing weight reduction are likely to be more prone to infection. In general, a broad-range multivitamin/mineral supplement is the best choice to support a restricted food intake, and this may also be suitable when travelling abroad in situations where food choices and quality may be limited.

- Eat several different fruits daily at least five times per week as regular fruit intake is associated with a lower incidence of the common cold.

- If the goal of doing exercise is not weight loss, and you plan to do a prolonged (90 minutes or more) moderate to high intensity exercise session, ensure adequate carbohydrate intake before and during exercise in order to limit the extent and severity of exercise-induced immune depression. Ingesting about 40 g carbohydrate per hour of exercise during prolonged workouts maintains blood sugar levels and lowers circulating stress hormones and so helps to limit immune function depression. A 500 mL bottle of a sports drink usually contains 30-40 g of carbohydrate.

- The consumption of beverages during exercise not only helps prevent dehydration (which is associated with an increased stress hormone response) but also helps to maintain saliva flow rate during exercise. Saliva contains several proteins with antimicrobial properties including immunoglobulin A, lysozyme, a-amylase, and defensins. Saliva secretion usually falls during exercise, but regular fluid intake (water is fine) during exercise can prevent this.

- The efficacy of most so-called dietary immunostimulants has not been confirmed. However, there is limited evidence that some flavonoids (e.g., quercetin at a dose of 1 g/day) or flavonoid containing beverages (e.g., non-alcoholic beer, green tea), and *Lactobacillus* and/or *Bifidobacterium* probiotics (daily doses of ~10^{10} live bacteria) can reduce respiratory infection incidence in physically active people or those under stress. Another potential benefit of probiotics could be a reduced risk of gastrointestinal infections – a particular concern when travelling abroad.

- High daily doses (up to 1000 mg) of vitamin C are not generally justified, but individuals engaged in intensive training and/or cold environments may gain some benefit for preventing respiratory infections.

- Avoid strenuous exercise for a few days when experiencing upper respiratory symptoms like sore throat, sneezing, runny, or congested nose. Avoid all exercise when experiencing symptoms like muscle/joint pain and headache, a chesty cough, fever (indicated by a resting body temperature of 38-40°C), and generalized feeling of malaise, diarrhea, or vomiting.

ALLERGIES AND INTOLERANCE

When the term **allergy** was first introduced in 1906, it meant an adverse reaction to a food or other substance not typically regarded as harmful or bothersome. For most people this is still what allergy means, although doctors use the word rather differently, and this can be both misleading and confusing. Doctors use the word allergy to mean an adverse reaction of the immune system to a substance not recognized as harmful by most people's immune systems. True allergies (for example, allergies to pollens, dust mites, fish, shellfish, or nuts) are typically associated with the formation of antibodies. Some people (doctors refer to these people as atopic) have an inherited tendency to this type of allergy, and they tend also to be prone to asthma, eczema, and hay fever; this condition is known as atopy. In certain circumstances, and especially during the first few years of life, atopic people may develop immunoglobulin E (IgE) antibodies when exposed to an allergy-inducing protein in a process called sensitization. When sensitization has occurred, the allergy-inducing protein is referred to as an allergen and the resulting **antibody** (also a protein) as allergen specific IgE. While doctors use the term allergy when referring to an adverse reaction that involves the immune system, the term **intolerance** is preferred when an adverse reaction shows no evidence of immune system involvement. The scientific term for intolerance is non-allergic hypersensitivity.

FOOD ALLERGY

A true gluten allergy—not to be confused with gluten sensitivity or **celiac disease**—is caused by gliadin, a glycoprotein that, along with another protein called glutenin, helps to form the gluten protein. Gluten is found in wheat and other similar cereal grains such as barley, oats, and rye. The symptoms of gluten allergy are similar to those of gluten intolerance but can be more severe. Gliadin is also one of the major allergens associated with wheat allergies and a known trigger for celiac disease, a serious autoimmune disorder of the small intestine. In a person with a gluten allergy, small amounts of gluten may be tolerated, but a person suffering from with celiac disease cannot tolerate any gluten at all. When a person with celiac disease eats gluten, the immune system initiates an unnecessary inflammatory response, and this eventually damages the lining of the small intestine. Celiac disease restricts absorption of nutrients and may lead to malnutrition and weight loss. Because celiac disease shares symptoms with a number of other disorders, including a gluten allergy, it is important that a test is conducted to confirm the condition. Gluten allergies and celiac disease are a major public health concern. It is estimated that 0.6% of children and 0.9% of adults in the USA have a gluten allergy while another 1% suffer from celiac disease.

A less common but dangerous allergy is to proteins in seeds or nuts. Each year there are several reported cases of fatalities due to a rapid, severe **anaphylactic shock** following ingestion of seeds or nuts, or more usually, to inadvertently eating foods (e.g., breads, curries, cakes, pastries, cookies) containing seeds, nuts, or nut extracts in people with seed or nut allergies.

FOOD INTOLERANCE

Food intolerance can occur when the body fails to produce a sufficient amount of a particular enzyme needed to digest a food component before it can be absorbed. For example, if a person suffers abdominal discomfort with flatulence and bloating or diarrhea every time they consume milk or milk-derived products (e.g., cream, yogurt, cheese), they may be suffering from lactose intolerance, a condition caused by lack of lactase, the enzyme that digests the main sugar in milk, a disaccharide called lactose. This is caused by the lactose not being absorbed but instead being fermented by the microbes in the intestine. Food intolerances are normally dose related, meaning the more you eat the worse the reaction is likely to be. There may also be a threshold amount required to be consumed before experiencing any symptoms, which can make it difficult to determine the specific cause.

A person with gluten sensitivity (also known as gluten intolerance) may also have symptoms such as bloating, abdominal pain, or diarrhea, but because the immune or autoimmune symptoms are not involved, it is not considered as serious a condition as celiac disease or gluten allergy. As many as 6% of people in the USA have gluten sensitivity.

If a person suffers nervous system symptoms because of an amount of caffeine in a mug of strong coffee that would be tolerated by most people, this person would be suffering from drug-like or pharmacological food intolerance. This can occur either because of an intolerance of chemicals naturally present in foods (such as theobromine in chocolate or tyramine in aged cheeses) or an intolerance of food additives such as sulfites or benzoates.

TOXIC FOOD REACTIONS

While enzymatic and pharmacological food intolerance reactions only affect some people, toxic food reactions affect everyone if an excessive amount of a particular food constituent is ingested. A good example is the false food allergy type of reaction that can occur when sufficient amounts of the substance called histamine accumulates in the flesh of spoilt (decayed) tuna (known as the scombroid reaction). As histamine is also the natural agent in the human body involved in allergic reactions, scombroid food poisoning often gets misidentified as a food allergy. This condition is named after the Scombridae family of fish, which includes tuna, mackerel, and bonito, because early descriptions of the illness noted an association with those species; however, other types of fish including mahi-mahi and amberjack are also known to cause this problem. Cooking the fish does not prevent illness, because histamine is not destroyed at normal cooking temperatures. None of the previous examples of food intolerance involve the immune system, and for this reason, none can result in life-threatening allergy or anaphylaxis, but they can result in severe abdominal discomfort.

With the exception of lactose intolerance, for which a conventional test exists, no reliable forms of testing exist for the types of food intolerance described previously. However, recent scientific studies are beginning to point to a delayed type food allergy in which the immune system is involved even though allergen-specific IgE is not present. For this reason, the controversial view that certain medically unexplained symptoms might be related to a delayed form of food allergy rather than being due to an unexplained or psychosomatic mechanism may yet prove to have some scientific worth. Studies that have used food exclusion followed by blinded and placebo-controlled food challenge have suggested that this kind of mechanism may apply in some cases of migraine, arthritis, and irritable bowel syndrome. However, with the exception of dietitian supervised food exclusion and food challenge, no validated test for this type of food allergy has so far emerged. Some practitioners use IgG (as opposed to IgE) blood tests when investigating such cases, but the general scientific consensus is that the data obtained from IgG blood tests is not scientifically robust, and most allergy specialists consider such tests to be unhelpful or misleading.

Key Points

- The immune system protects the body against potentially damaging microorganisms.

- People exposed to chronically stressful situations often have depressed immune function and suffer from an increased incidence of respiratory infections.

- Heavy, prolonged exertion is associated with numerous hormonal and biochemical changes, many of which potentially have detrimental effects on immune function leading to increased susceptibility to respiratory infection.

- Lack of sleep can also depress immunity and increase risk of infections. Getting less than seven hours sleep per night is associated with increased susceptibility to developing cold symptoms when exposed to a respiratory virus.

- Inadequate nutrition and in particular, dietary deficiencies of protein and specific micronutrients are associated with immune dysfunction.

- An adequate intake of iron, zinc, and B vitamins is particularly important, but the dangers of over-supplementation should also be considered. Many micronutrients given in quantities beyond a certain threshold reduce immune responses and may have other toxic effects.

- In general, supplementing individual micronutrients or consuming large doses of simple antioxidant mixtures is not recommended. Individuals should obtain complex mixtures of antioxidant compounds from consumption of fruits and vegetables. Supplementing vitamin D3 is an exception since many people exhibit inadequate vitamin D status during the winter months. Vitamin E supplements may be of benefit to the elderly in reducing their risks of infection.

- Some other supplements, including probiotics, plant polyphenols, and bovine colostrum may benefit immunity and reduce risks of infection if taken regularly in sufficient doses.

- Although countering the effects of all the factors that contribute to stress-induced immunodepression is an unrealistic target, minimizing many of the effects is possible. People can help themselves by eating a well-balanced, healthy diet that includes sufficient protein and carbohydrate to meet their energy requirements. Such a diet ensures an adequate intake of vitamins (with the possible exception of vitamin D), minerals, and trace elements without the need for special supplements.

- By adopting sound nutritional practice, reducing life stresses, maintaining good personal and food hygiene, and obtaining adequate sleep, people can reduce their risk of infection.

- The best defense against many infectious illnesses such as influenza, measles, mumps, cholera, typhoid, and yellow fever (but not the common cold) is vaccination.

Chapter 12

How to Maintain Healthy Senses, Tissues, and Organs

Objectives

After studying this chapter, you should:

- Appreciate why maintaining the health of your body is not just down to exercise, diet, sleep and hygiene

- Understand how particular aspects of your lifestyle and behavior can have a negative or positive impact on the health of your senses, tissues, and organs

- Understand the ways you can maintain and prolong the health of your senses, tissues, and organs and realize the consequences of not doing so

- Know the ways to protect the health of your eyes, ears, teeth and gums, bones, muscles and joints, skin, gut, brain, heart and circulation, lungs, kidneys and urinary tract, and reproductive organs

The previous chapters of this book have mostly been concerned with how regular exercise, a healthy diet, and good sleep quality can reduce your risk of developing chronic cardiovascular and metabolic diseases and reduce the risk of picking up infections. In the last chapter, you also learned about the importance of personal hygiene for reducing the transmission of pathogens that cause common illnesses such as the common cold and influenza. However, these are not the only ways in which you can protect the health of your body. The health of your specific body parts (figure 12.1) including your senses, tissues, and organs can be protected in other ways which mostly involve lifestyle and behavioral practices. This chapter explains the various ways that you can do this.

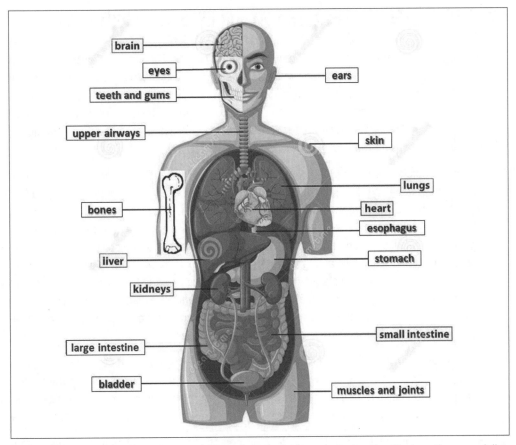

Figure 12.1: The various organs, tissues and parts of your body that you can keep healthy by eating a good diet, and other behavioral practices.

WAYS TO PROTECT THE HEALTH OF YOUR EYES AND SIGHT

Your eyes are an important part of your health and quality of life. There are many things you can do to keep them healthy and make sure your sight remains the best it can be. Some causes of failing sight are related to physical injury, type 1 diabetes, infection, and cancer but the major causes are type 2 diabetes and aging, which can lead to the development of **glaucoma**, diabetic retinopathy, and age-related **macular degeneration**. The following ten guidelines should be followed to help maintain the health of your eyes:

1. Have a comprehensive dilated eye examination every few years. This involves having drops in your eye that open up (dilate) the pupil so that the rear of your eye where light is detected (the retina) can be viewed and photographed by your optometrist. This can reveal the presence of blood vessel problems, glaucoma, **cataracts**, diabetic eye disease (known as retinopathy), and age-related macular degeneration, all of which can lead to partial or complete loss of vision and often have no advance warning signs. A dilated eye examination is the only way to detect these diseases in their early stages. You might think your vision is fine or that your eyes are healthy, but visiting your eye care professional for a comprehensive dilated eye exam is the only way to really be sure. Furthermore, when it comes to common vision problems, some people don't realize they could see better with glasses or contact lenses.

2. Know your family's eye health history. Talk to your family members about their eye health history so that you will know if anyone has been diagnosed with a disease or condition since many eye problems are hereditary. This will help to establish whether you are at higher risk for developing an eye disease or condition.

3. Ensure that your diet regularly includes the components that can help to protect your sight. You've probably heard before that carrots are good for your eyes and night vision in particular. But eating a diet rich in fruits and vegetables, particularly dark leafy greens such as spinach, kale, and collard greens, and eating fish high in omega-3 fatty acids (e.g., salmon, tuna, and mackerel) is also good for your eye health. Some supplements including lutein are also beneficial.

4. Avoid becoming overweight or obese as this increases your risk of developing diabetes and other systemic conditions, which can lead to loss of vision, such as diabetic eye disease or glaucoma.

5. Wear protective eyewear when swimming, playing certain sports such as squash, or doing activities that risk injuring your eyes around the home. Protective eyewear includes safety glasses and goggles, safety shields, and eye guards specially designed to provide the correct protection for a certain activity. Most protective eyewear lenses are made of polycarbonate, which is 10 times stronger than other plastics and protective eyewear can be purchased from many optician and sporting goods stores.

6. Quit smoking tobacco or preferably never start because smoking is as bad for your eyes as it is for the rest of your body. Smoking increases the risk of developing cataract, age-related macular degeneration, and optic nerve damage, all of which result in partial loss of vision and can lead to blindness.

7. Wear sunglasses on sunny days, especially in the spring and summer months when the ultraviolet (UV) sunlight is at its strongest. Sunglasses that block out 99-100% of both UV-A and UV-B radiation are the best ones for protecting your eyes from this harmful radiation. Also, never look at the sun directly, even when wearing sunglasses.

8. Give your eyes a rest, and use moistening eye drops (available without prescription from your local pharmacist) when your eyes feel dry. If you spend a lot of time at the computer or focusing on any one thing, you sometimes forget to blink, and your eyes can get fatigued, and the surface of the eye starts to dry out. Try adopting the 20-20-20 rule: Every 20 minutes, look away about 20 feet in front of you for 20 seconds as this can help reduce eyestrain.

9. Clean your hands regularly with soap and water, and avoid putting your fingers close to your eyes or rubbing your eyes with your hands as this risks eye infections such as conjunctivitis. Avoid people with this condition where possible as it is infectious. Clean your contact lenses properly, and always wash your hands thoroughly before putting in or taking out your contact lenses. Make sure to disinfect contact lenses as instructed and replace them as appropriate.

10. Practice workplace eye safety. Employers are required to provide a safe work environment. When protective eyewear is required as a part of your job, make a habit of wearing the appropriate type at all times.

WAYS TO PROTECT THE HEALTH OF YOUR EARS AND HEARING

Hearing loss or deafness is something to be avoided because once your hearing is damaged, it may be impaired permanently. It is important to be aware of the potential risks to your sense of hearing, the importance of early diagnosis, and what you can do to protect your hearing and take action to find a solution when you think your hearing is becoming worse. If you are finding it hard to hear the television or radio at normal volume or listening to others speaking, then take immediate action by going for a hearing test. Many optical stores now offer such tests for free or at very low cost. The following ten guidelines should be followed to protect your ears and your hearing health:

1. Keep away from loud noise as much as you can, and if unavoidably exposed to loud noise, use earplugs which are convenient and easy to obtain. They can be custom fitted for your ears by your local hearing healthcare provider. Clubs, concerts, lawnmowers, chainsaws, are generally sources of loud noise that is loud enough to create dangerous levels of sound. Generally, a noise is probably loud enough to damage your hearing if:

    • You have to raise your voice to talk to other people.

    • You can't hear what people nearby are saying.

    • It hurts your ears.

    • You have ringing in your ears or muffled hearing afterwards.

Noise levels are measured in decibels (dB): the higher the number, the louder the noise. Any sound over 85 dB can be harmful, especially if you're exposed to it for a long time. To get an idea of how loud this is: whispering is 30 dB, conversation is 60 dB, busy traffic is 70-85 dB, a motorbike is 90 dB, listening to music on full volume through headphones is 100-110 dB, a plane taking off is 120 dB.

2. Turn the volume of your speakers, earphones, or earbuds down. Listening to loud music through earphones and headphones is one of the biggest dangers to your hearing and according to the World Health Organization, over one billion teenagers and young adults worldwide are at risk for noise-induced hearing loss from unsafe use of audio devices. Earbuds are especially dangerous, as they fit directly next to the eardrum. If possible, opt for over-the-ear headphones.

   To help avoid damaging your hearing:

   - Use noise-cancelling earphones or headphones – don't just turn the volume up to cover up outside noise.

   - Turn the volume up just enough so you can hear your music comfortably, but no higher.

   - Don't listen to music at more than 60% of the maximum volume – some devices have settings you can use to limit the volume automatically.

   - Don't use earphones or headphones for more than an hour at a time – take a break for at least five minutes every hour.

   - Avoid being close to loud speakers at concerts and nightclubs.

   - Consider wearing musicians' earplugs that reduce the volume of music but don't muffle it and allow you to hear conversation.

3. Give your ears time to recover after being exposed to loud noises for a prolonged period of time, like at a concert or a dance club. If you can, step outside for five minutes every so often in order to let them rest. Your ears need an average of 16 hours of quiet to recover from one loud night out.

4. Don't use cotton swabs to dry or clean wax from your ears. A little bit of wax in your ears is not only normal, but it's also important to prevent dust and other harmful particles from entering the ear canal. Inserting anything inside your ear canals risks damaging your ear drum, and the damage is often permanent. If you have excess wax, you can clean around the canal very gently with a damp towel or you could use ear wax removal solution over the course of a few nights which will soften the wax so that it will eventually flow out on its own. If you have so much wax that it is blocking your ear canal and making you deaf, seek a professional opinion from your medical practitioner.

5. Take medications only as directed. Certain medications, such as non-steroidal anti-inflammatory drugs like aspirin, ibuprofen, and naproxen, if taken frequently, can sometimes contribute to hearing loss. Discuss medications with your doctor if you're concerned that they'll impact your hearing ability.

6. Keep your ears dry. Excess moisture can allow bacteria to enter and attack the ear canal. This can cause swimmer's ear or other types of ear infections, which can be dangerous for your hearing ability. Be sure you gently towel-dry your ears after bathing or swimming. If you can feel water in the ear, tilt your head to the side and tug lightly on the ear lobe to coax the water out. You can also ensure that your ears stay dry and healthy by using custom-fit swimmers' earplugs, which block water from entering the ear canal and have been shown to greatly reduce the risk of developing ear infections. Don't share your earplugs with anyone else.

7. Exercise is good for your ears as it gets the blood pumping to all parts of your body, including the ears. This helps the ears' internal parts stay healthy and working to their maximum potential. When cycling or horse riding, always wear a helmet. If you fall and hit your head, a concussion can harm your hearing.

8. Manage your stress and anxiety levels as these have been linked to both temporary and permanent **tinnitus** (a phantom ringing in the ears).

9. Protect your ears in loud workplaces. If you're exposed to loud noises through your work, you should speak to your employer who is obliged to make changes to reduce your exposure to loud noise such as:

    • Switching to quieter equipment if possible.

    • Making sure you're not exposed to loud noise for long periods.

    • Providing hearing protection, such as ear muffs or earplugs. Make sure you wear any hearing protection you're given.

10. Have a regular hearing check-up via your doctor or a hearing healthcare professional. That way, you'll be more likely to identify any early signs of hearing loss and take action as soon as you do. Taking action is important because untreated hearing loss, besides detracting from quality of life and interfering with your personal relationships, has been linked to other health concerns like depression, dementia, and heart disease.

WAYS TO PROTECT THE HEALTH OF YOUR TEETH AND GUMS

Good oral hygiene encompasses everything you do to keep your mouth, teeth, and gums healthy. Brushing your teeth regularly and protecting your teeth from long-term damage by eliminating or avoiding some potentially damaging dental habits will reduce the treatment you may need at the dentist and give you a whiter, brighter smile. Following these ten guidelines throughout life will improve your oral health and overall health:

1. Ideally, you should brush your teeth twice a day, and brushing before going to bed is crucial. Saliva helps fight the acid-forming bacteria that cause tooth decay, but you don't produce much saliva while you are sleeping.

2. Brush with proper technique which means brushing your teeth at a 45-degree angle and brush with both small back and forth strokes and up and down strokes. To clean behind your teeth and gums, place the bristles at a 45-degree angle again and repeat the brushing motion. You should be brushing your teeth for about two minutes in total, so spend 30 seconds on each quadrant of your mouth. Use only gentle pressure to prevent damaging your delicate gums, otherwise gum erosion and bleeding can occur. You should also gently brush your tongue (or use a tongue scraper) to help remove bacteria and prevent bad breath. Use a toothpaste with a flavor you like, and choose one containing fluoride (1350-1500 ppm is most effective) which protects teeth against decay. Some toothpastes are especially formulated for sensitive teeth, so use that sort if your teeth feel painful after consuming hot or cold foods.

3. Use the correct type of toothbrush. The American Dental Association recommends using a brush that has soft bristles and changing the brush every three months. An electronic toothbrush with a round head can be more effective for efficient plaque removal. It is important to keep your oral care equipment clean. Rinse off your toothbrush after use and store it in an upright position inside your medicine cabinet. Do not cover the brush head as this can lead to bacterial and fungal growth.

4. Floss occasionally if you have trapped meat fibers or food particles or other debris in-between your teeth that brushing cannot easily shift without damaging your gums. String floss can be harsh on gums, and most dentists now agree that its regular use poses too great a risk to the health of your gums. Dentists can repair damage to teeth caused by decay, but they cannot restore the health of your gums if they become damaged and infected. As we become older, the health of our gums is paramount; without healthy gums, we risk losing our teeth, and the underlying bones can become infected as well. A safer, gentler alternative to string or tape flosses are interdental brushes which come in a variety of sizes to suit the size of the gaps between your teeth. An oral water flosser or irrigator which sends a pulsed water jet to clean both in-between teeth and below the gum-line is another safer but effective option.

5. Avoid all tobacco products as not only does tobacco stain your teeth and cause bad breath, it can lead to oral cancer, gum disease (**gingivitis**), and abscesses. Of course, smoking tobacco has many other undesirable effects on your overall health including vital organs like your lungs and heart.

6. What you eat and drink influences the health of your teeth and gums. Reduce your consumption of sugary beverages, sweets, and cookies as sugar is converted into acid by the bacteria in your mouth, which can then lead to the erosion of the enamel of your teeth and the formation of cavities. Choose healthier options such as water, unsweetened tea, and low-calorie fruit juice. Although fruits are good for your general health, they can be harmful to teeth because of their acidity. This certainly does not mean avoiding fruit altogether, but fruit should be eaten at discrete meal times (e.g., with breakfast and as a dessert with dinner) and not snacked on throughout the day in order to limit the exposure of the teeth to acid. You should also reduce your consumption of carbonated drinks which are also harmful to your tooth enamel. Choose noncarbonated beverages instead and drink more water. Water won't stain your teeth or lead to cavities and it will actually help to prevent cavities

by washing away sugars and acids that could linger on your teeth. If you really can't do without your sugary carbonated drink, then consume it using a straw which will limit the exposure of your teeth to the fluid. Snack on crunchy vegetables such as celery and carrots which can help clear food residue from your teeth. Consume foods and beverages that are rich in calcium and vitamin D to help strengthen your teeth, bones, and help maintain healthy gums.

7. Use an antibacterial therapeutic mouthwash. A therapeutic mouthwash does more than mask bad breath. It can help reduce plaque, inflammation of the gums (gingivitis), cavities, and bad breath.

8. Visit your dentist regularly, at least twice per year. Regular trips to your dentist for a comprehensive oral exam can pinpoint any problems and keep them from getting worse. Your dentist or the dental hygienist will remove tartar, plaque, and make recommendations about how you can improve the care of your teeth and gums.

9. Don't ignore aches and pains. When you experience a toothache, gum sensitivity, or jaw pain, don't wait to visit your dentist; make an appointment immediately. Your dentist can discover the underlying cause and help prevent the issue from escalating into costly dental repair work.

10. Proper oral hygiene should begin at a very early age. Gently wipe your baby's gums when only a few weeks old. Brushing your baby's teeth should start as soon as the first tooth appears.

WAYS TO PROTECT THE HEALTH OF YOUR BONES

Bones are the support system of the body and are important to our mobility, so it is very important to keep them strong and healthy. Bones continuously undergo a small degree of turnover; that is, they are continuously being broken down and rebuilt in tiny amounts. Bones undergo growth and strengthening up to the age of 30 when we reach our peak bone mass. After that we tend to gradually lose bone mass, the bones become less dense, and the risk of fracture increases. As peak bone mass and density varies from person to person, those whose bones are not so strong at the age of 30 are more likely to get fractures in later life, particularly after the age of 60. Women generally have less bone mass and lower bone density than men, and at menopause, women no longer produce estrogen (which helps to maintain bone density), osteoporosis sets in, and the bones weaken at a faster rate than in men whose continued testosterone production maintains bone strength. Therefore, it is best to promote good bone development in our earlier years so that we end up with a relatively high bone mass and density at the age of 30, and then follow guidelines to help minimize our loss of bone as we age further. Although all this may seem a long way off to those who are relatively young now, it is important to realize that once osteoporosis sets in, it is extremely hard to reverse. The following ten guidelines should be followed to help maintain the health of your bones:

1. Know your family history because as with many medical conditions, family history is a key indicator of bone health. Those with a parent or sibling who has or had osteoporosis are more likely to develop it. So, find out whether your grandparents and great grandparents had any bone problems or a history of fractures.

2. Boost your dietary calcium consumption, as this mineral is essential for the proper development of teeth and bones. Vitamin D status is also important, as vitamin D helps the body absorb calcium in the gut and promotes bone development. Vitamin D is produced mostly in the skin via the action of sunlight and can also be obtained from the diet; good sources are oily fish, shrimp, egg yolk, mushrooms, dairy produce, and fortified foods such as milk and cereals. Foods that are good sources of calcium include yogurt, cheese, milk, spinach, and collard greens.

3. Avoid vitamin D deficiency. Many people in the northern hemisphere have low vitamin D status in the winter months because the sunlight is less and is not strong enough to produce vitamin D in the skin. A daily vitamin D3 supplement of 1,000 IU (25 µg) per day from October to March is usually sufficient to maintain vitamin D status at its high end-of-summer value during the winter months.

4. Vitamin K is important for normal blood clotting, but it also is thought to help the body make proteins for healthy bones and reduces the amount of calcium excreted in the urine. Good food sources of vitamin K include healthy greens such as kale, broccoli, Swiss chard, and spinach.

5. Diets high in potassium have been shown to improve bone health, possibly because potassium may neutralize acids that remove calcium from the body. Good food sources of potassium are sweet potatoes, white potatoes (with the skin on), yogurt, and bananas.

6. Regular exercise is key to maintaining many aspects of our health and our bone health is no exception. In fact, living a sedentary lifestyle is considered a risk factor for osteoporosis. Weight-bearing exercise such as walking, running, rope skipping, skiing, stair or hill climbing, and lifting weights strengthens bone, so these forms of exercise can have a positive effect on bone density. As we get older, the improved bone strength and balance we gain with regular exercise helps prevent falls (and the associated fractures) in those who are prone to develop osteoporosis.

7. Consume less caffeine, as too much of it can interfere with the body's ability to absorb calcium. One study showed that drinking more than two cups of coffee per day accelerated bone loss in subjects who also didn't consume enough calcium. So, drink coffee and cola drinks in moderation, and make sure to consume enough calcium, too.

8. As with caffeinated beverages, drink alcohol in moderation. Heavy alcohol consumption is known to cause bone loss (because it interferes with the actions of vitamin D). Moderate consumption (that's one drink per day for women, two per day for men) is fine, and recent studies actually show it may help slow bone loss.

9. Quit smoking, as numerous studies have shown that smoking can prevent the body from efficiently absorbing calcium, decreasing bone mass.

10. Avoid prolonged bed rest during periods of illness or through just being lazy and staying in bed all day. Avoiding weight-bearing physical activity, even by just not doing enough standing and walking, will result in loss of bone (and muscle mass – see below). In other words, use it or lose it! Astronauts in space experience prolonged periods of weightlessness and have been shown to lose up to 1% to 2% of their bone mass per month on a mission! Interestingly, some studies have found that supplemental vitamin K can help build back astronauts' lost bone, even more than calcium and vitamin D. That's just one more reason to eat your greens!

WAYS TO PROTECT THE HEALTH OF YOUR JOINTS

We need healthy joints in order to be able to move, run, jump, twist, and turn easily and without pain. There are just three types of joints in the body: fixed joints, slightly moveable joints and synovial joints. Fixed joints, like those that make up the skull, don't allow any movement and are held tightly together with fibrous connective tissue. Slightly moveable joints are joints that can move a little such as those between the vertebrae in the spine. Synovial joints are the most movable type of joint found in our bodies and include the elbow, hip and knee joints. They are composed of a joint capsule, lined by a membrane called the synovium that is filled with synovial fluid. Our joints are connected by ligaments and muscles for stability. They have a layer of smooth, white tissue called articular cartilage on the ends of the bones that helps to distribute compression forces, stops the bones from rubbing together, and permits smooth gliding when we move. The entire inner surface of the joint is lined by the synovial membrane (or synovium), except where the joint is lined with cartilage, and the interior of the joint capsule is filled with synovial fluid that acts as a lubricant (like the oil in your car) to reduce friction between the articular cartilage of joints during movement. Age, injury and everyday lifestyle habits can all contribute to the wear and tear of our cartilage, and unfortunately this damage is not readily repaired. Therefore, keeping your joints healthy to reduce the wear and tear on the cartilage is a key component to having an active lifestyle and continuing to play the sports you love. Healthy joints also play an important role in preventing the need for hip or knee joint replacement surgery. Here are ten steps you can take towards building healthier, stronger joints that will last a lifetime.

1. Keeping your weight within a healthy range is the best thing you can do for your joints. Weight-bearing joints, such as your back, hips, and knees have to support your body weight when you are upright. That's why so many overweight people have problems with these areas of the body. So, if you are overweight (see chapter 7 to know how to determine this), it is good to lose those extra pounds. Even losing a small amount of weight will give your knees some relief. Research has shown that if you lose 5 kg (11 lbs.) or more, you can halve your risk of developing **osteoarthritis** (when the protective cartilage on the ends of your bones wears down over time) in your knee joints.

2. Exercise is good for your joints and not only because it can help you lose extra pounds and maintain a healthy weight. Some research suggests that aerobic exercise can reduce the incidence of joint swelling because physical activity encourages circulation of the synovial fluid which allows bones to move past one another more smoothly. Furthermore, exercise triggers a biological process called autophagy which involves the removal of damaged cells in the joint. If your occupation requires you to be seated for long periods, it will put you in the high risk category for chronic joint pain because limited movement means more stiffness in your joints. So, change positions often, and take regular breaks from sitting; do some stretching, or take a short walk during scheduled work breaks. If you have to stay in the office, try taking phone calls while standing or walking around your desk. If your joints bother you, opt for exercises that won't give your joints a pounding. Instead of step aerobics or rope jumping, try some relatively low-impact exercises such as swimming or cycling. The key to a successful exercise program is variety. Completing a balance of aerobic, muscle strengthening, and flexibility exercises, along with keeping a healthy weight, will provide the base for good joint health for a lifetime. Take note of the following with regard to your physical activities:

- Cross-training adds variety to your exercise routine, because you do different activities each time you work out.

- Flexibility exercises allow you to maintain the full range of motion that healthy joints need to function optimally. Active stretching exercises such as yoga, tai chi, and Pilates all help our joints stay ready for more intense exercise. Stretching exercises should be performed before and after aerobic or resistance exercise workouts.

- Aerobic exercise activities should begin with relatively low intensity.

- As you age, you should avoid high-impact training such as jumping rope, step aerobics, or running on hard surfaces such as city streets. Low-impact exercises and sports such as bicycling, walking, and swimming are ideal and can be performed with minimal equipment. Useful gym equipment with low-impact loads on the legs include stair climbers or stationary cycle ergometers.

- Weight training keeps your muscles strong and allows for good joint stability. Performing weight training safely is critical, as is starting with low loads and higher repetitions for joint safety. Before starting a weight training program, you should seek the advice of a trained professional who can help to develop the optimal program for you and ensure that you learn to do the actions safely.

3. If the muscles in your limbs and around your joints are weak, your joints take more of a pounding, especially your spine, hips, and knees which support your body weight. Simple weight training exercises and adequate protein intake can help to build muscle and keep your muscles and surrounding ligaments strong. Try to focus on strengthening the muscles around the hip and knee joints, as these are the joints that need to support the entire body weight.

4. Always perform a warm up followed by stretching before doing any form of exercise. A warm-up is important for your joints as well as your muscles, so start with at least five minutes of gradual, low intensity preparation time before doing your planned exercise session. Do a few minutes of gentle stretching after the warm up and again after your exercise session has finished.

5. Certain exercises and activities can be tough on your joints and are best avoided. Examples include pounding exercises like kickboxing, step aerobics, and jumping as well as activities like roller blading and skate boarding which put a lot of stress on the ankle and knee joints. It is much easier on your joints if you opt for low-impact activities like cycling and swimming that offer the same calorie-burning benefits without the potentially damaging pounding.

6. Eating a healthy diet is good for your joints, because it helps build strong bones and muscles. You also need vitamin D to keep your joints in good health, and some studies suggest that dietary antioxidants such as vitamin C can help keep your joints healthy. Some foods have anti-inflammatory properties that can help to prevent joint pain caused by inflammation. Such foods include fruits, vegetables, and whole grains. Omega-3 fatty acids, found in oily fish, such as salmon and mackerel (and also available in capsules as supplements), have been shown to have effective anti-inflammatory actions, and some studies indicate that they can reduce the pain and inflammation of stiff joints in people with arthritis. Glucosamine, a supplement made from the shells of crab, lobster, and shrimp, has been shown to ease joint pain and stiffness, particularly in people with osteoarthritis of the knee, and some studies suggest that it may contribute to cartilage repair following joint injury.

7. Good posture is good for your joints, particularly in your spine and hips. If you stand and sit in a straight position, it will protect your joints and prevent your back muscles from becoming strained. Slouching puts extra pressure on your joints and can lead to pain in the neck, back, and shoulders. Having bad posture limits your range of motion and makes it so much harder for your muscles to take the load off your joints. Over time, poor posture can cause misalignment of the spine which eventually leads to even more joint stress and pain.

8. Adopting a good posture is also important when lifting and carrying. When lifting a heavy or bulky object, squat down and use the larger thigh muscles to raise the load by bending at your knees instead of having knees straight and bending your back. Use a back support if you lift objects regularly. If you use a backpack, be sure to use both straps placed over your shoulders instead of slinging it over one, as a lopsided weight puts more stress on your joints when you move. When you carry items by hand when on the move, use your arms instead of your hands and hold items close to your body, which is less stressful for your joints. Whenever possible, it is safer to slide heavy objects rather than lifting them.

9. To reduce the risk of joint injury, make sure you always wear protective gear when participating in high-risk activities, including leisure or work-related ones that involve repetitive kneeling or squatting. Consider wearing protective pads on your knees and elbows or elbow and wrist braces which can help reduce stress on your joints during activities. Always wear a helmet if there is a risk of falling (e.g., when cycling). Wear sensible shoes, and ladies, limit the time you spend in high heels, as all heels higher than one inch will put extra stress on your knees and may increase your risk of developing osteoarthritis.

10. If one of your joints feels sore after doing some form of activity, it is likely that you have incurred some damage which may lead to inflammation and swelling. In this situation try applying some ice wrapped in a towel to the affected area for no more than 15-20 minutes which will help to relieve the pain and reduce the inflammation. If you don't have ice available, try using a bag of frozen peas or corn wrapped in a light towel. Never apply ice directly to the skin.

WAYS TO PROTECT THE HEALTH OF YOUR MUSCLES

You have already heard a lot from me about the benefits of regular exercise for the health of your cardiovascular system, immune system, bones, and joints, but in order to be able to participate in physical activity, we need our muscles to be in good working order. If you exercise daily, it's important to maintain muscle health in order to avoid tears and strains. Keeping your muscles healthy will help you to be able to walk, run, play sports, and carry out all your daily activities including household chores. Healthy muscles are important as we get older in order to maintain good balance and reduce risk of falls and, of course, to remain independent. Exercising, getting enough rest, and eating a healthy balanced diet will help to keep your muscles in good shape for life.

Strong muscles also help to keep your joints in good shape. If the muscles around your joints, like your knee, get weak, you are more likely to suffer a joint injury which could leave you immobilized for weeks. Ligaments and joints can take a long time to heal after being damaged. As with bones, any period of immobilization lasting more than a few days will start to result in a loss of muscle tissue mass that can amount to as much as 30% over a period of six weeks. That will make your muscles become weaker, and this loss of strength will also be accompanied by a reduced capacity for fat oxidation and decreased endurance. So, it is important to say active. Furthermore, we all lose some muscle mass as we get older. Peak muscle mass and strength usually occurs around 25-30 years of age, and after that there is a small gradual decline which accelerates as we reach our 50s and 60s and beyond. The medics have a term for this which is "sarcopenia". In some individuals, particularly those who have led a sedentary lifestyle or just stopped doing much exercise when they reached middle-age, the loss of muscle mass can be so large that it compromises the ability to do everyday tasks that we normally take for granted. Like walking up a flight of stairs, standing up from a seated position in an armchair, or even getting up from the toilet seat! Things start to go rapidly downhill from there as you can imagine, often leading to loss of independence. The good news is that this sorry state is not inevitable, and even someone who was previously sedentary can reverse the process of sarcopenia by doing regular resistance exercises with both arms and legs and eating more protein at strategic times of the day. How to achieve this and some other tips to maintain your muscles follow:

1. Avoid prolonged bed rest during periods of illness or through just being lazy and spending too much time in bed all day. As with bone it's all about using it or losing it! Avoiding weight-bearing physical activity, even by just not doing enough standing and walking, will result in loss of muscle mass. That will make you weaker and less fit which then makes any exercise you do feel harder than before.

2. This may seem obvious, but doing regular exercise is very important for maintaining muscle health. People who exercise have stronger muscles than others in their age group. Practice weight-bearing exercises such as jogging, running, aerobics, and dancing. As long as you are not pregnant, you can include some step aerobics, squat jumping, jumping on the spot, or using a skipping rope (jolting exercises are best avoided during pregnancy). Higher muscle mass is associated with lower mortality, lower risk of type 2 diabetes, and lower incidence of disability in older age. Indeed, weight-bearing and resistance exercise are the most powerful ways to stave off muscle loss in aging and even disabled populations.

3. Before beginning any sort of physical activity, it's crucial to spend at least five minutes warming up. Focus on warming up the muscles you'll be using during your workout, and don't forget to do some gentle stretching before starting your exercise session. At other times, particularly in the mornings, do some brisk walking, light jogging, or light weight training, as this will help your muscles prepare for more intense activities such as a long run, sprints, or heavy weight training that you may do later in the day.

4. Spending a few minutes stretching your main muscle groups can drastically reduce the risk of muscle tears. Hold each stretch for 20 seconds to allow the muscles to become more flexible, and therefore less likely to sustain injury.

5. Stretching out your muscles also helps them reach their full range of motion. The best time to stretch is after your warm-up and before your intended activity. This way, your muscles will already be warm, and they will stretch better and with less risk of a tear. After exercising, it is a good idea to spend about 10 minutes cooling down. The cool-down process is similar to the warm-up process, except at a slower pace. Perform a less intense activity (e.g., walking or jogging rather than running at your usual pace) to allow your muscles to fully recover. A cool down will remove lactic acid from your working muscles more quickly than if you come to an abrupt halt after finishing your planned exercise session. Remember to allow enough time for both your warm up and cool down when planning your regular workouts.

6. What you eat greatly impacts the health of your muscles. Your diet can help your muscles to perform prolonged bouts of exercise, delay the onset of fatigue, adapt to increased demands, recover from exhausting exercise, grow and strengthen, repair themselves after damaging exercise, and function properly. Dietary carbohydrate is important for restoration of glycogen stores after prolonged exercise, and protein is essential for adaptation to training, maintaining muscle mass, and increasing it as desired when undertaking a program of resistance training. Good sources of dietary protein include meat, poultry, fish, shellfish, eggs, dairy products, beans, and other legumes. A healthy diet rich in lean protein is important for athletes who want to optimize their adaptation to training and perform to their full potential, and research shows that it's just as important for aging adults for maintaining or even increasing their muscle mass. In order to maximize the anabolic potential of resistance exercise training, it is recommended to ingest 20-25 g of protein with each meal of the day and have some additional protein, perhaps as a milk drink before going to bed. While we are asleep, muscle repair and growth can still take place but only if dietary protein is available. If you don't eat anything after your early evening meal, there is no protein to support synthesis

during the night, so on balance you actually lose muscle mass due to increased tissue protein breakdown while you sleep in the absence of nutrient intake.

7. Even with a great diet, it can be difficult to consume all of the nutrients you need to optimize muscle health. For instance, omega-3 fatty acids have been shown to have muscle-sparing effects in older people, but it can be difficult to get enough of these nutrients if you don't regularly consume oily fish such as mackerel, sardines, and salmon. The same is true for vitamin D, a nutrient your body synthesizes during sun exposure and which is now known to be important for muscle function in addition to its well-established effects on bone. Overall, fish oil, a vitamin D3 supplement, and a multivitamin tablet are great additions to a varied diet.

8. Almost everyone has experienced sore muscles, particularly the day after doing some unaccustomed exercise or working out too much. Some mild soreness can be a normal part of healthy exercise, but more severe soreness, often accompanied by stiffness and swelling, can occur after we have performed exercise in which the muscles are lengthened (stretched) while being activated. This form of activity is referred to as eccentric exercise, and it occurs during downhill running, squat jumping, bench stepping, decelerating from a sprint, and when we lower a weight such as a dumbbell. In some situations, muscles can become strained. Muscle strain can be mild (though still painful) such as when the muscle has just been stretched too much, but sometimes it can be severe, and the muscle actually tears. Contact sports like soccer, football, hockey, and wrestling can often cause strains. Sports in which you grip something (like a tennis racquet or golf club) can lead to strains in your wrist, forearm, or elbow. Range-of-motion exercises (such as stretching) are a good way to keep your muscles and ligaments flexible and including some simple resistance or static (isometric) exercises as part of your weekly exercise regimen will help to improve your muscle strength.

9. The tendons are fibrous connective tissues that connect the muscles to the bones. Tendons can be strained if they are pulled or stretched too much. The ligaments are also fibrous connective structures that connect bones to bones and stabilize joints. If they are stretched or pulled too much, the injury is called a sprain. Most people are familiar with the pain of a sprained ankle. The best immediate treatment is to apply ice wrapped in a towel to limit the inflammation, swelling, and pain.

10. Finally, it is important to allow your muscles to recover after doing a hard workout. Adaptation mostly takes place in the hours after the exercise has finished, not during the exercise. For recovery you need a long enough period of rest (e.g., a full night's sleep) and good post-exercise nutrition in the form of dietary carbohydrate to restore glycogen stores and protein to promote repair and adaptation. In addition, a relaxing massage or a warm bath can relieve muscle tension and help reduce fatigue. Leave ice baths to the professional athletes. They have limited benefit in reducing inflammation and soreness and can cause muscle cramping besides being distinctly uncomfortable!

WAYS TO PROTECT THE HEALTH OF YOUR SKIN

The skin is a protective layer that surrounds the body, and its condition is not only important to overall health but also affects how old you look. As well as protecting you against infection, your skin plays other important roles in your overall health. It helps keep you cool or warm, insulates you, stores energy, and provides sensation through touch, so you can interact with the outside world beyond what you see, hear, and smell. Good skin care and healthy lifestyle choices can help delay natural aging, prevent various skin problems, and keep you feeling and looking younger for longer. Here are ten guidelines for you to follow to maintain healthy skin:

1. Some exposure of the skin to sunlight is good because it allows the production of vitamin D3 which is needed for healthy bones, teeth, and an effective immune system to ward off infections. In the spring and summer months, about 20 minutes exposure to sunlight wearing shorts and T shirt is sufficient to get your daily dose of vitamin D. Too much sun over a lifetime can cause wrinkles, age spots, and other skin problems – as well as increase the risk of skin cancer. Therefore, one of the most important ways to take care of your skin is to protect it from the sun. For the most complete sun protection:

   - Use a broad-spectrum sunscreen with a sun protection factor (SPF) of at least 15. Apply sunscreen generously, and reapply every two hours – or more often if you're swimming or perspiring.

   - During the summer months, avoid sunbathing between 10 am and 3 pm when the sun's rays are strongest.

   - Protect your skin by wearing clothing that covers your skin (e.g., long-sleeved shirts, long pants, and wide-brimmed hats). Also consider laundry additives, which give clothing an additional layer of ultraviolet protection for a certain number of washings, or special sun-protective clothing – which is specifically designed to block ultraviolet rays.

2. Don't smoke, as smoking makes your skin look older and contributes to wrinkles. Smoking narrows the tiny blood vessels in the outermost layers of skin, which decreases blood flow and makes skin paler. This also depletes the skin of oxygen and nutrients that are important to skin health. Smoking also damages collagen and elastin, the fibers that give your skin its strength and elasticity. In addition, the repetitive facial expressions you make when smoking, such as pursing your lips when inhaling and squinting your eyes to keep out smoke, can contribute to wrinkles. In addition, smoking increases your risk of **squamous cell skin cancer**.

3. Limit the time you spend in the bath to no more than 10 minutes, and use warm rather than hot water. Hot water and long showers or baths remove oils from your skin. Avoid strong soaps. Strong soaps and detergents can strip oil from your skin. Instead, choose mild cleansers. To protect and lubricate your skin when shaving, apply shaving cream, lotion, or gel before shaving. For the closest shave, use a clean, sharp razor. Shave in the direction the hair grows, not against it. After washing or bathing, gently pat or blot your skin dry with a soft towel so that some moisture remains on your skin; avoid hard rubbing of the skin. If your skin is dry, use a moisturizer that suits your skin type. For daily use, consider a moisturizer that contains SPF 15 or 30.

4. A healthy diet can help you look and feel your best. Eat plenty of fresh fruits, green vegetables, whole grains, and lean meats to ensure sufficient protein and vitamins. A diet rich in vitamin C and low in fats and sugar promotes radiant skin. The association between diet and acne isn't clear, but some research suggests that a diet rich in fish oil or fish oil supplements and low in unhealthy fats and processed or refined carbohydrates might promote younger looking skin. Drinking plenty of water helps keep your skin hydrated.

5. Manage your stress levels because too much stress can make your skin more sensitive and trigger acne breakouts and other skin problems. Get enough sleep (seven to eight hours per night should be the norm for most people and getting your "beauty sleep" is not a myth). If you don't get enough good quality sleep, your skin gets tired just like you - it sags, and you get bags under your eyes. At the start of each day, set reasonable limits and expectations of what you can achieve in a day's work, and make time to do the things you enjoy.

6. Check your skin carefully and regularly. All men and women should examine their own skin periodically for spots, moles, warts, and unusual discoloring or growths that could turn out to be cancers. It is possible and advisable to have a health care professional perform a total body scan every few years to look for any signs of skin cancer. The most common cancers are **basal cell carcinoma**, squamous cell carcinoma, and **keratocanthoma** and are normally benign (i.e., they do not usually spread to the rest of the body and so are not life threatening), but they can be disfiguring and may require surgery to remove them and allow lab tests to confirm the diagnosis. However, some skin cancers, although far less common, are dangerous and can grow and spread to other tissues and organs and even be fatal if left untreated. The most common forms of these kinds of cancers are called **melanomas** and develop from melanocytes, the pigment-making cells of the skin. Melanocytes can also form benign (non-cancerous) growths called moles. Therefore, it is important to get any skin lesions checked out by your doctor as soon as possible after you notice them.

7. Protect your skin from dryness. The epidermis is made up of about 30% water, much of which is bound in the fats and oils that help prevent the water from evaporating. You can increase your skin's ability to bind water by using a good-quality moisturizer. Natural moisturizing ingredients include citrate, various minerals, urea, lactate, and amino acids.

8. Clean your skin properly. Water alone won't do it. You need something to clear out the oily residue that can clog pores and lead to pimples. Compounds that do this are called surfactants. However, avoid using harsh soaps on your face as most are alkaline, which can change the delicate pH balance of your skin and cause itching, redness, flaking, and dryness. Instead, opt for gentle soaps suitable for both your face and hands, liquid cleansers, and cleansing creams with natural ingredients like beeswax and mineral oil to dissolve dirt. Other moisture-replenishing ingredients include vegetable and fruit oils and less-irritating surfactants such as coconut oil (cocamidopropyl), amphoteric surfactants, alkyl ether sulfates, and alkyl glyceryl ether sulfonate.

9. Ditch the daily use of a rough exfoliating buffer or washcloth, and opt instead for just splashing warm water on your skin to remove the cleanser or using a soft cloth. A limited amount and frequency of exfoliation of your skin is desirable to remove the layers of dead skin, leaving you with a healthier glow and brighter skin. But don't overdo it, once every one or two weeks is fine. Make sure you always remove your makeup or sunscreen before going to bed. The skin needs to breathe overnight, and makeup prevents that meaning that leaving it on overnight clogs the pores which may cause blemishes and/or blackheads.

10. Exercising regularly will improve the circulation to your skin which helps to keep it healthy. Remember to drink plenty of water to stay well hydrated.

WAYS TO PROTECT THE HEALTH OF YOUR GUT AND DIGESTIVE ORGANS

Your digestive system breaks down the foods you eat into the nutrients that the cells of your body can absorb and use. Your digestive health is directly impacted by the foods you eat and the lifestyle you live. There are various steps you can take to improve your digestive health, which can actually improve your overall health and sense of well-being. Your gut, particularly the large intestine (colon), is home to about 1 kg of bacteria which live on undigested food such as fiber that reaches them. The size and composition of the bacterial population in your gut (known as the gut microbiota) has some important influences on your health and is affected by your diet, some drugs (e.g., antibiotics), and probiotics. Follow these 10 guidelines to help ensure the health of your digestive system:

1. Eat a diet that is high in fiber and rich in fruits, vegetables, legumes, and whole grains to maintain or improve your digestive health. A high-fiber diet speeds up the rate at which food moves through your digestive tract, making you less likely to get constipated and can also help to prevent various digestive conditions, such as **diverticulosis**, **hemorrhoids**, and **irritable bowel syndrome** (IBS). In addition, it can help you achieve or maintain a healthy weight.

2. Consume both insoluble and soluble types of fiber as they help your digestive system in different ways. Humans lack the enzymes needed to digest insoluble fiber (roughage), and therefore it helps add bulk to the stools whereas soluble fiber (which is also indigestible) draws in water and can help prevent stools being too watery. Good sources of insoluble fiber include leafy green vegetables, legumes, whole grains, wheat bran, nuts, and seeds.

3. Limit foods that are high in fat because fatty foods tend to slow down the digestive process, making you more prone to **constipation**. You should not try to avoid fat altogether because some is essential, and also it contains fat-soluble vitamins, but you can pair-up fatty foods with high-fiber foods which will make them easier on your digestive system.

4. Choose lean rather than fatty meats, and use cooking methods that remove much of the saturated fat such as grilling or roasting. Fatty meats like pork belly or streaky bacon can lead to slow and uncomfortable digestion. When you eat meat, choose lean cuts, such as pork loin, beef steak, chicken breast, or thigh with the skin removed, and don't eat the fat on steaks and chops. Also make sure that you chew your food well by taking small bites and keep chewing until the mouthful is liquefied or has lost all its flavor. Then swallow it completely before you take another bite.

5. Include probiotics into your diet by eating foods that contain them or taking a probiotic supplement like Yakult or Actimel. Probiotics contain some of the same kind of healthy bacteria that are naturally present in your digestive tract. Probiotics, either from foods such as yogurt, sauerkraut, kimchi, kefir, kombucha, tempeh, and fermented pickles or as supplements help keep the body healthy by combating the effects of a poor diet, antibiotics, and stress. In addition, probiotics can strengthen immune function by interactions with the immune cells in your gut, and possibly even help treat IBS. Probiotics can help to prevent diarrhea when taking antibiotic drugs to treat a bacterial infection. Many antibiotic medications do not discriminate between the good and bad bacteria and can end up killing a significant proportion of your gut microbiota. Taking a probiotic supplement after antibiotic medication can help restore your healthy population of gut bacteria. Otherwise there is a big risk that your gut will become colonized by harmful bacteria like *E. coli* which can cause significant health problems. Numerous studies indicate that daily ingestion of a probiotic can reduce the incidence of gastrointestinal infections and improve gut and immune health in general. Aim for ones that contain *Lactobacillus* and/or *Bifidobacterium* species in a daily dose of 10 billion (10^{10}) live bacteria (known as colony forming units or CFU).

6. Your digestive system functions best when you consume your meals on a regular schedule, so aim to sit down for breakfast, lunch, and dinner around the same time each day, and limit eating of snacks between meals. In fact, if you eat appropriately at meal times, there is actually no need whatsoever for snacks unless you are very physically active. Leave about 10-12 hours between dinner and breakfast with only a light lunch or snack in between what should be your two main meals of the day. The gut lining consists of a single layer of cells that are replenished every two to three days, but this repair cannot take place as effectively if your gut is working hard on digestion most of the time. Leaving 10-12 hours between meals gives a clear period for the gut to focus on repair and replenishment.

7. Staying well hydrated by drinking plenty of water is good for your digestive health. Fiber draws water into the colon to create softer, bulkier stools, allowing them to pass through more easily which reduces the risk of constipation.

8. Avoid the bad habits such as smoking tobacco and consuming too much caffeine or alcohol as all these can interfere with the functioning of your gastrointestinal tract, and lead to problems like stomach ulcers and heartburn.

9. Exercise regularly as this helps keep foods moving through your digestive system, reducing constipation, as well as helping you to maintain a healthy weight, which is good for your digestive health. Do your exercise before meal times but not shortly after a heavy meal.

10. Too much stress can be bad for your digestion, so try to manage the sources and consequences of stress in your life by finding stress-reducing activities that you enjoy and practice them on a regular basis. Calm down and relax for at least 10 minutes before you eat any meal as your arousal-based sympathetic nervous system will interfere with your digestive function and likely result in bloating and discomfort after eating.

Some Common Gut Problems and Their Solutions

Food intolerance: You don't have to be suffering from celiac disease to react to gluten. Many people have a detectable reaction to gluten that doesn't cause the amount of inflammation and damage to the inner lining of the intestines that would class them as celiac. This less severe form of intolerance to gluten is called non-celiac gluten sensitivity, and it is far more common than celiac disease. Listen to your body; if you eat food that contains gluten, and it doesn't agree with you, it probably doesn't. The same goes for other foods: if something doesn't agree with you, then stop eating it and look for alternatives.

Heartburn: After chewing and swallowing food, the esophogeal sphincter opens to allow entry of the food into the stomach. The sphincter then closes, so that food can be retained in the stomach while the acid and digestive enzymes do their job. Many people who suffer from a form of indigestion known as acid reflux or heartburn think it is because they produce too much stomach acid, but it is just as likely that they don't produce enough. This can cause a change in pressure in the stomach which allows the esophogeal sphincter at the top to open, letting the contents pass back out into the esophagus where it causes irritation, inflammation, and pain. Eating some protein at each meal and chewing your food well both raise acid production. Sauerkraut is also a strong stimulant for your body to produce stomach acid, so try eating some of this at the start of your meal.

Constipation: If you have not pooed for over 24 hours, it does not necessarily mean that you are constipated. You don't need to poo daily. The idea that you need a daily bowel movement is simply not true for most of us. Normal bowel activity is classed as anything more than three times a week and fewer than three times a day, and it does not have to be a "perfectly formed" stool – normality is anything from putty to firm consistency. So long as you pass it easily it is OK.

Antibiotic-associated diarrhea: Antibiotic medications kill bacteria including those in your gut. One week of taking daily oral antibiotics can wipe out a large proportion of your resident gut bacteria (microbiota). Consuming probiotic foods (e.g., fermented dairy products such as yogurt) or probiotic supplements (e.g., Yakult, Actimel) for a few weeks after completing your course of antibiotics can help restore your population of healthy gut bacteria and prevent your gut from being colonized by undesirable bacteria which can cause infection and diarrhea.

Leaky gut leading to endotoxemia: Leaky gut is a common condition in people with poor digestive health, and it is caused by inflammation of the gut lining making it much more permeable than normal to the passage of large molecules such as proteins from the gut directly into the bloodstream which are then viewed as antigens by the immune system. In some cases, gut bacteria or their toxins can also slip through into the blood stream causing **endotoxemia** and fever-like symptoms. One of the most powerful treatment strategies for this problem is the Gut And Psychology Syndrome (GAPS) diet. It is a very restrictive dietary regimen, avoiding all grain, starchy vegetables, and most sugars, focusing instead on liquid foods such as soups and broths. Research indicates that daily bovine colostrum supplements (about 20 g/day) can also be effective in treating a leaky gut.

WAYS TO PROTECT THE HEALTH OF YOUR HEART AND CIRCULATION

Coronary heart disease is a major cause of premature death and other circulatory problems include thrombosis (an unwanted blood clot that lodges in a blood vessel such as a vein in your leg or your lungs), peripheral vascular disease, high blood pressure, and stroke. Here are ten ways to keep your heart and circulation healthy and working well:

1. Eating well is always your best medicine. Choose some foods from the following list every day. The active ingredients in these foods are well documented in preventing heart disease:

   - Garlic, onions, and chives contain organic compounds called allyl sulfides that prevent excessive blood clotting.

   - Berries of all kinds, especially the European blueberry (bilberry), are high in flavonoids that reduce risk of atherosclerosis.

   - Green and black teas contain polyphenols that help stop the accumulation of low-density lipoprotein (LDL, the so-called bad cholesterol) and reduce the risk of atherosclerosis.

   - Turmeric and cumin are two spices high in anti-inflammatory curcumin, which reduce the inflammation that is assumed to be another cause of heart disease. Curcumin also prevents excessive cholesterol accumulation.

   - Vegetables such as broccoli, cabbage, sprouts, cauliflower, kale, and mustard greens are all high in compounds such as indoles that help improve cholesterol metabolism.

   - Citrus fruits contain not only vitamin C but also numerous bioflavonoids such as quercetin that are reported to reduce inflammation and cholesterol levels.

   - Flaxseed, hempseed oil, and oily fish (especially salmon, catfish, mackerel, and trout) have high levels of omega-3 fatty acids that reduce inflammation, lower cholesterol and triglycerides, raise high-density lipoprotein (HDL, or good cholesterol), and reduce blood clotting.

- Cultured soy products such as tofu, tempeh, and miso are high in genistein and other **isoflavones** known for their cholesterol-lowering effects.

- Foods rich in β-carotenes (which are natural antioxidants) are good for the health of your heart. These foods include carrots, cabbage, winter squash, sweet potatoes, dark leafy greens like spinach, apricots, and seaweed.

2. Never smoke or quit smoking now as smokers are three to four times more likely to experience fatal heart attack than non-smokers. If you are a smoker and you stop now, within one year of quitting, your risk of heart attack will be halved. For a comparison of smoking tobacco products versus vaping, see the sidebar.

Why Vaping Is Safer Than Smoking

Scientific studies indicate that failing to quit smoking strongly increases the risk of lung cancer and cardiovascular disease. Cutting down the number of cigarettes smoked per day helps, but the risk of both cancer and cardiovascular disease compared with a non-smoker is still considerably higher. Indeed, one recent study meta-analysis of 141 cohort studies found that even one cigarette a day equated to a 48% increased risk of coronary heart disease for men and 57% for women. Although this risk is about half of that for smoking 20 cigarettes per day, it is still significant, so the only answer is to stop smoking completely. People who smoke are addicted to nicotine, and a safer alternative is to switch to vaping with electronic cigarettes (e-cigs) instead. Vaping liquids contain the nicotine that satisfies the cravings associated with addiction to cigarettes, but they are thought to be far less harmful to health. The good news is that there is conclusive evidence that completely substituting e-cigs for combustible tobacco cigarettes reduces users' exposure to numerous toxic and carcinogenic substances that are present in tobacco. In 2015 Public Health England issued a report stating that "e-cigarettes are 95% less harmful than tobacco". In 2017, a Cancer Research UK-funded study was the first to show evidence that long term e-cigarette users had far lower levels of key harmful toxins in their bodies than tobacco smokers. Vaping also avoids the potential problem for non-smokers of inhaling secondary smoke from someone who is smoking a tobacco product in their vicinity (e.g., someone walking in front of them or stood close by).

3. Avoid all convenience, fried, and processed foods like chips, and fast foods that can lead to atherosclerosis. Also limit your consumption of sugar, sweetened foods, and soft drinks as heart disease is strongly linked to sugar consumption.

4. Physical activity exercises your heart as well as your muscles, and that leads to improvements in its blood and oxygen supply and makes it fitter and stronger and much less prone to the development of coronary heart disease. A minimum of 30 minutes per day of aerobic exercise will improve your aerobic capacity and help prevent diseases affecting your cardiovascular system. Aerobics, brisk walking, hill walking, jogging, cycling, swimming, canoeing, kayaking, and cross-country skiing are all suitable forms of aerobic exercise.

5. Reducing mental stress and anxiety enhances cardiovascular health. Moderate the impact of stress on your heart by working to improve relationships; take more vacations; practice yoga, meditation, or tai chi; and seek psychotherapy for unresolved problems and acupuncture to relieve chronic pain.

6. Drink alcohol only in moderation. You don't need to cut out alcohol altogether; a glass of red wine each day with dinner will provides you with some polyphenols that help to prevent heart disease. Drinking more than this amount will not give additional benefits and could be detrimental to the health of your heart and other organs. For those who do not want to drink wine, you can also get the polyphenols from red grape juice and cranberry juice. Choose the no added sugar versions of these.

7. Consume caffeinated products like coffee only in moderation. Drinking one or two cups of coffee a day will do no damage and acts as a useful mental stimulant, but excessive amounts of caffeine (which also comes from dark chocolate, cola drinks, and energy drinks) may be too stimulating and lead to heartbeat irregularities, higher-than-optimal blood pressure, and a greater risk of stroke. Drink green tea instead.

8. While cholesterol is thought to be a risk factor in heart disease, ask your health care provider to test for other compounds periodically, especially if you have a family history of heart disease or type 2 diabetes. Test for blood levels of glucose, glycated hemoglobin, homocysteine, fibrinogen, and C-reactive protein. High levels of any of these compounds in the blood are associated with a higher risk of heart problems and can be corrected by diet changes and nutritional supplements, or medication if necessary. Low levels of thyroid hormone and high levels of cortisol can also increase risk of heart disease.

9. Check your blood pressure regularly using a battery-operated portable blood pressure monitor designed for use at home. They are inexpensive, and anyone can learn to use one. Sit down and relax for 10 minutes before taking a reading and repeat one or two more times. Alternatively, use the blood pressure monitor at your local doctor's surgery. If your blood pressure consistently exceeds 140 mmHg (systolic) or 90 mmHg (diastolic), let your medical practitioner know immediately as this indicates that you may have hypertension that can be treated effectively with prescription medication.

10. Forget supplements as you will get all the micronutrients you need if you eat a healthy balanced and varied diet. You do need adequate amounts of iron, vitamin C (which assists nonheme iron absorption from green vegetables), vitamin B12, and folic acid in order to produce normal amounts of red blood cells and the hemoglobin (the oxygen carrying pigment in your blood cells that gives blood its red color) that they contain. Deficiencies of iron or these vitamins result in anemia (a lower than normal blood hemoglobin concentration) which makes you feel tired and listless; in this situation iron supplements may be warranted.

WAYS TO PROTECT THE HEALTH OF YOUR LUNGS

We often don't consider the important role our lungs play in keeping us strong and well. But we certainly take notice when we start to experience problems with our breathing. Breathing provides us with the oxygen that the cells of our body need. Problems in oxygen delivery arise if we don't have enough red cells or hemoglobin in our blood (a condition known as anemia), if our heart is failing, or when our lungs are not doing their job of getting the oxygen in the atmosphere into our blood. The latter can occur if we are suffering from a severe respiratory illness such as **asthma**, **pneumonia**, **chronic obstructive pulmonary disease**, **emphysema**, or c**hronic bronchitis**. These conditions can cause blockage or narrowing of our airways and/or a thickening of the respiratory membranes across which oxygen must pass to get from the air in our lungs into the blood.

Just like the muscles, bones, heart, and circulation, our lungs benefit from regular movement and activity. Everyday breathing in the resting state or even when performing most light daily activities will only cause the lungs to function at less than 30% of their full capacity. Our resting rate of lung ventilation is about 10 liters of air passing in and out of the lungs per minute. During moderate exercise (e.g., jogging) this increases to around 50 liters per minute, and during exercise close to aerobic capacity this can increase up to 100-150 liters per minute depending on fitness. Since regular day-to-day activity doesn't help you use your lungs to full capacity, you need to occasionally challenge the lungs by doing some intense physical activities. This will also help to rid your lungs of the toxins and tar that accumulate due to the presence of pollutants, allergens, dust, and smoke (including secondary smoke you have inhaled from people smoking cigarettes around you) in the atmosphere. The level of these pollutants can be particularly high in the big cities. Follow these 10 guidelines to improve your lung health and keep these vital organs going strong throughout your life:

1. To help keep your lungs functioning properly, you can do some simple breathing techniques. These techniques can be performed by healthy people as well as those who are suffering from breathing problems related to asthma, emphysema, and chronic bronchitis etc. One effective technique is known as "diaphragmatic breathing". This uses your conscious awareness of the diaphragm muscle, which is the large flat muscle separating the abdominal cavity from the lungs and heart in the chest. By concentrating on lowering your diaphragm as you breathe in, you'll get a much deeper inhalation. This technique is used by many professional singers to increase their lung capacity.

2. If you simply perform slower and deeper breathing than normal, it can help you get closer to reaching your lungs' full capacity. Slowly and continuously inhale over a period of about 5-10 seconds while consciously lowering your diaphragm and expanding your rib cage, allowing the floating ribs to open like wings. Finally, allow the upper chest to expand and lift, filling your lungs with air as fully as you can. After this, breathe out slowly but as completely as possible by letting the chest fall, then contracting the ribs and, finally, contracting the muscles in the wall of your abdomen (that's what we call the "abs") to lift the diaphragm and expel the last bit of air. Relax with normal breathing for 30 seconds and then repeat the whole procedure 5-10 times.

3. You can also increase your lung capacity by increasing the length of your breathing movements in and out. Begin by counting how long a natural breath takes. Inhalation and exhalation generally take the same amount of time, so if it takes three seconds to inhale, it should take three seconds to exhale. Once you've determined the duration for your average breath, add one more second to each inhalation and exhalation until you can comfortably extend the length of time it takes to fill and empty your lungs. Take care to avoid straining or causing discomfort; it should be a gradual and easy process.

4. Your posture affects your lung function and capacity because the lungs are soft structures, and they can only expand to take up the room that you make for them. You can make more room for your lungs and increase their capacity by occasionally standing or sitting tall and extending your arms overhead (as if attempting to reach the ceiling) while breathing in deeply. If you are sitting on a chair (make sure it is a very stable one!), lean back slightly, raise your arms, lift your chest, and open the front of your body as you breathe deeply. These postural changes will allow you to expand your lungs more fully.

5. Staying well hydrated is important for the lungs as it is for the rest of the body. It helps to keep the film of protective liquid than lines the mucosa of the airways thin which helps the lungs function better.

6. Regular moderately intense physical activities are great for the lungs and your respiratory muscles just as it is for your heart.

7. Laughing is another great exercise to work the abdominal muscles and increase lung capacity. It will also clear out your lungs by forcing stale air out and allowing fresh air to enter into more areas of your lungs.

8. If you smoke, you should stop altogether to improve the condition of your lungs. Cigarette smoke contains thousands of harmful chemicals, some of which can cause health problems including serious lung diseases like lung cancer and chronic obstructive pulmonary disease. Cigarette smoke causes damage and inflammation of the airways which narrows their diameter making breathing more difficult. The same applies for smoke from cigars and pipe tobacco. With time, tobacco smoke can destroy lung tissues, which in turn increases your risk of lung cancer. If you suffer from any kind of lung disease, giving up smoking can help manage your condition and improve your quality of life, so be determined to quit smoking and get help from professionals if needed. Smoking also markedly increases the risk of cardiovascular disease.

9. Non-smokers should always try to avoid exposure to second-hand smoke to improve the condition of their lungs. Second-hand smoke is toxic and can damage your lungs and your overall health. Here are some things you can do to avoid second-hand smoke:

    - Do not allow other people to smoke in your home, car, or workplace.

    - Support businesses and activities that are smoke-free.

    - Avoid public places that permit smoking.

    - Stay at smoke-free hotels when traveling to avoid residual smoke from previous patrons.

10. In addition to cigarette smoke, there are various other pollutants present in the air that are harmful for your lungs as well as overall health. Even the synthetic fragrances used in various laundry products and air fresheners emit toxic chemicals. There are several things you can do to improve the quality of the air that you breathe:

- Avoid highly polluted and industrialized areas.

- Do your bit to minimize outdoor pollution and help create a cleaner environment by walking or cycling instead of driving whenever possible.

- When building or remodeling your house, opt for eco-friendly options like formaldehyde-free cabinetry, linoleum instead of vinyl flooring, nonvolatile paints, adhesives, etc.

- In your home, have at least two houseplants per 10 square meters of space. These plants should be in 25-30 cm pots. Use indoor plants such as a fern, spider plant, peace lily, bamboo palm, aloe vera, English Ivy, dracaena etc. Make sure to keep the foliage dust-free, and do not overwater the plants as it may lead to mold growth.

- Minimize the use of harsh cleaners and cleaners with strong fragrances.

- Avoid using aerosol sprays.

- Ensure adequate ventilation.

WAYS TO PROTECT THE HEALTH OF YOUR KIDNEYS, BLADDER, AND URINARY TRACT

The best way to prevent urinary tract infection complications is to keep the kidneys and the entire urinary system healthy. This can be done through proper diet and nutrition. Our kidneys are responsible for filtering out waste products such as ammonia, uric acid, and urea, but also helps to regulate our blood volume and pressure by excreting more or less water, salt, and potassium according to the body's needs. The more acidic the food we consume, the greater is the strain on our kidneys for getting rid of that waste. Many healthcare experts recommend eating 80% alkaline foods with only 20% acidic food, but the Western diet is the exact opposite as it is rich in wheat flour and meat products which create an acidic environment which research studies have shown to be detrimental to kidney health. However, the good news is that research is also showing that by eating more fruits and vegetables (which are alkaline foods), we can counter these undesirable effects. Here are ten ways in which you can help to maintain the health of your kidneys, bladder and urinary tract.

1. Drink at least 1.5 liters of water each day to flush out waste products and avoid high concentrations of toxins or drugs you have taken building up in your kidney tubules. This will also keep you well hydrated.

2. Exercise regularly for at least 30 minutes per day. Maintain a healthy weight according to your age to avoid putting excess strain on all bodily systems.

3. Avoid taking too many drugs, especially pain medicines or drugs containing nonsteroidal anti-inflammatory drugs such as ibuprofen. Drugs and toxins get about five times as concentrated in the kidney tubules compared with the blood, so any compounds that are harmful to cells will likely damage the cells that line the kidney tubules first. This is why kidney failure is always a risk with drug overdoses.

4. Get a routine physical exam by your medical practitioner if you are prone to recurrent **urinary tract infections** (UTIs), and consider getting urine culture tests done every few months. If untreated, these UTIs can spread to the bladder and kidneys.

5. Eat a healthy diet and avoid high intakes of red meat. Eat more fresh fruits and cruciferous vegetables like cauliflower, cabbage, and broccoli. Choose foods low in sodium, sugar, and fats but high in fiber content. Drinking cranberry juice (with no added sugar) can help to prevent urinary tract infections.

6. Pay close attention to personal hygiene – clean your private parts regularly with fresh water but avoid harsh soaps and make sure to shower thoroughly after swimming in pools or lakes. And don't share a bath with anyone else.

7. If you have high blood pressure, then your risk of developing kidney related issues is greater. So, talk to your doctor about angiotensin converting enzyme (ACE) inhibitors which are known to reduce these risk factors. Daily ingestion of a glass of concentrated beetroot juice is a natural way to reduce your blood pressure as it has high nitrate content. The nitrate gets converted into nitric oxide in your body which is a vasodilator (it opens up blood vessels as so reduces blood pressure). The other main modifiable risk factors for developing chronic kidney disease are being overweight or obese, having high levels of blood cholesterol and triglyceride, being type 2 diabetic, and smoking. These are all things you can modify by adopting appropriate lifestyle behaviors.

8. If you are prone to getting UTIs frequently, get them treated immediately. Procrastinating treatment can complicate matters. See an expert urologist to rule out other complicated health conditions that could be the underlying cause behind frequent UTIs. Don't wait too long to use the restroom. Withholding urination can put added pressure on your bladder which can lead to infection.

9. Avoid foods and beverages that may irritate your bladder. If you have an overactive or sensitive bladder, avoid caffeinated foods and beverages and alcoholic drinks. Drinking excess alcohol can damage the kidneys (and liver) so avoid binge drinking.

10. If you suffer from diabetes, exercise control over blood sugar. Follow all medical advice given by your doctor about the disease, regarding your diet, taking insulin, and other medications etc. Diabetes (both type 1 and type 2) is a major risk factor for chronic kidney disease.

WAYS TO PROTECT THE HEALTH OF YOUR REPRODUCTIVE ORGANS

The female reproductive system is one of the systems in the body that serves many vital functions, but its ability to create new life comes to a stop after the menopause (around the age of 40-50 years) when the ovaries stop producing estrogen. It is a different scenario for men who remain capable of bearing children until very late in life. Although men's testosterone production may decline with aging, reproductive function is generally maintained. Most of the time, women are more conscious of reproductive and sexual health than men. But this should not be the case. The well-being of a person's reproductive system is vital, both for men and women. Learning about this during adolescence will ensure that as a person grows older, there's a lesser likelihood of developing complications and diseases. There are some ways to ensure the health of the reproductive system that are common to both men and women are there are others that are specific to men or women. Ten of the common ones are listed below and the gender specific ones are shown in the sidebar:

1. The very first step to taking care of one's reproductive health is exercising, eating healthily, and getting sufficient quality sleep. These steps will not only keep the reproductive system healthy, but it will also keep the whole body healthy too. Keeping the proper weight is essential. People who are obese or overweight experience hormone imbalances which can impair their reproductive function.

2. Avoid stress or try to minimize stress in your life. Stress which can be mental, emotional, physical, or environmental can have negative effects on the reproductive system. In men, too much stress can cause erectile dysfunction, lower the sperm count, and even cause impotence. In women, on the other hand, too much stress can disrupt or even put a stop to the menstrual cycle. Both these situations can result in other associated health problems.

3. When it comes to sexual intercourse, it's crucial to choose one's partner(s) wisely. Especially for women, it's imperative to find someone who will respect her boundaries. It's best to look for sexual partners who are conscious about their sexual health too. Aside from this, maintaining reproductive health also entails making regular visits to the doctor. Do this to check whether everything is OK, and make sure to be screened for sexually transmitted diseases and cancer of the cervix (women) or prostate gland (men).

4. It's also important to watch out for any changes in the body. Most of the time, people are the best ones to judge whether there's something wrong with their body or not. There may be times when a person feels embarrassed admitting to any problems with their reproductive system. But when a person notices something off, he or she should immediately seek advice from a medical professional. It's always best to catch symptoms of illnesses and diseases early on when they are still treatable. Keeping things secret may lead to more severe consequences.

5. Be aware that sex comes with different health risks. These are typically linked to diseases and infections. Many people think there are only two or three sexually transmitted diseases (STDs) – syphilis, gonorrhoea, and the human immunodeficiency virus (HIV) that causes the acquired immunodeficiency syndrome (AIDS). In fact, there are many other diseases that can be spread through sexual contact, including chlamydia, genital warts (caused by the human papilloma virus), herpes, vaginitis, and viral hepatitis. When a person knows how to take care of their reproductive system, they are more likely aware of the risks and understand how to protect themselves better. For a person to take care of their reproductive health, they must take some proactive steps to guard against STDs.

6. Avoid unhealthy habits such as smoking. People who want to keep their reproductive systems healthy should quit this habit altogether. Smoking affects the reproductive systems of both genders. Smoking also clogs arteries and causes vasospasm. These conditions eventually lead to erectile dysfunction.

7. Avoid drinking too much alcohol as this is also very harmful to the reproductive system. Alcohol can interfere with the function of the hypothalamus in the brain, the pituitary gland, the testes in males, and the ovaries in females, thereby causing impotence and infertility. In the testes, alcohol can adversely affect the Leydig cells, which produce and secrete the hormone testosterone resulting in reduced testosterone levels in the blood. Alcohol also decreases the production, release, and/or activity of luteinizing hormone and follicle-stimulating hormone, two hormones with critical reproductive functions in both men and women.

8. Vitamin D is especially vital for reproductive health. Although there are some foods rich in vitamin D and vitamin D3 supplements are cheap and readily available, it's better to get your vitamin D from sunlight exposure, but be sure to do this safely. You only need about 20 minutes exposure per day in the spring and summer wearing shorts and T shirt. You only usually need to consider supplements in the autumn and winter months when the sunlight is too weak to produce vitamin D in your skin.

9. It is important to be medically fit as there are many different conditions which may have a negative effect on a person's reproductive health. These include thyroid problems, eating disorders, malnutrition, anatomical problems, and even diabetes. Keeping these conditions in check will help a person improve his or her health overall. And when the whole body is healthy, so is the reproductive system.

10. Occupational hazards can be harmful to reproductive function, especially for men and can result in infertility. When a person is exposed to excess heat, chemicals (e.g., pesticides, herbicides and industrial solvents), and radiation, it will be detrimental to their reproductive health. So, try to avoid these hazards.

Gender-Specific Tips for Maintaining Reproductive Health for Men and Women

Specific tips for women:

Women have a lot more to do regarding keeping the reproductive system healthy. For women, the reproductive system is one of the most important in the body. It's the place where new life is formed, and so it's important to keep it safe at all times. Here are some special tips for women to keep in mind:

- Eat right, exercise, maintain a healthy body weight, and get enough sleep – keeping these habits in your lifestyle is still is the best way to keep the reproductive system healthy. Being overweight/underweight may cause problems with pregnancy.

- Another thing to remember is that stress affects the normal menstrual cycle and encourages an imbalance of hormones that may cause problems later on. Too much stress can even put a stop to the menstrual cycle which can also result in other associated health problems.

- Tone the pubococcygeus muscle (which supports the pelvic bowl) by simply squeezing the pubococcygeus muscle again and again for about 10 minutes. Doing this is extremely beneficial for a woman's sexual and reproductive health. Practice this exercise regularly, and it will also enhance the sensitivity of the vagina as well as its ability to stay lubricated. Keeping the muscle strong and healthy also prevents urinary incontinence and a prolapsed uterus.

- Increase magnesium and calcium intake. Calcium helps lower the effects of premenstrual fatigue. It also reduces depression and cravings which come with the menstrual cycle. Magnesium, on the other hand, aids in reducing sugar cravings. It also eases headaches, dizziness, and low blood sugar which are linked to premenstrual syndrome. Good sources of these minerals are leafy green vegetables, seaweed, nuts, lentils, coconut, avocado, and sesame seeds.

- Visit the gynecologist regularly and have regular cervical smear tests. Whenever a woman notices anything out of the ordinary, it's important to visit the gynecologist immediately. This is especially important when discovering an infection. It's important to find the issue and solve it before any other issues come up.

- Exercise regularly, preferably outdoors as research shows that being active and spending time outdoors is extremely beneficial, especially for women. When a woman exercises at least three to five times a week and gets enough sun, it can help lower the occurrence of menstrual cramps. Vitamin D is also vital for the body to absorb calcium and magnesium better.

- Orgasm regularly as this will keep the whole reproductive system toned and healthy. It also helps women de-stress and sleep better. Intense and prolonged orgasms are especially beneficial. They make a woman feel more blissful and sexually fulfilled.

- Find natural treatments for menstrual cramps. Menstrual cramps are horrible, especially since they come at a time when a woman feels most sensitive and vulnerable. To be able to reduce the effects, here are some natural remedies to try:

  - Drink some herbal tea every 15 minutes or so until the cramps go away.

  - Avoid cold food and beverages. These can worsen the menstrual cramps.

  - To enhance circulation, alternate cold and hot footbaths when the menstrual cycle starts.

- Stop smoking because research shows that smoking often alters the ovaries, the uterus, and other parts of the female reproductive system. In addition, smoking during pregnancy increases the risk of your baby developing congenital malformations.

- Engage in safe sex – safe sex is paramount to preventing disease. There are some sexually transmitted diseases that are incurable, such as human papilloma virus (HPV), human immunodeficiency virus (HIV), herpes and these conditions may change your life forever. Before engaging in any sexual intercourse, having your partner tested is a fool-proof way to know whether he is safe, or simply using a condom can prevent transmission.

Specific tips for men:

The male reproductive system is one of the most important parts of the body, and maintaining good reproductive health is essential to sexual development and procreation. However, many men often tend to overlook their reproductive health, and as a result this can lead to numerous complications and diseases. Good reproductive health depends on diet, lifestyle, medical conditions, occupational exposures, and many other factors. Below are some practical tips for men to keep in mind:

- If you are currently sexually active and engage in unprotected sex with more than one partner, it is important that you undergo regular screening for HIV and other sexually-transmitted diseases (STDs). Make sure that you use condoms when engaging in sexual activity to reduce your risk from contracting a sexually-transmitted disease.

- Practice good personal hygiene by washing your genitals regularly using water and a mild soap or shower gel to prevent the accumulation of dirt and germs in your genitalia that can potentially cause infection. Also be sure to wear clean underwear by changing them often.

- Maintain a healthy lifestyle by eating a healthy diet, exercising regularly, and maintaining a healthy body weight. You may be surprised to know just how important a proper diet and exercise are towards maintaining proper reproductive health. Eating a nutritious diet rich in nutrients, low in fats, and engaging in regular physical activity will help to ensure that your reproductive system is functioning at peak efficiency.

- Quit smoking because smoking can be a major contributing factor to sexual dysfunction in men. Previous research has shown that a high proportion of men who suffered from erectile dysfunction were smokers. Smoking contributes to the development of vascular problems which can cause blockage of the small arteries that feed blood into the penis making it difficult to attain an erection during sexual intercourse.

- Make sure that you have a physical examination by your doctor at least once a year. Your doctor will be able to screen for any abnormalities or irregularities and take immediate steps to remedy the issue. You can also discuss with your doctor any concerns that you may have regarding your reproductive health. If you find any symptoms that indicate a problem with your reproductive system, it is important to seek medical advice. Detecting and identifying any problem in its early stage will increases the chances that it can be corrected and will not progress to something worse.

- Avoid excessive drinking of alcohol which can directly and indirectly act and affect the hypothalamus in the brain, the pituitary gland, and the testes. Alcohol reduces the amount of testosterone in the blood as well.

- Minimize sources of stress in your life as this can adversely affect testosterone production, lower the sperm count, and even be the cause of impotence.

- Be aware that your occupation can have a direct effect on your reproductive health. Occupational hazards are the most important reason for most of the male infertility cases. Avoid exposure to radiation, chemicals, and constant or excess heat. Avoid exposure to chemicals such as pesticides, herbicides and industrial solvents as it will affect your reproductive health.

WAYS TO PROTECT THE HEALTH OF YOUR BRAIN AND MENTAL HEALTH

Finally, let's not forget about our brains! Mental well-being is an important component of our health, and we should be aiming to have optimal mental well-being (i.e., feeling as good as we can be) as part of our overall aim to have optimal health. Mental well-being includes our emotional, psychological, and social well-being and it affects how we think, feel, and act. It also influences how we react to stress and cope with problems, how we communicate with others, and the decisions and choices that we make in our daily lives. In some cases, good mental well-being can even prevent the onset or relapse of a physical or mental illness. For example, it is known that effective stress management can have a positive impact on delaying coronary heart disease and stroke. However, our brains change as we age, and mental function changes along with it. Mental decline is common, particularly loss of short-term memory, cognitive function, and problem solving abilities, and it's one of the most feared consequences of aging. But cognitive impairment is not inevitable; it can be prevented or at least delayed. Here are ten ways you can help maintain your brain function and mental capacity:

1. We all know that what we eat has a big impact on our physical well-being, but it also affects your mental happiness. As the old saying goes "a healthy body makes a healthy mind", so follow the guidelines for healthy eating described in chapter 4. Eating a good breakfast, a light lunch, and an evening meal will keep your energy levels up and keep you feeling good all day long. Research indicates that people who eat a Mediterranean style diet that emphasizes fruits, vegetables, fish, nuts, and olive oil are less likely to develop depression, cognitive impairment and dementia. Whether this is a direct result of the diet or the fact that it has a low content of sugar and processed foods has not been established.

2. While a lot of people drink alcohol and caffeine to boost their mood, the effect is only temporary. When the feelings of energy or excitement fade you will often feel a lot worse than before you drank, which has a big effect on your mental well-being. Most people only drink alcohol or caffeine in moderation which can often be good for you. However, some people carry on drinking to delay the onset of these negative feelings, or to escape underlying feelings of nervousness or depression. This is very dangerous and can cause long-term health problems or cover up existing conditions. Try to drink no more than two units of alcohol per day and try not to drink caffeinated beverages after 7 pm so that you will sleep well.

3. Doing some exercise every day has mental as well as physical benefits. Exercise is a distraction and can help to take your mind off things that are making you feel stressed, and the exhilaration you feel during and after exercise can boost your mood for hours. As you adapt to regular exercise most everyday activities like cleaning, gardening, and climbing stairs will feel easier, which in turn will also make you feel better about yourself. Research has shown that doing regular exercise protects against the development of dementia. However, if you are planning to take up cycling or physical contact sports, be sure to protect your head. Moderate to severe head injuries, with or without concussion, increase the risk of cognitive impairment.

4. Having supportive social networks, good relationships, and regular communication with family and friends has positive effects on your mental health. Many mental health problems have their roots in trouble with communication and can be helped or even prevented by keeping in touch with others.

5. Taking a break from work or your normal day-to-day routine, enjoying some pastimes or cultural activities, and taking a holiday are ways to improve your mood and take your mind off things. Think of it as giving your mind some time to relax as well as your body.

6. So much of our time nowadays is taken up by the pressures of work that we can sometimes forget about what we enjoy. Maybe you love to paint, play a musical instrument, complete a jigsaw, or build model aircraft. Whatever it is, taking some time out to dedicate just to yourself will help you cope with stress, focus your mind, and allow you to express yourself.

7. Many people are unhappy or self-conscious about their appearance, the way they speak or their background, comparing themselves unfairly to others they see in magazines, the cinema or on television. These kinds of feeling can lead to an entrenched sense of worthlessness or even bring about debilitating conditions such as depression and eating disorders. So just accept that like everyone else you are a unique individual with certain weaknesses and strengths. Nobody is perfect! Being happy provides a great boost to our mental well-being. For many people, happiness comes from knowing you are loved, valued, respected, or cared for by others and the enjoyment that comes from doing things we like such as being outdoors in good weather, going on holidays, playing with children, or pets. So do whatever it takes to make yourself feel happy.

8. Caring for other people or pets can be very rewarding and boost your mood, making you feel good about yourself and valued by those you care for and help out. Really caring for others can help greatly improve your mental health and allow you to understand why other people care for you and why you should care for yourself. In fact, just being nice to others can make you feel good, too.

9. Just like the rest of your body, your brain needs exercise too in order to stay healthy. Research indicates that brainy activities stimulate new connections between nerve cells and may even help the brain generate new cells, developing neurological "plasticity", and building up a functional reserve that provides a hedge against future cell loss as we get older. Any mentally stimulating activity should help to build up your brain and improve your mental well-being. Read, take courses, try "mental gymnastics," such as word puzzles or math problems Experiment with things that require manual dexterity as well as mental effort, such as drawing, painting, other crafts, crosswords, and even computer games. Learning a new language or just learning a new word (buy yourself a dictionary) every day is also a good way of making sure your memory stays in full working order, which will help as you get older as well as in day-to-day life by improving your vocabulary and ability to communicate with other people.

10. People who are anxious, depressed, sleep-deprived, or exhausted tend to score poorly on cognitive function tests. Poor scores don't necessarily predict an increased risk of cognitive decline in old age, but good mental health and restful sleep are certainly important goals.

Key Points

- Maintaining the health of your body is not just down to exercise, diet, sleep and hygiene. Although these aspects of your lifestyle are extremely important there are other specific things you can do to maintain and prolong the health of your body's various tissues and organ systems.

- Particular aspects of your lifestyle and behavior can have a negative or positive impact on the health of your senses, tissues, and organs.

- There are various ways by which you can reduce specific disease risks or avoid certain behaviors which risk the health of your senses, tissues, and organs.

- The quality of your life, particularly in your later years, will be detrimentally affected if the function of your senses, tissues, and organs are not maintained as well as they can be, so act now.

- Think what your life would be like if you lost your senses of sight or hearing. What you would do if you broke your hip or had heart or lung problems that meant you could not enjoy an outdoor active life? Or you could no longer enjoy safe sex with your partner? Or you lost your memory or had other mental problems. Many diseases, injuries, and physical disabilities that you can avoid by being proactive could mean the loss of your independence or place a heavy burden on your loved ones. Nobody wants that.

Chapter 13

How to Achieve Effective Weight Loss With a Personalized Plan Combining Multiple Diets and Your Choice of Exercise

Objectives

After studying this chapter, you should:

- Be aware of the most common mistakes when undertaking a weight loss plan

- Understand why combining dieting and exercise for body fat loss is more effective than dieting alone

- Appreciate the importance of setting goals and defining your weight loss strategies

- Realize that you do not have to stick to just one method of dieting and that using multiple methods will help keep up your motivation to achieve your weight loss goals

- Understand how to modify your diet and exercise habits to maintain your weight loss after finishing your weight loss plan

In this chapter, I will describe a personalized weight loss plan which I guarantee will be effective for body weight and fat loss. What's more is that it is a plan that is much easier to stick to than those that use a single diet strategy. My plan involves using multiple diets (a different one every week) and you can choose your own preferred type of physical activity to further promote fat burning, minimize loss of lean tissue, and help to maintain your resting metabolic rate. Keeping to my weight loss plan for 10 weeks should see the average overweight person lose about 8 kg (18 lbs.).

The first step in the process of losing weight should always be to define the goals: Is weight loss really required, and if so, how much and over what period of time? With goals established, various strategies can be put in place to achieve the weight loss. In the process of attempting to achieve weight loss, several mistakes can be made, and these will be explained first.

COMMON MISTAKES

When trying to lose weight, people often make some of the following mistakes:

- *Trying to lose weight too rapidly.* Most people are impatient about weight loss. They want to see results within a couple of weeks, but unfortunately this expectation is not realistic. Although rapid weight loss is possible, the initial reduction of body weight on low-carbohydrate or very low energy diets is mostly dehydration as water that is combined with glycogen is lost as the body's carbohydrate reserves become depleted. Only a small part of the weight loss will be fat, and it will be restored as soon as normal eating resumes.

- *Not eating breakfast.* Another weight loss approach that people try is skipping breakfast and sometimes even skipping lunch as well. Although this approach may work for some, it increases hunger feelings later in the day, and one large evening meal can easily compensate for the daytime reduction in food intake. In addition, missing breakfast may make you feel tired during the day and less inclined to exercise later on after your occupational work has finished.

- *Cutting down on protein intake as well as carbohydrate or fat.* When losing body weight (being in negative energy balance), you also risk losing muscle mass. But this risk can be reduced by consuming sufficient amounts of protein. Indeed, the proportion of protein in your diet should increase at the expense of carbohydrate or fat to assist with your weight loss.

DEFINING GOALS

It is essential to decide on your weight loss goals right at the start. These goals should be carefully thought out and realistically achievable. Goals also have to be defined with a time schedule in mind. How much weight must be lost and how soon? A realistic expectation is a weight loss of about 1 kg (2.2 lbs.) every two weeks, so to lose 3 kg at least six weeks are needed. Achieving this particular goal means generating, on average, a 500 kcal (2 MJ) energy deficit per day. While this could be achieved by dieting alone, you have already learned that weight loss becomes gradually more difficult due to the lowering of resting metabolic rate. Therefore, it makes more sense to try to achieve the desired weight loss through exercise or – and this is probably the best option – to do it via a combination of exercise and dieting. This will give you scope to lose more weight, more quickly, and with a smaller impact on your appetite than with dieting alone while maintaining your muscle mass and improving your fitness and overall health.

ESTABLISHING THE STRATEGY

The next step is to establish a strategy that will help you lose weight. The following general tips about dieting will help you successfully achieve weight loss:

- Determine a realistic body-weight goal. Define the weight you want to reach and stick to it.

- Do not try to lose more than about 0.5-1.0 kg/week (about 1-2 lbs./week), and do not restrict dietary energy intake by more than 500 to 750 kcal/day on consecutive days.

- Eat more fruit and non-starchy vegetables to achieve a low energy dense diet.

- Avoid snacking between your regular meals. If you really feel the need for a snack, choose low-fat and low-carbohydrate food items; raw celery, spring onion, shredded carrots, and watermelon are excellent choices.

- Study food labels, and try to find substitutes for high-fat foods. Look not only at fat content but also at the energy content per serving.

- Limit fat add-ons such as sauces, sour cream, coleslaw, and high-fat salad dressings, or choose the low-fat versions of these products. Better still, use a sprinkle of dried mixed herbs instead to add extra flavor without the calories.

- Avoid drinking sugar-sweetened beverages; choose the low energy versions with artificial sweeteners and no added sugar. In fact, there several food and drink items that you really should avoid if your diet is going to work (see the sidebar for which ones to remove from your kitchen before you start dieting so that you are not tempted to have them).

- Try to structure your eating into three smaller meals each day.

- Avoid eating any extremely large meals. Try using a smaller diameter plate; for example, use one that is 23 cm (9 inches) in diameter rather than the usual 28 cm (11 inches).

- Make sure that protein intake is the same or higher than normal, and consume a high-protein meal at breakfast and for your main meal in the evening. High-protein items (which can include beans, fish, and egg as well as meat) should cover about one quarter of your plate.

- Limit your intake of bread and starchy vegetables like potatoes by serving these on only two or three days of the week.

- Use higher fiber carbohydrate sources like brown rice and legumes, and limit these to no more than one quarter of your plate, and fill half your plate with low energy density vegetables like gourds, carrots, broccoli, and leafy greens.

- Use only skimmed or semi-skimmed milk (or soya milk) and reduced fat versions of yogurt, coleslaw, etc.

- Add some beetroot, beansprouts, red cabbage, or sauerkraut to your main meals for added bulk fiber and flavor but very few added calories.

- Add a sprinkle of dried herbs, chili bits, curry powder, ground pepper, garlic granules, or fine sea salt to your meals to add flavor without calories

- Eat slowly, savor your food, and begin your main meal by eating the high-protein and low energy density food items first. Finish with the higher carbohydrate items.

- Try to stop eating when you feel 80% rather than 100% full. Do you really want dessert?

- If you do have dessert, stick to fruit such as chopped apple, melon, or pear with one tablespoon of low-fat yogurt.

- Avoid drinking alcoholic beverages. If you don't want to cut out alcohol altogether, then compensate by doing more exercise: one small (125 mL) glass of wine or a half pint (235 mL) of beer both contain about 100 kcal and you will have to walk or jog one mile (1.6 km) to burn that off.

- A multivitamin and mineral supplement may be useful during periods of energy restriction to guard against possible deficiencies. This is the only supplement you will need.

- Remember that to lose weight, dieting is not the only answer. Increase your energy expenditure by doing more exercise. It will improve your fitness and health and help to maintain your muscle mass when you are in negative energy balance.

- Measure your body weight weekly and obtain measurements of body fat regularly (every 1-2 months). Keep a record of the changes.

Foods to Avoid and Get Rid of When Dieting to Lose Weight

There are several foods that you really should avoid eating if your weight loss diet is going to work. These food and drink items are listed next. If you have any stored in your cupboards, fridge, or freezer, it is best to get rid of them before starting your diet so that you are not tempted to have them. Don't just rely on your willpower for this; the temptation to eat them will always be there, and old habits can be hard to break. So do yourself a favor: give these foods away or simply put them in the trash bin. If they are not there, you can't be tempted to have them. You will quickly realize that this list includes foods that are high in calories, added sugar, and fat. Alcohol is also on the list as it provides energy but little else. Switch to zero alcohol beverages such as non-alcoholic beer and low-calorie soft drinks (e.g., diet cola, ginger beer, or lemonade). Here is the list of 10 items to avoid:

- Breakfast cereals that contain added sugar (go for plain oats, Weetabix, or no-added sugar muesli instead).

- Cookies, cakes, and candy which are all high sugar items.

- Milk chocolate (you can still have the occasional small piece of dark chocolate which has lower sugar and higher cocoa content).

- Snack foods such as potato chips, peanuts, pretzels, breakfast cereal bars, and dried fruit.
- Ready meals and sauces which are usually high in added sugar.
- White bread, flatbread, naan bread, garlic bread, and crackers.
- High-fat food items such as cream, cheese, butter, margarine, fatty cuts of meat, skin-on poultry, burgers, and sausages.
- Sweet tropical fruits like mango, peaches, nectarines, and papaya (choose apple, melon, pear, grapes, and berries instead which have a lower energy density and contain less carbohydrate and more water).
- Sugar-sweetened beverages, fruit juices, smoothies, milk shakes, and cordials (choose diet, light, or low-calorie versions of soft drinks instead).
- All kinds of alcoholic drinks.

THE COMBINATION 100 GPD WEIGHT LOSS PLAN

This is my idea of an effective weight loss plan. The "100 GPD" means the aim is to lose, on average 100 **G**rams of fat **P**er **D**ay which will mean losing the same or slightly greater amount of body weight. Your initial goal is to adhere to the 100 GPD weight loss plan for 10 weeks. By the end you should have lost about 7 kg (15 lbs.) of body fat and 8 kg (18 lbs.) of body weight. The originality of the plan lies in how I suggest this is achieved.

It is not done by dieting alone but by combining dieting with more exercise. But that is not all: the really clever and novel aspect of the plan is that you do not stick to just one diet for 10 weeks; in fact, you change the diet each week. To lose 100 g of body fat per day you will need a daily total energy deficit of about 800 kcal. So, a reasonable aim is to reduce your dietary energy intake by 400 kcal per day and burn off an additional 400 kcal per day with exercise.

THE DIETARY ENERGY RESTRICTION PART OF THE WEIGHT LOSS PLAN

You can personalize this part of the plan as there is no need to stick to the same diet every week for 10 weeks to achieve your goal. Of course, virtually all the books and articles you will have read before will almost certainly have promoted one particular diet because the author has had this one idea and wants to sell it (and their book!) to you. Forget it. You will soon get bored with eating the same foods and probably give up. Instead give yourself some variety. Chapter 7 described several different diets that can achieve the 400-kcal energy deficit that you are aiming for here. Table 13.1 below illustrates exactly what you have to do to achieve this with the different diets.

So why not choose a different diet each week? You can choose the diets that suit you best according to your personal preferences and that fit with what you are doing that week. This is a very simple approach, and you won't get bored; every week will be different from the previous one. You can follow the suggested sequence in table 13.1 which ensures you will be having different foods each week, or you can come up with your own sequence. To achieve the desired weekly dietary energy deficit, you won't need to diet every day of the week as indicated by the frequency needed column in table 13.1. On the other days you can eat normally, but don't over compensate by eating more than usual. Whenever possible, on the normal eating days adhere to the principles of healthy eating that I described in chapter and the strategy guidelines listed at the beginning of this chapter. You could try out the Mediterranean or Japanese diet (described in chapter 4) on these days to add further healthy variety to your eating plan.

Table 13.1: What you have to do to achieve an average of 400 kcal/day (2,800 kcal/week) energy deficit with different diets in overweight adults and my suggestion of which weeks during your 10-week plan to apply the diets

Diet	What it involves	Frequency needed	Week number of your 10-week plan
Low-carbohydrate (Atkins)	1,500 kcal/day (6.3 MJ/day) with <20 g carbohydrate daily	5-6 days per week	Weeks 1 and 6
Low-fat	1,500 kcal/day (6.3 MJ/day) with <10% fat	5-6 days per week	Weeks 2 and 7
High-protein with low energy density	1,500 kcal/day (6.3 MJ/day) with 30% protein	5 days per week	Weeks 3 and 8
5:2	Only 500 kcal (2.1 MJ) on 2 days/week	2 days per week	Weeks 4 and 9
Skip lunch	No 500 kcal (2.1 MJ) lunch	6 days per week	Week 5
Low energy density	1,400 kcal/day (5.8 MJ/day) with 25% protein	7 days per week	Week 5 (alternative)
Very low energy	800 kcal/day (3.4 MJ/day) with 30% protein	4 days per week	Week 10
4:3	Only 500 kcal (2.1 MJ) on 3 days/week	3 days per week	Week 10 (alternative)

Assumes that you normally consume 2,000 kcal/day to achieve energy balance.

As indicated in the footnote to table 13.1, the figures are based on the assumption that your daily energy intake is normally 2,000 kcal. This amount of food energy is the number of calories you need to achieve energy balance if your resting daily energy expenditure is 2,000 kcal/day. You should calculate your own personal resting daily energy expenditure as described in chapter 5 and adjust the energy intakes shown in table 13.2 accordingly to achieve the desired 400 kcal/day energy deficit.

The sequence of diets over the 10 weeks I have suggested in table 13.1 does have its advantages: Starting with a low-carbohydrate diet in week one will get you off to a good start, and the reduced carbohydrate availability should speed up your exercise training adaptations by promoting the molecular signals that lead to increases in the numbers of mitochondria and increasing your ability to oxidize fat (as explained in chapter 9). You follow this in week two with a switch to a low-fat diet which means you get to eat more carbohydrate which is what you will have been missing most in week one. Next up in week three is a high-protein diet with low energy density, which again will be good for training adaptation. Week four brings the 5:2 intermittent fasting diet, where you get to eat normally for five days of the week followed by week five, where you just eliminate lunch for six days. For the next five weeks you can simply repeat this sequence of diets or, if you want to finish with a flourish in week 10, you can go for the more extreme very low energy diet (on four alternate days of the week) or the 4:3 diet on three days of the week instead of the skipping lunch option.

I have devised the 100 GPD Weight Loss Plan because it will be suitable for most people, safe, and provides a good outcome in a reasonable amount of time. The multiple diets and the variety of the dieting strategy each week largely eliminates increases in appetite and cravings for particular foods compared with a weight loss plan that uses a single diet such as Atkins, but it is just as, if not more, effective for weight loss. On a low-carbohydrate diet like Atkins, you will dying for some bread, rice, potato, pasta, or sweets after only a few weeks, and similarly on a low-fat diet you will soon be missing the texture and taste of fatty foods such as cheese, pizza, burgers, and sausages.

THE EXERCISE PART OF THE WEIGHT LOSS PLAN

Now for the exercise part of the weight loss plan to burn that extra 400 kcal per day. The best choice of exercise is going to be one that you want to do and that you will enjoy. There is no point in choosing to run for 30 minutes if you don't really like running and will put off going or make excuses for not going. If the thought of doing one activity continuously is too much to handle, then why not split it up. Do one activity for half that amount of time and burn 200 calories and then change activity, or later in the day do a different activity until you have worked off another 200 calories. That way you will have some variety and will be training different muscle groups. Selecting which exercises you want to do, and determining the duration and frequency of the sessions in a day is one way of personalizing your plan to suit you. The exercises I have suggested in table 13.2 are all predominantly aerobic forms of exercise which is the best way to burn fat, but it is also a good idea to include some additional resistance exercise (say three 10- to 15-minute sessions per week) in order to help maintain or even increase muscle mass in the face of the energy deficit.

The calories you burn in the activities listed in table 13.2 are all approximate and based on a person weighing 70 kg (154 lbs.). The number of calories you burn will depend on your weight and how much effort you are putting into it. If you are heavier, then you will burn more calories. If you are laid back and taking the activity easy you will burn less calories than if you push yourself harder and work at a higher intensity.

Table 13.2: Duration of exercise needed to expend 400 kcal

Activity	Exercise time (minutes)
Aerobics	45
Badminton	49
Circuit training	53
Cycling 15 km/h (10 mph)	61
Running 10 km/h (6 mph)	27
Walking 4 km/h (2.5 mph)	87
Swimming	34

There are, of course, some fairly equivalent (in terms of calorie burn) alternatives to the activities listed in table 13.2. You could do dancing instead of aerobics, soccer or tennis instead of badminton, rowing instead of cycling, or have a game of golf instead of a long walk. Remember that everything you do burns calories, even vacuuming or mopping the floor, dusting, mowing the lawn, cleaning the car, walking up the stairs, and just standing up rather than sitting or lying down uses more calories. Although these activities alone do not burn many calories, it all helps so next time you need to do housework or chores think of them as additional ways to burn calories. You can also take advantage of the opportunities to do exercise that arise when you are out and about. For example, you can walk to the shops rather than using motorized transport or take the stairs rather than the elevator in the mall or the department store.

If possible, stick to the exercise part of the plan every day of the week. Don't worry if circumstances mean that you have to miss out on exercise on one or two days of the week; it will not have a significant impact on your weight loss over 10 weeks, and you may be able to make up for it by exercising a little more than usual on the day after your off-exercise day.

The amount of body fat and weight you will lose will vary slightly from one week to the next, but this is not a concern. Keep in mind that you will achieve the overall goal of the plan after the 10 weeks is up. Sticking to the plan means you should expect to lose, on average, about 700 g (1.5 lbs.) of body fat per week. Keep that up for 10 weeks and you will have lost 7 kg (15 lbs.) of body fat, which should equate to an 8-9 kg (17-20 lbs.) drop in body weight.

It is a good idea to record what you do in terms of physical activity and what you eat on a daily basis using a simple weekly food and activity chart such as the one created by the UK National Health Service, which is available to download for free at the website **https://www.nhs.uk/ Tools/Documents/WEIGHT LOSS-PACK/week-1.pdf**.

You don't necessarily have to use this or include so much detail, but it does no harm to celebrate what you are achieving by noting in a diary what you have eaten and what amount and type of exercise you have done each week. This may help to further strengthen your resolve to continue with your weight loss plan.

WHAT IF YOU WANT TO LOSE MORE WEIGHT THAN THIS?

I appreciate that the 100 GPD Weight Loss Plan may not be suitable for everyone's goals. If you want to lose more than 7 kg (15 lbs.) of body fat, then you could continue with the plan for another 5-10 weeks. However, if you want to lose more weight in the same 10-week period, then you could try using the more extreme dieting plan that is summarized in table 13.3. In this plan your average daily dietary energy deficit is 550 kcal (which is 3,850 kcal/week). The plan still uses the strategy of varying the diet each week, but there is a little more variation in the energy deficit from week to week as it ranges between 3,500-4,500 kcal/week. If you also up the volume (session duration) of your daily exercise to burn 550 kcal as indicated in table 8.4, your total average daily energy deficit will be 1,100 kcal. That is 7,700 kcal/week, and that should allow you to lose 1.0 kg (2.2 lbs.) of body fat per week or 10 kg (22 lbs.) after 10 weeks. That should be about 12-13 kg (26-29 lbs.) of weight loss. As with this plan, you should lose about 1,000 grams of body fat per week; I'm calling it the 1000 GPW Weight Loss Plan.

Table 13.3: What you need to do to achieve an average of 550 kcal/day (3,850 kcal/week) energy deficit with different diets in overweight adults and which weeks to apply the diet

Diet	What it involves	Frequency needed	Week number of your 10-week plan
Low-carbohydrate (Atkins)	1,500 kcal/day (6.3 MJ/day) with <20 g carbohydrate daily	7 days per week	Weeks 1 and 6
Low-fat	1,500 kcal/day (6.3 MJ/day) with <10% fat	7 days per week	Weeks 2 and 7
Very low energy	800 kcal/day (3.4 MJ/day) with 30% protein	4 days per week	Weeks 3 and 8
High-protein with low energy density	1,500 kcal/day (6.3 MJ/day) with 30% protein	7 days per week	Weeks 4 and 9
4:3	Only 500 kcal (2.1 MJ) on 3 days/ week	3 days per week	Week 5
All day fast	No food, only drink water or low-calorie beverages	2 days per week	Week 10

Assumes that you normally consume 2,000 kcal/day to achieve energy balance.

Table 13.4: Duration of exercise needed to expend 550 kcal

Activity	Exercise time (minutes)
Aerobics	62
Badminton	67
Circuit training	73
Cycling 15 km/h (10 mph)	84
Running 10 km/h (6 mph)	37
Walking 4 km/h (2.5 mph)	120
Swimming	47

WEIGHT MAINTENANCE FOLLOWING SUCCESSFUL WEIGHT LOSS

Having put in the hard work in achieving successful weight loss, it would be a shame to put the weight back on in the months that follow. So be aware of the pitfalls. Remember that losing body weight usually becomes increasingly difficult as weight loss progresses because the body responds to weight loss by becoming more efficient, which is usually referred to as "food efficiency". With the 100 GPD and 1000 GPW weight loss plans that combine dieting and exercise, it should not be an important issue, but it is still likely that your resting metabolic rate will drop slightly, so when resuming your normal pattern of food intake, it is best to employ some of the strategies you have learnt such as continuing to exclude high-fat processed foods and sugar sweetened beverages in favor of low-fat or low-calorie equivalents and generally aim to maintain a low energy density diet with adequate protein and lots of fruit and vegetables. In other words, make sure that your altered eating habits stay altered, at least to some degree.

The concept of food efficiency fits in with the theory that the body has a weight set point. Although interindividual differences in body weight of humans are large, the body weight of an individual is usually fairly constant and typically varies only ±0.5% over periods of 6 to 10 weeks (±350 g for an individual with a body mass of 70 kg). If rats are given an energy-restricted diet for several weeks, they lose body mass rapidly. Upon being permitted to eat freely again, they restore this body mass within weeks, and their weight becomes identical to their counterparts who had free access to food for the entire period. A similar change happens when rats are overfed. Evidence also exists for such a set point for body weight in humans: In a well-designed study, maintenance of a 10% reduction in body weight induced by a period of underfeeding (800 kcal/day for 4-7 weeks) was associated with a 6% reduction in total energy expenditure in non-obese subjects (see figure 13.1). Resting energy expenditure and non-resting energy expenditure both each decreased to a similar extent. Maintenance of a 10% higher than normal body weight induced by overfeeding (5,000-8,000 kcal/day for 4-6 weeks) was associated with an 8% increase in total energy expenditure. Therefore, maintenance of a reduced or elevated body weight is associated with compensatory changes in energy expenditure, which oppose the

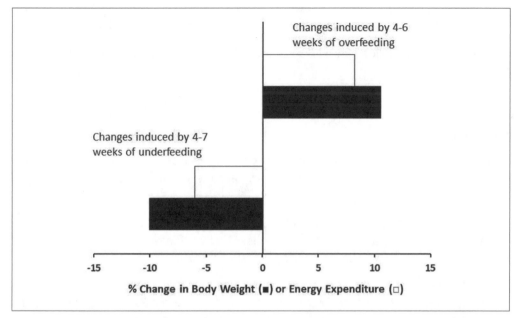

Figure 13.1: Changes in daily energy expenditure in response to weight loss or weight gain. A 10% reduction in body weight induced by underfeeding resulted in a 6% decrease in energy expenditure, and a 10% gain in body weight induced by overfeeding resulted in an 8% increase in energy expenditure. This finding shows that the body has compensatory mechanisms that try to maintain a normal body weight. Data from Leibel et al. (1995).

maintenance of a body weight that is different from the usual weight. This study shows that the body has compensatory mechanisms that try to maintain a normal body weight.

Often, the considerable effort applied to achieve weight loss is exceeded by the effort required to maintain the new lower body weight. After the weight is lost, it can be regained in a relatively short period. This effect is usually referred to as the yo-yo effect. Studies in animals have documented this pattern of weight cycling. After a period of food restriction and weight reduction, animals tend to regain the weight quickly if they are allowed free access to food. Several prospective studies have shown that weight fluctuation (gain–loss or loss–gain) or weight variability is associated with increased mortality, independent of the direction of weight change. When taking limited account of preexisting disease, however, studies show little evidence of negative side effects of weight cycling. Thus, from your own health perspective, the risks from overweight and obesity far exceed the potential risks of weight cycling.

Unfortunately, if you have been overweight for quite some time, your body's perceived normal weight may have been adjusted upwards of your true normal healthy weight. So, bear this in mind after achieving your desired weight loss, and don't succumb to cravings to eat more or go back to unhealthy eating habits

Finally, to maintain the long-term health benefits of exercise you need to keep exercising. What you did activity-wise 5, 10 or 20 years ago will not protect you in later life if regular exercise is not maintained. If you do some exercise, it means you can afford some indulgences, such as a nice glass of wine with dinner or some ice cream with your fruit for dessert without risking a return to a positive energy balance and cumulative weight gain. Always remember that doing exercise is good for your health in so many ways. It makes no sense whatsoever to avoid it.

The final chapter that follows provides some example meal plans for the various diets listed in tables 13.1 and 13.3.

Key Points

- When attempting to lose weight, the most common mistakes are trying to lose weight too rapidly, not eating breakfast, and cutting down on protein intake as well as carbohydrate or fat.

- It is essential to decide on your weight loss goals right at the start. These goals should be carefully thought out and realistically achievable. Goals also have to be defined with a time schedule in mind. How much weight must be lost and how soon?

- General advice for weight loss includes: eating more fruit and vegetables to achieve a low energy density diet, selecting low-fat and low-carbohydrate snacks, finding substitutes for high-fat foods, limiting fat add-ons such as sauces, creams, and dressings or using the low-fat versions of these products, not eating any large meals, avoiding drinks that are sugar-sweetened or contain alcohol beverages, and making sure that protein intake is the same or higher than normal.

- The 100 GPD Weight Loss Plan generates an 800 kcal per day energy deficit using a combination of diet and exercise. The multiple diets and the variety of the dieting strategy each week largely eliminates increases in appetite and cravings for particular foods compared with single diet such as Atkins but is just as, if not more, effective for weight loss. With the 100 GPD Weight Loss Plan, you should lose about 7 kg (15 lbs.) of body fat in 10 weeks.

- For larger weight loss within a 10-week period the 1000 GPW Weight Loss Plan generates a 1,100 kcal per day energy deficit using a combination of diet and exercise which should result in a loss of about 10 kg (22 lbs.) of body fat in 10 weeks.

- Weight maintenance following weight loss requires that you continue to employ some of the strategies you have learnt, such as continuing to exclude high-fat processed foods and sugar sweetened beverages in favor of low-fat or low-calorie equivalents and generally aim to maintain a low energy density diet with adequate protein and lots of fruit and vegetables.

- By remaining physically active, you will reap the benefits of a healthier life as you get older as well assisting with your weight maintenance.

Chapter 14

Example Meal Plans for Different Weight Loss Diets

Objectives

After studying this chapter, you should:

- Be able to plan suitable meals for the very low energy diet and "fasting days" on the 4:3 and 5:2 diets

- Be able to plan suitable meals for the low-carbohydrate (Atkins) diet

- Be able to plan suitable meals for the low-fat diet

- Be able to plan suitable meals for the high-protein diet

- Be able to plan suitable meals for the low energy density diet

- Appreciate that you can vary many of the meal plans to some degree to suit your personal food and taste preferences

- Appreciate the value of adding low energy density foods and natural flavorings to your meals when dieting

- Know what to drink and what to avoid drinking when dieting

If you are planning to follow any of the weight loss diets described in chapter 8 or the multi-diet 100GPD or 1000GPW weight loss plans described in chapter 13, then you need to know some example meal plans for breakfasts, lunches, and evening dinners for these diets. This chapter provides some example meal plans, but you can vary them to some degree to suit your personal food and taste preferences, substituting like for like for the meats, green vegetables, legumes, breads, and pasta items that are mentioned below. For example, it is perfectly fine to use turkey instead of chicken; lean pork or non-oily fish like cod instead of beef; spring greens, leeks, cabbage, or green beans instead of spinach; sweet potato, corn or rice instead of potato; peas or butter beans instead of red beans or baked beans; and penne pasta, macaroni, or noodles instead of spaghetti. Just stick to the guideline amounts in grams and the calorie (kcal) amounts will not be very different.

It is also worth remembering that some tasty vegetables such as sauerkraut, beansprouts, pickled silver-skin onions, red cabbage, and beetroot can be used as an accompaniment to most lunches or dinners on all the diets because they have a low energy density and contain very few calories (typically only 5-15 kcal in a 50 g serving) but provide flavor, fiber, and bulk which will make your food on the plate look more substantial and make you feel fuller and more satisfied. These foods, along with other vegetables such as spinach, kale and cabbage are particularly useful on the very low energy diets, semi-fasting days on the intermittent diets, and the low-carbohydrate diets where the usual filling carbohydrate staples like potatoes, rice, pasta, and bread are severely restricted or absent altogether. They are also an absolutely essential part of the low energy density diet.

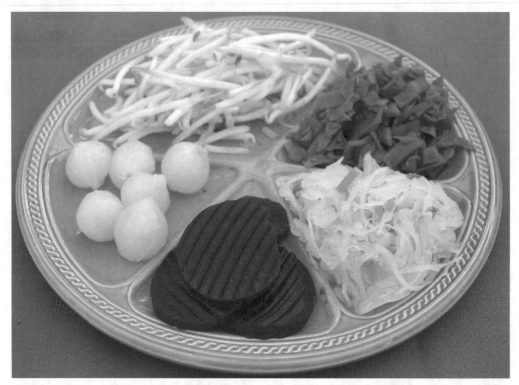

Photo 14.1: A selection of 50 g portions of low-calorie accompaniments to main meals

Another useful tip is to enhance the flavor of the food you eat by adding a teaspoon of dried mixed herbs, dried chili bits, ground garlic or ginger powder, turmeric or paprika powder to your cooking in casseroles, stews, soups, and roast meat dishes. These can provide a huge boost to flavor but only add five calories per teaspoon at most.

Another important point is to be careful with what you choose to drink. For all the diets described in this chapter, you don't want to add extra calories from hot or cold beverages. That means cutting out altogether any sugar sweetened beverages such as energy drinks, sports drinks, flavored soft drinks, and cordials, and avoiding milkshakes and creamy or milky hot drinks like coffee and cocoa. Obviously, water is fine, but there is an excellent selection of artificially sweetened fruit flavored soft drinks, mixers, and cordials. Look for the "low-calorie", "diet" or "light" versions on the supermarket shelves. You can still drink coffee or tea but use a zero-calorie artificial sweetener instead of sugar and skimmed or semi-skimmed milk instead of whole milk or cream. Finally, you should not drink any alcoholic beverages like wine, beer, or spirits on most of the diets although you could allow yourself no more than one glass of wine or beer on the non-fasting days of the intermittent fasting diets.

MEALS FOR DAYS ON THE VERY LOW-ENERGY DIET AND "FASTING DAYS" ON THE INTERMITTENT FASTING 4:3 AND 5:2 DIETS

On a very low energy diet, it is common practice to take nutrition in the form of liquid, high-protein meals supplemented with vitamins and minerals, but this is only really necessary if this type of diet is being kept up for more than two to three weeks. Liquid meals are usually in the form of a soup or a milk-based beverage (with or without added egg) in the form of a shake or smoothie. Milk-based shakes are available as powders that are reconstituted with water and come in a variety of flavors, including banana, strawberry, chocolate, cookie, toffee, and vanilla. Each 50 g serving of a shake or smoothie provides about 200 kcal, 6-8 g fat, 15-20 g carbohydrate, 15-20 g protein, about 5 g fiber and 1 g salt together with vitamins and minerals. Consuming three or four of the 50 g servings will usually provide sufficient micronutrients and protein to meet recommended daily intakes. It is usually recommended to consume these four times per day, at regular intervals, three to four hours apart. Alternatively, half a can (200 g) of soup normally provides 100-130 kcal, so three of these can be consumed per day together with some mixed leaf salad, sauerkraut, beansprouts, or shredded carrot or beetroot, and one slice of wholemeal bread (70 kcal) per serving.

However, in both the 100 GPD and 1000 GPW weight loss plans, the very low-calorie diet is only employed for one week, so normal foods can be consumed, just as they can for the intermittent semi-fasting diets such as the 4:3 and 5:2 diets.

Meals for the "fasting days" on Intermittent Fasting Diets such as 4:3 and 5:2 should amount to no more than 500 kcal/day (for women) and 600 kcal/day (for men), whereas for days on the very low-calorie diet, the calorie intake should not exceed 800 kcal/day. Simply pick and mix from the meal and snack options shown below or read food labels and use the same principles to come up with your own meal ideas. In order not to add extra calories from drinks consumed with meals have water, mineral water or low-calorie (diet) versions of fruit juices or cordials, tonic water, cola, lemonade etc. If you cannot do without your tea or coffee with every meal, use skimmed or semi-skimmed milk rather than whole milk and artificial low-calorie sweeteners instead of sugar. Avoid all alcohol on these low-calorie intake days. The very low energy intake on the semi-fasting days of intermittent fasting diets is limited to 500-600 kcal/day and will almost certainly not provide sufficient protein and micronutrients to meet minimum daily requirements. This can be compensated for by having a high-protein dinner on the day before the semi-fasting day and a high-protein breakfast on the day after. A multivitamin and mineral supplement is advised if you intend to stay on one of these types of diet for a month or more.

Some example breakfasts, lunches, dinners, and snacks are as follows:

Breakfasts Containing About 125 kcal

- *Spinach or Tomato omelet*

  One medium egg: 78 kcal

  60 g fresh spinach or two tomatoes: 16 kcal

  Add salt and a sprinkling of herbs (e.g., chives, oregano, parsley, sage or a mixture) to the omelet for more flavor

  Cup of tea or coffee with semi-skimmed milk: 23 kcal

  Total kcal = 117

- *Blueberries, cranberries, raisins, or sultanas with Greek yogurt and almonds or walnuts*

  One tablespoon blueberries/cranberries/raisins/sultanas: 42 kcal

  Three tablespoon fat-free Greek yogurt: 24 kcal

  Four whole almonds or two walnuts with skin crushed: 28 kcal

  Cup of tea or coffee with semi-skimmed milk: 23 kcal

  Total kcal = 117

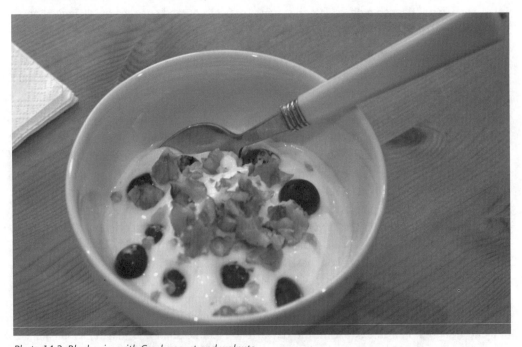

Photo 14.2: Blueberries with Greek yogurt and walnuts

Breakfasts Containing About 250 kcal

- *Grapefruit and a blueberry or cherry muesli*

  Half a pink grapefruit: 55 kcal

  35 g swiss style muesli (no added sugar): 110 kcal

  75 mL semi-skimmed milk: 36 kcal

  20 blueberries or four pitted chopped red cherries: 16 kcal

  150 mL glass of low-calorie cranberry juice: 10 kcal

  Cup of tea or coffee with semi-skimmed milk: 23 kcal

  Total kcal = 250

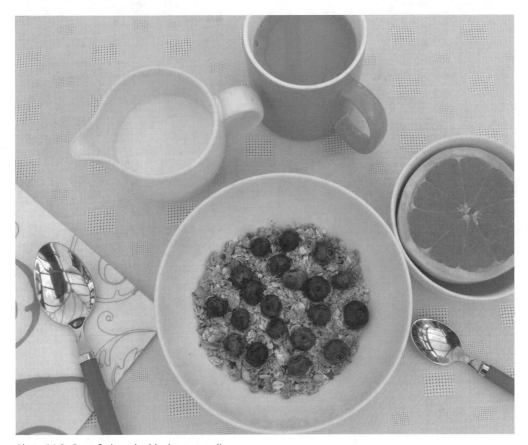

Photo 14.3: Grapefruit and a blueberry muesli

- *Orange or Grapefruit and all bran cereal with sliced banana*

  Half a large orange or a small pink grapefruit: 45 kcal

  35 g all bran cereal (no added sugar): 102 kcal

  75 mL semi-skimmed milk: 36 kcal

  Half a small banana, chopped into 10 thin slices: 44 kcal

  Cup of tea or coffee with semi-skimmed milk: 23 kcal

  Total kcal = 250

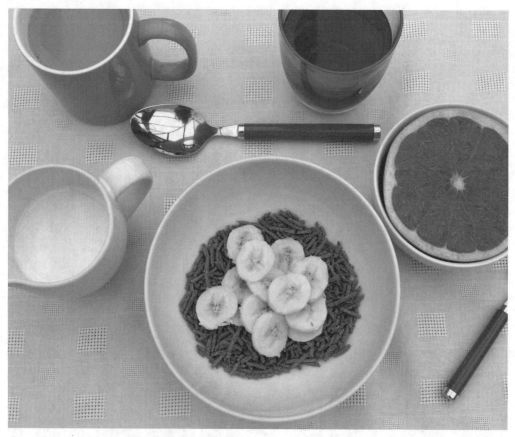

Photo 14.4: Grapefruit and all bran cereal with sliced banana

Lunches Containing About 125 kcal

- *Soups*

  Hot soups are also a suitable alternative for some meals. Half a can of soup (200 g) such as pea and ham, lentil and bacon, chicken and vegetable, mulligatawny, minestrone, tomato or mushroom normally contains about 100-130 kcal, 3-5 g fat, 10-20 g carbohydrate, 5-10 g protein, about 3-5 g fiber and 1 g salt. The soups that contain a mixture of meat and vegetable tend to be the most nutritious.

- *Salads (without salad cream, mayonnaise, or coleslaw)*

  Lettuce/Rocket/Watercress/Spinach/Mixed (60 g): 15 kcal

  Celery (two stalks, 100 g): 20 kcal

  Tomato (one medium size, 120 g): 22 kcal

  Thin sliced cooked ham/chicken/turkey (two slices, diced, 50 g): 60 kcal

  Juice from half a squeezed lime or lemon: 5 kcal

  Total kcal = 122

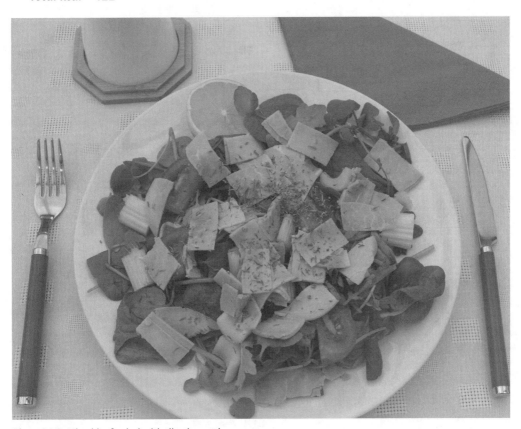

Photo 14.5: Mixed leaf salad with diced roast ham

Lunches Containing About 250 kcal

- *Tasty substantial soups with bread*

  As we have already seen, hot soups are an excellent option, but you can also have some bread, and a little extra protein can be added in the form of small pieces of sliced cold cooked meats (about 25 g) to help ensure that daily protein requirements are met. Use wholegrain or wholemeal bread as these contain more micronutrients than processed bread. You can add up to 100 mL water to increase the volume of the soup and adding a small amount (e.g., one teaspoon) of red or green pesto will help to thicken it and add extra flavor.

  Soup such as pea and ham, chicken and mushroom, lentil and bacon, or beef and tomato (200 g): 125 kcal

  Thin sliced cooked ham/chicken/turkey/beef (1 slice, diced, 25 g): 30 kcal

  One teaspoon red or green pesto: 20 kcal

  Add sprinkle of mixed herbs or chili bits to add flavor

  Wholemeal bread (one slice, 30 g): 70 kcal

  Total kcal = 245

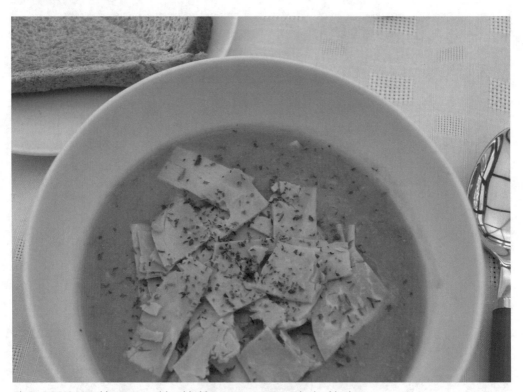

Photo 14.6: Pea and ham soup with added ham, green pesto and mixed herbs

- *Salads (without salad cream, mayonnaise or coleslaw; add salt, herb, lemon juice to flavor) with bread*

Lettuce/Rocket/Watercress/Spinach/Mixed (60 g): 15 kcal

Celery (two stalks, 100 g): 20 kcal

Tomato (one medium size, 120 g): 28 kcal

Five spring onions (small size, 10 cm long, 60 g): 25 kcal

Five pitted green olives: 25 kcal

Thin sliced cooked ham/chicken/turkey (two slices, diced, 50 g): 60 kcal

Juice from half a squeezed lime or lemon: 5 kcal

Toasted wholemeal bread (one slice, 30 g): 70 kcal

Total kcal = 248

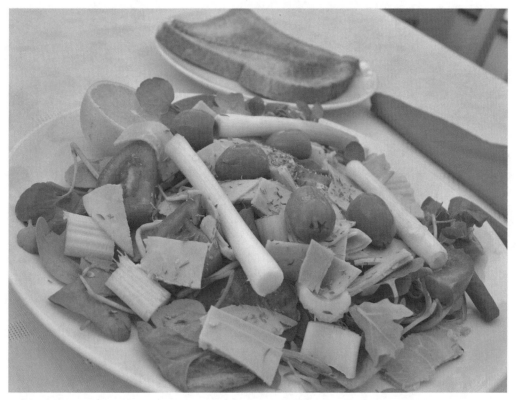

Photo 14.7: Mixed leaf salad with spring onion, green olives, and diced roast ham with a slice of toasted wholemeal bread

Dinners Containing About 250 kcal

60 g steamed spinach: 15 kcal

Celery (two stalks, chopped, and steamed): 20 kcal

100 g lean skinless chicken breast or lean beefsteak (grilled): 135 kcal

100 g steamed new potatoes: 75 kcal

Two slices of pickled beetroot: 5 kcal

Total kcal = 250

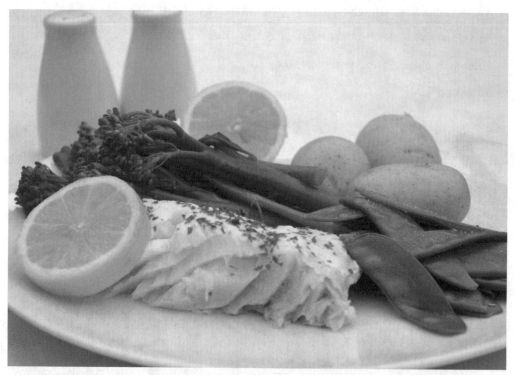

Photo 14.8: Oven-baked cod loin with lemon and parsley accompanied by tenderstem broccoli, mangetout, and new potatoes

60 g steamed mangetout: 15 kcal

130 g steamed tenderstem broccoli: 35 kcal

100 g cod fillet or cod loin (oven baked with lemon and parsley): 125 kcal

100 g steamed new potatoes: 75 kcal

Total kcal = 250

Dinners Containing About 400 kcal

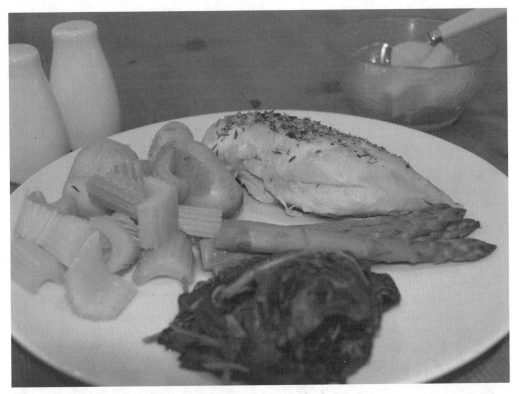

Photo 14.9: Chicken breast and vegetables with chopped mango for dessert

60 g steamed spinach: 15 kcal

One celery stalk, chopped and steamed: 10 kcal

Four asparagus spears (medium size, 15 cm long, steamed): 12 kcal

150 g lean skinless chicken breast, lean beef steak, or lamb steak (grilled or pan fried): 200 kcal

100 g steamed new potatoes: 75 kcal

80 g chopped mango: 73 kcal

Total kcal = 400

- *Chicken saag curry*

  150 g skinless, boneless chicken breast or thighs chopped into 6 pieces: 200 kcal

  One tablespoon medium strength curry powder: 20 kcal

  100 g tomato puree: 40 kcal

  80 g onions peeled: 30 kcal

  60 g mushrooms, sliced: 15 kcal

  One red pepper (100 g), cut into chunks: 40 kcal

  One stalk of celery, cut into chunks: 10 kcal

  60 g spinach: 15 kcal

  300 mL (10fl oz) water plus one chicken stock cube: 5 kcal

  Serve with 100 g fresh beansprouts: 30 kcal

  Total kcal = 400

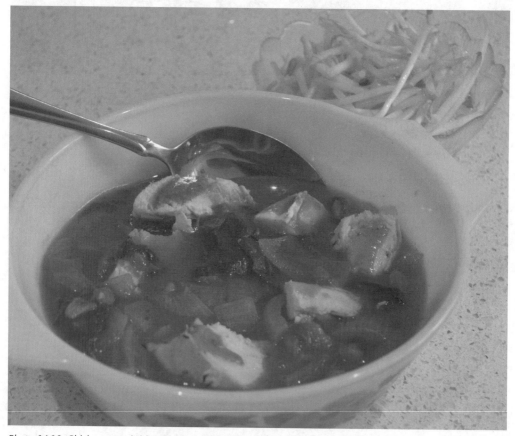

Photo 14.10: Chicken saag (with added spinach) curry served with beansprouts

- *Chicken and bacon casserole*

  150 g skinless, boneless chicken breast or thighs chopped into 6 pieces: 200 kcal

  50 g lean bacon, chopped: 35 kcal

  100 g tomato puree: 30 kcal

  80 g small onions or shallots, whole and peeled: 30 kcal

  60 g mushrooms, sliced: 15 kcal

  120 g carrots, cut into chunks: 50 kcal

  One stalk of celery, cut into chunks: 10 kcal

  Sprinkle of mixed herbs (oregano, thyme, parsley, black peppercorns): 5 kcal

  300 mL (10fl oz) water plus one chicken stock cube: 20 kcal

  Serve with 50 g sauerkraut: 5 kcal

  Total kcal = 395

For further meal ideas see: **https://www.goodtoknow.co.uk/recipes/538311/5-2-diet-meal-plans-what-to-eat-for-500-calorie-fast-days**.

MEALS FOR THE LOW-CARBOHYDRATE (ATKINS) DIET

The low-carbohydrate diet typically supplies a total of 1,500 kcal/day with less than 20 g/day carbohydrate. The following breakfasts contain about 300 calories, the lunches provide 300-400 calories, and the dinners contain 400-500 calories. For beverages, drink tea or coffee (use artificial sweeteners not sugar), water, low-calorie fruit squash, or low-calorie carbonated drinks such as cola, lemonade or tonic water.

Breakfasts

Two egg omelet with 30 g grated cheese and 50 g sliced red pepper

100 g smoked salmon with half a sliced ripe avocado and two tablespoon cream cheese, sprinkled with black pepper

One slice bacon, one poached egg, one tomato and 50 g sauerkraut

One 80 g pork or beef sausage (with less than 3 g carbohydrate), one fried egg, one tomato and 50 g sauerkraut

Two slices of Serrano (or Parma) ham, two fried eggs, and one tomato

Two scrambled eggs with four steamed or fried, chopped asparagus spears, and one slice of bacon

Lunches

Goat's cheese salad made with 80 g salad leaves, five olives, four cherry tomatoes, half a sliced ripe avocado, 50 g cubed cucumber, and 50 g crumbled goat's cheese. Drizzled with one teaspoon extra virgin olive oil

One 150 g baked chicken thigh served over mixed salad leaves, half a chopped red pepper, and four cucumber slices. Topped with 30 g grated cheese

Two celery stalks each filled with 30 g cottage cheese and wrapped in thin sliced 25 g piece of roast chicken, ham or beef and served with 30 g beansprouts.

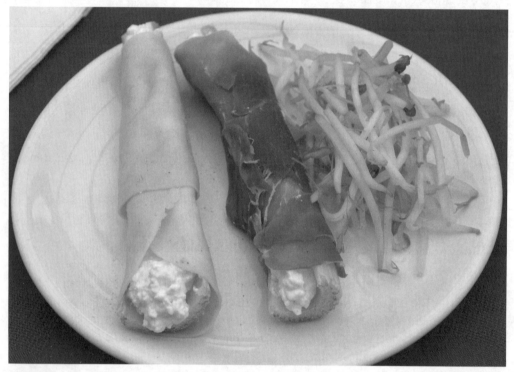

Photo 14.11: Celery stalks filled with 30 g cottage cheese and wrapped in thin sliced 25 g piece of roast chicken and Parma ham and served with 30 g beansprouts

Greek salad including five olives, 100 g baby spinach, half a sliced ripe avocado, half a chopped red onion, 50 g cubed cucumber and 30 g feta cheese. Drizzled with one teaspoon olive oil

One small tin of salmon served over 100 g baby spinach leaves, five cherry tomatoes, one quarter of thinly sliced cucumber. Drizzled with one teaspoon extra virgin olive oil

One small tin of mackerel in brine, drained, served over 100 g spinach leaves, 30 g crumbled feta cheese, and half a chopped red pepper

Two scrambled eggs cooked with 50 mL milk, served with five steamed asparagus spears, and three slices of Serrano (or Parma) ham

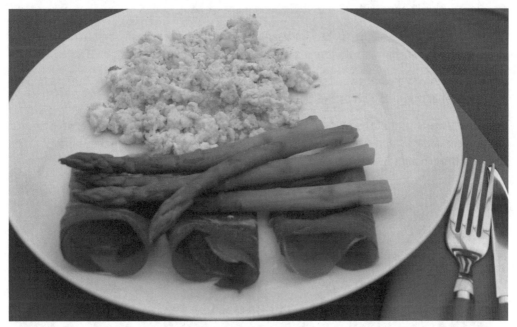

Photo 14.12: Scrambled eggs with asparagus spears and Serrano ham

Dinners

200 g pork tenderloin served with 100 g broccoli, and 100 g cauliflower mashed with one teaspoon butter. Topped with 30 g grated cheddar cheese

Two smoky chorizo sausages cooked and served with 80 g green beans and 100 g chopped steamed leek or cauliflower, with topping of one tablespoon cream cheese

Chicken breast wrapped in two slices of Serrano (or Parma) ham. Served with 100 g chopped leeks or celeriac, mashed with one teaspoon butter

Beef stir-fry made with 200 g beef rump steak strips, 100 g beansprouts, five sliced mushrooms, half a sliced red or green pepper, and 50 g chopped onions or 30 g water chestnuts. Stir-fried with two tablespoon soya sauce

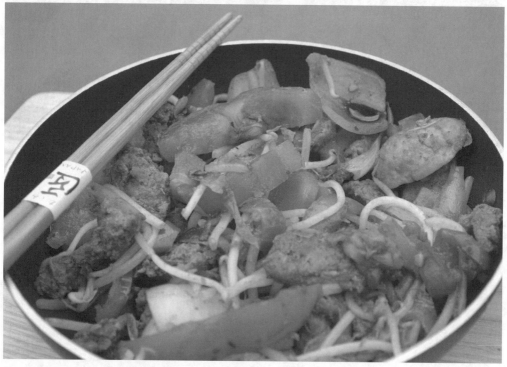

Photo 14.13: Beef stir-fry made with beef rump steak strips, beansprouts, mushrooms, pepper, onions, and soya sauce

130 g salmon baked in foil topped with one teaspoon butter and 1 teaspoon parsley. Served with 100 g steamed cauliflower and 80 g sautéed kale cooked in one tablespoon olive oil with one finely chopped slice of lean bacon

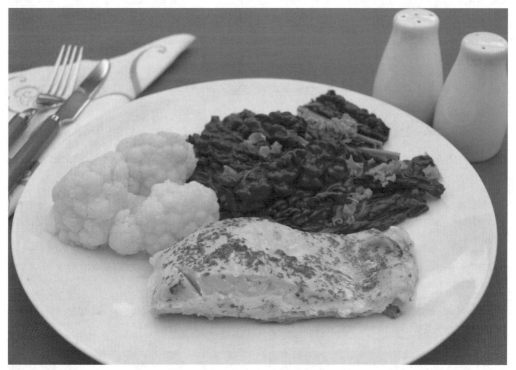

Photo 14.14: Oven baked salmon with butter and parsley served with steamed cauliflower and sautéed kale cooked in olive oil with bacon bits

MEALS FOR THE LOW-FAT DIET

The low-fat diet typically provides a total of 1,500 kcal/day with less than 10% fat or less than 20 g/day fat. From the listed meals below, choose one breakfast, one lunch, and one dinner per day.

Breakfasts

Two whole wheat biscuits (such as Shredded Wheat, Weetabix, or Oatibix) with semi-skimmed milk

Porridge made with skimmed milk and topped with a spoon of honey and 20 raisins

Fruit smoothie – one ripe banana, cranberry juice, and frozen red fruit blended together and served with an English muffin toasted and spread with a "light" spread or marmite

Lean bacon sandwich – two slices of lean back bacon, trimmed of all fat and grilled or microwaved. Served between two slices of wholemeal bread or in a toasted bun with one finely chopped tomato

Kedgeree made from 100 g poached smoked haddock, 100 g boiled rice, and curry paste or red pesto topped with hard-boiled egg quarters

Muesli (40 g) with rolled oats, wheat flakes, and a variety of dried fruits (e.g., cranberries, raisins, sultanas) served with low-fat yogurt and topped with a strawberry

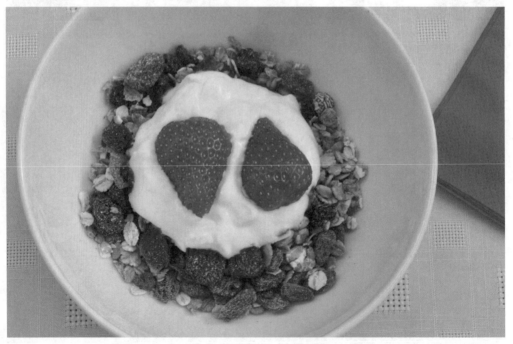

Photo 14.15: Muesli with rolled oats, wheat flakes, dried raisins and sultanas, served with low-fat yogurt and topped with a strawberry

Lunches

One jacket potato served with 30 g cottage cheese, sauerkraut, and a side salad with squeezed lemon or lime dressing

Chunky vegetable soup and a wedge of crusty wholegrain bread

Sandwich consisting of two slices of wholemeal bread with lean roast ham, mustard, and watercress, or tinned tuna and cucumber

Half a can of baked beans on toast, or for something different, try mashed banana on toast

Pasta with tomato sauce and finely chopped roast ham or chicken pieces

Chicken pasta salad

Dinners

Poached or grilled white fish (180 g) served with new potatoes and peas

Cottage pie made with Quorn or very lean minced beef (150 g), mashed potato, and served with red cabbage

Stir fried 150 g pork tenderloin with chopped onion, green pepper, mushrooms, and noodles

Burger made with lean mince (150 g) and finely chopped onion with chili sauce and sauerkraut

Mixed vegetable rice risotto

Chicken saag curry (see earlier recipe) with 50 g beansprouts, and with 120 g boiled brown or white rice

Fish cake served with mixed leaf salad, tomato, and a sweet chili sauce

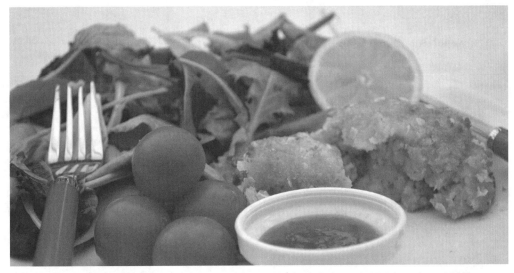

Photo 14.16: Cod and prawn Thai-style fishcake with mixed leaf salad, cherry tomatoes, and sweet chili sauce

DAILY MEAL PLANS FOR THE HIGH-PROTEIN DIET

The high-protein diet typically provides a total of 1,500 kcal/day with 30-35% protein or 110-130 g/day protein. The sample daily meal plans below each provide about 110 grams of protein per day. However, you can adjust the portions to meet your needs.

Meal Plan 1

Breakfast

Three eggs, one slice whole grain toast with one tablespoon almond butter and a pear.

Lunch

Fresh avocado and cottage cheese salad with orange segments.

Dinner

170 g grilled beef steak or lamb steak, one medium sweet potato, and 150 g grilled sliced zucchini (courgette).

Meal Plan 2

Breakfast

Low-fat yogurt, shredded dessicated coconut, and strawberries.

Lunch

120 g canned salmon, mixed greens, olive oil and vinegar, and an apple.

Dinner

170 g grilled chicken with quinoa and Brussels sprouts.

Meal Plan 3

Breakfast

Oatmeal and one cup plain Greek yogurt with a quarter of a cup of chopped pecans.

Lunch

120 g grilled chicken mixed with half a chopped ripe avocado and red bell pepper and a peach.

Dinner

Chili con carne made with 150 g beef cubes or lean mince, one chopped onion, 100 g red kidney beans, half a can of chopped tomatoes, and one tablespoon chili powder served with 120 g boiled white or brown rice.

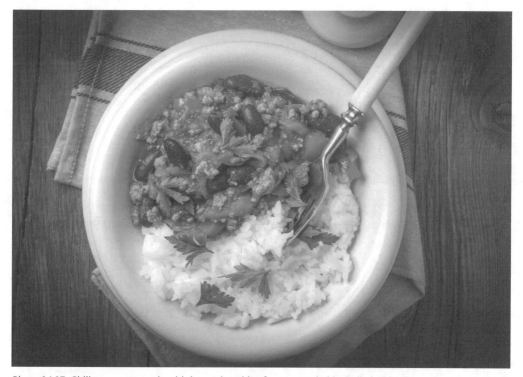

Photo 14.17: Chili con carne made with lean minced beef accompanied by boiled white rice

Meal Plan 4

Breakfast

Spanish omelet made with three eggs, 30 g cottage cheese, chili peppers, black olives, salsa, and an orange.

Lunch

Two celery stalks each filled with 30 g cottage cheese and wrapped in thin sliced 25 g piece of roast chicken, ham, or beef.

Dinner

180 g halibut, lentils, and broccoli.

Meal Plan 5

Breakfast

One cup of cottage cheese with a quarter of a cup of chopped walnuts, diced apples, and cinnamon.

Lunch

120 g canned salmon mixed with one tablespoon low-fat yogurt on sprouted grain bread, and carrot sticks.

Dinner

150 g Chicken meatballs with Marinara Sauce, spaghetti squash, and raspberries.

Meal Plan 6

Breakfast

Frittata made with three eggs, 30 g cottage cheese, and half a cup of diced potatoes.

Lunch

75 g thin sliced cooked ham with tomato, and mixed salad leaves with an apple.

Dinner

100 g shrimp fajitas with grilled onions and bell peppers, guacamole, one cup of black beans on a corn tortilla.

Meal Plan 7

Breakfast

Two scrambled eggs made with 50 mL milk, and one chopped green pepper.

Lunch

One cup plain Greek yogurt mixed with a quarter of a cup of chopped mixed nuts and pineapple.

Dinner

180 g grilled salmon, potatoes, and sautéed spinach.

DAILY MEAL PLANS FOR THE LOW-ENERGY DENSITY DIET

The low energy density diet provides a total of 1,300 to 1,500 kcal/day with an energy density of less than 1.5 kcal/g. The diet contains 25-30% protein with low-fat (less than 30 g/day) and limited carbohydrate (less than 130 g/day). Here are some low energy density meals that you might like to try. You could also try adapting your own favorite dishes to reduce their energy density too. The main principle is to avoid fatty foods or use reduced fat versions of foods like cheese and milk, use only lean meat and fish, and include lots of fruit and non-starchy vegetables. Most vegetables have an energy density less than 1.0 kcal/g (e.g., salad leaves and spinach are only 0.2 kcal/g, carrots and most gourds are 0.4 kcal/g and beans are about 0.9 kcal/g). Using the principles of energy density, you can achieve a lower calorie intake which will help towards weight loss, while allowing you to continue to enjoy generous portions of food and get an overall balanced diet. Essentially you are reducing the number of calories in a meal and increasing the size of it by weight (total grams of food on your plate) and volume by lowering the amount of fat in a meal and by increasing the amount of water and fiber rich ingredients.

Breakfasts With Low Energy Density and Fewer Than 250 kcal

- *Half a pink grapefruit.*
  35 g swiss style muesli (no added sugar) with 75 mL semi-skimmed milk and 20 blueberries or six seedless green grapes

- *Half a large orange.*
  35 g all bran cereal (no added sugar) with 75 mL semi-skimmed milk and six seedless red grapes.

- *Cup of seedless grapes.*
  Two Weetabix with 75 mL semi-skimmed milk.

- *Fruit smoothie*
  300 mL (11 fl oz) fruit smoothie made with fruit, nonfat yogurt, and crushed ice.

Lunches With Low Energy Density and Fewer Than 250 kcal

Half a can of soup (200 g) such as pea and ham, lentil and bacon, chicken and vegetable, mulligatawny, minestrone, tomato, or mushroom. Add small pieces (about 40 g) of sliced cold meats (e.g., ham, turkey, chicken or beef) to help ensure that daily protein requirements are met. Serve with one slice of wholegrain or wholemeal bread as these contain more micronutrients than processed bread.

Macaroni cheese made with low-fat cheddar and chopped steamed asparagus and broccoli.

Half a small tin of chopped tuna in pitta bread stuffed with mixed salad leaves and chopped tomato

Sandwich made with wholemeal bread with hummus or lean sliced meat, and plenty of vegetables like lettuce, cucumbers, and tomatoes.

Salad with 10 g mixed salad leaves (e.g., lettuce, rocket, spinach, watercress), two celery stalks, two tomatoes, five spring onions, and five pitted green olives served with two diced slices of cold meat (e.g., ham, chicken, turkey, or beef), and drizzled with juice from half a squeezed lime or lemon.

Dinners With Low Energy Density and Fewer Than 800 kcal:

Spaghetti Bolognese made with 200 g lean mince, reduced calorie Bolognese sauce, 60 g cannellini beans, half a can of chopped tomatoes, garlic, and 150 g boiled spaghetti.

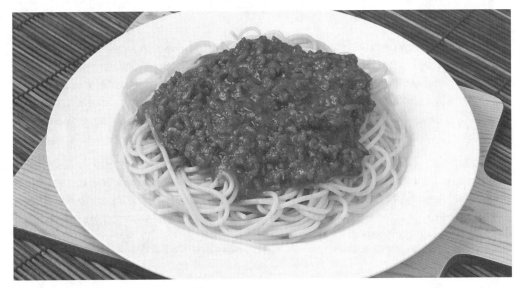

Photo 14.18: Spaghetti Bolognese

200 g grilled lean meat (e.g., beefsteak, chicken breast, pork tenderloin) with your choice of three of the following steamed vegetables: cauliflower, broccoli, aubergine, mangetout, zucchini (courgette), spinach, cabbage, kale. Serve with 120 g penne pasta or boiled brown rice.

Chili con carne made with 150 g beef cubes or lean mince, one chopped onion, 100 g red kidney beans, half a can of chopped tomatoes, and one tablespoon chili powder served with 120 g boiled white or brown rice.

180 g oven baked cod fillet or cod loin with lemon and parsley accompanied by 60 g steamed mangetout, 130 g steamed tenderstem broccoli, and 100 g steamed cauliflower.

Chicken saag curry (see recipe described earlier in this chapter) served with 50 g beansprouts and 120 g boiled brown rice.

For desserts have fruit (e.g., grapes, plums, chopped apple, melon, or mango) topped with low-fat yogurt.

Key Points

- Very low energy diets with specially formulated liquid meals are designed to provide about 800 kcal/day with sufficient protein and micronutrients to meet minimum daily requirements.

- The energy intake on the semi-fasting days of intermittent fasting diets is limited to 500-600 kcal/day and will almost certainly not provide sufficient protein and micronutrients to meet minimum daily requirements. This can be compensated for by having a high-protein dinner on the day before the semi-fasting day and a high-protein breakfast on the day after. A multivitamin and mineral supplement is advised if the intention is to stay on this type of diet for more than one month.

- Other diets that supply a total of 1500 kcal/day and are high in one particular macronutrient (i.e., fat, carbohydrate or protein) should provide sufficient protein and micronutrients to meet minimum daily requirements.

- For the low energy density diet, you reduce the number of calories in a meal and increase the size of it by weight (total grams of food on your plate) and volume by lowering the amount of fat in a meal, and by increasing the amount of water and fiber rich ingredients like fruit and non-starchy vegetables. An advantage of low energy density foods is that the fewer calories a food contains, the more of it you can eat. This helps keep you from the hunger pangs that are many a diet's downfall.

- When dieting you should avoid drinking any sugar sweetened beverages, milkshakes, creamy or milky hot drinks, and alcohol. Stick to water, artificially sweetened the "low-calorie", "diet" or "light" versions of fruit flavored soft drinks, mixers, and cordials. You can still drink coffee or tea, but use a zero-calorie artificial sweetener instead of sugar, and skimmed or semi-skimmed milk instead of whole milk or cream.

Appendix

Table A.1: Recommended daily intakes for North America

	MEN		WOMEN	
	19-70 years	Over 70 years	19-70 years	Over 70 years
Biotin (µg)*	30	30	30	30
Choline (mg)*	550	550	425	425
Folate (µg)	400	400	400	400
Niacin (mg)	16	16	14	14
Pantothenic Acid (mg)*	5	5	5	5
Riboflavin (mg)	1.3	1.3	1.1	1.1
Thiamin (mg)	1.2	1.2	1.1	1.1
Vitamin B6 (mg)	1.3	1.7	1.3	1.5
Vitamin B12 (µg)	2.4	2.4	2.4	2.4
Vitamin A (µg)	900	900	700	700
Vitamin C (mg)	90	90	75	75
Vitamin D (µg)	15	20	15	20
Vitamin E (mg)	15	15	15	15
Vitamin K (µg)*	120	120	90	90
Calcium (mg)	1,000	1,200	1,000	1,200
Chloride (g)*	2.3	1.8	2.3	1.8
Chromium (µg)*	35	30	25	20
Copper (µg)	900	900	900	900
Fluoride (mg)*	4	4	3	3
Iodine (µg)	150	150	150	150
Iron (mg)	8	8	18	8
Magnesium (mg)	420	420	320	320
Manganese (mg)*	2.3	2.3	1.8	1.8
Molybdenum (µg)	45	45	45	45
Phosphorus (mg)	700	700	700	700
Potassium (g)*	4.7	4.5	4.7	4.7
Selenium (µg)	55	55	55	55
Sodium (g)*	1.5	1.2	1.5	1.2
Zinc (mg)	11	11	8	8
Protein (g)	56	56	46	46

Values are recommended daily allowances (RDAs) or adequate intakes (AIs). The latter are denoted with asterisks. NS = Not specified.

Data from The National Academies of Science, Engineering and Medicine, Health and Medicine Division, *Dietary Reference Intakes Tables and Application*, Washington, DC: National Academies of Science, 2011.

Table A.2: Recommended daily intakes for United Kingdom

	MEN		WOMEN	
	19-70 years	Over 70 years	19-70 years	Over 70 years
Biotin (µg)	NS	NS	NS	NS
Choline (mg)	NS	NS	NS	NS
Folate (µg)	200	200	200	200
Niacin (mg)	17	16	13	12
Pantothenic Acid (mg)	NS	NS	NS	NS
Riboflavin (mg)	1.3	1.3	1.1	1.1
Thiamin (mg)	1.0	0.9	0.8	0.8
Vitamin B6 (mg)	1.4	1.4	1.2	1.2
Vitamin B12 (µg)	1.5	1.5	1.5	1.5
Vitamin A (µg)	700	700	600	600
Vitamin C (mg)	40	40	40	40
Vitamin D (µg)	10	10	10	10
Vitamin E (mg)	NS	NS	NS	NS
Vitamin K (µg)	NS	NS	NS	NS
Calcium (mg)	700	700	700	700
Chloride (g)	2.5	2.5	2.5	2.5
Chromium (µg)	NS	NS	NS	NS
Copper (mg)	1.2	1.2	1.2	1.2
Fluoride (mg)	NS	NS	NS	NS
Iodine (µg)	140	140	140	140
Iron (mg)	8.7	8.7	14.8	8.7
Magnesium (mg)	300	300	270	270
Manganese (mg)	NS	NS	NS	NS
Molybdenum (µg)	NS	NS	NS	NS
Phosphorus (mg)	550	550	550	550
Potassium (g)	3.5	3.5	3.5	3.5
Selenium (µg)	75	75	60	60
Sodium (g)	1.6	1.6	1.6	1.6
Zinc (mg)	9.5	9.5	7	7
Protein (g)	55.5	53.3	55.5	53.3

Values are recommended daily allowances (RDAs) or adequate intakes (AIs). The latter are denoted with asterisks. NS = Not specified.

Data from *Dietary Reference Values for Food Energy and Nutrients in the United Kingdom: Report of the Panel on Dietary Reference Values of the Committee on Medical Aspects of Food Policy,* London: Her Majesty's Stationary Office, 1991.

Table A.3: Recommended daily intakes of vitamins, minerals and protein for Australia and New Zealand

	MEN		WOMEN	
	19-70 years	Over 70 years	19-70 years	Over 70 years
Biotin (μg)	NS	NS	NS	NS
Choline (mg)	NS	NS	NS	NS
Folate (μg)	400	400	400	400
Niacin (mg)	16	16	14	14
Pantothenic Acid (mg)	NS	NS	NS	NS
Riboflavin (mg)	1.3	1.6	1.1	1.1
Thiamin (mg)	1.2	1.2	1.1	1.1
Vitamin B6 (mg)	1.3	1.7	1.3	1.5
Vitamin B12 (μg)	2.4	2.4	2.4	2.4
Vitamin A (μg)	900	900	700	700
Vitamin C (mg)	45	45	45	45
Vitamin D (μg)	NS	NS	NS	NS
Vitamin E (mg)*	10	10	7	7
Vitamin K (μg)	NS	NS	NS	NS
Calcium (mg)	1000	1300	1000	1300
Chloride (g)	NS	NS	NS	NS
Chromium (μg)	NS	NS	NS	NS
Copper (mg)	NS	NS	NS	NS
Fluoride (mg)	NS	NS	NS	NS
Iodine (μg)	150	150	150	150
Iron (mg)	8	8	18	8
Magnesium (mg)	420	420	320	320
Manganese (mg)	NS	NS	NS	NS
Molybdenum (μg)	NS	NS	NS	NS
Phosphorus (mg)	1000	1000	1000	1000
Potassium (g)*	3.8	3.8	2.8	2.8
Selenium (μg)	70	70	60	60
Sodium (mg)*	460-920	460-920	460-920	460-920
Zinc (mg)	14	14	8	8
Protein (g)	64	81	46	57

Values are recommended daily allowances (RDAs) or adequate intakes (AIs). The latter are denoted with asterisks. NS = Not specified.

Data from National Health and Medical Research Council, Australia, 2014 **(https://www.nrv.gov.au/resource/nrv-summary-tables)**.

Glossary

absorption—The transport of nutrients from the intestine into the blood or lymph system.

acceptable macronutrient distribution range (AMDR)—The range of intake for a particular energy source (i.e., carbohydrate, fat, and protein) that is associated with reduced risk of chronic disease while providing intakes of essential nutrients.

ad libitum—Having as much as you desire of something such as food.

adenosine triphosphate (ATP)—A high-energy compound that is the immediate source for muscular contraction and other energy-requiring processes in the cell.

adequate intake (AI)—Recommended dietary intake comparable to the RDA but based on less scientific evidence.

adipocyte—An adipose tissue cell whose main function is to store triglyceride (fat).

adipokine—Chemical messenger molecule secreted from adipose (white fat) tissue.

adipose tissue—White fatty tissue that stores triglyceride.

aerobic—Occurring in the presence of free oxygen.

aerobic capacity—The highest rate of oxygen consumption by the body that can be determined in an incremental exercise test to exhaustion. Also known as maximal oxygen uptake.

alcohol—A colorless liquid that has depressant and intoxicating effects. Ethyl alcohol or ethanol (C_2H_5OH) is the alcohol found in wines, spirits, and beers.

allergy—An adverse reaction of the immune system to a substance not recognized as harmful by most people's immune systems.

Alzheimer's disease—A progressive mental deterioration that can occur in middle or old age, due to generalized degeneration of the brain. It is the commonest cause of premature senility.

amino acid (AA)—The chief structural molecule of protein, consisting of an amino group (NH_2) and a carboxylic acid group (CO_2H) plus another so-called R-group that determines the properties of the amino acid. Twenty different amino acids can be used to make proteins.

amylopectin—A branched-chain starch (polymer of glucose).

amylose—A straight-chain starch that is more resistant to digestion compared with amylopectin.

anabolic—A constructive metabolic process whereby simple body compounds are formed into more complex ones (e.g., when protein is synthesized from many amino acids).

anaerobic—Occurring in the absence of free oxygen.

anaphylactic shock—An extreme, often life-threatening allergic reaction to an antigen (foreign molecule) to which the body has become hypersensitive. Symptoms include dizziness, loss of consciousness, labored breathing, swelling of the tongue and airways, blueness of the skin, low blood pressure, heart failure, and death.

anemia—A condition defined by an abnormally low blood hemoglobin content resulting in lowered oxygen carrying capacity. The most common cause is iron deficiency.

angiogenesis—The physiological process through which new blood vessels are formed from pre-existing vessels to improve blood supply to a tissue.

anorexia nervosa— An eating disorder characterized by abnormally small food intake and refusal to maintain a normal body weight (according to what is expected for gender, age, and height), a distorted view of body image, an intense fear of being fat or overweight and gaining weight or "feeling fat" when clearly the person is below normal weight.

antibody—Soluble protein produced by B lymphocytes with antimicrobial effects. Also known as immunoglobulin.

antioxidant—Molecules that can prevent or limit the actions of free radicals, usually by removing their unpaired electron and converting them into something far less reactive.

apolipoprotein—Proteins that bind fats (lipids) to form a complex of triglycerides, cholesterol, and protein called lipoproteins that are used to transport fats through the lymphatic and circulatory systems.

appetite—A desire for food for the purpose of enjoyment that is developed through previous experience. Controlled in humans by an appetite center in the hypothalamus.

arteriosclerosis—Hardening of the arteries. Also known as atherosclerosis.

arthritis—A common condition that causes pain and inflammation in a joint. Can be caused by a form of autoimmune disease.

asthma—A respiratory condition in which sufferers get occasional attacks of spasm in the smooth muscle lining the upper airways (bronchi) of the lungs, causing narrowing of the airways and severe difficulty in breathing. It is usually connected to allergic reaction or other forms of hypersensitivity.

Atkins diet—A very low-carbohydrate diet which is used for weight loss.

atom—The smallest unit of an element that retains all the properties of the element. The atoms of all elements can be broken down physically into the same subatomic particles: protons, neutrons, and electrons. Hence, the atoms of the various elements differ only in the numbers of protons, neutrons, and electrons that they contain.

atrophy—A wasting away, a diminution in the size of a cell, tissue, organ, or part.

Atwater factor—The average net energy values for carbohydrate, fat, and protein, named after Wilbur Olin Atwater: 17 kJ/g (4 kcal/g) for carbohydrate, 37 kJ/g (9 kcal/g) for fat, and 17 kJ/g (4 kcal/g) for protein.

autoregulatory feedback—A process within many biological systems, resulting from an internal adaptive mechanism that works to adjust that system's response to maintain homeostasis (i.e., a stable internal environment) when something forces a change. Sensory mechanisms may detect the change and feed this information back to a central controller so that appropriate adjustments can be made to restore stability.

average daily metabolic rate (ADMR)—The average energy expenditure over 24 hours.

basal cell carcinoma—The most common type (> 80%) of all skin cancers and usually benign. Most common cause is excess sun exposure.

basal metabolic rate (BMR)— Energy expenditure under basal, overnight fasted conditions representing the energy needed to maintain life under these basal conditions.

beriberi—A disease caused by deficiency of vitamin B1 (thiamin) which is characterized mainly by damage to peripheral nerves, wasting, and congestive heart failure.

binge eating disorder—An eating disorder in which a person feels compelled to consume a lot of food in a short period of time and is accompanied by feelings of loss of control, and in many cases, guilt and embarrassment.

bioavailability—In relation to nutrients in food, the amount that may be absorbed into the body.

bioelectrical impedance analysis (BIA)—A method to calculate percentage of body fat by measuring electrical resistance due to the water content of the body.

body mass index (BMI)—Body mass in kilograms divided by height in meters squared (kg/m^2). An index used as a measure of obesity.

bomb calorimeter—An instrument to measure the energy content in which food is completely oxidized and the resulting heat production is measured.

brain-gut peptides—These are peptide hormones that are involved in the control of digestion, appetite, and satiety.

branched-chain amino acid (BCAA)—Three essential amino acids that can be oxidized by muscle. Includes leucine, isoleucine, and valine.

bulimia nervosa—An eating disorder characterized by repeated episodes of binge eating (consumption of large amounts of usually energy-dense foods) followed by purging of the stomach contents, allowing insufficient time for most of the nutrients from the heavy meal to be absorbed.

caffeine—A stimulant drug found in many food products such as coffee, tea, and cola drinks. Stimulates the central nervous system and used as an ergogenic aid to improve sport performance. Caffeine also improves concentration and cognitive function when fatigued.

calorie (cal)—Traditional unit of energy. One calorie expresses the quantity of energy (heat) needed to raise the temperature of 1 g (1 mL) of water 1 °C (e.g., from 14.5 °C to 15.5 °C).

cancer—An abnormal growth of cells that have the ability to invade or spread to other parts of the body.

capillary—The smallest vessel in the cardiovascular system. Capillary walls are only one cell thick. All exchanges of molecules between the blood and tissue fluid occur across the capillary walls.

carbohydrate (CHO)—A compound composed of carbon, hydrogen, and oxygen in a ratio of 1:2:1 (e.g., CH_2O). Carbohydrates include sugars, starches, and dietary fibers.

carboxyl group (COOH or CO2H)—Acidic group of amino acids, fatty acids, and components of the tricarboxylic acid (TCA) or Krebs cycle.

carcinogenic—A cancer-inducing substance.

catalyst—A substance that accelerates a chemical reaction, usually by temporarily combining with the substrates and lowering the activation energy and is recovered unchanged at the end of the reaction (e.g., in the body enzymes act as catalysts).

cataract—A clouding of the lens in the eye which leads to a decrease in vision. Cataracts often develop slowly and can affect one or both eyes. Over time these patches usually become bigger causing blurry, misty vision, and eventually blindness.

catechin—A type of natural plant phenol and antioxidant that belongs to the flavanol group of compounds, part of the chemical family of flavonoids.

celiac disease—An immune reaction to eating gluten, a protein found in wheat, barley, and rye. If you have celiac disease, eating gluten triggers an immune response in your small intestine which causes it to become inflamed and unable to absorb nutrients. It can cause a range of symptoms including diarrhea, abdominal pain, and bloating.

cell—The smallest discrete living unit of the body.

cellulose—A major component of plant cell walls and the most abundant nonstarch polysaccharide. Cannot be digested by human digestive enzymes.

cerebrospinal fluid (CSF)—The fluid found in the brain and spinal cord.

cholecystokinin (CCK)—A hormone secreted by the duodenum that acts to stimulate the secretion of enzymes in pancreatic juice. Also induces satiety via actions in the hypothalamus of the brain.

cholesterol—A lipid transported in the blood in high- and low-density lipoproteins (HDL and LDL, respectively). High HDL levels are somewhat protective against coronary heart disease. Cholesterol is also found in cell membranes and is a precursor of steroid hormones.

chronic bronchitis—Disease of the upper airways (bronchi) in which the inflamed bronchial tubes produce a lot of mucus. This leads to coughing and difficulty breathing. Cigarette smoking is the most common cause, but it can also arise due to prolonged exposure to polluted or dusty air.

chronic disease—Disease that develops over time such as type 2 diabetes, peripheral vascular disease, and coronary heart disease. Often associated with unhealthy lifestyle behaviors.

chronic obstructive pulmonary disease (COPD)—Disease in which the airways become blocked causing breathing difficulties.

chylomicrons—A class of lipoproteins that transport exogenous (dietary) cholesterol and triglycerides from the small intestine to tissues after meals.

cirrhosis—A degenerative disease of the liver. The most common cause is excessive consumption of alcohol.

cis—A prefix indicating the geometrical isomer in which the two like groups are on the same side of a double bond with restricted rotation (e.g., in unsaturated fatty acids in which the hydrogen ions are on the same side of the double bond).

coefficient of digestibility—The percentage energy of food ingested that is digested, absorbed, and available for metabolic processes in the body.

coenzyme—Small molecules that are essential in stoichiometric amounts for the activity of some enzymes. Examples include nicotinamide adenine dinucleotide (NAD), flavin adenine dinucleotide (FAD), pyridoxal phosphate (PLP), thiamin pyrophosphate (TPP), and biotin.

colon—The large intestine. This part of the intestine is mainly responsible for forming, storing, and expelling feces.

colorectal cancer—The development of cancer in the colon or rectum (parts of the large intestine); also known as bowel cancer and colon cancer. This part of the intestine is mainly responsible for forming, storing, and expelling feces.

complex carbohydrates—Foods containing starch and other polysaccharides as found in bread, pasta, cereals, fruits, and vegetables in contrast to simple carbohydrates such as glucose, milk sugar, and table sugar.

conditionally essential—A nutrient that becomes indispensable in certain situations.

constipation—Hard stools in rectum making defecation difficult.

coronary heart disease (CHD)—Narrowing of the arteries supplying the heart muscle that can cause heart attacks.

cortisol—A steroid hormone secreted from the adrenal glands in response to stress or low blood sugar.

cytokine—Protein released from cells that acts as a chemical messenger by binding to receptors on other cells. Cytokines include interleukins (IL), tumor necrosis factors (TNF), colony-stimulating factors (CSF), and interferons (IFN).

cytoplasm—The fluid found inside a cell.

daily reference value (DRV)—Recommended daily intakes for the macronutrients (carbohydrate, fat, and protein) as well as cholesterol, sodium, and potassium. On a food label, the DRV is based on a 2,000 kcal (8.4 MJ) diet.

daily value (DV)—A term used in food labeling that is based on a daily energy intake of 2,000 kcal (8.3 MJ) and for the food labeled. Gives the percentage of the RDI and the DRV recommended for healthy people in the US.

dental caries—Erosion or decay of tooth caused by the effects of bacteria in the mouth.

dementia—An overall term that describes a wide range of symptoms associated with a decline in memory or other thinking skills severe enough to reduce a person's ability to perform everyday activities. Alzheimer's disease accounts for 60 to 80 percent of cases.

deoxyribonucleic acid (DNA)—The compound that forms genes (i.e., the genetic material).

diabetes mellitus—A disorder of carbohydrate metabolism caused by disturbances in production or utilization of insulin. Causes high blood glucose levels and loss of sugar in the urine.

diarrhea—Frequent passage of a watery fecal discharge because of a gastrointestinal disturbance or infection.

diastolic—The filling phase of the cardiac cycle when the ventricles are relaxed.

dietary reference intake (DRI)—The term used to encompass the latest nutrient recommendations by the Food and Nutrition Board of the National Academy of Sciences.

dietary (or daily) reference value (DRV)—Recommended daily intakes for the macronutrients (carbohydrate, fat, and protein) as well as cholesterol, sodium, and potassium. On a food label, the DRV is based on a 2,000 kcal (8.3 MJ) diet.

diet-induced thermogenesis (DIT)—The energy needed for the digestion, assimilation, and metabolism of food that is consumed (also referred to as thermic effect of food, or TEF).

diffusion—The movement of molecules from a region of high concentration to one of low concentration, brought about by their kinetic energy.

digestion—The process of breaking down food to its smallest components so that it can be absorbed in the intestine.

disaccharide—Sugars that yield two monosaccharides on hydrolysis. Sucrose, the most common, is composed of glucose and fructose.

diverticulosis—The condition of having multiple pouches (diverticula) in the colon that can become inflamed. These are outpockets of the colonic mucosa and submucosa through weaknesses of muscle layers in the colon wall. They typically cause no symptoms but can cause abdominal pain and bloating with complications that can include rectal bleeding, abdominal infections, and constipation, or diarrhea.

dopamine—A catecholamine neurotransmitter and hormone formed by decarboxylation of dehydroxyphenylalanine (dopa). A precursor of epinephrine (adrenaline) and norepinephrine (noradrenaline).

dual energy X-ray absorptiometry (DEXA)—A special type of X-ray scan that measures bone mineral density. This type of scan may also be called a DXA scan.

eating disorder—A psychological disorder centering on the avoidance or purging of food, such as anorexia nervosa and bulimia nervosa.

efficiency—The ratio of the useful work performed by a machine or a person to the total energy expended.

eicosanoids—Derivatives of fatty acids in the body that act as cell-to-cell signaling molecules. They include prostaglandins, thromboxanes, and leukotrienes.

electrolyte—A substance that, when dissolved in water, conducts an electric current. Electrolytes, which include acids, bases, and salts, usually dissociate into ions carrying either a positive charge (cation) or a negative charge (anion).

element—The smallest units into which a substance can be broken down chemically are the elements, each of which has different and unique properties. At least 94 elements are known to exist, but only about 12 are common in living organisms. The most abundant are oxygen, carbon, hydrogen, and nitrogen (in that order). Those four elements constitute 96% of the mass of a human.

elevated post-exercise oxygen consumption (EPOC) — The amount of oxygen our body consumes following completion of a bout of exercise that is in excess of the pre-exercise oxygen consumption baseline level. Essentially, our body uses more oxygen after exercise than before exercise, and we expend more calories during our recovery from exercise than we do before exercise. This effect is fairly small but can last for several hours.

emphysema—A long-term, progressive disease of the lungs that causes shortness of breath due to over-inflation of the alveoli (air sacs in the lung). In people with emphysema, the lung tissue involved in exchange of gases (oxygen and carbon dioxide) is impaired or destroyed.

endocrine—Ductless glands that secrete hormones into the blood.

endotoxemia—The presence of toxins from bacteria in the blood, which may cause hemorrhages, kidney damage, and shock.

energy—The ability to perform work. Energy exists in various forms, including mechanical, heat, and chemical energy.

energy balance—The balance between energy intake and energy expenditure.

energy density—The amount of energy (or calories) per gram of food. Lower energy density foods provide fewer calories per gram of food – this means that you can have satisfying portions of these foods with relatively low-calorie content.

energy expenditure (EE)—The energy used per unit of time to produce power.

energy expenditure for activity (EEA)—The energy cost associated with physical activity (exercise).

enzyme—A protein with specific catalytic activity. They are designated by the suffix -ase frequently attached to the type of reaction catalyzed (e.g., oxidase, lipase). Virtually all metabolic reactions in the body are dependent on and controlled by enzymes.

epinephrine—A hormone secreted by the adrenal gland in response to acute stress. It is a stimulant, prepares the body for fight or flight, and is an important activator of fat and carbohydrate breakdown during exercise. Also known as adrenaline.

erythrocyte—Red blood cell that contains hemoglobin and transports oxygen.

esophagus—Part of the intestinal tract located between the mouth and the stomach.

essential amino acids—Amino acids that must be obtained in the diet and cannot be synthesized in the body. Also known as indispensable amino acids.

essential fatty acids—Unsaturated fatty acids that cannot be synthesized in the body and must be obtained in the diet (e.g., linoleic acid and α-linolenic acid).

essential nutrient—A food component that provides energy or promotes growth and repair of tissues and must be obtained from the diet as a deficiency of it will result in ill-health.

estimated average requirement (EAR)—Nutrient intake value estimated to meet the requirements of an average individual in a certain age and gender group.

extracellular fluid (ECF)—Body fluid that is located outside the cells, including the blood plasma, interstitial fluid, cerebrospinal fluid, synovial fluid, and ocular fluid.

fatty acid (FA)—A type of fat having a carboxylic acid group (COOH) at one end of the molecule and a methyl (CH_3) group at the other end, separated by a hydrocarbon chain that can vary in length. A typical structure of a fatty acid is $CH_3(CH_2)_{14}COOH$ (palmitic acid or palmitate). Also known as free fatty acid or nonesterified fatty acid.

fasting—Starvation; abstinence from eating that may be partial or complete.

fat—Fat molecules contain the same structural elements as carbohydrates, but they have little oxygen relative to carbon and hydrogen and are poorly soluble in water. Fats are also known as lipids (derived from the Greek word *lipos*), and fat is a general name for oils, fats, waxes, and related compounds. Oils are liquid at room temperature, whereas fats are solid.

fat-free mass—Lean body mass (or weight of body components excluding all fat).

Fatmax—The exercise intensity at which the rate of whole-body fat oxidation is highest.

feces—The excrement discharged from the intestines, consisting of bacteria, cells from the intestines, secretions, and a small amount of food residue.

fat-free mass (FFM)—Lean mass of a tissue or the whole body.

fiber—Indigestible carbohydrates.

fish oil—Oils high in unsaturated fats extracted from the bodies of fish or fish parts, especially the livers. The oils are used as dietary supplements.

flavonoid—A diverse group of phytonutrients (plant chemicals) found in almost all fruits and vegetables. Along with carotenoids, they are responsible for the vivid colors in fruits and vegetables. Like many other phytonutrients, flavonoids are powerful antioxidants with anti-inflammatory and immune system benefits. They are not classed as essential but are needed for optimal health.

flexitarian diet—A semi-vegetarian diet which is primarily a plant-based diet but includes meat, dairy, eggs, poultry, and fish on occasion or in small quantities.

food efficiency—The adaptive decrease in resting metabolic rate in response to prolonged dietary energy restriction and weight loss.

food group—A collection of foods that share similar nutritional properties or biological classifications. Nutrition guides typically divide foods into food groups and recommend daily servings of each group for a healthy diet. Common examples of food groups include dairy, meat, fruit, vegetables, grains, and beans.

free radical—An atom or molecule that possesses at least one unpaired electron in its outer orbit. Important free radicals include the superoxide ($\cdot O_2$-), hydroxyl ($\cdot OH$), and nitric oxide ($\cdot NO$) radicals. They are highly reactive and may cause damage to lipid membranes, causing membrane instability and increased permeability. Free radicals can also cause oxidative damage to proteins, including enzymes, and damage to DNA.

fructose—A six-carbon sugar found in fruits. It is converted to glucose in the liver.

ganglioside—A class of galactose-containing glycolipid (meaning a complex of carbohydrate and fat) known as cerebrosides and found in the tissues of the central nervous system (i.e, brain and spinal cord).

gastrointestinal tract—Gastrointestinal system or alimentary tract. The main sites in the body used for digestion and absorption of nutrients. It consists of the mouth, esophagus, stomach, small intestine, large intestine, rectum, and anus.

gene—A specific sequence in DNA that codes for a particular protein. Genes are located on the chromosomes. Each gene is found in a definite position (locus).

ghrelin—Peptide hormone secreted by cells of stomach that promotes hunger and appetite.

gingivitis—Infection and inflammation of the gums.

glaucoma—A common eye condition where the optic nerve, which connects the eye to the brain, becomes damaged. It's usually caused by fluid building up in the front part of the eye, which increases pressure inside the eye. Glaucoma can lead to loss of vision if it isn't diagnosed and treated early.

glucagon—A peptide hormone produced in the pancreas that has the opposite action to insulin. Glucagon secretion increases when the blood sugar level falls below normal and stimulates the liver to break down stored glycogen into glucose which is released into the circulation.

gluconeogenesis—The synthesis of glucose from noncarbohydrate precursors such as glycerol and amino acids.

glucose—Blood sugar.

glycemic index (GI)—Increase in blood glucose and insulin in response to a meal. The GI of a food represents how much blood glucose rises over a two-hour period after eating a certain food item containing 50 g carbohydrate and is expressed against a reference food, usually glucose.

glycemic load (GL)—Increase in blood glucose and insulin response to a meal (like the GI) but takes into account the amount of that food that is normally consumed. The GL is obtained by multiplying the GI value by the carbohydrate content of the food and then dividing by 100.

glycerol—Three-carbon molecule that is the backbone structure of triglycerides.

glycogen—Polymer of glucose used as a storage form of carbohydrate in the liver and muscles.

glycolysis—The sequence of reactions that converts glucose (or glycogen) to pyruvate.

glycoprotein—A protein that is attached to one or more sugar molecules.

high-density lipoprotein (HDL)—A protein-lipid complex in the blood plasma that facilitates the transport of triglycerides, cholesterol, and phospholipids.

high-density lipoprotein cholesterol (HDLC)—Cholesterol that is transported in the blood in the form of HDL particles.

high-quality protein—Dietary proteins that contain all the essential amino acid in a proportion needed by the human body. Also known as complete proteins.

hemicellulose—A form of dietary fiber found in plants. Differs from cellulose in that it can be hydrolyzed by acid outside of the body.

hemoglobin—The red, iron-containing respiratory pigment found in red blood cells. Hemoglobin is important in the transport of oxygen and in the regulation of blood pH.

hemorrhoids—Swellings containing enlarged blood vessels found inside or around the bottom (the rectum and anus). In many cases, hemorrhoids (also known as piles) don't cause symptoms and some people don't even realize they have them. But when symptoms do occur, they may include: bleeding after defecation and lumps hanging outside the anus as well as a sore and painful bottom.

high intensity interval exercise (HIIE)—Repeated bouts of heavy dynamic exercise such as sprinting separated by short recovery intervals.

high intensity interval training (HIIT)—Repeated bouts of heavy dynamic exercise such as sprinting separated by short recovery intervals that are performed regularly (i.e., at least three times per week).

homeostasis—The tendency to maintain uniformity or stability of the internal environment of the cell or of the body.

hormone—An organic chemical produced in cells of one part of the body (usually an endocrine gland) that diffuses or is transported by the blood circulation to cells in other parts of the body, where it regulates and coordinates their activities.

hydration status—Refers to body fluid levels. Euhydration is the normal state of body water content (typically about 40 liters). Hypohydration (or dehydration) is detrimental to both exercise performance and health and should be prevented by provision of fluids to match water loss.

hypertension—Higher than normal blood pressure, usually above a threshold of 140/90 mmHg.

hypertrophy—Increase in size of a tissue such as muscle.

hypoglycemia—Drop in the blood glucose concentration below 3 mmol/L that causes symptoms of faintness, dizziness, disorientation, and fatigue.

hyponatremia—Below-normal plasma sodium concentration (i.e., below 140 mmol/L).

hypothalamus—Region at base of brain responsible for integration of sensory input and effector responses in regulation of body temperature. Also contains centers for control of hunger, appetite, and thirst.

immune system—Cells and soluble molecules involved in tissue repair after injury and in the protection of the body against infection.

immunodepression—Lowered functional activity of the immune system.

intracellular fluid—The fluid inside cells also known as cytoplasm.

intramuscular triglyceride (IMTG)—Storage form of fat found in muscle fibers.

inflammation—The body's response to injury, which includes redness (increased blood flow) and swelling (edema) caused by increased capillary permeability.

insoluble fiber—Fiber that does not dissolve in water.

insomnia—Difficulty with sleeping.

insulin—A hormone secreted by the pancreas involved in carbohydrate metabolism, particularly in the control of the blood glucose concentration. Insulin stimulates glucose uptake from the blood by muscle, liver, and adipose tissue.

insulin resistance—A condition that occurs when target tissues such as muscle, liver, and adipose tissue become less responsive to the actions of insulin. It is strongly associated with being overweight and having signs of chronic low-level inflammation. Precedes the onset of type 2 diabetes.

interleukin—Type of cytokine produced by leukocytes and some other tissues. Acts as a chemical messenger, rather like a hormone, but usually with localized effects.

intermittent fasting diet (IFD)—A form of dieting that involves fasting or very low-calorie intake in between periods of normal eating (e.g., fasting or only eating about 500 kcal on two or three days of the week).

interstitial fluid—The fluid that fills any spaces that lie between cells.

intolerance (to food)—A condition in which symptoms of abdominal discomfort with flatulence and bloating or diarrhea occur every time a particular food is consumed. Usual cause is when the body fails to produce a sufficient amount of a particular enzyme needed to digest a food component before it can be absorbed.

irritable bowel syndrome (IBS)—A common condition that affects the digestive system that causes symptoms like stomach cramps, bloating, diarrhea, and constipation. These tend to come and go over time, and can last for days, weeks or months at a time. It is usually a lifelong problem, with no cure, although diet changes and medicines can often help control the symptoms. The exact cause is unknown, but it has been linked to things like food passing through your gut too quickly or too slowly, oversensitive nerves in your gut, stress, and a family history of IBS.

isoflavone—An estrogen-like compound, an isomer of flavone (a type of plant flavonoid), found in soybeans and used to reduce cholesterol levels, maintain bone health, etc.

jejunum—The middle and longest part of the small intestine where a lot of the absorption of nutrients takes place. The jejunum is approximately one to two meters long.

joule (J)—Unit of energy according to the Systeme Internationale. One joule is the amount of energy needed to move a mass of 1 g at a velocity of 1 m/s.

keratocanthoma—Type of benign skin cancer arising from hair follicles.

ketone bodies (or ketones)—Acidic organic compounds produced during the incomplete oxidation of fatty acids in the liver. Contain a carboxyl group (-COOH) and a ketone group (-C=O). Examples include acetoacetate and β-hydroxybutyrate.

kilocalorie (kcal)—Unit of energy equal to 1,000 calories.

kilojoule (kJ)—Unit of energy equal to 1,000 joules.

kwashiorkor—A pure protein deficiency, mainly in children, characterized by a bloated belly caused by edema as well as muscle wasting and impaired immunity with increased susceptibility to infections.

lactic acid—Metabolic end product of anaerobic glycolysis.

lactose—Milk sugar, a disaccharide linking a molecule of glucose and a molecule of galactose.

low-density lipoprotein (LDL)—A protein-lipid complex in the blood plasma that facilitates the transport of triglycerides, cholesterol, and phospholipids. High blood levels are associated with increased incidence of coronary heart disease.

low-density lipoprotein cholesterol (LDLC)— Cholesterol that is transported in the blood in the form of LDL particles.

lean body mass (LBM)—All parts of the body, excluding fat.

legume—The high-protein fruit or pod of vegetables, including beans, peas, and lentils.

leptin—Regulatory hormone produced by adipose tissue. When released into the circulation, it influences the hypothalamus to control appetite.

leukocyte—White blood cell. Important in inflammation and immune defense.

linoleic acid—An essential fatty acid.

α-linolenic acid—An essential fatty acid.

lipid—A compound composed of carbon, hydrogen, oxygen, and sometimes other elements. Lipids dissolve in organic solvents but not in water and include triglyceride, fatty acids, cholesterol, and phospholipids. Lipids are commonly called fats.

lipoprotein—A complex of lipid (fat) in the form of triglyceride, cholesterol and phospholipid with protein that is used for fat transport in the circulation.

long-chain fatty acid (LCFA)—Part of triglycerides. Long-chain fatty acids have hydrocarbon chains with 12 or more carbon atoms and are the most abundant type of fatty acid. Palmitic acid and oleic acid are the most abundant long-chain fatty acids in humans.

long-chain triglyceride—Storage form of fat consisting of glycerol and three long-chain (12 carbon atoms or more) fatty acids

lutein—A naturally occurring plant carotenoid found in high quantities in green leafy vegetables such as spinach, kale and yellow carrots. It is thought to help prevent eye diseases including age-related macular degeneration, cataracts, and retinitis pigmentosa.

lymphocyte—Type of white blood cell important in the acquired immune response. Includes both T cells and B cells. The latter produce antibodies.

macromineral—Dietary elements essential to life processes that each constitute at least 0.01% of total body mass. The seven macrominerals are potassium, sodium, chloride, calcium, magnesium, phosphorus, and sulfur.

macronutrients—Nutrients ingested in relatively large amounts (carbohydrate, fat, protein, and water).

macrophage or monocyte—Type of white blood cell that can ingest and destroy foreign material and initiate the acquired immune response.

macular degeneration—A chronic eye disease that causes blurred vision or a blind spot in your visual field. It is generally caused by abnormal blood vessels that leak fluid or blood into the macula which is the part of the retina responsible for central vision.

maltodextrin—A glucose polymer (commonly containing 6 to 12 glucose molecules) that exerts lesser osmotic effects compared with glucose and is used in a variety of sports drinks as the main source of carbohydrate.

maltose—A disaccharide that yields two molecules of glucose upon hydrolysis.

marasmus—A protein deficiency resulting from a total dietary energy deficiency, characterized by extreme muscle wasting.

medium-chain fatty acid (MCFA)—A fatty acid with 8 to 10 carbon atoms.

megadose—An excessive amount of a substance in comparison to a normal dose (such as the RDA). Usually used to refer to vitamin supplements.

melanoma—A malignant type of cancer that develops from the pigment-containing cells known as melanocytes. Melanomas typically occur in the skin, but may rarely occur in the mouth, intestines, or eye.

meta-analysis—A type of study or report that uses a statistical approach to combine the results from multiple studies in an effort to increase power (over individual studies), improve estimates of the size of the effect and/or is used to resolve uncertainty when reports disagree.

metabolic syndrome—The co-occurrence of several known cardiovascular disease risk factors, including insulin resistance, obesity, high blood cholesterol and high blood pressure (hypertension).

metabolizable energy—The net energy remaining of ingested food energy after fecal and urinary energy losses are subtracted from the chemical energy of the food. The metabolizable energy represents the energy available for growth or reproduction and for supporting metabolic processes such as work (locomotion), biosynthesis, thermoregulation, maintenance metabolism, etc.

metalloenzyme—An enzyme that needs a mineral component (e.g., copper, iron, magnesium, or zinc) to function effectively.

methyl group—CH_3 group.

microbiota—The population of micro-organisms that are found in a particular environment or location such those that occupy the gut or the skin.

micromineral—Dietary elements essential to life processes that each make up less than 0.01% of total-body mass and are needed in quantities of less than 100 mg a day. Among the 14 microminerals (also known as trace elements) are iron, zinc, copper, chromium, and selenium.

micronutrients—Organic vitamins and inorganic minerals that must be consumed in relatively small amounts in the diet to maintain health.

millimole—One thousandth of a mole which is the amount of a chemical compound whose mass in grams is equivalent to its molecular weight, which is the sum of the atomic weights of its constituent atoms.

mineral—An inorganic element found in nature though the term is usually reserved for those elements that are solid. In nutrition, the term mineral is usually used to classify dietary elements essential to life processes. Examples are calcium and iron.

mitochondrion—Oval or spherical organelle containing the enzymes of the tricarboxylic acid cycle and electron-transport chain. Site of oxidative phosphorylation (resynthesis of ATP involving the use of oxygen).

mitochondrial biogenesis—The process by which cells increase their numbers of mitochondria to increase the capacity for aerobic ATP production.

mol (molar)—Unit of concentration (nmol: nanomolar = 10^{-9} mol; mmol: micromolar = 10^{-6} mol; mmol: millimolar = 10^{-3} mol).

mole—The amount of a chemical compound whose mass in grams is equivalent to its molecular weight, which is the sum of the atomic weights of its constituent atoms.

molecular epidemiology studies—The patterns and causes of disease in defined populations.

molecule—An aggregation of at least two atoms of the same or different elements held together by special forces (covalent bonds) and having a precise chemical formula (e.g., O_2, H_2O, $C_6H_{12}O_6$).

monoglyceride—Glycerol molecule linked to one fatty acid.

monosaccharide—A simple sugar that cannot be hydrolyzed to smaller units (e.g., glucose, fructose, and galactose).

monounsaturated fatty acid—Fatty acids that have one double bond in the fatty acid hydrocarbon chain with all of the remainder carbon atoms being single-bonded.

morbidity—The condition of being ill, diseased, or unhealthy. One morbidity may lead to another morbidity (e.g., having type 2 diabetes may lead to the development of cardiovascular disease).

mortality—The condition of being dead. You usually hear of mortality in terms of the number of deaths in a population over time, either in general (e.g., all-cause mortality) or due to a specific cause.

myoglobin—A protein in muscle that functions as an intracellular respiratory pigment that is capable of binding oxygen and releasing it only at very low partial pressures.

MyPlate—The current nutrition guide published by the USDA Center for Nutrition Policy and Promotion, a food circle (i.e., a pie chart) depicting a place setting with a plate and glass divided into five food groups.

MyPyramid—From 2005 to 2011 it was the American food guide pyramid produced by the USDA Center for Nutrition Policy and Promotion. In June 2011 it was replaced by the USDA's MyPlate.

neurotransmitters—Signaling molecules that transfer information from one nerve ending to the next (e.g., acetyl choline, dopamine, serotonin).

nitrate—A small molecule (NO_{-3}) that is naturally abundant in beetroot and rhubarb. It is used by athletes (usually in the form of concentrated beetroot juice) to improve endurance performance as it reduces the oxygen cost of exercise. It can also lower resting blood pressure so can be used as a remedy to treat mild hypertension.

non–insulin-dependent diabetes mellitus (NIDDM)—Also known as type 2 diabetes.

nonessential amino acids—Amino acids that can be synthesized in the body.

nonnutritive sweetener—A substance that can enhance the flavor and/or texture of food or beverages but are very low in calories or contain no calories at all.

nutrient—Substances found in food that provide energy or promote growth and repair of tissues.

nutrient density—Amount of essential nutrients expressed per unit of energy in the food.

nutrient reference value (NRV)—A replacement term for the recommended daily allowance (RDA). The NRVs provide recommended intakes for energy, protein, carbohydrate, fiber, fats, vitamins, minerals and other nutrients based on age, sex and life stages.

nutrition—The total of the processes of ingestion, digestion, absorption, and metabolism of food and the subsequent assimilation of nutrient materials into the tissues. Also used as a general term meaning the food and beverages that we consume.

obesity—An excessive accumulation of body fat. The term obesity is usually reserved for people who are 20% or more above the average weight for their size or have a BMI of 30 kg/m^2 or more.

oleic acid—A monounsaturated fatty acid that is the most widely distributed and abundant fatty acid in nature; it contains 18 carbon atoms.

oligosaccharide—A short chain carbohydrate polymer consisting of up to 10 monosaccharides (simple sugars) linked together by glycosidic bonds.

optimal health—Not just the absence of illness or disease but the best your health can be and a state which is associated with reduced risk of developing chronic disease.

osteoarthritis—The most common form of arthritis. It occurs when the protective cartilage on the ends of your bones wears down over time. Although osteoarthritis can damage any joint in your body, the disorder most commonly affects joints in your hands, knees, hips, and spine.

osteoporosis—A weakening of the bone structure that occurs when the rate of demineralization exceeds the rate of bone formation.

palatability—Pleasure provided by foods or fluids that are agreeable to the palate (sensed by taste buds on the tongue), which often varies relative to the homeostatic satisfaction of nutritional, water, or energy needs.

Paleo diet—A dietary plan based on foods similar to what might have been eaten during the Paleolithic era, which dates from approximately 2.5 million to 10,000 years ago. A Paleo diet typically includes lean meats, fish, fruits, vegetables, nuts, and seeds – foods that in the past could be obtained by hunting and gathering. A Paleo diet avoids or limits foods that became common when farming emerged about 10,000 years ago such as dairy products, legumes, and grains.

palmitic acid—The most common saturated fatty acid found in animals and plants; it contains 16 carbon atoms.

pancreas—An organ located below and behind the stomach. It secretes insulin and glucagon (involved in plasma glucose regulation) and pancreatic enzymes involved in the digestion of fats and protein in the small intestine.

pathogen—Microorganism that can cause symptoms of disease. A pathogen can be a bacterium or a virus.

peptide—Small compound formed by the bonding of two or more amino acids. Larger chains of linked amino acids are called polypeptides or proteins.

peptide bond—The bond formed by the condensation of the amino group and the carboxyl group of a pair of amino acids. Peptides are constructed from a linear array of amino acids joined together by a series of peptide bonds.

peripheral vascular disease—A disease of blood vessels outside the heart. Peripheral vascular disease affects the arteries or veins of the peripheral circulation, as opposed to the cardiac circulation.

phospholipids—Fats containing a phosphate group that on hydrolysis yield fatty acids, glycerol, and a nitrogenous compound. Lecithin is an example. Phospholipids are important components of membranes.

phytonutrients—Certain organic components of plants that are thought to promote human health but are non-nutrients. They differ from vitamins because they are not considered an essential nutrient, meaning that without them, people will not develop a nutritional deficiency. Examples include the carotenoids, flavonoids and coumarins.

plasma—The liquid portion of the blood in which the blood cells are suspended. Typically accounts for 55% to 60% of the total blood volume. Differs from serum in that it contains fibrinogen, the clot-forming protein.

pneumonia—A severe respiratory illness caused by bacterial or viral infection, in which the lungs become inflamed and the air sacs fill with pus making breathing difficult. A potentially fatal condition if not treated quickly.

polypeptide—A peptide that, upon hydrolysis, yields more than two amino acids.

polyphenols—A large class of naturally occurring compounds that includes the flavonoids, flavonols, flavonones, and anthocyanidins. These compounds contain a number of phenolic hydroxyl (-OH) groups attached to ring structures, which confers them with powerful antioxidant activity.

polysaccharide—Polymers of (arbitrarily) more than about 10 monosaccharide residues linked together by glycosidic bonds in branched or unbranched chains. Examples include starch and glycogen.

polyunsaturated fatty acid (PUFA)—Fatty acid that contains more than one carbon–carbon double bond in the hydrocarbon chain.

power—Work performed per unit of time.

pre-clampsia—A condition that affects some pregnant women, usually during the second half of pregnancy (from around 20 weeks) or soon after their baby is delivered. Early signs are developing high blood pressure (hypertension) and protein in the urine (proteinuria). In some cases, further symptoms can occur, including swelling of the feet, ankles, face and hands, severe headache, vision problems and pain just below the ribs. Although many cases are mild, the condition can lead to serious complications for both mother and baby if it's not monitored and treated.

probiotic—A supplement usually derived from dairy foods or a dietary supplement containing live bacteria that replace or add to the beneficial bacteria normally present in the gut.

prospective cohort study—A longitudinal study that follows over time a group of similar individuals (known as a cohort), who differ with respect to certain factors under investigation (e.g., their daily fruit intake), to determine how these factors affect rates of a certain outcome (e.g., cancer).

protein—Biological macromolecules composed of a chain of covalently linked amino acids. Proteins may have structural or functional roles (e.g., as enzymes, receptors and membrane transporters).

recommended dietary allowance (RDA)—Recommended intake of a particular nutrient that meets the needs of nearly all (97%) healthy individuals of similar age and gender. The RDAs are established by the Food and Nutrition Boards of the National Academy of Sciences.

reference daily intake (RDI)—Nutrient intake standards set by the FDA based on the 1968 RDA for various vitamins and minerals. RDIs have been set for infants, toddlers, people over four years of age, and pregnant and lactating women.

reference intake—The UK equivalent to the daily value (DV) shown on North American food packaging. Reference intakes are useful guidelines on the amount of energy and nutrients you need for a healthy balanced diet each day. The %RI tells you how much of your daily healthy maximum is in the portion of the product and is based on the following values: 2,000 kcal energy, 70 g fat, 20 g saturated fat, 90 g sugars, and 6 g salt (or 2.4 g sodium).

reference nutrient intake (RNI)—Defined as the level of intake required to meet the known nutritional needs of more than 97.5% of healthy persons. In the United Kingdom the RNI is similar to the original RDA.

resistance exercise—Exercise in which a muscle contraction is opposed by force. The resistance is often applied by using weights. Regular resistance exercise results in increased muscle size, strength, and power.

resting energy expenditure (REE)—Energy expenditure under resting conditions. The REE includes the resting metabolic rate plus the small (10-30%) transient increases in energy expenditure that occur following feeding.

resting metabolic rate (RMR)— The energy required for the maintenance of normal body functions and homeostasis in resting conditions. The RMR is the largest component of daily energy expenditure in a relatively inactive person.

saccharide—Generic name for sugars including monosaccharides such as glucose and disaccharides such as sucrose.

saccharin—An artificial sweetener made from coal tar.

salt—Sodium chloride: a white crystalline substance which gives seawater its characteristic taste and is used for seasoning or preserving food. In chemistry a salt is any chemical compound formed from the reaction of an acid with a base, with all or part of the hydrogen of the acid replaced by a metal or other cation.

sarcopenia—Loss of muscle mass that occurs with aging.

satiety—Sensation of fullness and satisfaction following eating that inhibits further desire to consume food.

saturated fat—A type of fat containing a high proportion of fatty acid molecules with only single bonds and no double bonds; it is considered to be less healthy in the diet than unsaturated fat.

scurvy—A disease caused by a lack of vitamin C. The typical characteristics of the condition are general weakness, anemia, gum disease, and dry, scaly, and bruised skin.

serotonin—A brain neurotransmitter. Also known as 5-hydroxytryptamine (5-HT).

short-chain fatty acid (SCFA)—A fatty acid containing six or fewer carbon atoms. Produced by bacteria in the gut from the fermentation of undigested food.

sleep efficiency—A measure of sleep quality, it is the ratio of the total time spent asleep (total sleep time) in a night compared to the total amount of time spent in bed.

sodium—A silvery-white chemical element (symbol Na) which combines with other chemicals. Salt is a sodium compound in which the sodium is combined with chlorine (Cl) to form sodium chloride (NaCl).

soluble fiber—Fiber that dissolves well in water.

solvent—A liquid medium in which particles can dissolve.

squamous cell skin cancer—A cancer of the keratinocyte cells in the outer layer of the skin. It is the second most common type of skin cancer in the UK. Most people treated for it are completely cured with simple treatment.

starch—A carbohydrate made of multiple units of glucose attached together by bonds that can be broken down by human digestion processes. Starch is also known as a complex carbohydrate.

steroid—A complex molecule derived from the lipid cholesterol containing four interlocking carbon rings.

sucrose—A disaccharide consisting of a combination of glucose and fructose; table sugar from cane or beet.

sugar—Any of the class of soluble, crystalline, typically sweet-tasting carbohydrates found in plant and animal tissues and exemplified by glucose and sucrose.

sugar-sweetened beverage—A drink that contains added sugars for sweetness and energy.

superfood—This term is actually a marketing term for food with supposed health benefits as a means to sell more products. Scientists do not use the term and nutritionally speaking, there is no such thing as a superfood.

Systeme Internationale (SI)—International Unit System, a worldwide uniform system of metric units.

systolic—Indicating the maximum arterial pressure during contraction of the left ventricle of the heart.

thermic effect of exercise (TEE)—The energy required for exercise. Increased muscle contraction increases energy expenditure and heat production due to the inefficiency of energy transformations.

thermic effect of food (TEF)— The increased energy expenditure following feeding that is due to the energy needed for the digestion, assimilation, and metabolism of food after it is consumed (also referred to as diet-induced thermogenesis).

thermogenesis—The production of heat. Metabolic processes in the body generate heat constantly.

time-restricted feeding—A daily eating pattern in which all your food is eaten within an 8- to 12hour timeframe every day, with no deliberate attempt to alter nutrient quality or quantity.

tinnitus—The term for hearing sounds that come from inside your body, rather than from an outside source. It is often described as "ringing in the ears", although several sounds can be heard, including buzzing, humming, whistling, and hissing.

tissue—An organized association of similar cells that perform a common function (e.g., muscle tissue).

toxoplasmosis—An infection caused by a single-celled parasite named *Toxoplasma gondii* that may invade tissues and damage the brain, especially of the fetus and newborn.

trace element—Dietary elements essential to life processes that each make up less than 0.01% of total-body mass and are needed in quantities of less than 100 mg a day. Among the 14 trace elements (also known as microminerals) are iron, zinc, copper, chromium, manganese, molybdenum, and selenium.

trans—A prefix indicating that geometrical isomer in which like groups are on opposite sides of a double bond with restricted rotation.

***trans* fatty acids**—Unsaturated fatty acids that contain at least one double bond in the *trans* configuration.

transit time—The time that food stays in the gastrointestinal tract.

triacylglycerol—The storage form of fat composed of three fatty acid molecules linked to a three-carbon glycerol molecule. Also known as triglyceride.

tricarboxylic acid (TCA) cycle—A series of reactions that are important in energy metabolism and take place in the mitochondrion. Also known as the Krebs cycle (after Hans Adolf Krebs, who first described the reactions involved) or the citric acid cycle, because citrate is one of the key intermediates in the process.

triglyceride—The storage form of fat composed of three fatty acid molecules linked to a three-carbon glycerol molecule. Also known as triacylglycerol.

type 1 diabetes mellitus—Insulin-dependent diabetes mellitus. A chronic condition in which the pancreas produces little or no insulin. Usually a consequence of an autoimmune destruction of the β cells in the pancreas at an early age.

type 1 fibers—Small-diameter muscle cells that contain relatively slow-acting myosin ATPases and hence contract slowly. Their red color is caused by the presence of myoglobin. These fibers possess a high capacity for oxidative metabolism, are extremely fatigue resistant, and are specialized for the performance of repeated contractions over prolonged periods.

type 2 diabetes mellitus—Non-insulin-dependent diabetes mellitus. Usually a consequence of being overweight or obese and not doing enough regular exercise. Prevalence increases with age.

type 2 fibers—Muscle cells that are much paler than type 1 fibers because they contain little myoglobin. They possess rapidly acting myosin ATPases, and so their contraction (and relaxation) time is relatively fast. A high activity of glycogen phosphorylase and glycolytic enzymes endows type 2 fibers with a high capacity for rapid (but relatively short-lived) ATP production.

unit of alcohol—One unit equals 10 milliliters or 8 grams of pure alcohol, which is the amount of alcohol the average adult can process in an hour. The number of units in a drink is based on the size of the drink, as well as its alcohol strength. For example, a pint of strong lager contains three units of alcohol, whereas the same volume of low-strength lager has just over two units. One glass of wine contains about 1.5 units.

unsaturated fatty acid (UFA)—Fatty acid (FA) containing at least one double bond within its hydrocarbon chain.

upper intake level (UL)—The highest level of daily nutrient intake likely not to pose a health problem.

upper respiratory tract infection (URTI)—Viral or bacterial infections of the throat and upper airways like colds and flu.

urea—End product of protein metabolism. Chemical formula: $CO(NH_2)_2$

urinary tract infection (UTI)—A bacterial infection of the urinary tract (i.e., the urethra and/or bladder).

urine—Fluid produced in the kidney and excreted from the body. Contains urea, ammonia, and other metabolic wastes.

vegan—Vegetarian who eats no animal products.

vegetarian—One whose food is of vegetable or plant origin. Some versions of the diet allow the consumption of dairy products (e.g., milk, cheese, yogurt) and/or eggs.

visceral fat—Body fat that is stored within the abdominal cavity and is therefore stored around a number of internal organs such as the intestines, liver and pancreas. It is commonly known as belly fat and is associated with increased risks of a number of health problems including type 2 diabetes.

vitamin—An organic substance necessary in small amounts for the normal metabolic functioning of the body. Must be present in the diet because the body cannot synthesize it (or an adequate amount of it).

waist-to-height ratio—The circumference around the waist in centimeters divided by the height in meters.

waist-to-hip ratio (WHR)—The circumference around the waist in centimeters divided by the circumference around the hips in centimeters.

water—The universal solvent of life (H_2O). The body is composed of 60% water.

watt (W)—Unit of power or work rate (J/s).

weight cycling—A cycle in which the considerable effort applied to achieve weight loss is exceeded by the effort required to maintain the new lower body weight. After the weight is lost, it is regained in a relatively short period. Also referred to as the yo-yo effect.

white blood cell—Important cells of the immune system that defend the body against invading microorganisms. Also known as a leukocyte.

yo-yo effect—See weight cycling.

Zone diet— The Zone Diet is about eating a certain balance of macronutrients to get in a "zone" for specific health benefits and to facilitate weight loss. To get into the zone you have to eat a specific ratio of 40% carbohydrate, 30% protein, and 30% fat. As part of the diet, carbohydrates should have a low glycemic index, protein should be lean, and fat should be mostly monounsaturated.

References

This is a list of reference sources I have used in putting together this book. You can find the journal articles on the PubMed website **(https://www.ncbi.nlm.nih.gov/pubmed)**. PubMed is a search engine that comprises more than 27 million papers and review articles for biomedical literature from Medline, life science journals, and online books. Just type in the title of the article or a few author surnames to bring up a 250-word abstract of the article; for many articles you can click on a link to get the full article. The other reference sources in the list below are books and websites where you will find helpful information on particular topics.

First, here are my top 10 recommended websites (in alphabetical order) for information relevant to general healthy living advice:

American College of Sports Medicine (ACSM). **https://www.acsm.org**

British Heart Foundation. **https://www.bhf.org.uk/**

Everyday Health. **https://www.everydayhealth.com/**

Harvard Health. **https://www.health.harvard.edu/topics/staying-healthy**

Mayo Clinic. **https://www.mayoclinic.org/**

My Fitness Pal. **https://www.myfitnesspal.com/**

National Health Service (NHS) UK 111. **https://www.111.nhs.uk/**

National Institutes of Health (NIH) USA. **https://www.nih.gov/**

Sport2Health. **https://www.sport2health.com/**

Web MD. **https://www.webmd.com/**

LIST OF REFERENCES

Abbott, Howard, Christin, et al. (1988). Short-term energy balance: Relationship with protein, carbohydrate and fat balances. *Am J Physiol 255* (3 Pt 1): E332-E337.

Achten, Gleeson and Jeukendrup. (2002). Determination of the exercise intensity that elicits maximal fat oxidation. *Med Sci Sports Exerc 34* (1): 92-97.

Achten, Venables and Jeukendrup. (2003). Fat oxidation rates are higher during running compared to cycling over a wide range of intensities. *Metabolism 52* (6): 747-752.

Action on Hearing Loss website. https://www.actiononhearingloss.org.uk/

Afshar, Richards, Mann, et al. (2015). Acute immunomodulatory effects of binge alcohol consumption. *Alcohol 49* (1): 57-64.

Age UK website. https://www.ageuk.org.uk/

Allergy UK website. https://www.allergyuk.org/

Alzheimer's Society website. https://www.alzheimers.org.uk/

American Alliance for Health, Physical Education, Recreation and Dance (AAHPERD) website. https://www.aahperd.org

American College of Obstetricians and Gynecologists website. https://www.acog.org/Patients

American College of Sports Medicine (ACSM) website. https://www.acsm.org

American College of Sports Medicine. (2007). Exercise and fluid replacement. *Med Sci Sports Exerc 39*: 377-390.

American College of Sports Medicine. (2015). Protein intake for optimal muscle maintenance. https://www.acsm.org/docs/default-source/brochures/protein-intake-for-optimal-muscle-maintenance.pdf

American Dietetic Association. (1997). Health implications of dietary fiber. Am Diet Assoc 97:1157-1160.

American Heart Association website. https://www.heart.org/

American Lung Association website. https://www.lung.org/

American Physiological Society website. https://www.the-aps.org

American Psychiatric Association. (2013). *Diagnostic and Statistical Manual of Mental Disorders.* 5th ed. Washington, DC: American Psychiatric Association.

Andersen. (1990). Diagnosis and treatment of males with eating disorders. In Andersen (Ed.), *Males With Eating Disorders*, pp. 133-162. New York: Brunner/Mazel.

Andersen. (1995). Eating disorders in males. In Brownell and Fairburn (Eds.), *Eating Disorders and Obesity: A Comprehensive Handbook*, pp. 177-192. London: Guildford Press.

Andrews, Balart and Bethea. (1998). *Sugarbusters.* London: Vermillion.

Anton, Hida, Heekin, et al. (2017). Effects of popular diets without specific calorie targets on weight loss outcomes: Systematic review of findings from clinical trials. *Nutrients 9* (8): E822.

Aranow. (2011). Vitamin D and the immune system. *J Invest Med 59*: 881-886.

Armbruster, Evans and Sherwood-Laughlin. (2018). *Fitness and Wellness*. Champaign, IL: Human Kinetics.

Asthma and Allergy Foundation of America website.www.aafa.org/

Atkins: Low Carb Diet Program and Weight Loss Plan website. https://www.atkins.com/

Atkins. (1992). *Doctor Atkins' New Diet Revolution*. New York: Avon Books.

Atkinson, Foster-Powell and Brand-Miller. (2008). International table of glycemic index and glycemic load values: 2008. *Diab Care 31* (12): 2281-2283.

Aune, Giovannucci, Boffetta, et al. (2017). Fruit and vegetable intake and the risk of cardiovascular disease, total cancer and all-cause mortality: A systematic review and dose-response meta-analysis of prospective studies. *Int J Epidemiol 46* (3): 1029-1056.

Australian Dietary Guidelines. (2015). https://www.eatforhealth.gov.au/guidelines/about-australian-dietary-guidelines.

Australian Food, Supplement and Nutrient (AUSNUT) Database. https://www.foodstandards.gov.au/science/monitoringnutrients/ausnut/foodnutrient/

Australian National Nutrient Database. https://www.foodstandards.gov.au/science/monitoringnutrients/ausnut/ausnutdatafiles/Pages/foodnutrient.aspx

Bachman, Deitrick and Hillman. (2016). Exercising in the fasted state reduced 24-hour energy intake in active male adults. *J Nutr Metab 2016*: 1984198, Epub.

Bailey, Winyard, Vanhatalo, et al. (2009). Dietary nitrate supplementation reduces the O2 cost of low-intensity exercise and enhances tolerance to high-intensity exercise in humans. *J Appl Physiol 107* (4): 1144-1155.

Ballor and Keesey. (1991). A meta-analysis of the factors affecting exercise-induced changes in body mass, fat mass and fat-free mass in males and females. *Int J Obes 15* (11): 717-726.

Barnosky, Hoddy, Unterman and Varady. (2014). Intermittent fasting vs daily calorie restriction for type 2 diabetes prevention: A review of human findings. *Transl Res 164* (4): 302-311.

Barrett. (2003). Medicinal properties of Echinacea: Critical review. *Phytomedicine 10*: 66-86.

Barrett, Brown, Locken, et al. (2002). Treatment of the common cold with unrefined Echinacea: A randomized, double-blind, placebo-controlled trial. *Ann Intern Med 137*: 939-946.

Baumgartner, Chumlea and Roche. (1990). Bioelectric impedance for body composition. *Exerc Sport Sci Rev 18*: 193-224.

Bell, McHugh, Stenenson and Howatson. (2014). The role of cherries in exercise and health. *Scand J Med Sci Sports 24* (3):477-490.

Bender and Bender. (1997). *Nutrition. A Reference Handbook*. Oxford: Oxford University Press.

Bendik , Friedel, Roos, et al. (2014). Vitamin D: A critical and essential micronutrient for human health. *Front Physiol 5*: 248.

Bennell, Matheson and Heevwisse. (1999). Risk factors for stress fractures. *Sports Med 28*: 91-122.

Bermon, Castell, Calder, et al. (2017). Consensus statement: Immunonutrition and exercise. *Exerc Immunol Rev 23*: 8-50.

Beumont (1995). The clinical presentation of anorexia and bulimia nervosa. In Brownell and Fairburn (Eds.), *Eating Disorders and Obesity: A Comprehensive Handbook*, pp. 151-158. London: Guildford Press.

Bischoff-Ferrari, Orav, Willett and Dawson-Hughes. (2014). The effect of vitamin D supplementation on skeletal, vascular, or cancer outcomes. *Lancet Diabetes Endocrinol 2* (5): 363-364.

Blaak. (2001). Gender differences in fat metabolism. *Curr Opin Clin Nutr Metab Care 4* (6): 499-502.

Blair, Kohl, Paffenbarger, et al. (1989). Physical fitness and all-cause mortality: a prospective study of healthy men and women. *J Am Med Assoc 262*: 2395-2401.

Bloomfield. (2001). *Optimizing bone health: Impact of nutrition, exercise and hormones. Sports Sci Exch #82 14* (3). https://www.gssiweb.com /en/sports-science-exchange/Article/sse-82-optimizing-bone-health-impact-of-nutrition-exercise-and-hormones.

Blot. (1997). Vitamin/mineral supplementation and cancer risk: International chemoprevention trials. *Proc Soc Exp Biol Med 261*: 291-296.

Blundell, Gibbons, Caudwell, et al. (2015). Appetite control and energy balance: impact of exercise. *Obes Rev Suppl 1*: 67-76.

Blundell, Stubbs, Hughes, et al. (2003). Cross talk between physical activity and appetite control: Does physical activity stimulate appetite? *Proc Nutr Soc 62* (3): 651-661.

Booth, Huggins, Wattanapenpaiboon and Nowson. (2015). Effect of increasing dietary calcium through supplements and dairy food on body weight and body composition: A meta-analysis of randomised controlled trials. *Br J Nutr 114* (7): 1013-1025.

Borchers, Selmi, Meyers, et al. (2009). Probiotics and immunity. *J Gastroenterol 44* (1): 26-46.

Bouchard. (1994). Genetics of obesity: Overview and research directions. In Bouchard (Ed.), *The Genetics of Obesity*, pp. 223-233. Boca Raton, FL: CRC Press.

Bouchard, Tremblay, Despres, et al. (1990). The response to long-term overfeeding in identical twins. N Engl J Med 322(21):1477-1482.

Bouchard, Tremblay, Després, et al. (1994). The response to exercise with constant energy intake in identical twins. *Obes Res 2* (5): 400-410.

Boutcher. (2011). High-intensity intermittent exercise and fat loss. *J Obesity* 2011: 868305, Epub.

Bradbury, Appleby and Key. (2014). Fruit, vegetable and fiber intake in relation to cancer risk: Findings from the European Prospective Investigation into Cancer and Nutrition (EPIC). *Am J Clin Nutr 100* (Suppl 1): 394S-398

Brilla and Landerholm. (1990). Effect of fish oil supplementation on serum lipids and aerobic fitness. *J Sports Med Phys Fitness 30*: 173-180.

British Association of Sport and Exercise Sciences (BASES) website. https://www.bases.org.uk

British Heart Foundation website. https://www.bhf.org.uk/

British Lung Foundation website. https://www.blf.org.uk/

British Society for Allergy and Clinical Immunology (BSACI) website. https://www.bsaci.org.uk

British Society for Immunology (BSI) website. https://www.immunology.org

Brouwer, Wanders and Katan. (2010). Effect of animal and industrial trans fatty acids on HDL and LDL cholesterol levels in humans: A quantitative review. *PLoS One 5* (3): e9434.

Brown and Gordon. (2003). Fungal beta-glucans and mammalian immunity. *Immunity 19*: 311-315.

Brutsaert, Hernandez-Cordero, Rivera, et al. (2003). Iron supplementation improves progressive fatigue resistance during dynamic knee extensor exercise in iron-depleted, nonanemic women. *Am J Clin Nutr 77*: 441-448.

Burgomaster, Howarth, Phillips, et al. (2008). Similar metabolic adaptations during exercise after low volume sprint interval and traditional endurance training in humans. *J Physiol 586* (1): 151-160.

Buscemi, Vandermeer, Hooton, et al. (2005). The efficacy and safety of exogenous melatonin for primary sleep disorders: A meta-analysis. *J Gen Intern Med 20* (12): 1151-1158.

Buttriss, Welch, Kearney and Lanham-New (Eds.). (2017). *Public Health Nutrition*, 2nd Edition. London: Wiley-Blackwell.

Byrne and Byrne. (1993). The effect of exercise on depression, anxiety and other mood states: A review. *J Psychosomatic Res 37*: 565-574.

Calder. (2006). N-3 polyunsaturated fatty acids, inflammation and inflammatory diseases. *Am J Clin Nutr 83*: 1505S-1519

Calle, Thun, Petrelli, et al. (1999). Body-mass index and mortality in a prospective cohort of US adults. *N Engl J Med 341* (15): 1097-1105.

Cancer Research UK website. https://www.cancerresearchuk.org/

Chan and Mantzoros. (2005). Role of leptin in energy-deprivation states: Normal human physiology and clinical implications for hypothalamic amenorrhea and anorexia nervosa. *Lancet 366* (9479): 74-85.

Centers for Disease Control and Prevention. (2013). Alcohol and Public Health: Alcohol-Related Disease Impact (ARDI). Average for United States 2006–2010 Alcohol-Attributable Deaths Due to Excessive Alcohol Use. Available at: https://www.nccd.cdc.gov/DPH_ARDI/Default/Report

Centers for Disease Control and Prevention. (2017). National Diabetes Statistics Report, 2017. Available at https://www.cdc.gov/diabetes/pdfs/data/statistics/national-diabetes-statistics-report.pdf

Cohen, Doyle, Alper, et al. (2009). Sleep habits and susceptibility to the common cold. *Arch Intern Med 169* (1): 62-67.

Cumming. (1996). Exercise-associated amenorrhoea, low bone density and oestradiol replacement therapy. *Arch Intern Med 156*: 2193-2195.

Curatolo and Robertson. (1983). The health consequences of caffeine. *Ann Intern Med 98* (5 Pt1): 641-653.

Davis, Murphy, McClellan, et al. (2008). Quercetin reduces susceptibility to influenza infection following stressful exercise. *Am J Physiol 295* (2): R505-R509.

de Castro. (1987). Macronutrient relationships with meal patterns and mood in the spontaneous feeding behavior of humans. *Physiol Behav 39* (5): 561-569.

de Castro and Elmore. (1988). Subjective hunger relationships with meal patterns in the spontaneous feeding behavior of humans: Evidence for a causal connection. *Physiol Behav 43* (2): 159-165.

de Koning, Malik, Kellogg, et al. (2012). Sweetened beverage consumption, incident coronary heart disease and biomarkers of risk in men. *Circulation 125*: 1735-1741.

Depaola, Faine and Pamer. (1999). Nutrition in relation to dental medicine. In Shils, Olson, Shike and Ross (Eds.). *Modern Nutrition in Health and Disease*, pp. 1099-1124. Baltimore: Williams and Wilkins.

Devries, Sithamparapillai, Brimble et al. 2018. Changes in kidney function do not differ between healthy adults consuming higher- compared with lower- or normal-protein diets: a systematic review and meta-analysis. *J Nutr 148* (11): 1760-1775.

Diabetes UK website. https://www.diabetes.co.uk/

Diaz, Krupka, Chang, et al. (2015). Fitbit®: An accurate and reliable device for wireless physical activity tracking. *Int J Cardiol 185*: 138-140.

Doherty and Smith. (2005). Effects of caffeine ingestion on rating of perceived exertion during and after exercise: A meta-analysis. *Scand J Med Sci Sports 15* (2): 69-78.

Dohm, Beeker, Israel and Tapscott. (1986). Metabolic responses after fasting. *J Appl Physiol 61* (4):1363-1368.

Douglas, Hemila, Chalker and Treacy. (2007). Vitamin C for preventing and treating the common cold. *Cochrane Database Syst Rev 18* (3): CD000980.

Dulloo and Jacquet. (1998). Adaptive reduction in basal metabolic rate in response to food deprivation in humans: A role for feedback signals from fat stores. *Am J Clin Nutr 68* (3): 599-606.

Durnin and Womersley. (1974). Body fat assessed from total body density and its estimation from skin fold thickness: Measurements on 481 men and women aged from 16 to 72 years. *Br J Nutr 32* (1): 77-97.

Edwards, Margaria and Dill. (1934). Metabolic rate, blood sugar and the utilization of carbohydrate. *Am J Physiol 108*: 203-209.

Eshak, Iso, Kokubo, et al. (2012). Soft drink intake in relation to incident ischemic heart disease, stroke and stroke subtypes in Japanese men and women: The Japan Public Health Centre–based study cohort *Am J Clin Nutr 96*: 1390-1397.

European Association of Allergy and Clinical Immunology (EAACI) website. https://www.eaaci.org

European College of Sports Science (ECSS) website. https://www.sport-science.org

Evenson, Goto and Furberg. (2015). Systematic review of the validity and reliability of consumer-wearable activity trackers. *Int J Behav Nutr Phys Act 12*: 159.

Everyday Health website. https://www.everydayhealth.com/

Fast Diet website. https://www.thefastdiet.co.uk/

Ferguson, Rowlands, Olds and Maher. (2015). The validity of consumer-level, activity monitors in healthy adults worn in free-living conditions: A cross-sectional study. I*nt J Behav Nutr Phys Act 12*: 42.

Ferreira and Behnke. (2011). A toast to health and performance! Beetroot juice lowers blood pressure and the O2 cost of exercise. *J Appl Physiol 110* (3): 585-586.

Field, Byers, Hunter, et al. (1999). Weight cycling, weight gain and risk of hypertension in women. *Am J Epidemiol 150* (6): 573-579.

Flatt. (1995). Use and storage of carbohydrate and fat. *Am J Clin Nutr 61*: 952S-959

Fogelholm, Koskinen and Laasko. (1993). Gradual and rapid weight loss: Effects on nutrition and performance in male athletes. *Med Sci Sports Exerc 25*: 371-377.

Fontani, Corradeschi, Felici, et al. (2005). Cognitive and physiological effects of Omega-3 polyunsaturated fatty acid supplementation in healthy subjects. *Eur J Clin Invest 35*: 691-699.

Food and Nutrition Board. (2005). *Dietary Reference Intakes for Energy, Carbohydrate, Fiber, Fat, Fatty Acids, Cholesterol, Protein and Amino Acids (Macronutrients)*. Washington, DC: National Academies Press.

Fung, Malik, Rexrode, et al. (2009). Sweetened beverage consumption and risk of coronary heart disease in women. *Am J Clin Nutr 89* (4): 1037-1042.

Galbo. (1983). *Hormonal and Metabolic Adaptation to Exercise.* New York: Verlag.

GBD 2016 Alcohol Collaborators. (2018). Alcohol use and burden for 195 countries and territories, 1990–2016: a systematic analysis for the Global Burden of Disease Study 2016. *Lancet 392* (10152): 1015-1035.

Gearhardt, Corbin and Brownell. (2009). Preliminary validation of the Yale Food Addiction Scale. *Appetite 52*: 430-436.

Gearhardt, White, Masheb, et al. (2012). An examination of the food addiction construct in obese patients with binge eating disorder. *Int J Eating Disorders 45*: 657-663.

Geleijnse, Launer, Van der Kuip, et al. (2002). Inverse association of tea and flavonoid intakes with incident myocardial infarction: The Rotterdam Study. *Am J Clin Nutr 75* (5): 880-886.

Gibala and McGee. (2008). Metabolic adaptations to short-term high-intensity interval training: A little pain for a lot of gain? *Exerc Sport Sci Rev 36* (2): 58-63.

Gibney, Macdonald and Roche (Eds.). (2008). *Nutrition and Metabolism* (the Nutrition Society textbook). Oxford: Blackwell Science.

Gibson. (1996). Are high-fat, high-sugar foods and diets conducive to obesity? *Int J Food Sci Nutr 47* (5): 405-415.

Gill and Panda. (2015). A smartphone app reveals erratic diurnal eating patterns in humans that can be modulated for health benefits. *Cell Metab 22*: 789-798.

Girgis, Clifton-Bligh, Turner, et al. (2014). Effects of vitamin D in skeletal muscle: Falls, strength, athletic performance and insulin sensitivity. *Clin Endocrinol 80*: 169-181.

Gleeson. (2013). Exercise, nutrition and immunity. In Calder and Yaqoob (Eds.), *Diet, Immunity and Inflammation*, pp. 652-685. Cambridge: Woodhead Publishing.

Gleeson. (2015). Effects of exercise on immune function. *Sports Sci Exch 28* (151): 1-6.

Gleeson. (2016). Immunological aspects of sport nutrition. *Immunol Cell Biol 94*: 117-123.

Gleeson, Bishop, Stensel, et al. (2011). The anti-inflammatory effects of exercise: Mechanisms and implications for the prevention and treatment of disease. *Nat Rev Immunol 11*: 607-615.

Gleeson, Bishop and Walsh. (Eds.). (2013). *Exercise Immunology*. Abingdon: Routledge.

Going, Massett, Hall, et al. (1993). Detection of small changes in body composition by dual-energy x-ray absorptiometry. *Am J Clin Nutr 57* (6): 845-850.

GoodtoKnow website. https://www.goodtoknow.co.uk

Graudal, Galloe and Garred. (1998). Effects of sodium restriction on blood pressure, renin, aldosterone, catecholamines, cholesterols and triglyceride: A meta-analysis. *JAMA 279* (17): 1383-1391.

Hall, Moore, Harper and Lynch. (2009). Global variability in fruit and vegetable consumption. *Am J Prev Med 36* (5): 402-409.

Hall, Bemis, Brychta, et al. (2015). Calorie for calorie, dietary fat restriction results in more body fat loss than carbohydrate restriction in people with obesity. *Cell Metab 22* (3): 427-436.

Hall, Chen, Guo, et al. (2016). Energy expenditure and body composition changes after an isocaloric ketogenic diet in overweight and obese men. *Am J Clin Nutr 104* (2): 324-333.

Hall and Guo. (2017). Obesity energetics: Body weight regulation and the effects of diet composition. *Gastroenterology 152* (7): 1718-1727.

Halson. (2013). Nutritional interventions to enhance sleep. *Sports Sci Exch 26* (116): 1-5.

Hamilton. (2010). Vitamin D and human skeletal muscle. *Scand J Med Sci Sports 20*: 182-190.

Hao, Lu, Dong, et al. (2011). Probiotics for preventing acute upper respiratory tract infections. *Cochrane Database Syst Rev* (September 7): CD006895.

Hargreaves. (1995). *Exercise Metabolism*. Champaign, IL: Human Kinetics.

Harper. (1999). Nutritional essentiality: Evolution of the concept. *Nutr Today 36*: 216-222.

Harvard Health website. https://www.health.harvard.edu/topics/staying-healthy

Haskell, Lee, Pate, et al. (2007). Physical activity and public health: Updated recommendation for adults from the American College of Sports Medicine and the American Heart Association. *Med Sci Sports Exerc 39*: 1423-1434.

Hausswirth, Louis, Aubry, et al. (2014). Evidence of disturbed sleep and increased illness in overreached endurance athletes. *Med Sci Sports Exerc 46* (5): 1036-1045.

Hawley, Burke, Phillips and Spriet (2011). Nutritional modulation of training-induced skeletal muscle adaptations. *J Appl Physiol 110*: 834-845.

He, Aw Yong, Walsh and Gleeson. (2016). Is there an optimal vitamin D status for immunity in athletes and military personnel? *Exerc Immunol Rev 22*: 42-64.

Health website. https://www.health.com/

Healthline website. https://www.healthline.com/

HelpGuide website. https://www.helpguide.org/articles/

Hemila. (2011). Zinc lozenges may shorten the duration of colds: A systematic review. *Open Resp Med J 5*: 51-58.

Henry, Lightowler, Stirk, et al. (2005). Glycaemic index and glycaemic load values of commercially available products in the UK. *Br J Nutr 94*: 922-930.

Hertog, Feskens, Hollman and Katan. (1993). Dietary antioxidant flavonoids and risk of coronary heart disease: The Zutphen elderly study. *Lancet 342*: 1007-1011.

Hickson. (2015). Nutritional interventions in sarcopenia: A critical review. *Proc Nutr Soc 74* (4): 378-386.

Hinton, Giordano, Brownlie and Haas. (2000). Iron supplementation improves endurance after training in iron-depleted, nonanemic women. *J Appl Physiol 88*: 1103-1111.

Holloszy and Coyle. (1984). Adaptations of skeletal muscle to endurance exercise and their metabolic consequences. *J Appl Physiol 56* (4): 831-838.

Hooper, Martin, Abdelhamid and Davey Smith. (2015). Reduction in saturated fat intake for cardiovascular disease. *Cochrane Database Syst Rev* (June 10): CD011737.

Hoppeler and Fluck. (2003). Plasticity of skeletal muscle mitochondria: Structure and function. *Med Sci Sports Exerc 35*: 95-104.

Howatson, Bell, Tallent, et al. (2012). Effect of tart cherry juice (Prunus cerasus) on melatonin levels and enhanced sleep quality. *Eur J Nutr 51* (8): 909-916.

Howell and Kones. (2017). "Calories in, calories out" and macronutrient intake: The hope, hype and science of calories. *Am J Physiol Endocrinol Metab 313* (5): E608-E612.

Hoy, Goldman and Sebastian (2016). Fruit and vegetable intake of US adults estimated by two methods: What We Eat in America, National Health and Nutrition Examination Survey 2009-2012. *Public Health Nutr 19* (14): 2508-2512.

Hoy and Goldman. (2014). Fiber Intake of the US Population: What We Eat in America, National Health and Nutrition Examination Survey 2009-2010. Food Surveys Research Group Dietary Data Brief No. 12. Available at https://www.ars.usda.gov/ARSUserFiles/80400530/pdf/DBrief/12_fiber_intake_0910.pdf

Hu, Huang, Wang, et al. (2014). Fruits and vegetables consumption and risk of stroke: A meta-analysis of prospective cohort studies. *Stroke 45* (6): 1613-1619.

Hubert, King and Blundell. (1998). Uncoupling the effects of energy expenditure and energy intake: Appetite response to short-term energy deficit induced by meal omission and physical activity. *Appetite 31*: 9-19.

Hultman. (1967). Physiological role of muscle glycogen in man, with special reference to exercise. *Circ Res 10*: I99-I114.

Hunt, Chakaravorty, Annan, et al. (1994). The clinical effects of vitamin C supplementation in elderly hospitalized with acute respiratory infections. *Int J Vit Nutr Res 64*: 202-207.

Hunt and Donald. (1954). The influence of volume on gastric emptying. *J Physiol 126*: 459-474.

Institute of Biology website. https://www.iob.org

International Federation of Sports Medicine (FIMS) website. https://www.fims.org

International Glycemic Index (GI) Database (Sydney University, Australia). https://www.researchdata.ands.org.au/international-glycemic-index-gi-database/11115 and https://www.glycemicindex.com/foodSearch.php

International Society of Exercise and Immunology (ISEI) website. https://www.isei.dk

Jackson and Pollock. (1978). Generalized equations for predicting body density of men. *Br J Nutr 40* (3): 497-504.

Jagetia and Aggarwal. (2007). "Spicing up" of the immune system by curcumin. *J Clin Immunol 27* (1): 19-35.

Jeffery, Hellerstedt, French and Baxter. (1995). A randomized trial of counseling for fat restriction versus calorie restriction in the treatment of obesity. *Int J Obes Relat Metab Disord 19* (2): 132-137.

Jeppesen and Kiens. (2012). Regulation and limitations to fatty acid oxidation during exercise. *J Physiol 590* (5): 1059-1068.

Jeukendrup. (2002). Regulation of skeletal muscle fat metabolism. *Ann N Y Acad Sci 967*: 217-35.

Jeukendrup and Gleeson. (2018). *Sport Nutrition.* 3rd ed. Champaign, IL: Human Kinetics.

Johnstone. (2007). Fasting—The ultimate diet? *Obesity Rev 8*: 211-222.

Jones, Cameron, Thatcher, et al. (2014). Effects of bovine colostrum supplementation on upper respiratory illness in active males. *Brain Behav Immun 39*: 194-203.

Kagan, Harris, Winkelstein, et al. (1974). Epidemiologic studies of coronary heart disease and stroke in Japanese men living in Japan, Hawaii and California: Demographic, physical, dietary and biochemical characteristics. *J Chronic Dis 27* (7-8): 345-364.

Kaiser, Shikany, Keating and Allison. (2013). Will reducing sugar sweetened beverage consumption reduce obesity? Evidence supporting conjecture is strong, but evidence when testing effect is weak. *Obes Rev 14*: 620-633.

Kandelman. (1997). Sugar, alternative sweeteners and meal frequency in relation to caries prevention: New perspectives. *Br J Nutr 77* (Suppl 1): S121-S128.

Keesey and Hirvonen. (1997). Body weight set-points: Determination and adjustment. *J Nutr 127* (9): 1875S-1883S

Keys, Menotti, Karvonen, et al. (1986). The diet and 15-year death rate in the seven countries study. *Am J Epidemiol 124* (6): 903-915.

King, Burley and Blundell. (1994). Exercise-induced suppression of appetite: Effects on food intake and implications for energy balance. *Eur J Clin Nutr 48* (10): 715-724.

King, Caudwell, Hopkins, et al. (2007). Metabolic and behavioral compensatory responses to exercise interventions: Barriers to weight loss. *Obesity (Silver Spring) 15* (6): 1373-1383.

Kit, Fakhouri, Park, et al. (2013). Trends in sugar-sweetened beverage consumption among youth and adults in the United States: 1999-2010. *Am J Clin Nutr 98* (1): 180-188.

Kivimaki, Luukkonen, Batty, et al. (2017). Body mass index and risk of dementia: Analysis of individual-level data from 1.3 million individuals. *Alzheimer's and Dementia* 1-9.

Knapik, Meredith, Jones, et al. (1988). Influence of fasting on carbohydrate and fat metabolism during rest and exercise in men. *J Appl Physiol 64* (5): 1923-1929.

Kohrt. (1995). Body composition by DXA: Tried and true? *Med Sci Sports Exerc 27* (10): 1349-1353.

Kopp-Hoolihan. (2001). Prophylactic and therapeutic uses of probiotics: A review. *J Am Diet Assoc 101*: 229-238.

Kumanyika and Cutler. (1997). Dietary sodium reduction: Is there cause for concern? *J Am Coll Nutr 16* (3): 192-203.

Laaksi. (2012). Vitamin D and respiratory infection in adults. *Proc Nutr Soc 71*: 90-97.

Laaksi, Ruohola, Mattila, et al. (2010). Vitamin D supplementation for the prevention of acute respiratory tract infection: A randomized, double-blinded trial among young Finnish men. *J Infect Dis 202*: 809-814.

Lanou and Barnard. (2008). Dairy and weight loss hypothesis: An evaluation of the clinical trials. *Nutr Rev 66* (5): 272-279.

Lansley, Winyard, Fulford, et al. (2011). Dietary nitrate supplementation reduces the O_2 cost of walking and running: A placebo-controlled study. *J Appl Physiol 110* (3): 591-600.

Larsen, Schiffer, Borniquel, et al. (2011). Dietary inorganic nitrate improves mitochondrial efficiency in humans. *Cell Metab 13* (2): 149-159.

Lassale, Batty, Baghdadli, et al. (2018). Healthy dietary indices and risk of depressive outcomes: a systematic review and meta-analysis of observational studies. *Mol Psychiatry doi*: 10.1038/s41380-018-0237-8. [Epub ahead of print – 26 September 2018].

Layman and Walker. (2006). Potential importance of leucine in treatment of obesity and the metabolic syndrome. *J Nutr 136* (1 Suppl): 319S-323S.

Lean, Leslie, Barnes, et al. (2018). Primary care-led weight management for remission of type 2 diabetes (DiRECT): an open-label, cluster-randomised trial. *Lancet 391* (10120): 541-551.

Ledikwe, Blanck, Kettel Khan, et al. (2006). Dietary energy density is associated with energy intake and weight status in US adults. *Am J Clin Nutr 83* (6): 1362-1368.

Leibel, Rosenbaum and Hirsch. (1995). Changes in energy expenditure resulting from altered body weight. *N Engl J Med 332* (10): 621-628.

Lichtenstein. (2014). Dietary trans fatty acids and cardiovascular disease risk: Past and present. *Curr Atheroscler Rep 16* (8): 433.

Lichtenstein, Ausman, Jalbert and Schaefer. (1999). Effects of different forms of dietary hydrogenated fats on serum lipoprotein cholesterol levels. *N Engl J Med 340* (25): 1933-1940.

Lin, Rexrode, Hu, et al. (2007). Dietary intakes of flavonols and flavones and coronary heart disease in US women. *Am J Epidemiol 165* (11): 1305-1313.

Linde, Barrett, Wolkart, et al. (2006). Echinacea for preventing and treating the common cold. *Cochrane Database Syst Rev* CD000530.

Liu, Liu, Huang, et al. (2017). Dietary total flavonoids intake and risk of mortality from all causes and cardiovascular disease in the general population: A systematic review and meta-analysis of cohort studies. *Mol Nutr Food Res 61* (6).

Longo and Panda. (2016). Fasting, circadian rhythms, and time-restricted feeding in healthy lifespan. *Cell Metab 23*: 1048–1059.

Macknin. (1999). Zinc lozenges for the common cold. *Cleveland Clin J Med 66*: 27-32.

Malik, Pan, Willett and Hu. (2013). Sugar-sweetened beverages and weight gain in children and adults: a systematic review and meta-analysis. *Am J Clin Nutr 98*: 1084-1102.

Malik, Schulze and Hu. (2006). Intake of sugar-sweetened beverages and weight gain: A systematic review. *Am J Clin Nutr 84*: 274-288.

Mann and Truswell. (2002). *Essentials of Human Nutrition*. Oxford: Oxford University Press.

Marshall. (2000). Zinc for the common cold. *Cochrane Database Syst Rev 2*: CD001364.

Martin, Heilbronn, de Jonge, et al. (2007). Effect of calorie restriction on resting metabolic rate and spontaneous physical activity. *Obesity (Silver Spring) 15* (12): 2964-2973.

Matthews, Ockene, Freedson, et al. (2002). Moderate to vigorous physical activity and the risk of upper-respiratory tract infection. *Med Sci Sports Exerc 34*: 1242-1248.

Matthews. (1999). Proteins and amino acids. In Shils, Olson, Shike and Ross (Eds.). *Modern Nutrition in Health and Disease*, pp. 11-30. Baltimore: Williams and Wilkins.

Maughan and Gleeson. (2010). *The Biochemical Basis of Sports Performance*. 2nd ed. Oxford: Oxford University Press.

Maughan, Gleeson and Greenhaff. (1997). *Biochemistry of Exercise and Training*. Oxford: Oxford University Press.

Mayo Clinic website. https://www.mayoclinic.org/

McMurray, Ben-Ezra, Forsythe and Smith. (1985). Responses of endurance-trained subjects to caloric deficits induced by diet or exercise. *Med Sci Sports Exerc 17* (5): 574-579.

Medical News Today website. https://www.medicalnewstoday.com/

MedicineNet website. https://www.medicinenet.com/

MedlinePlus website. https://www.medlineplus.gov/

Meeusen, Duclos, Foster, et al. (2013). Prevention, diagnosis and treatment of the overtraining syndrome: Joint consensus statement of the European College of Sport Science and the American College of Sports Medicine. *Med Sci Sports Exerc 45* (1): 186-205.

Melkani and Panda. (2017). Time-restricted feeding for prevention and treatment of cardiometabolic disorders. *J Physiol 595* (12): 3691-3700.

Meneton, Jeunemaitre, de Wardener and MacGregor. (2005). Links between dietary salt intake, renal salt handling, blood pressure and cardiovascular diseases. *Physiol Rev 85*: 679-715.

Mengheri. (2008). Health, probiotics and inflammation. *J Clin Gastroenterol 42* (2): S177-S178.

Mental Health Foundation website. https://www.mentalhealth.org.uk/

Michalska, Szejko, Jakubczyk and Wojnar. (2016). Nonspecific eating disorders: A subjective review. *Psychiatr Pol 50* (3): 497-507.

Mickleborough, Head and Lindley. (2011). Exercise-induced asthma: Nutritional management. *Curr Sports Med Rep 10* (4): 197-202.

Mikkelsen, Toubro and Astrup. (2000). Effect of fat-reduced diets on 24-h energy expenditure: Comparisons between animal protein, vegetable protein and carbohydrate. *Am J Clin Nutr 72* (5): 1135-1141.

Minocha. (2009). Probiotics for preventive health. *Nutr Clin Prac 24* (2): 227-241.

Mishell. (1993). Non-contraceptive benefits of oral contraceptives. *J Reprod Med 38*: 1021-1029.

Moore, Churchward-Venne, Witard, et al. (2015). Protein ingestion to stimulate myofibrillar protein synthesis requires greater relative protein intakes in healthy older versus younger men. *J Gerontol Ser A Biol Sci Med Sci 70*: 57-62.

Mosley. (2019). *The Fast 800. How To Combine Rapid Weight Loss And Intermittent Fasting For Long-Term Health.* Short Books: London, UK.

Mosley and Spencer. (2014). *The Fast Diet: Lose Weight, Stay Healthy, Live Longer.* New York: Atria Books.

Mursu, Voutilainen, Nurmi, et al. (2008). Flavonoid intake and the risk of ischaemic stroke and CVD mortality in middle-aged Finnish men: The Kuopio Ischaemic Heart Disease Risk Factor Study. *Br J Nutr 100* (4): 890-895.

My Fitness Pal website. https://www.myfitnesspal.com/

MySportScience website. https://www.mysportscience.com/

National Cancer Institute website. https://www.cancer.gov/

National Health Service (NHS) UK 111 Online website. https://www.111.nhs.uk/

National Health Service (NHS) UK Choices website. https://www.nhs.uk/

National Health Service (NHS) UK Weight loss plan. https://www.nhs.uk/live-well/healthy-weight/start-the-nhs-weight loss-plan/

National Institute for Health Care and Excellence UK website. https://www.nice.org.uk/

National Institutes of Diabetes and Digestive and Kidney Diseases (NIDDK) website.

https://www.niddk.nih.gov/

National Institutes of Health (NIH) USA website. https://www.nih.gov/

National Kidney Foundation website. https://www.kidney.org/

National Osteoporosis Foundation website. https://www.nof.org/patients/

National Sleep Foundation website. https://www.sleepfoundation.org/

Nieman. (1994). Exercise, infection and immunity. *Int J Sports Med 15* (Suppl 3): S131-S141.

Nieman, Henson, Austin and Sha. (2011). Upper respiratory tract infection is reduced in physically fit and active adults. *Br J Sports Med 45*: 987-992.

Nieman, Johansen, Lee and Arabatzis. (1990). Infectious episodes in runners before and after the Los Angeles Marathon. *J Sports Med Phys Fitness 30*: 316-328.

Nilsson and E Hultman. (1973). Liver glycogen in man; the effects of total starvation or a carbohydrate-poor diet followed by carbohydrate feeding. *Scand J Clin Lab Invest 32*: 325-330.

Nissen and Sharp. (2003). Effect of dietary supplements on lean mass and strength gains with resistance exercise: A meta-analysis. *J Appl Physiol 94* (2): 651-659.

Nitzke, Freeland-Graves and American Dietetic Association. (2007). Position of the American Dietetic Association: Total diet approach to communicating food and nutrition information. *J Am Dietetic Assoc 107* (7): 1224-32.

Noakes, Goodwin, Rayner, et al. (1985). Water intoxication: A possible complication during endurance exercise. *Med Sci Sports Exerc 17*: 370-375.

Noakes and Windt. (2017. Evidence that supports the prescription of low-carbohydrate high-fat diets: A narrative review. *Br J Sports Med 51* (2): 133-139.

Nutrition Society website. https://www.nutritionsociety.org

Olsen and Heitmann. (2009). Intake of calorically sweetened beverages and obesity. *Obes Rev 10*: 68-75.

Oral Health Foundation website. https://www.dentalhealth.org/

Paffenbarger, Hyde, Wing and Hsieh. (1986). Physical activity, all-cause mortality, and longevity of college alumni. *N Engl J Med 314*: 605-613.

Pannemans, Wagenmakers, Westerterp, et al. (1998). Effect of protein source and quantity on protein metabolism in elderly women. *Am J Clin Nutr 68* (6): 1228-1235.

Pedersen and Febbraio. (2008). Muscle as an endocrine organ: Focus on muscle-derived interleukin-6. *Physiol Rev 88*: 1379-1406.

Pendergast, Horvath, Leddy and Venkatraman. (1996). The role of dietary fat on performance, metabolism and health. *Am J Sports Med 24* (6): S53-S58.

Perry and Wang. (2012). Appetite regulation and weight control: The role of gut hormones. *Nutr Diabetes 2* (1): e26.

Perry, Heigenhauser, Bonen and Spriet. (2008). High-intensity aerobic interval training increases fat and carbohydrate metabolic capacities in human skeletal muscle. *Appl Physiol Nutr Metab 33* (6): 1112-1123.

Perusse and Bouchard. (2000). Gene-diet interactions in obesity. *Am J Clin Nutr 72* (5 Suppl): 1285S-1290

Phillips. (2011). The science of muscle hypertrophy: Making dietary protein count. *Proc Nutr Soc 70*: 100-103.

Phillips. (2015). Nutritional supplements in support of resistance exercise to counter age-related sarcopenia. *Adv Nutr 6* (4): 452-460.

Phinney, Horton, Sims, et al. (1980). Capacity for moderate exercise in obese subjects after adaptation to a hypocaloric, ketogenic diet. *J Clin Invest 66*: 1152-1161.

Physiological Society website. https://www.physoc.org

Polivy and Herman. (1995). Dieting and its relation to eating disorders. In Brownell and Fairburn (Eds.), *Eating Disorders and Obesity: A Comprehensive Handbook*, pp. 83-86. London: Guildford Press.

Poppitt and Prentice. (1996). Energy density and its role in the control of food intake: Evidence from metabolic and community studies. *Appetite 26* (2): 153-174.

Prietl, Treiber, Pieber and Amrein. (2013). Vitamin D and immune function. *Nutrients 5* (7): 2502-2521.

Public Health England. Composition of foods integrated dataset (CoFID). https://www.gov.uk/government/publications/composition-of-foods-integrated-dataset-cofid

PubMed website. https://www.ncbi.nlm.nih.gov/pubmed/

QuickStats. (2017). Percentage of total daily kilocalories consumed from sugar-sweetened beverages among children and adults, by sex and income level: National Health and Nutrition Examination Survey, United States, 2011-2014. *MMWR Morb Mortal Wkly Rep 66* (6): 181.

Rankinen, Perusse, Weisnagel, et al. (2002). The human obesity gene map: The 2001 update. *Obes Res 10* (3): 196-243.

Ren, Semenkovich, Gulve, et al. (1994). Exercise induces rapid increases in GLUT4 expression, glucose transport capacity and insulin-stimulated glycogen storage in muscle. *J Biol Chem 269* (20): 14396-14401.

Rennie. (2005). Body maintenance and repair: How food and exercise keep the musculoskeletal system in good shape. *Exp Physiol 90*: 427-436.

Rimm, Katan, Ascherio, et al. (1996). Relation between intake of flavonoids and risk for coronary heart disease in male health professionals. *Ann Intern Med 125* (5): 384-389.

Rippe and Angelopoulos. (2016). Sugars, obesity and cardiovascular disease: Results from recent randomized control trials. *Eur J Nutr 55* (Suppl 2): 45-53.

Ristow, Zarse, Oberbach, et al. (2009). Antioxidants prevent health-promoting effects of physical exercise in humans. *Proc Natl Acad Sci 106* (21): 8665-8670.

Robertson, Kato, Rhoads, et al. (1977). Epidemiologic studies of coronary heart disease and stroke in Japanese men living in Japan, Hawaii and California: Incidence of myocardial infarction and death from coronary heart disease. *Am J Cardiol 39* (2): 239-243.

Romeo, Warnberg, Nova, et al. (2007). Moderate alcohol consumption and the immune system. A review. *Br J Nutr 98* (1): S111-S116.

Ross, Manson, Abrams, et al. (2011). The 2011 report on dietary reference intakes for calcium and vitamin D from the Institute of Medicine: What clinicians need to know. *J Clin Endocrinol Metab 96*: 53-58.

Ross. (2000). Functional foods: The Food and Drug Administration perspective. *Am J Clin Nutr 71* (6 Suppl): 1735S-1738

Roxas and Jurenka. (2007). Colds and influenza: A review of diagnosis and conventional, botanical and nutritional considerations. *Alt Med Rev 12* (1): 25-48.

Royal National Institute of Blind People (RNIB) website. https://www.rnib.org.uk/

Rugg-Gunn. (2013). Dental caries: Strategies to control this preventable disease. *Acta Med Acad 42* (2): 117-130.

Scherr, Nieman, Schuster, et al. (2012). Nonalcoholic beer reduces inflammation and incidence of respiratory tract illness. *Med Sci Sports Exerc 44* (1): 18-26.

Schlundt, Hill, Pope-Cordle, et al. (1993). Randomized evaluation of a low-fat ad libitum carbohydrate diet for weight reduction. *Int J Obes Relat Metab Disord 17* (11): 623-629.

Schoenfeld, Aragon and Krieger. (2013). The effect of protein timing on muscle strength and hypertrophy: A meta-analysis. *J Int Soc Sports Nutr 10*: 53.

Schulte, Avena and Gearhardt. (2015). Which foods may be addictive? The roles of processing, fat content, and glycemic load. *PLoS One 10* (2): e0117959.

Schwellnus, Soligard, Alonso, et al. (2016). How much is too much? (Part 2) International Olympic Committee consensus statement on load in sport and risk of illness. *Br J Sports Med 50* (17): 1043-1052.

Sears. (1995). *The Zone: A Dietary Road Map.* New York: Harper Collins.

Seidelmann, Claggett, Cheng, et al. (2018). Dietary carbohydrate intake and mortality: a prospective cohort study and meta-analysis. *Lancet Public Health 3* (9): e419-e428.

SELF Nutrition Data website. https://www.nutrition data.self.com

Senate Select Committee on Nutrition and Human Needs. (1977). *Dietary Goals for the United States.* Washington, DC: US Government Printing Office.

Shan, Ma, Xie, et al. (2015). Sleep duration and risk of type 2 diabetes: a meta-analysis of prospective studies. *Diabetes Care 38* (3): 529-537.

Sheppard, Kristal and Kushi. (1991). Weight loss in women participating in a randomized trial of low-fat diets. *Am J Clin Nutr 54* (5): 821-828.

Shils, Olson, Shike, et al. (Eds.). (2005). *Modern Nutrition in Health and Disease.* Baltimore: Williams and Wilkins.

Silber and Schmitt. (2010). Effects of tryptophan loading on human cognition, mood and sleep. *Neurosci Biobehav Rev 34* (3): 387-407.

Skeaff and Miller. (2009). Dietary fat and coronary heart disease: Summary of evidence from prospective cohort and randomised controlled trials. *Ann Nutr Metab 55* (1-3): 173-201.

Slyper. (2013). The influence of carbohydrate quality on cardiovascular disease, the metabolic syndrome, type 2 diabetes and obesity: An overview. *J Pediatr Endocrinol Metab 26* (7-8): 617-629.

Snijders, Res, Smeets, et al. (2015). Protein ingestion before sleep increases muscle mass and strength gains during prolonged resistance-type exercise training in healthy young men. *J Nutr 145*: 1178-1784.

Snow-Harter. (1994). Bone health and prevention of osteoporosis in active and athletic women. *Clin Sport Med 13*: 389-404.

Sport2Health website. https://www.sport2health.com/

Somerville, Braakhuis and Hopkins. (2016). Effect of flavonoids on upper respiratory tract infections and immune function: A systematic review and meta-analysis. *Adv Nutr 7*: 488-497.

Stackpool, Porcari, Mikat, et al. (2014). The accuracy of various activity trackers in estimating steps taken and energy expenditure. *J Fitness Res 3*: 32-48.

Stubbs, Harbron and Prentice. (1996). Covert manipulation of the dietary fat to carbohydrate ratio of isoenergetically dense diets: Effect on food intake in feeding men ad libitum. *Int J Obes Relat Metab Disord 20* (7): 651-660.

Stubbs, Ritz, Coward and Prentice. (1995). Covert manipulation of the ratio of dietary fat to carbohydrate and energy density: Effect on food intake and energy balance in free-living men eating ad libitum. *Am J Clin Nutr 62* (2): 330-337.

Symons, Sheffield-Moore, Wolfe and Paddon-Jones. (2009). A moderate serving of high-quality protein maximally stimulates skeletal muscle protein synthesis in young and elderly subjects. *J Am Diet Assoc 109*: 1582-1586.

Tappy. (1996). Thermic effect of food and sympathetic nervous system activity in humans. *Reprod Nutr Dev 36* (4): 391-397.

Tappy and Lê. (2010). Metabolic effects of fructose and the worldwide increase in obesity. *Physiol Rev 90* (1): 23-46.

Tappy and Lê. (2015). Health effects of fructose and fructose-containing caloric sweeteners: Where do we stand 10 years after the initial whistle blowings? *Curr Diab Rep 15* (8): 54.

Te Morenga, Mallard and Mann. (2013). Dietary sugars and body weight: Systematic review and meta-analysis of randomized controlled trials and cohort studies. *BMJ 346*: e7492.

Temple, Bernard, Lipshultz, et al. (2017). The safety of ingested caffeine: A comprehensive review. *Front Psychiatry* (May 26): 80.

Thorning, Raben, Tholstrup, et al. (2016). Milk and dairy products: Good or bad for human health? An assessment of the totality of scientific evidence. *Food Nutr Res 60*: 32527.

Thorogood. (1996). Nutrition. In Lawrence, Neil, Mant and Fowler (Eds.), *Prevention of Cardiovascular Disease: An Evidence-based Approach*, pp. 54-66. Kings Lynn: Oxford University Press.

Threapleton, Greenwood, Evans, et al. (2013). Dietary fibre intake and risk of cardiovascular disease: Systematic review and meta-analysis. *BMJ 347*: f6879.

Tippett and Cleveland (Eds.). (1999). How current diets stack up: Comparison with dietary guidelines. *Agriculture Information Bulletin 750*: 51-70.

Tipton. (2013). Dietary strategies to attenuate muscle loss during recovery from injury. *Nestle Nutr Inst Workshop Ser 75*: 51-61.

Trapp, Chisholm, Freund and Boutcher. (2008). The effects of high-intensity intermittent exercise training on fat loss and fasting insulin levels of young women. *Int J Obesity 32* (4): 684-691.

Tudor-Locke, Han, Aguiar, et al. (2018). How fast is fast enough? Walking cadence (steps/min) as a practical estimate of intensity in adults: a narrative review. *Br J Sports Med 52*: 776–788.

UK Food Standards Agency. (2013). Food Hygiene: A Guide For Businesses. © Crown Copyright 2013. Available at https://www.food.gov.uk/business-industry/food-hygiene/

UK Food Standards Agency website. https://www.food.gov.uk/

UK Government Dietary Recommendations. (2016). Government dietary recommendations: The Eatwell Guide. https://www.gov.uk/government/publications/the-eatwell-guide

UK Food Standards Agency website. https://www.food.gov.uk/business-industry/food-hygiene.

UK National Diet and Nutrition Survey Rolling Programme for 2008/2009 to 2011/2012. (2014). https://www.gov.uk/government/collections/national-diet-and-nutrition-survey.

UK National Diet and Nutrition Survey Rolling Programme for 2012/2013 to 2013/2014. (2016). https://www.gov.uk/government/uploads/system/uploads/attachment_data/file/551352/NDNS_Y5_6_UK_Main_Text.pdf.

UK National Nutrient Database. Composition of foods integrated dataset (CoFID). https://www.gov.uk/government/publications/composition-of-foods-integrated-dataset-cofid

US Department of Agriculture. (2000). Dietary Guidelines for Americans, 2000. https://www.health.gov/dietaryguidelines/dga2000/document.

US Department of Agriculture. (2003). USDA national nutrient database for standard reference. https://www.nal.usda.gov/fnic/foodcomp/Data/index.html.

US Department of Agriculture. (2005). Dietary Guidelines for Americans, 2005. https://www.health.gov/dietaryguidelines.

US Department of Agriculture. (2015). 2015-2020 Dietary Guidelines for Americans. https://health.gov/dietaryguidelines/2015/guidelines.

US Department of Agriculture Food Composition and Branded Food Products Databases. https://www.ndb.nal.usda.gov/ndb/

US Food and Drug Administration Food Products Database. https://www.fda.gov/food/resourcesforyou/consumers/ucm274593.htm

US Food and Drug Administration website. https://www.fda.gov/Food/default.htm

van Vliet, Burd and van Loon. (2015). The skeletal muscle anabolic response to plant- versus animal-based protein consumption. *J Nutr 145* (9): 1981-1991.

Walsh, Gleeson, Pyne, et al. (2011). Position statement part two: Maintaining immune health. *Exerc Immunol Rev 17*: 64-103.

Walsh, Gleeson, Shephard, et al. (2011). Position statement part one: Immune function and exercise. *Exerc Immunol Rev 17*: 6-63.

Web MD website. https://www.webmd.com/

Weck, Bornstein and Blüher. (2012). Strategies for successful weight reduction: Focus on energy balance. *Dtsch Med Wochenschr 137*: 2223-2228.

Weigle, Breen, Matthys, et al. (2005). A high-protein diet induces sustained reductions in appetite, ad libitum caloric intake and body weight despite compensatory changes in diurnal plasma leptin and ghrelin concentrations. *Am J Clin Nutr 82* (1): 41-48.

Westerterp. (2013). Metabolic adaptations to over-and-underfeeding: Still a matter of debate? *Eur J Clin Nutr 67*: 443-445.

Westerterp, Donkers, Fredrix and Boekhoudt. (1995). Energy intake, physical activity and body weight: A simulation model. *Br J Nutr 73*: 337-347.

Weyers, Mazzetti, Love, et al. (2002). Comparison of methods for assessing body composition changes during weight loss. *Med Sci Sports Exerc 34* (3): 497-502.

What to expect website. https://www.whattoexpect.com/pregnancy/

WHO. (1996). *Trace Elements in Human Nutrition and Health.* Geneva: WHO Press.

WHO. (2015). *Guideline: Sugars Intake for Adults and Children.* Geneva: WHO Press.

WHO. (2015). Healthy Diet Factsheet. https://www.who.int/mediacentre/factsheets/fs394/en.

Willems, van den Heuvel, Schoemaker, et al. (2017). Diet and exercise: a match made in bone. *Curr Osteoporos Rep 15*: 555-563.

Willett. (2000). Diet and cancer. *Oncologist 5*: 393-404.

Women's Health website. https://www.womenshealthmag.co.uk/

Wynne, Stanley, McGowann and Bloom. (2005). Appetite control. *J Endocrinol 184*: 291-318.

Yin, Jin, Shan, et al. (2017). Relationship of sleep duration with all-cause mortality and cardiovascular events: a systematic review and dose-response meta-analysis of prospective cohort studies. *J Am Heart Assoc 6* (9): e005947.

Zeisel, Da Costa, Franklin, et al. (1991). Choline, an essential nutrient for humans. *FASEB J 5* (7): 2093-2098.

Zemel. (2004). Role of calcium and dairy products in energy partitioning and weight management. *Am J Clin Nutr 79* (5): 907S-912S.

Zemel, Richards, Mathis, et al. (2005). Dairy augmentation of total and central fat loss in obese subjects. *Int J Obes (Lond) 29* (4): 391-397.

Zemel, Shi, Greer, et al. (2000). Regulation of adiposity by dietary calcium. *FASEB J 14* (9): 1132-1138.

Zone Diet website. https://www.zonediet.com/the-zone-diet/

CREDITS

Cover and interior design:	Annika Naas
Cover photo:	© AdobeStock
Interior photos:	© AdobeStock, © Micheal Gleeson
Illustrations:	© Michael Gleeson, unless otherwise noted
Typesetting:	www.satzstudio-hilger.de
Managing editor:	Elizabeth Evans
Copyeditor:	Joshua Brazee

People Analytics

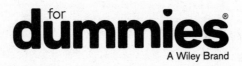

for dummies®

A Wiley Brand

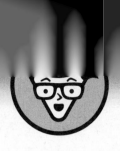

People Analytics

by Mike West

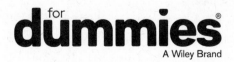

A Wiley Brand

People Analytics For Dummies®

Published by: **John Wiley & Sons, Inc.**, 111 River Street, Hoboken, NJ 07030-5774, www.wiley.com

Contents at a Glance

Table of Contents

Introduction

You might already be familiar with how the power of data analytics has transformed the fields of marketing, sales, supply chain management, or finance. You may also be familiar with the idea that people are a company's greatest investment. Well, like peanut butter and chocolate eventually found their way into a delicious treat, these two ideas found their way together, too — the happy result is called *people analytics.*

Welcome to *People Analytics For Dummies*, a book written for people open to the idea that there need not be any contradiction between what makes companies great places to work and great at producing business results. People analytics is built on the premise that what makes companies great is people, and that what can make more companies great when it comes to people is data analysis. Not any kind of analysis — specifically, the analysis of people at work.

In this book, you'll find an introduction to the data, metrics, and analysis at the basis of this new field called people analytics. Because it's a new field, this may be the first time you're hearing anything at all about it or, like most of the people doing the work today, you're figuring it out as you go along. In any case, even if you're familiar with people analytics already, this book may introduce you to new ways of approaching your work and may also provide you with some tips on how best to explain to others exactly what you do. (It never hurts to be able to express clearly and succinctly to others the importance of the work you do.)

About This Book

This is a book about making important management decisions about people by using data analysis rather than whim or instinct. This is a book about getting great business results while at the same time creating a great place for people to work. This is a book about finding a way to be a great company that relies on continuous feedback and learning rather than a mediocre company that's satisfied with either doing it the way it's always been done or that tries to keep up by slavishly copying the competition. This book is the recipe for getting the highest possible individual, team, and company performance while also making employees happier!

In *People Analytics For Dummies*, I talk about the ways that analysis can connect human resources decisions to business strategy as well as offering an overview of some of the nuts-and-bolts of how to do the analysis. You'll find out about gathering data about your employees at different stages of their careers, detecting patterns from the data, making predictions, and measuring the consequences of the actions you take. You'll find out how to use data to continuously improve the methods you use to attract, activate, and retain talented people so that you can achieve higher levels of productivity.

When I can, I include real-world examples from companies I have worked with — big and small — so that you can learn from the real world how to collect and analyze data in ways that can help you make better business decisions across a wide variety of human resources management topics: recruiting, performance, rewards, learning and development, leadership, diversity, and attrition. These examples show you the broad variety of opportunities for a smart application of people analytics.

Whether you're an executive, a human resources professional, or an analyst, you'll find something in this book for you.

Foolish Assumptions

To get the most from this book, I assume that you

>> Have worked for, are working for, or want to be working for a company large enough that establishing better decisions about how you manage people can add value

>> Are willing to let data help you make decisions about how you identify, select, pay, develop, and manage people

>> Are willing to try something different than what you have done in the past or than what other companies are doing

>> Are comfortable reading about business strategy, systems, science, and statistics

>> Have access to some people data or at least want to collect and analyze people data

>> Are looking, of course, for an accessible source that keeps it as simple as possible and provides practical advice about how to get started in the real world, as opposed to what you might find in an academic textbook or scientific journal

Icons Used in This Book

Throughout this book, you'll see these little graphical icons to identify useful paragraphs:

TIP

The Tip icon marks tips and shortcuts that you can take to make a specific task easier.

REMEMBER

The Remember icon marks the information that's especially important to know. To siphon off the most important information in each chapter, just skim these paragraphs.

TECHNICAL STUFF

The Technical Stuff icon marks information of a highly technical nature that you can safely skip over without harm.

WARNING

The Warning icon tells you to watch out! It marks important information that may save you headaches. Warning: Don't skip over these warnings!

How This Book is Organized

The book is arranged into five self-contained parts, each composed of several self-contained chapters. By *self-contained,* I mean that I do my best to tell you everything you need to know about a single topic inside each chapter. But I admit that more than a few times I had to put references to other parts of the book when it wasn't reasonably possible to cover in one chapter everything that's important to know.

The possibilities for adventure are truly endless, but start where you are right now. Whether you're an executive, HR professional, or analyst, you'll find something worth reading in *People Analytics For Dummies.*

Here is an overview:

Part 1: Getting Started with People Analytics

These early chapters serve as a primer on people analytics. In this part, you learn to walk before you run, but what you find here lays the foundation for all that comes later. You'll see my definition of people analytics and find an introduction to its important concepts, applications, and options. You may be especially pleased at the nontechnical nature of the first part. Not much bit-bytes or psychobabble is necessary because, as you see in Part 1, people analytics is about business first, people second, analysis third, and systems last.

Part 2: Elevating Your Perspective

It is unfortunate that most people think of analytics as something that is necessarily abstract, complex, or foreign to what they do. In the beginning of Part 2, you get to see how simply counting people up in different ways and looking at the results can help you gain new perspectives on things you do all the time. The fact is, the methods of people analytics need not be abstract, complex, or foreign — they can just be empirically valid ways of better doing what you always do.

If you read the entire part, you'll have learned some basic methods to get more perspective on how people produce value for businesses (or don't), have gained insight into why results vary, and have seen how, with careful attention to the right level of detail, you can focus your efforts to get value out of analytics faster. The absence of a business value orientation leads analytics into dead ends and trivial pursuits.

Part 3: Quantifying the Employee Journey

In this part, I define a universal measurement framework for human resources centered around two different but related concepts: the *employee journey* and something I call the *triple-A framework"*

>> **Employee journey:** I call the stages employees go through from the day they become aware of the job opportunity to the day they eventually exit the company the *employee journey*. Taking this holistic, long-term point of view implied by this term helps you see patterns you would not otherwise have seen had you organized your analysis in any other way. Also, seeing the company through the eyes of employees can help you see the world in a totally new and different way. Sounds clichéd, but it's true.

>> **Triple-A framework:** The employee perspective is important, but for obvious reasons it has to be paired with the needs of the business as well. The triple-A framework provides the fundamental measurements and analysis for the three big people-related problems each company needs to solve if they hope to grow as a business: attracting talent, activating talent, and controlling the rate of talent exit (attrition).

The combination of the employee journey and the triple-A framework can unify otherwise disparate and competing efforts by providing a single, unified measurement framework that relates employee and company needs with data.

After an introduction to the employee journey in Chapter 8, you'll find more detail on the methods of measurement and analysis in each of the three A's that follow: attraction (Chapter 9), activation (Chapter 10), and attrition (Chapter 11).

Part 4: Improving Your Game Plan with Science and Statistics

Analytics are all about using data to increase certainty. This is rooted in, at a minimum, math and science, but the analysis of people builds on the knowledge of diverse methods and caveats developed from hundreds of years of research in psychology, sociology, social psychology, and behavioral economics. Most of the current writing on people analytics is either so high-level as to not include any mention of how-to specifics or is pretty difficult to read if you don't already have an extensive background in systems, behavioral science, or statistics. I can't do justice to anything that is typically taught in a 6- to-8-year PhD program for the aforementioned topics, but I have carefully selected a few versatile tools that can get you started on your journey and that you can keep using for a lifetime of contributions.

Part 5: The Part of Tens

If you have ever read another book in the *For Dummies* series, this part of the book is like seeing an old friend again — the friend might be wearing a different outfit, but you will recognize the person right away. The Part of Tens is a collection of interesting people analytics learnings, advice, and warnings broken out into ten easy-to-digest chunks. There are ten misconceptions, ten pitfalls, ten design principles and the like. These chapters crystalize some concepts you get a chance to read in the rest of the book, or a way to get right to the concepts that matter if you haven't.

Beyond the Book

It used to be that a book started on the first page and ended on the last — not any more. The digital revolution has not just changed the way we buy books, it has also changed the way we write and read books. I have created a plethora of online resources that go together with this book to assist you on your people analytics journey. These items fit more readily on the World Wide Web than they do between the covers of the book (and in doing so saves a few trees in the process). Importantly, these resources can be updated, searched, shared, cut and paste from and downloaded as pdfs.

Two resources I am the most excited about sharing are the HR Metric Definitions Guide and a guide to great sample employee survey questions. At the current time, these are the most comprehensive mainstream sources for obtaining information in this format.

Extras: All *People Analytics For Dummies* online support resources are accessible for easy download at www.dummies.com/go/peopleanalyticsfd.

>> **HR Metric Definitions Guide:** Find hundreds of HR metric definitions following a standard convention, organized by topic (Appendix A).

>> **Great Employee Survey Questions:** Find hundreds of great employee survey questions that follow a standard convention, organized by topic (Appendix B).

>> **Job Analysis:** Get started with the crucial task of job analysis (Appendix C).

>> **Competency Analysis:** Learn how to measure competencies with competence (Appendix D).

>> **Ten Things to Set You On the Right Path When You Analyze Attraction:** Here's a great Part of Tens we just couldn't get fit in the book. (Appendix E).

>> **Ten Counterintuitive but Unifying People Analytics Design Principles:** And the fun never stops! Yet another Part of Tens for your reading pleasure! (Appendix F).

Cheat Sheet: If you are looking for the traditional *For Dummies* Cheat Sheet, visit www.dummies.com and type **People Analytics For Dummies Cheat Sheet** in the Search box.

People analytics is a vast domain containing a lot to learn — human resource management, behavioral science, technology systems and statistics, for starters. Unfortunately, one book cannot do justice to all of these topics, but fortunately that's why there is more than one book in this world (and people to help write them).

Aside from an introduction to something you may not have known much about before, what I aim to do in this book is cover that area of knowledge necessary for a successful application of people analytics not already covered by other books. I provide a unique (if not sometimes strange) point of view about what *really* matters, honed over many years of practical experiences in the field. What I have to say often isn't what people thought they would find, but I have seen success and I have seen failure, and I stand by what I think is important enough to share in this format. If you are looking to obtain more depth in a specific technical domain, there are plenty of resources you can turn to in order to go deeper — not the least of which are other *For Dummies* books.

Other For Dummies books: You can use a number of related books to drill down into topics I could only briefly touch on in this book — for example, *Data Warehousing For Dummies* (by Thomas C. Hammergren), *Business Intelligence For Dummies* (by Swain Scheps), *SQL All-in-One For Dummies* (By Allen G. Taylor), *Python For Dummies* (by Stef and Aahz Maruch), *Predictive Analytics For Dummies* (by Anasse Bari, Mohamed Chaouchi, and Tommy Jung), *Data Science For Dummies* (by Lillian Pierson), *Business Statistics For Dummies* (by Alan Anderson), *R For Dummies* (by Andrie de Vries and Joris Meys), *Statistical Analysis with R For Dummies* (by Joseph Schmuller), *Social Psychology For Dummies* (by Daniel Richardson), *Excel Dashboards & Reports For Dummies* (by Michael Alexander), *Data Visualization For Dummies* (by Mico Yuk and Stephanie Diamond), *Tableau For Dummies* (by Molly Monsey and Paul Sochan), and *Agile Project Management For Dummies* (by Mark C. Layton and Steven J. Ostermiller), all published by Wiley. Any and all of these books can produce valuable knowledge, skills, and abilities that can be used to become a more effective leader, implementer, and consumer of people analytics.

Where to Go from Here

You don't need to read this book from cover to cover. You can, if that strategy appeals to you, but it's set up as a reference guide, so you can jump in wherever you need to. Looking for something in particular? Take a peek at the table of contents or index, find the section you need, and then flip to the page to resolve your problem.

1

Getting Started with People Analytics

Chapter **1**

Introducing People Analytics

A business consists of people who work on behalf of the company (employees) doing things for other people who don't work for the company (customers). Business decisions about people working for the company — who to hire, where to find them, what to pay them, what benefits to provide, whom to promote, and countless other decisions — have a substantial unseen impact on the company's capability to meet customer needs, bottom-line performance, and reputation.

Traditionally, the way the leaders of companies have made human resources-related decisions has been based on gut instinct, copying what other companies are doing, tradition, or compliance with government mandates.

Today, many business decisions are now being made with data. What customer segments to focus on, what product feature improvements to make, what projects to invest in, and where to put a new store are just a few of countless examples of important business decisions that are increasingly made with data. If you go into a board meeting or participate in an investor phone call, you will see that the most important parts of the discussion are all about a series of important numbers recorded in the balance sheet, what the company is seeing in other numbers that suggest actions that may impact the balance sheet, and whether or not previous actions that promised to impact the numbers in the balance sheet have actually done so. The conversation may drift from abstract to tangible and back to abstract again, but numbers serve the purpose of keeping the conversation anchored to what is real and to drive accountability for real results.

Fortunately, now you can use data for human resources-related decisions, too. Thanks to the prevalence of human resource information systems, plus the wide-scale accessibility of modern data collection, analysis, and presentation tools, human resources-related decisions can be made with data just like countless other business decisions.

In this chapter, I define the term *people analytics* and talk about some of the ways that companies I've worked with have used a human resource approach informed by data to solve real-life business problems. Then I describe how you also can add people analytics to your arsenal — and increase your people data savvy, too.

Defining People Analytics

At a high level, *people analytics* consists simply of applying evidence to manage-ment decisions about people.

More specifically people analytics lives at the intersection of statistics, behavioral science, technology systems, and the people strategy.

REMEMBER

People strategy means making deliberate choices among differing options for how to manage a group of people.

Figure 1-1 illustrates how people analytics joins together these four broad con-cepts (statistics, science, systems, and strategy) to create something new that didn't exist before.

Many forward-thinking companies are already realizing the benefits of evidence-based decision making in human resources. To identify what other people think people analytics is, I rounded up 100 job descriptions related to people analytics from job boards. To summarize, I created a word cloud from the words in those job descriptions; it appears in Figure 1-2.

If you're not already familiar with word clouds, this is how they work: The more frequently a word appears in the text that you're analyzing, the bigger and darker that word looks in the word cloud. You can tell from the figure that *data, analytics, human resources (HR),* and *business* must be central concepts to people analytics.

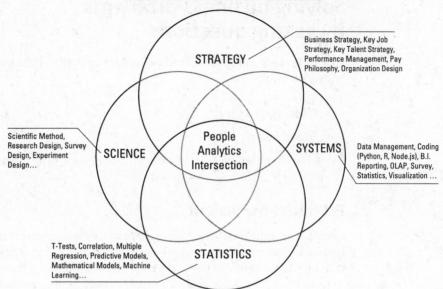

FOUR S PEOPLE ANALYTICS FRAMEWORK

STRATEGY

Business Strategy, Key Job Strategy, Key Talent Strategy, Performance Management, Pay Philosophy, Organization Design

Scientific Method, Research Design, Survey Design, Experiment Design…

SCIENCE

People Analytics Intersection

SYSTEMS

Data Management, Coding (Python, R, Node.js), B.I. Reporting, OLAP, Survey, Statistics, Visualization …

T-Tests, Correlation, Multiple Regression, Predictive Models, Mathematical Models, Machine Learning…

STATISTICS

FIGURE 1-1:
People analytics is what happens when human resources professionals realize the power that a good dataset gives them.

People Analytics Job Description Word Cloud

ability (715) advanced (290) analyses(215) analysis (811) analyst (340) analytics (1718) analyze (205) applications (215) areas (225) build (225) business (1589) capital (227) clients (228) communication (515) company (444) consulting (384) create (306) customers (259) data (1062) decision (292) degree (330) demonstrated (227) description (223) design (410) development (956) drive (223) effectively (386) employee (362) ensure (221) environment (232) excel (395) executive (273) experience (1132) functional (402) global (271) hr (1840) human (644) identify (279) implementation (234) improvement (261) including (547) information (414) initiatives (211) insights (263) internal (308) job (540) key (348) knowledge (373) lead (320) leaders (319) leadership (252) level (301) management (1514) metrics (476) modeling (307) needs (348) operations (310) opportunity (253) organization (397) organizational (312) partners (353) people (383) performance (460) planning (561) position (333) preferred (295) present (301) problem (216) processes (612) products (221) programs (346) project (655) provide (720) related (456) reporting (1272) required (733) research (467) resources (521) responsibilities (430) role (222) senior (242) service (339) skills (637) solutions (267) statistical (483) strategic (240) strategy (361) strong (417) successful (210) support (689) systems (466) talent (551) team (710) technology (227) tools (415) trends (253) understanding (271) work (961) workforce (836) years (488)

FIGURE 1-2:
Creating a word cloud is a kind of data analysis to identify and visualize trends in vocabulary.

These 100 job descriptions are from Human Resources department that are ahead of the pack in using hard data and analysis as decision-making tools. The insights data is providing these companies gives them an advantage over companies that do not yet know how to do these things. A vast majority of companies do not yet have people analytics and most people do not even know what people analytics is. That being the case, you, by learning about people analytics, will be in a great position to differentiate yourself among your peers (and your company among its competitors).

Solving business problems by asking questions

Like all business analysis disciplines, people analytics offers businesses ways to answer questions that:

>> Produce new insight

>> Solve problems

>> Evaluate the effectiveness of solutions and improve going forward

Produce new insight

Donald Rumsfeld once said, "*There are known knowns; there are things we know we know. We also know there are known unknowns; that is to say we know there are some things we do not know. But there are also unknown unknowns — the ones we don't know we don't know.*" Donald Rumsfeld can get his words a little twisted up, but to finish his point for him: the most perilous things in this world for you are the things you should know but don't know you should know. One of the great contributions people analytics can make to you is to reveal some of the perilous things you don't know and don't even know you should know but in fact should know.

This unknown unknowns' problem can be epitomized by an experience I had with a large pharmaceutical company. This company was very successful. It had an over hundred-year history of scientific achievement and business success. This company was a leader and financial powerhouse in its industry, if not all industries. They were a great company and they knew it.

With a smart, scientifically-oriented management team, the company tried to measure nearly everything. As a result, it was among some of the first companies to apply rigor to human resources with data. This is how I got stared in the field of people analytics before we even called it people analytics. After working at this company, I went on to do this work at other companies, but work in the people analytics field was few and far between back in the early days.

One of the earliest data-oriented human resource activities at this great pharmaceutical company was to participate in a common employee survey conducted across many companies, facilitated by a consulting firm that would provide confidentiality to everyone involved. This survey allowed the company to compare itself as an employer against a selection of the highest-performing companies across all industries across roughly 50 aspects of the employee experience using roughly 100 survey items. A few examples of the categories of employee experience the survey measured were: employee opinion about the company's prospects for future success, leadership, managers, pay, benefits, opportunities for learning and development as well as attitudes such as overall satisfaction, motivation, and commitment to the company.

In reviewing the results, it was no surprise to all that this well-run company performed above other high-performing companies in nearly all categories of the survey. Employees at this company were on average more committed, more motivated, and happier than employees at other companies and all of this could be validated statistically.

What was surprising to everyone was that the company performed slightly below other high-performing companies in a set of questions the survey referred to categorically as Speaking Up. The Speaking Up category represented agreement or disagreement with statements that indicated employees felt the company provided a safe environment for them to express their concerns or disagreements with their superiors. This finding seemed odd, because everyone talked about how the company had a history of making decisions by consensus. When young, intelligent scientists joined the company, they were told to be aware of the importance of consensus in the company's culture and should therefore expect to work together with others more than they might have had to do in previous environments.

Given the seeming oddness of the Speaking Up finding, and that the company had performed well on all other questions on the survey, no substantive new actions were decided. There was some concern expressed by the head of human resources about the Speaking Up items, but at the time there was an ongoing debate among the executive leadership team about whether or not the company should intentionally break its culture of consensus decision-making in order to keep up with new competitors. At the time, the assessment of the leadership team was that, overall, the survey results were good and the Speaking Up issue must have just been echoes of their effort to change the culture for the better.

No one at the time foresaw the connection between the survey findings and the disaster that would ensue next. Around that time, a previously successful but bull-headed research director had disregarded the concerns of some scientists about a possible safety issue with a drug. The safety issue was not crystal clear at that time, but the issue should have received more attention. The executive had a reputation for having a big ego, but he also delivered results for the company, so the company let him win this argument. Time and attention costs money. The scientists' concerns about the drug were squelched in favor of progress. The result of rushing ahead was a drug that later had to be recalled — a foolish mistake that risked lives, cost the company billions of dollars, and nearly took down the company for good. At the direction of the bullheaded director, the company pushed through a pharmaceutical product that should have been scrutinized further. Specifically, no scientists should have been made to feel unsafe to express their opinion and all credible concerns should have been researched more thoroughly before taking the drug to market.

What this example shows is that even simple early efforts in people analytics — a seemingly trivial employee survey — can deliver new insight that is not obvious or trivial. The result in this case may not be the best example of successful people analytics, but it illustrates the potential in ways that success wouldn't have. Unfortunately, at the time nobody knew that the weakness identified in the survey was so important. The survey produced an insight that blew in the opposite direction of what the executives believed and so the weakness that had been correctly identified was disregarded. Mysteriously, the employee survey had actually predicted the reason for the company's near demise — it was providing access to an unknown unknown. In short, the survey was warning us about something the company otherwise could not have known was important. Had the company taken the Speaking Up issue more seriously, executives could have put in place a way for the concerned scientists to express themselves so the bullheaded director could have been checked, preventing the giant mistake. Now I know how important it is to take even a basic employee survey effort very seriously, because you don't know what you don't know, but when you ask a lot of questions you have a flying chance of finding out what you don't know.

Solve problems

Data can also help you devise solutions to known problems.

A children's hospital knew that the attrition rate for nurses in their first year was 25 percent. This means that 1 in 4 nurses hired would leave the company in the first year they were employed by the company. In contrast, the average employee attrition rate was only 10 percent, meaning 1 in 10 people overall would leave the company in a given year. Therefore, early tenure nurse attrition was 2.5 times worse than average attrition. Even worse, early tenure attrition is a self-reinforcing problem, because if you change nothing there was a fairly high chance the replacement may also leave as quickly and around and around you go.

For good reasons, the hospital wanted to bring that early tenure nurse attrition rate down. Each nurse exit in the first year had to be replaced by another nurse that had to be identified, hired, onboarded, and trained. Of course, hiring and training new nurses' costs money, but, more importantly, new nurses are less familiar with how to deal with complex situations and more likely to make mistakes than experienced nurses.

Some analysis of applicant and employee history data showed that the hospital could hire nurses more likely to stay by simply hiring more experienced nurses, rather than nurses straight out of nursing school. Seems obvious to say now, but they didn't really know how much of a difference it would make for them operationally until they looked at the data. While more experienced hires have to be paid more, the data showed they were also more likely to be successful and they were more likely to stay with the children's hospital beyond their first year. By focusing on hiring the candidates with the characteristics that predicted longevity, the data showed the hospital could reduce the overall first-year attrition rate from 25 percent to 15 percent. The reduction in attrition on the cost of recruiting and training would more than offset the cost of spending more money to hire experienced nurses from the outset. As time went on, the attrition rate of nurses decreased, costs went down, and patient safety measures went up.

Evaluate solutions and plan to improve

You also can use data to evaluate the effectiveness of solutions on a small scale so you can make sure the solutions will actually work before implementing them more broadly. Experiments can provide a dataset that allows testing ideas in ways that prevent costly mistakes (facilitating improvement) before rolling out ideas more broadly.

A pet store chain had a history of keeping track of standard retail measures, like same store sales and customer satisfaction, as well as people-related measures, like employee enthusiasm and knowledge of pet-related topics. Measuring both kinds of data together helped the pet store chain uncover correlations between how it hired, trained, and rewarded employees in the stores and the goals it was trying to achieve: increased customer loyalty and increased store sales.

By looking at the employee and customer data together, the company knew many things that other companies could only dream of knowing. For example, the pet retailer knew that the more employees in the stores knew about a pet topic, the more the store would sell in that pet topic area. For example, if people in the store knew a lot about frogs, they would sell more frogs. If they knew less about birds, they sold less birds and bird-related supplies, and so on and so forth across every category of pet. If store employees had the knowledge necessary to capture the imagination of the customers as well as help the customer solve their pet problems, the customer would, over time, spend more money at the store. As a result of this information, the pet retailer consciously hired, trained, and rewarded employees in ways designed to increase employee knowledge about pet topics. The pet retailer also used test results to identify stores that needed training, measure the results of that training, and assess its impact on the bottom line.

Despite their best efforts, however, the pet store chain was seeing increased competition from big-box retailers, grocery stores, and online retailers, which made it difficult to grow revenue profitably. Big-box retailers, grocery stores, and online retailers were starting to stock many of the same items as the pet retailer and they could offer these items at a lower cost. If the pet retailer decided to compete on cost, it would put pressure on the profit margins of the pet retailer because the pet retailer didn't have other items they could mark up to make up for the losses in the items they marked down to compete. To make matters worse, this was in a period of economic downturn and increasing gas costs. Customers were condensing their shopping trips to as few store locations as possible and they were selecting the lowest-priced locations with the largest range of products. The bottom line is that less customers coming into the pet stores meant less sales.

The pet store needed to get a handle on its situation, and so it embarked on some new store-level experimentation and analysis. One of the experiments the pet retailer embarked on was to use some of the square footage available in some of the stores to offer pet services in addition to pets and pet supplies. Examples of pet services include: dog grooming, doggie daycare, dog training, and pet health clinics. The theory was that services would provide a reason to draw more people into the stores and, just as increasing pet knowledge increased sales, the pet retailer hoped that offering services would do the same. But no one really knew if this was true.

In the beginning, the services were not offered at all pet store locations. The expertise required to offer these services required new company training and the employees hired to perform these roles needed to be more skilled, which meant they also needed to be paid more. The company had to learn how to source, hire, train, and pay entirely new types of people for entirely new types of jobs than they were accustomed to in the past. Rolling this idea out to all stores — without a period of observation and learning — could bankrupt the company. By choosing a small number of stores to start with, the company could measure the impact of the changes, assess their performance, and assess what to do next. If the experiment with the new services was working, the services could be expanded to more stores — if not, then the service program could be modified or abandoned. If the company had implemented the services in all stores, then it would not be able to assess if they were working or not and it would be very risky.

The way to analyze data from an experiment of this nature is straightforward. The pet retailer chose a small set of stores to usher in the new pet services and chose another set of stores without the services to act as a comparison. With relatively simple math, the pet retailer was able to identify the impact of the services on customer store visits, sales, and loyalty using the same data and metrics they had already been using just by comparing locations to each other. The experiment validated that adding services in fact increased store visits, overall customer spending, and customer loyalty in the stores that offered services versus those stores that did not. It may seem obvious that when people went to the pet store to get Fido groomed that they also would be more likely to purchase other items. A less obvious finding was that those customers that got Fido groomed also spent more on Fido over the entire lifetime of Fido, not just at those visits when Fido and the pet parent were in the store together for the grooming. By offering services, the pet retailer was both attracting and creating better lifetime customers. The inevitable result is increased sales.

Through its analysis, the pet retailer was able to validate the fact that its investment in people to provide services was working. The stores where services were available produced more of the business outcomes the company was looking for and those stores that did not provide services did not. The solution for the company then became more certain — expand the program. Additional research questions included the mix of services to offer in the stores and how to scale the services to more stores with equal quality, but the company knew enough to proceed and could evaluate these more complex questions as they worked services into more stores in differing packages.

Further analysis of the store-level employee data over time indicating that the satisfaction and retention (reduction of attrition) of the new service employees in the store had more impact on customer loyalty and sales than that of other types of store employees — cashiers or stockers for example. Across all jobs, the more distinct pet-related knowledge for the job required, the more impact attrition in that job had on the pet retailer's success. With this information, the company prioritized how it allocated its people budget to reduce attrition in key jobs, as opposed to spreading their resources out thinly across all jobs, which might produce inferior results — or no results — while spending the same amount of money. The pet retailer learned that employee attrition matters more in certain key jobs and, since profit margins were thin, they had to prioritize where to spend their money to get the best results.

REMEMBER

Many people do not like to talk about differences in pay, but the reality is that there are always differences in pay based on many factors. Job responsibility is a valid criterion for differentiating pay. It is natural, in everyone's best interest, and generally agreed to be fair, for each company to focus its resources on the unique jobs and people that make it successful. Furthermore, any entry level store worker that wanted to learn a more lucrative service job had the opportunity to apply — and frequently they did. Having a ladder of jobs of increasing skill and pay made working for the pet retailer more of a long-term career opportunity to potential employees, rather than just a fun, short-term job fix. By adding higher-paying services roles, the pet retailer was able to make themselves more attractive to both the customers and employees it wanted to attract for the long term.

Using people data in business analysis

People are the face, heart, and hands of your company. All companies depend on people in every aspect of their business because people

>> Empathize with customers wants, pains, and problems

>> Create and improve products and services

>> Design, manage, and execute the strategies, systems, and processes that help everyone work together toward a productive enterprise

Considering how important people are to the performance of each company, it's amazing that more companies don't study employee data for insight into their businesses. Your company probably hires experts with advanced skills to analyze your finances, equipment, and workflows, so why isn't anyone studying the people who use these things?

Part of the reason is that, until recently, the pool of available employee data was pretty shallow. When companies had only physical file folders full of employee data stored in the file cabinet, the opportunities for deep, meaningful analysis were few. Over the past couple of decades, though, the amount of electronic data that companies keep (intentionally and unintentionally) about their employees has quietly been building.

Today, your company probably has a flood of electronic employee data, whether you realize it or not. You'll find some of this data in obvious places, but you might not have thought about the data available from some of the sources I list here:

>> Employee resource planning systems (ERP)

>> Human resources information systems (HRIS)

>> Payroll systems

>> Applicant tracking systems (ATS)

>> Learning management systems (LMS)

>> Performance management systems

>> Market pay benchmark surveys

>> Employee surveys

>> Email and calendar system data

>> Corporate intranet (internal websites) traffic data

>> Job boards

>> Social network comments

>> Government Census and Department of Labor data

The good news is that businesses do seem to know that their employees are their greatest asset. What businesses don't seem to know is how to analyze data about their employees to improve their business outcomes. In the chapters in this book, I demonstrate how you can do just that.

Applying statistics to people management

All managers think they're above average at making decisions, but at least half of them are wrong! I've just demonstrated the wide variety of data that human resources managers have available to them, but they need the right tools and methodologies to interpret and make decisions based on that data. If you misinterpret your data, the option that seems right can turn into a disaster for your company.

That's where statistics come in. You might think of statistics in terms of the procedures a statistician uses, like t-tests and regressions, but analyzing data with statistics isn't just a mechanical operation. My favorite book on statistics, *The Nature of Statistics*, by Allen Wallis and Harry Roberts, defines *statistics* as "a body of methods for making wise decisions in the face of uncertainty." The field of statistics offers the tools, but you need to wisely apply those tools to produce useful insight from data.

Combining people strategy, science, statistics, and systems

As a relatively new field, people analytics feels a lot like what I imagine the Wild West of American folklore must have felt like: There aren't a lot of rules, and everyone's making their own way to some unclear new opportunity.

If you asked a group of people analysts to describe their work, the answers you'd hear would likely be quite different from each other and depend a lot on the background of the individual person. Here are some examples of how the categorically different types of people you find working in the field of people analytics think categorically differently about what they do.

>> **Human resources:** Someone with this background might describe people analytics as "the decision science of HR" or "the datafication of HR." Put a different way, as customer analytics is to sales, people analytics is to human resources. The focus of a person with a human resources or management strategy background is likely on the implications of data on how the company manages people or human resources conducts its work, with less emphasis on the nuances of how the data was produced.

>> **Behavioral science:** A person who comes from a scientific background is likely to describe people analytics as simply a new term referring to the near century old practice among university professors and graduate student research to study people in the workplace in fields as wide ranging as: psychology, sociology, anthropology, and economics. This crowd carries the all-important distinction of three letters behind their name, (PhD) or two letters before their name (Dr.). The focus of the doctors is on the application of science to human behavior to produce new learning, less so on the day-to-day processes to efficiently collect, store, and use the data. Scientists

are best at identifying new data that should be collected and developing a reliable and valid means to collect that data, but probably not best at how to do that efficiently.

>> **Statistics or data science:** These folks might describe people analytics as using statistical methods and machine learning algorithms to infer insights about the people aspects of businesses from data. Their focus is on mathematics and technical processes to produce insight from an existing dataset, with less emphasis on the determination of what data should be collected or how to apply the findings from data to produce change.

>> **Information technology:** Someone in this camp probably would focus on those systems that would make reporting and analysis more efficient to produce. Their focus is typically more on the overall data architecture and systems than the analysis itself. From an information technology standpoint, people analytics is nothing more than the application of reporting (sometimes referred to as *business intelligence)* to the specific domain of human resources, as opposed to something new and different.

The answer, of course, is that people analytics is all of these things, and a dozen things in between. You can apply the tools of people analytics to many purposes. Just like in the Wild West, rugged individualism is a common characteristic among people analysts, but we still stand to gain a lot by listening to and learning from each other.

Blazing a New Trail for Executive Influence and Business Impact

The human resources organization that endeavors to incorporate people analytics into its processes stands to benefit in many ways. Not only does mathematical analysis of data add weight and seriousness to the proposals to deliver to your executive team, but the results you get from programs you based on data are also better for the employees and the company.

Taking on new analytical responsibilities isn't something you can do lightly, though. For human resources professionals who are accustomed to the ways of "old HR," people analytics methods might seem very strange at first. However, learning these new tricks is definitely worth your while.

Moving from old HR to new HR

For human resources practitioners, learning new problem-solving approaches based on data and analytics doesn't mean abandoning the soft skills they've developed over their careers. People analytics simply adds more tools to your human resources tool belt.

I tell you in the following list about some of the differences I've seen between organizations that use only the "old HR" approach and those that have also incorporated the "new HR" tools and methodologies — the benefits of expanding your toolset will speak for themselves:

>> **Old HR focuses on creating policies based on how we have done it before or based on a concept known as *best practices*.** *Best practices* is the idea that your company can achieve greatness simply by copying the practices of other successful companies. The concept of best practices assumes that the selected best practices are what resulted in those other companies' success, without any scrutiny of whether or not that is actually true or if the presumed benefits of the new practices can be replicated from one situation to another. Instead, New HR uses data to evaluate what was working or not working for you already in the past, scrutinize assumptions underlying proposed changes, predict what will happen if changes are implemented, and evaluate if the predictions made were correct or not.

>> **Old HR produces overworked HR professionals.** The old way was to implement all possible ideas that might matter and keep adding to this each year without scrutinizing what worked or didn't in the past, and therefore resulted in adding a lot of new activities without taking any old activities away. The old way resulted in too many commitments and not enough time or resources to achieve consistent results in any one area. New HR uses data to direct time and resources on what matters most and reducing time and resources on those things that do not matter at all or as much.

>> **Old HR directs HR professionals to deliver programs, practices, processes, and policies in functional focus silos such as Talent Acquisition, Compensation and Benefits, Employee Relations, Diversity.** New HR uses data to identify system-level results coming from cross-functional inputs and collaboration on big picture problems.

>> **Old HR assumes that success consists of staying busy with activity.** New HR doesn't confuse motion with progress.

>> **Old HR often focuses on the questions of how to increase the consistency of HR activity or how to reduce the operating costs of HR activity.** New HR focuses on the question of how to increase the value of HR activity through evaluation of business impact.

>> **Old HR is a service provider to the rest of the company.** New HR is a trusted business partner.

Using data for continuous improvement

Continuous improvement is an old business topic that is more important today than it was even in the past. People analytics is a great tool for iteratively evaluating your policies and processes for continuous improvement. Looking at people data lets you get a high-level view of the organization and then dive down to scrutinize tiny details.

Using analytics, you can narrow the sea of opportunities into a refined focus on what are the most important problems for you to work on right now. Because you're prioritizing based on correlations to business outcomes data, you know that the problems you're working on are important ones in your organization — ones that make a difference to the people you work with as well as your customers. You can really tell whether your solutions are working — it's all right there in the data.

You've probably encountered (or even initiated yourself!) programs, policies, and practices that no longer serve the company, or maybe ones you're not sure ever really worked in the first place. With the data behind you, you can confidently make the call to let go of those that don't work.

People analytics provides support to your objective of differentiating your company in the market in decisions ranging from the type and quality of talent you want to hire to the way work gets done in your organization to the employee culture you want to create to how you handle pay to what unique benefits you provide to how you express messages to employees and potential employees and to countless other decisions. Human resources professionals who can use data analysis to direct, evaluate, and modify all these human resources-related decisions to the advantage of the company in the market become more valued members of the company's leadership team.

Accounting for people in business results

In a June 2005 article for *Harvard Business Review* titled "The Surprising Economics of a 'People Business'," Felix Barber and Rainer Strack encapsulate the growing awareness of the effect that people have on business outcomes:

In order to identify where and how value is being created — or squandered — people-intensive businesses need people measures that are as rigorous as financial measures, but that help to understand the productivity of people rather than of capital. The distinct but generally unappreciated economics of people-intensive businesses call not only for different metrics but also for different management practices. For instance, because even slight changes in employee productivity have a significant impact on shareholder returns, "human resources management" is no longer a support function but a core process for line managers.

The companies I worked for early in my career were large companies that spent billions of dollars on people: large pharmaceuticals companies, large retail companies, large technology companies, and large hospitals. These large, successful companies had already achieved advantages by paying careful attention to the people they hired and how they managed them, and it just made sense for them to be on the cutting edge of people analytics in their search to multiply their sizable people advantages.

As time has gone on, I have worked with smaller companies in a more diverse range of industries that want to reduce the advantage large companies in their industry have over them or find a new edge by applying people analytics, too. Today, people analytics work is not limited to a specific industry or company size; it offers opportunities that span across and within companies of nearly all types and sizes.

Competing in the New Management Frontier

Data analysis in the field of finance was once the frontier of business management, and the first companies who used it gained a distinct advantage over their competition. In turn, data analysis in the field of marketing was once a competition wrecking differentiator. Over time, though, these techniques became so widely used that their benefits no longer offered a leg up on the competition. Instead, using these kinds of analysis is just the price of entry into the game of big-time business.

Today, I believe that the business world is seeing the rise of data analysis in the field of human resources as the latest example of this trend. Eventually, everyone will need to use people analytics to keep up, but for now, forward-thinking companies have a chance to use it to realize a true advantage.

Now that you're convinced, your first task is to figure out where to get started. To do that, you need to choose a project. As you will see through the methods and examples I share in this book, people analytics can help you use data to broadly find:

» Where your company's people strengths and people weaknesses lie

» How to drive change with data

» How to prioritize and allocate scarce resources and time

Specifically, you'll have to determine where to look to find the best return on investment for your effort in people analytics.

>> Is it in applying data to the recruiting process to find ways to increase recruiter output, reduce hiring time, reduce hiring cost, or increase hiring quality?

>> Is the best use of your time in listening more carefully to employees to understand what obstacles are preventing them from doing their best work or using data to identify hidden undercurrents that may be a threat to the company's future success? Is a bad manager, missing tools and resources, arguments among employees, a lack of competitive pay and benefits, or other issues preventing optimum productivity, resulting in a decline in employee motivation and commitment?

>> Is the best use of your time to identify meaning from patterns in data about who stays and who goes? Is it in challenging the common assumptions about what makes an employee stay or leave the company, identifying what employee characteristics or conditions makes employee exit more predictable, determining what actions can management take to reduce the likelihood of its best employees leaving, or evaluating if the actions management is taking are working?

These are just a sample of questions from three broad categories of exploration where you can apply your time and resources in people analytics, among thousands of possibilities.

REMEMBER

The analysis that is most beneficial to one company may not be beneficial at all to another company. Without knowing more about your company, I cannot tell you where you should begin for you to have the biggest impact. To avoid an overcomplicated list of options (and a thousand-page book), I have reduced the range of possible focus into three core people problems that all companies must solve: employee attraction, employee activation, and employee attrition. There will be much more about the concepts, measures, and methods of analysis for these topics in the book to come. A careful review of each of the three high-level areas of focus (attraction, activation, and attrition) provided here in this book will help you determine where your attention will have the most impact for your company.

There is no shortage of opportunities of what you can learn about these topics or places your initial work may take you, so let's get you started!

Chapter **2**

Making the Business Case for People Analytics

The view that people matter to business results is consistent across industries and over large and small companies alike, yet when push comes to shove — when each executive's annual initiatives and priorities are set — people (along with the HR departments tasked with helping these people succeed) are usually an afterthought. Companies spend fortunes updating their equipment, buying and assimilating other companies, launching new marketing campaigns, extending product lines, and carrying out other miscellaneous strategic initiatives, but when it comes to putting real management time and resources into getting really good at acquiring, activating, and retaining people who are the best in the world at carrying out the stated business strategies, very few companies come up with anything of any noteworthy difference. Why is that?

In large part, the answer to this question lies in the short-term financial view rewarded by Wall Street's quarterly earnings report cycles. Little thought is put into the people-intensive activities that occur over the long term. Yet, if you're committed to improving your financial results for the long term, you must work to improve the underlying drivers that produce those results — including employee acquisition, experience, engagement, and retention.

How do you make a convincing argument for these people-oriented initiatives? You need to demonstrate a basic value model that illustrates where the results your company aspires for stem from and how people connect to that. (Figure 2-1 shows what a model like this would look like.)

BUSINESS VALUE CREATION MODEL

People Results	Process Results	Customer Results	Financial Results
"To achieve our vision, what capabilities must we grow and how must we learn and change?"	"To achieve our vision, what must we be good at?"	"To win, what are we going to be best at - how must we look to our customers?" Text	"If we succeed, how will we look to our shareholders?"

FIGURE 2-1: Business value creation model.

After more than 20 years of working with dozens of different companies of different sizes and in all sorts of industries, I have never heard anyone dispute the logic of the diagram shown in Figure 2-1. So why don't leaders pay more attention to all the inputs, including people, rather than focus only on the outputs? The likely reason is that improving HR sounds boring. Also, achieving results in the people sphere — managing talent attraction, activation, and attrition — require significant substantive effort over a long period.

REMEMBER

Sustained and substantive work devoted to building success through people — even when proven to move the financial needle — is not often the strength of those who have managed to work their way to the top. They made their own way through what has traditionally been a sink-or-swim world in a fly-by-the-seat-of-their-pants manner, so managing other people over the long term can be a complete blind spot. Nevertheless, someone in senior leadership has to be convinced of how to harness the power of people as a group; otherwise, it will never be a priority.

TIP

Unless you have a business sponsor who believes in the usefulness of people analytics from the start, you'll have to find some mathematical supports for your arguments. Few busy executives will "take it on faith" that totally changing their approach to people is the best solution for reaching financial Shangri-La.

So, how do you demonstrate that what you can do with HR will help the bottom line? Simple: by using data. And yet, it has become a question of which came first — the chicken or the egg? You need data in order to sell your plan to get the resources you need in order to collect the data, but you can use the data only after getting the resources necessary to collect and evaluate the data.

Somehow you need to make an argument for people analytics even when you haven't received any support to collect data and apply people analytics yet. I give you the best plays I have to get out of this pickle.

Getting Executives to Buy into People Analytics

Executives are open to new possibilities that change the way they do things when (and only when) they believe those things meet their needs. To boil down many years of economic and psychological theory, every action that people take is because of a dissatisfaction. People feel dissatisfied in their current condition, for some reason. Because of this dissatisfaction, they are internally motivated to take an action to relieve it. Think of it like going to the refrigerator to get a drink when you're thirsty or quickly jerking your hand from the stove when the pan is still hot. The discomfort triggers action to relieve the pain and to achieve an expected state of increased happiness.

Getting started with the ABCs

An easy-to-understand theory known as the ABC model spells out how to get people to do anything you want them to. (See Figure 2-2.) The letters *ABC* stand for *a*ntecedents, *b*ehaviors, and *c*onsequences.

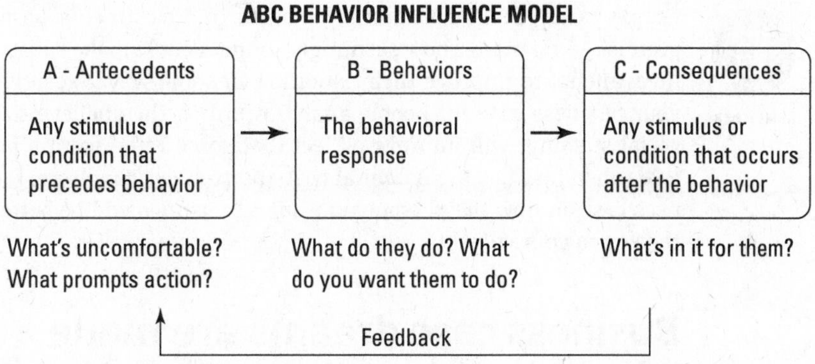

ABC BEHAVIOR INFLUENCE MODEL

A - Antecedents	B - Behaviors	C - Consequences
Any stimulus or condition that precedes behavior	The behavioral response	Any stimulus or condition that occurs after the behavior
What's uncomfortable? What prompts action?	What do they do? What do you want them to do?	What's in it for them?

Feedback

FIGURE 2-2: The ABC behavior influence model.

In the context of the business case for people analytics, the antecedents (A) represent the first part of the story that supports why you want people analytics. The A part can consist of the previous experiences and feelings of the executives you're trying to convince. Sometimes, that involves some pain they are experiencing with employees. Sometimes, what propels executives forward are the observations they make about another company's efforts in people analytics. Sometimes, what propels executives forward is the convincing arguments of the salespeople who want to sell your executives a new system or service. The A part gets the process started, but it usually isn't enough to get you all the way there.

Skipping to the last letter in the theory, the consequences (C) represent what the people you're trying to convince want to happen. What are the consequences of engaging in people analytics or not engaging in people analytics? (In my experience, C is probably driving 80 percent of the motivation to buy into your business case.) The consequences have to be sufficiently large enough to pull people through the costs or hard work of B.

The middle letter, B, refers to the behaviors that are necessary to move from antecedents to consequences. Members of your executive team may need to change the way they make decisions, they may need to invest some money in some systems, or they may have to be willing to let you go collect some data. Given that B involves taking a risk and making some changes, A and C had better be quite compelling.

Creating clarity is essential

One reason for the lack of interest in people analytics among the higher-ups is that the people you want to convince don't understand how they will be better off with people analytics than without. To put it bluntly, executives don't see how the supposed benefits justify the cost or the trouble that's caused by moving from the current state to the proposed state that people analytics offers.

REMEMBER

People rarely make substantial changes or investments based on an abstract premise — no matter how seemingly sound. People make substantial changes and investments to improve their condition in some way. Executives won't buy into your business case for people analytics unless they believe that their results or social standing will improve or feel that some relief from a previous obligation more than justifies the potential cost and trouble. Therefore, focusing your business case on how the person you want to convince will be better off in the end is the key to your success.

Business case dreams are made of problems, needs, goals

Contrary to popular belief, solutions in themselves really have no value. Solutions derive their value from the problems they were meant to solve. I know there's a good chance that the reason you picked up this book is that you already sense that you have a problem that people analytics will help you with; you just haven't fully baked that problem definition until it has crispy edges. Your business leaders probably haven't defined the problem yet, either — much less realized that it's a people problem you can solve with analytics. At this point, most business leaders still aren't accustomed to looking to data to solve HR or management problems that relate to people, let alone looking to HR for data.

The first step in making a business case for people analytics is the same as the first step in starting a people analytics project: Clearly define the problem. People analytics is a solution, and solutions derive their value from the problems they solve. Without a problem, a solution has zero value, so people analytics isn't the starting point of your business case.

First, you need to understand the problem. It starts with demonstrating that you have a deep understanding of the pain the business generally (and the business leader personally) faces. However, developing that deep understanding takes some serious work and a lot of conversation.

Here are some questions for you to work on answering:

>> What problem can people analytics solve for the person you want to buy into it?

>> What is the need that people analytics will satisfy for the person you want to convince?

>> What goals can be achieved by people analytics to help the person you want to convince?

>> What is the pain that people analytics will take away?

If you can answer one or more of these questions with absolute clarity, you have a good chance of getting your business case approved. If you can't, you're on thin ice.

If you don't have absolute clarity, go meet with more executives and ask them to specify their problems, needs, goals, and pains.

TIP

If the executives want to turn the conversation to what you do, don't go there. It's better to keep them talking about what *they* see as problems than to have them focus on what you see as problems. Stay away from what they think you want to hear — always return the attention to them and their problems.

Tailoring to the decision maker

Here's a scenario: If you were proposing people analytics to a CEO whom you know values a fully engaged workforce and is concerned about productivity levels across the enterprise, you might start with the problem that the company needs to learn more about — why employee engagement is down in some groups and up in some others and how to control it. Therefore, you want to study the drivers of employee engagement. You are using your CEO's language.

Knowing what's important to the decision-maker you're trying to convince and using that person's own language to help them understand your pitch are good strategies. If your CEO believes (or can be easily convinced) that employee engagement is a problem, either generally speaking or in some specific group, this could serve as your opening.

Alternatively, your CEO may believe that employee engagement does matter but may not perceive it to be a problem. In this case, you have more work to do. Then you need to find out what your CEO perceives to be a problem. After you understand that, you can explore whether he or she would be interested in looking for the people connections to help him solve that problem using a new approach that we call *people analytics*.

In addition to identifying the problem that's important to your CEO, you also have to understand how she or he makes decisions. People have different preferences for evidence. For some people, the evidence that other successful companies are using people analytics already may be a compelling enough reason for your company to do it too. Other people may have higher standards. They may need to be convinced with a different argument, like this: "Management is important to our future, and management is about people; therefore, people analytics can help us manage better." Finally, some people may be convinced only by a spreadsheet showing a specific dollar ROI per program.

Keep digging until you figure out the right way to talk to each particular decision-maker that you need to persuade to proceed.

TIP

Influence = IQ × EQ²

To influence the stakeholders who will decide whether your project proceeds, you need the perfect balance of offering solid ideas (Intelligence Quotient/IQ) and offering them in a way that connects with other people (Emotional Quotient/EQ). If EQ represents "people smarts," it represents both the solution you present and the way you present it, so I squared it.

Your challenge is to define that problem for yourself and articulate it in a way that your potential executive sponsors can understand. Doing this requires, in effect, that you peel the onion. For more on that, see the next section.

Peeling the onion

The particular business problem you're dealing with depends on circumstances. At first the business problem may not sound like it has to do with people at all, but if you ask the question "why?" enough times consecutively, you usually arrive at some point where the behaviors of people (or the actions they do or don't take) prove crucial.

Think about all the ways people matter to business results:

>> People invent products and services.

>> People interact with customers.

>> People do the right things for each other and for the world — or they do the wrong things.

All the things that people do or don't do have consequences. The thoughts, attitudes, and behaviors of people affect business results. With this concept in mind, it seems obvious that people analytics — a method designed to understand people — is useful at some level. However, though you and I are convinced, you aren't done yet. Now your work starts.

Have you ever heard some variant of this statement: "A problem well-defined is a problem half-solved" - John Dewey? The truth quotient is high for this one. The more you understand the problem, the more you and others can see how people analytics can help solve the problem.

In this context, "peeling the onion" means that, after you identify a problem, you continue asking probing questions to uncover evidence of the problem. The evidence is useful in putting together a compelling business case.

The evidence

>> Proves or disproves the problem.

>> Demonstrates the magnitude of the problem.

>> Provides a measurable expression of the problem for analysis.

>> Assists you in identifying measures you can correlate with other measures.

>> Provides a starting point to measure progress.

I've found these questions useful in conversation to peel the onion:

>> How do you know that this is a problem?

>> What measurements show evidence of this problem?

>> What is the situation right now? What would you prefer it to be?

>> What do you think causes this problem?

- Which causes do you think matter most?
- Where, specifically, does this problem show up?
- Whom does this problem affect most? Whom does it affect least?
- When does this problem occur most often?

If this exercise fails to produce any compelling problem for people analytics, your next option is to show the person you are trying to convince a problem that they didn't know about. They didn't realize that they have a problem with people, but maybe they should. For this, you need to find a way to collect a little data without much investment. Lure them in with a free taste test to see whether they decide to buy.

Identifying people problems

You often need more than a high-level argument to sway others to a people analytics way of thinking about people. Part of the problem is that everybody has an opinion about people, and most folks are unwilling to change their own opinions; when faced with an opposing view, many retreat to their corner and say, "Well, you have your opinion, and I have mine." To progress beyond such a stalemate, you need more than just opinions about people — you also need some *facts* about them.

In my professional experience, executives who have had a small taste of data-derived insights about people cannot resist wanting more, particularly about people at their own company. There are many ways to tempt executives, but you can hardly go wrong with these four metrics:

- **Win/loss ratio of hires and exits to your top competitors:** If the majority of number-one picks whom you contact from your competitors reject your recruiters' inquiries, that's a problem. If you lose 20 percent of your offers to candidates to Facebook, Amazon, Apple, Netflix, or Google (known collectively as FAANG), that's a problem.

  Maybe FAANG isn't bothering you but a large portion of your employees in key jobs are being poached by the same competitor. That's a problem. This info isn't difficult to find — it and could prove to be quite an eye-opener for the executive team.

- **Voluntary employee attrition rate by business segment:** You can look at division, job function, performance rating, tenure, and region (and any other segment that interests your executives). When you start to look at data like this, you inevitably see something that inspires the interest of executives (or strikes fear deep into their hearts).

>> **Engagement percent by business-relevant segments:** *Engagement* is an index of survey questions that measures the degree to which employees are committed to the company and motivated to apply discretionary effort. Research shows a large percentage of employees are so frustrated at work that they're just standing by and collecting a paycheck, with no motivation to do anything more than the bare minimum. An executive who can see data from the company's own people indicating a problem may be open to pursuing a people analytics strategy to resolve the situation.

>> **Likelihood to pursue a new job opportunity in the next 12 months and/or likelihood to recommend the company as an employer:** Again, you can learn many things from a simple survey question. You would be shocked to realize what people will divulge. These questions have been found to correlate with actual outcomes and with business performance.

These basic insights are not expensive or difficult to acquire, and they're great entry points to start generating interest and questions to which to apply more advanced people analytics. Most importantly, these insights can elevate problems to the attention of executives — problems they may not have otherwise known about.

REMEMBER

After you have identified problems, needs, goals, or pains, you have a good start — but you still have to figure out the best angle to persuade the executive to invest money and time. To answer this, you have to understand how the executive you want to persuade is motivated.

In the following sections, I give you three options: driven by feelings, driven by time or money, and driven by the need to lead.

Taking feelings seriously

One of the most important discoveries to come out of recent marketing research is that people buy the feeling they anticipate enjoying as a result of purchasing and using the product or service. Counterintuitively, people don't actually buy your product or service based on a logical assessment of the product's features; instead, they buy based on the emotion or psychic satisfaction that they imagine it will trigger or stimulate. This is why product quality, service, and relationships are important product differentiators.

To put a marketing research spin on things, what is the feeling that an executive will experience after buying into this idea of people analytics? What you need to do is present the executive with a picture of how people analytics will generate deep feelings of security, comfort, status, prestige, warmth, or personal connection.

ADDING DESIRE AND FEAR TO THE MIX

Some people believe that only two basic motivations underlie all action: the desire for gain and the fear of loss.

Here's a fear-based argument: Imagine, if you will, that if you do nothing to correct certain trends in your enterprise, there's an increasing risk of diverse candidates bringing an adverse-impact lawsuit against the company at some inopportune moment. The business case for people analytics may be simply this: "Don't let the company fail to do the right things, resulting in an embarrassing and expensive loss in court. Instead, let's get ahead of this thing with people analytics to find ways to remove bias from our decision processes."

If you would rather make a positive business case, what you say may be more nuanced. It may be sharing a summary of all the ways that Google and other well-branded companies are using people analytics to revolutionize their HR efforts. They're deriving business advantages from people analytics, and you don't want your company to be left behind.

Keep in mind that the promise of good outcomes is more motivating to some people, and that the fear of bad outcomes is more motivating to others.

Note: Keep an eye out for the consequences of inaction as well. Another way to convince a stakeholder is to talk about what will happen if you don't do something to solve the problem.

Think about what lies under the surface of the executive's emotions. Does the person want to feel the pride of being on the leading edge? Feel superior to his or her competitors? Avoid being left behind competitively? Feel more certainty and control?

TIP

Outside of general feelings about people, it's an advantage to know about the problems in the company that this executive is consumed with at the moment. If you talk about that business problem and pose the question "why?" enough times, generally it comes back to a people issue.

Saving time and money

Some people like those business cases that are all about saving the company time or money. In business, you pay for time, so time and money are basically interchangeable.

The business cases that are used for business intelligence and data science teams usually stress the fact that the company is already spending a substantial amount of time and money preparing reports and analysis for executives; they're just doing it inefficiently. The business case isn't centered on whether the company should be preparing the reports — the business case is based on an argument that implementing a system or a centralized team, or both, will reduce the time and money spent generating the same information.

A similar argument can be made for HR, if reporting and analysis work in which executives already find value is already occurring. The business case for making a change is that they can get the same information more efficiently if they give you the money. (This may work in situations where you're already doing something with data, but probably won't work in situations where you aren't.)

TIP

You may be better off pointing out that the company is already making a lot of HR-related decisions without data and that using data will allow the company to make these decisions better or faster or for less money than using the archaic decision-making processes.

Leading the field (analytically)

At a high level, you essentially have these three options to run HR:

>> **Low cost (don't even try to compete):** You can go for a low-cost, low-frills HR operating model where you're just expecting your HR people to run basic processes legally and as efficiently as possible. You're running plays that have been run by large companies for over 100 years, so what could go wrong? You're abiding by government legislation and "pushing paper" as accurately and as fast as you can. If it doesn't seem to be going well, you're not going to know why, but do feel free to fire the head of HR and try again.

>> **High quality (follow the leader):** You aspire to be like the best companies in the world, so you copy the things they do in HR. If they change their 401k match, you change your 401k match. If they go to open-office floor plans, you go to open-office floor plans. If they give employees beanbags and ping-pong tables, you give your employees beanbags and ping-pong tables. If they give free lunches — well, maybe you can't do that, but you give one free lunch per week or you discount the company cafeteria or do something related. These are simple examples of "best practices." You aspire for high quality, and you're fine with copying, but you don't want to invent it.

Best practices might sound great, but the problem is that you don't have unlimited time and money, so you still have to choose. And there's the rub: How are you actually supposed to choose? You don't really know why the other company does what it does. You don't know positively whether it really works. You don't really know whether it's profitable. You don't really know whether it was designed to solve a problem that you don't have. You don't know whether it creates other, unforeseen problems. That's a lot of you-don't-knows. How do you choose?

» **Innovation:** If you do the hard work of asking important questions about how people connect to business results and the best way to manage people, you'll find your way to answers using data and experimentation. You'll run your HR department more like a curious science teacher would rather than like a hard-liner hall monitor. You'll look for empirical certainty about the decisions you make that impact workers' lives — from whom to hire to how much to pay employees to which benefits to offer.

If you choose the third option, you'll need some data. Maybe that's what your executives want you to create. Can you paint a compelling picture of what this will look like? If so, this in itself may be enough to be convincing, given the alternatives.

People Analytics as a Decision Support Tool

The increasing use of technology, enterprise systems, and online recruiting platforms like LinkedIn is generating more information and data than ever before. There's a common understanding that something in this data might be useful but that, as with a messy closet, people struggle to find what they're looking for.

The solutions you implement in people analytics are intended to cut through the accumulations of data to find the insight you need in order to make better decisions and improve performance.

Decisions about people are some of the most important and impactful decisions a company can make. Think about all the decisions that are made about people in a business:

» What type of people to hire

» When to hire people

» How to hire people

» How many people to hire

» Whom to hire

» How much to pay

» How to reward

>> What to train

>> When to train

>> How to train

And so on. The sum of these decisions made about people for a business are demonstrated in the large amount of money that businesses spend on people, as reflected in their ledgers. Certainly, the quality of these decisions impacts the quality of the results of all those expenditures. Important and expensive decisions will be made regardless; with people analytics, you're just better able to connect the dots.

How well decisions are made comes back to the quality of the thinking of the people who make the decision and the information they have to make it. Those who apply data and analysis to making decisions have an advantage. Most business areas where crucial decisions are made — finance, marketing, and operations, for example — have already learned and applied this simple fact. Not applying data to human resources puts HR executives at a substantial disadvantage in obtaining support and resources on a relative basis to leaders of finance and marketing. It also puts the company at a substantial disadvantage to other companies.

If you want to get down to brass tacks, here's the deal: People analytics allows you to measure company performance at a much deeper level than you could before — right down at the people level — which by necessity allows you to

>> **Learn from the past to improve results in the future:** Whether you're talking about information gleaned from the hiring process or employee surveys or employee exit interview data or some other type of data, people analytics allows you to learn what is working or not working more quickly so that you can make the adjustments you need to improve performance. People analytics provides the measurement feedback to hold everyone accountable for the effectiveness of the actions we decide to take.

>> **Predict future performance with greater accuracy:** Before the world had a deep appreciation for biology and medicine, it used to be that, when a person fell ill, doctors (if you want to call them that) had a hard time predicting what would happen. After science helped doctors develop more insight into what was occurring inside the body, doctors could do a better job of predicting what would happen when they observed certain patterns. Often, these predictions allow humans to take actions that change their future or the future of others. (For example, if your blood pressure is high, you do something about it with an intent to change the course of a future impending heart attack.) With people analytics, you are doing the same thing by looking deeper

into the body of the company, which allows you to measure the health of the company, thus increasing your ability to predict future company outcomes and ultimately enable you to suggest actions that provide more control over company outcomes.

>> **Focus efforts to improve on things that will have the most impact per dollar input and let go of things that have no significant impact:** Many people management and HR practices are based on myths, falsehoods, incompatible ideas, ideas that never really worked, and other actions that worked before but no longer do. People analytics ushers in a new way of being for HR that directs it to apply resources to actions that will have the most impact and take away actions that do not.

>> **Manage in a more effective way:** With people analytics, you can bring forward data, spot problems, and work together to solve problems with enlightened collaborative group participation rather than an authoritarian "gut instinct" management style.

>> **Know that you're doing the right thing (and be able to defend that you're doing the right thing):** People analytics can help you make employment-related decisions that are less biased and that provide ongoing transparent feedback, which by nature will result in a more diverse, inclusive, and ethically managed company. These same analytics can be used to defend the decisions that were made with both internal and external stakeholders.

>> Reports and analyses can be used when the company is taken to court or to meet the stated requirements of the Equal Employee Opportunity Commission (EEOC).

Formalizing the Business Case

What kind of business case you create depends on the characteristics of the decision-makers, formal processes established to make decisions, and the culture of your company. Some places might require a formal report and a polished presentation in the boardroom. Other companies might be satisfied with a slide show presentation, a short memo, or even an email. The requirements probably vary, depending on the magnitude of resources you're asking for.

Regardless, a great habit to form as you begin your people analytics journey is to assemble the following (if for no other reason than the clarity of your own thinking):

- » **Problem:** The clear definition of the problem that you worked so hard to define at the beginning.

- » **Problem evidence:** The symptoms demonstrating that the problem is real.

- » **Problem impact:** The effects that this problem has on the business.

- » **Solution:** The scope and substance of the solution you propose. Create a vision of how good the situation will be after you implement the solution.

- » **Solution evidence:** The criteria that determine that the solution fixed the problem.

- » **Solution impact:** The benefits that the company stands to gain.

- » **Process:** The steps you'll need to complete in order to implement the solution.

- » **Cost:** Estimates of the funding the project needs.

- » **Timeline:** Dates and milestones for completing the process steps.

You might also want to include a summary of the other solutions you considered, the criteria you used to choose the solution, the methods you used to estimate the gains the company will realize, and other specifics from your notes. If you're presenting this report to executives, though, you should put that detail in appendixes at the end. One-page summaries on the front of a lengthy document aren't called executive summaries for nothing!

Presenting the Business Case

The business case itself lays out the problem and the proposed solution. Presenting the business case to stakeholders is an opportunity to evaluate that business case. You confirm that the problem is a real pain point in the company and that the solution you proposed is sound. If you've been bouncing ideas off the stakeholders throughout the process, this part of the presentation should yield no surprises.

The presentation also gives the stakeholders the chance to dive into specifics, such as making sure there's money in the budget for software licenses and confirming the availability of executives, human resources and IT to work on the project.

TIP

Build a modular presentation with time for questions between modules. A monolithic speech that never stops for air will lose your audience. Also, it wouldn't hurt to preview the business case with a few meeting participants to build support so that you have allies in the room. Choose carefully, though; if your stakeholder does not support your business case, they will have time to poke holes in it.

I like to structure my business case presentations like this:

1. Thank everyone in the meeting for the time they have invested to this point. Let them know it was helpful in developing the business case you're about to present.

2. Remind the room of everyone's mutual self-interests.

3. State the objectives for the presentation. Say something like this: "Our objective today is to find out whether the people analytics approach we are suggesting will meet your needs. If not, we want to understand what would have to change." Leave the door open to try again if they don't love your business case.

4. Review the big picture around the problem.

5. Review the problem evidence and problem impact. Ask the stakeholders to make sure you didn't leave anything out. Let them add, modify, or delete.

6. Review the solution evidence and solution impact. Ask them to make sure you got it right and that you didn't leave anything out. Let them add, modify, or delete.

7. Discuss the decision criteria. Does the proposal have to show how the project aligns to an existing company objective? Is there a maximum budgetary requirement? Is there a particular return on investment (ROI) requirement? Is this project in competition with other projects for resources? Is there a particular way you want the business case presented? Essentially, if you have come all this way to ask others to support the work you believe in, you should be able to ask them, "Wouldn't it be fair for you to tell me how you make this important decision, so I can speak to that now or come back with something better next time I come up here to talk to you about the work I am proposing?"

8. Propose the solution steps, costs, and timeline.

9. Review how the proposed solution addresses the problems and satisfies the decision criteria.

10. Decide to proceed (if all goes well).

11. Discuss the specifics of timing, who's doing what, and project funding.

Ultimately, the business case presentation gives the stakeholders the opportunity to decide that this is a good project to start and that now is a good time to start it. If you've defined the problem well and really sold the solution, you'll soon be starting your first people analytics project.

» **Deciding on a method of planning and mode of operation**

» **Designing a solution that will give you what you need**

Chapter 3

Contrasting People Analytics Approaches

Too commonly, I hear that a company has spent years setting up an advanced data dashboard and visualization system only to discover it doesn't give executives what they want or need. It is said in different ways. Some examples include:

» "We implemented a self-service dashboard environment, but nobody uses it."

» "We have lots of data — we're *drowning* in data now — but what we really need are insights."

» "We have people working on reporting, but now we are looking for ways to get more business impact from our data."

The good news is that these problems are avoidable if you determine what you're looking for, design each people analytics project to give you what you need, and communicate with others accordingly.

To simplify the enigma of people analytics possibilities, I offer three of your main project considerations with two options each.

Figuring Out What You Are After: Efficiency or Insight

Here's the first question to ask when it comes to your own people analytics project: What are you looking to achieve? In my experience, companies embark on people analytics projects primarily to either increase efficiency when answering many different common questions (reporting) or to answer new questions (developing new insight).

Either objective can bring your company value and both are important, but mixing up the two in a single project is a recipe for disappointment. Figure 3-1 shows an overview of the two approaches, with the efficiency-oriented data project emphasizing systems design and the insight-oriented data project emphasizing analysis design. In the following sections, I talk about each one so that you can decide what is your primary focus for each project.

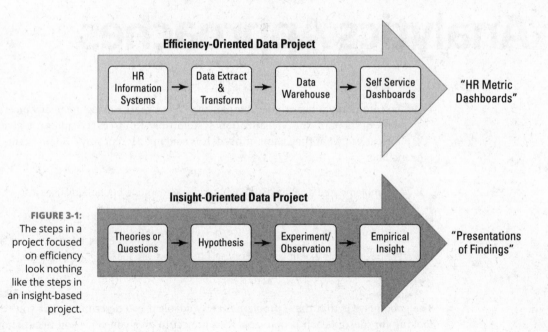

FIGURE 3-1: The steps in a project focused on efficiency look nothing like the steps in an insight-based project.

Efficiency

The classic example of an efficiency objective is that you want to use a system to automate reports that someone is already regularly producing on desktop software application like Excel, Tableau or R. For example, you or someone you work with may work for 40 hours per month to produce a regular update to data visualizations of Headcount, Headcount Growth Rate, Hire Rate, Exit Rate, Promotion

Rate and Time to Hire, all of which go into a slide deck for the executive management team. These represent seven out of over one hundred possible HR metrics. The process to achieve the visualizations is cumbersome, time consuming and error prone because of the human effort required to get the data necessary to produce the metrics from systems, bring it together, perform calculations, and then make it into graphs. You are able to perform this effort for a limited number of metrics and segments, rather than for all relevant metrics and segments for your company (say, by division, business unit, location, job, tenure, or gender). To increase the number of metrics and segments you can produce each month, you will have to hire more people to perform the work.

Most modern dashboard and visualization systems can automate the actions required to produce hundreds of HR metrics and make them available to a wide number of different users on visual dashboards that can be segmented or filtered so the user can get just what they need or want — say, by division, business unit, location, job, tenure, or gender. If you are hoping to implement data architecture and systems to eliminate the hard work to get the data you or others need — or make it happen with less effort – this is an efficiency objective.

When you pursue an efficiency objective, your most significant choices relate to the data architecture and reporting systems you will use to replace human effort with machine (automation).

Reporting systems continually evolve, so that even the most cutting-edge systems seem out of date within a few years. Once you begin on this path, you will likely feel pressure to overhaul regularly to keep up with cool new features, but frankly, today's reporting systems perform the same fundamental objective they did 20 years ago: produce the metrics we need all the time with as little human effort necessary, given the current state of technology. That's to say their primary objective is efficiency; the rest is just the outfit you put on it.

If increasing the efficiency of your analytics effort is of more immediate and pressing interest to you than discovering new insights, you have many resources to learn more about this. Books like *Business Intelligence For Dummies* (by Swain Scheps) and *Data Warehousing For Dummies,* 2nd Edition (by Thomas C. Hammergren), all from Wiley Publishing, can be quite helpful for understanding the high-level concepts and choices you have to make.

Insight

An emphasis on problems and questions is a hallmark of an insight-oriented people analytics project. You start with a problem you want to work on and then use data to answer questions that you believe will help you better understand that problem.

When you are looking for new insight, your most significant efforts relate to defining the problem focus, the questions that you want answered and the design of an analysis workflow that will offer some insight to resolve the questions. The best insight projects are rooted in the scientific method. You begin with ideas and collect the specific data you need to confirm or reject those ideas, as opposed to hoping to stumble upon an idea you find buried in data accidentally collected in some system designed for other reasons. Though you might find data in systems or you might even set up systems to continue collecting a particular set of data over time, the problem you are analyzing dictates the data you collect and the systems you store it in, not the other way around. The scientific method directs your attention to the particular data that matters for that problem — as a result, the scientific method has many advantages over alternatives. However, the scientific method requires a way of problem solving that may be foreign to people who are not trained in science.

TIP

The scientific method doesn't necessarily require much or any technology. In some cases, though, statistical applications can be a big help. Minitab, R, SAS, SPSS, and Stata are some popular choices. In the right hands, they can help you use advanced statistical methods to help you tease meaning from the data you collected, in the process increasing your certainty about the insights gained.

A people analytics initiative to achieve insight is better at addressing specific problems and helping with specific decisions.

Having your cake and eating it too

You are interested in both efficiency and insight for different reasons. Sometimes you are looking for answers to new questions, which may require new data and new approaches (developing new insight) and other times you are just looking to improve the workflow you use to get answers to common questions that occur over and over again (developing efficiency).

By forcing you to choose, I have offered a simplified view of a complex continuum of options and decisions. The best data environment for people analytics is designed to meet some aspects of both efficiency and insight needs. That is to say that the best data environment addresses standard reporting needs and can also be leveraged in investigative analysis to produce new insights as well. However, even with a data environment designed to do both, you cannot automatically assume that implementing a reporting system will do both from the get-go.

You also should not assume that projects designed to implement systems that produce reporting efficiency should necessarily precede projects designed to produce insights. If designing a standardized reporting environment will take you one to two years and a several million dollar investment to build, and you can do analysis that will produce insights of immediate value to your company without that architecture, then don't wait. When performing work that others value, you may produce the justification you need to get agreement to make investments to automate the repetitive actions in a system so they can be performed more efficiently in the future. On the other hand, if the effort to produce a new insight only needs to be performed once or fails altogether then automation is unnecessary. For this reason, I promote the sometimes-counterintuitive idea that it is better to start with insight projects.

Deciding on a Method of Planning

Another question to answer in your people analytics project is about how you plan to manage it: with a waterfall approach or an agile approach.

Waterfall project management

Waterfall project management describes a method that is linear and sequential toward a known outcome. The plan includes every stage of development from the beginning, and those stages do not change. No stage can start until the preceding stage completes. It's the traditional project management approach.

Imagine a waterfall on the cliff of a steep embankment. Once the water flows over the edge of the embankment and begins its journey down the side, it's too late to choose a different embankment to fall over. It's the same situation with waterfall project management: Once a phase of development is completed, the development proceeds to the next phase, and there's no turning back. Figure 3-2 illustrates the steps that can appear in a waterfall project plan.

TIP

In a waterfall project, you have to determine correctly all the stakeholders' needs, preferences, and requirements from the outset. Therefore, waterfall is best suited to scenarios where everyone already knows the solution, such as common standardized reports. When you are able to determine precise project requirements up front, the waterfall approach is fine. If the standard reports and data visualizations that other companies have already implemented successfully suit your needs, then waterfall is a fine approach, if for no other reason than the fact that it is broadly understood and respected.

Agile project management

In contrast to a waterfall approach, *agile* project management describes a process in which you make a little progress, pause to evaluate the situation and adjust the plan, progress a little more, adjust some more, and so on. Each plan, design, build, and text iteration is known as a *sprint*.

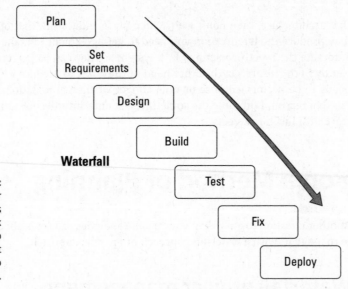

Waterfall

Plan

Set Requirements

Design

Build

Test

Fix

Deploy

FIGURE 3-2:
Once the water (project) has fallen over a rock on the cliff (step in the project plan), there's no going back.

REMEMBER

If you know at the outset where you are going, mapping the path of the waterfall is obvious. However, if you don't know exactly where you want to go, or if you know conditions will likely change along the way, the waterfall strategy makes you commit to too many important design decisions up front.

For example, at one major technology company, I was intent upon studying employee commitment, defined as the likelihood a given employee or group of employees would stay or leave in a one-year time frame. I developed an employee survey with an intent to understand what explains, drives, and predicts employee commitment by mathematically correlating employee responses to a series of independent items with how the same people respond to an Intent to Stay item (which I would eventually validate by a precise analysis using actual exit data). The problem to resolve was that at the outset, I could not possibly know what really drives commitment, and therefore I would not know what should not be on the survey. Is it managers? Is it pay? Is it the employee's reaction to the nature of the mission of the company? Is it the perception of the benefits program? Is it linked to positive or negative interactions with work colleagues? Is it some element of culture? Is it the job design? Is it the organization design? Is it the leadership? Depending on whose research I was reading or who I spoke to, I would get a different answer. The list just kept getting longer and longer. Eventually I arrived at the conclusion that I could not reasonably ask everything that might matter on one survey. The questions I add to the survey would imply that I already know things I clearly don't know. An agile project design allowed me to test several preliminary random sample surveys, modifying between each survey, until I had reached a reasonable conclusion on what questions would be best to include in a broader and more permanent survey effort. With each iteration of the survey,

I removed some questions my data analysis showed were not useful and added some new questions to test by the space freed up from the last test.

REMEMBER

The *agile* nature of the project I describe here was the iterative design. At the outset, I did not know how many tries I would need to arrive at the ultimate design. I kept going until I could reasonably conclude I had arrived at a sufficient number of items significant enough to explain, predict, and possibly control employee exit in the future.

REMEMBER

The problems with people can be uncertain, can appear as one thing but be another, or can start in one place and move to another. Each problem requires a different analysis and different data to solve it, so you don't know specifically what additional data and analysis you will require until you get into the work. More importantly, your full understanding of what the real problem is may not develop until you progress well into a project.

The agile approach calls for breaking down projects into smaller pieces, releasing segments of the project as they are finished, and requiring closer collaboration between technical and nontechnical stakeholders. It is well suited to the investigative methods you use to gain insights. By employing a more rapid deployment of features, you can evaluate the impact on the behavior and experience of users quickly, reevaluate where you are, and choose your next direction. Figure 3-3 shows a visualization of the iterations in an agile project.

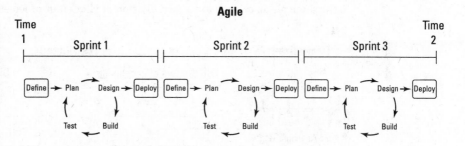

FIGURE 3-3: In an agile project, you complete a segment and then "come up for air" before starting on the next sprint.

An agile project requires technical and nontechnical teammates to evaluate their work together as they move through the process. The shorter time intervals separating conversations between technical and nontechnical stakeholders create valuable learning opportunities for everyone. The agile approach works beautifully for learning: It recognizes the value of everyone, accepts early failures with a constructive attitude, and facilitates a means to work together to solve problems.

An agile approach requires you to temporarily accept an imperfect or incomplete outcome; however, over the long term, it can get you where you need to go faster and at a lower risk of large-scale failure than the waterfall approach. You don't want your systems people to labor for a year before you find out that you didn't need those features or that this report just wasn't as useful as you thought it would be. Agile helps you find this out sooner rather than later.

Choosing a Mode of Operation

One characteristic of people analytics that I need to talk about is whether you have a centralized team that takes responsibility for the projects or whether you instead ask people across the company to pitch in. One of the questions I hear most frequently is this: If it is thought to be a new job, where should the person or persons in this new job report to?

Some companies have a team of people analytics professionals focused on and embedded in each business division, such as sales, engineering, and operations. Others have people analytics professionals that are embedded in and support the different sub-functions of Human Resources (talent acquisition, compensation, benefits, employee relations, diversity, learning and development, and so) Others have a central team of people analytics professionals focused on the whole company from one team. Figure 3-4 illustrates how people analytics teams might all report to the same place, or each to its own division or HR Center of Excellence head.

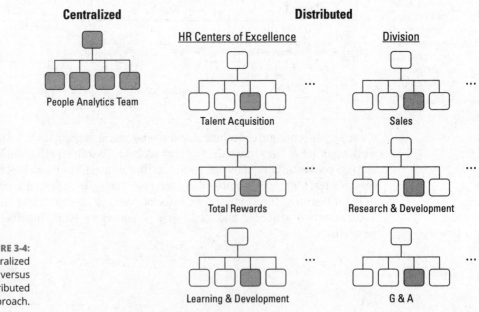

FIGURE 3-4:
A centralized approach versus a distributed approach.

TIP

If you're in a smaller company, you likely have fewer options, simply because you have fewer resources. Your company might not even have enough roles for it to make sense to have a dedicated team of specialized analysts. Engaging local college professors, grad students, consultants or analysts in other parts of the company (marketing, finance, IT, and so on) to fill in the skills gaps is always an option.

A company that starts with a loosely formed group might decide to centralize that function and invest in more dedicated resources as people analytics proves its value to the company over time. However, both approaches have pros and cons, of course, and the distributed approach offers its own benefits even if you can afford many dedicated resources.

Centralized

Centralizing the people analytics function lets a company reduce the inefficient redundancies of distributed mode.

Leaders of companies that centralize the effort tend to hire people with advanced degrees in niche analytical skill sets — superhero nerds, you might say. Focused analysts have the benefit of a full-time dedication to a clear objective. They get to work with a team that was hand-picked to bring all the skills to the table.

A centralized people analytics team also has a perspective that spans the entire company. Though a team dedicated to a single business division or HR center of excellence (a team dedicated to a single area of HR, such as recruiting, training, or employee relations) can focus tightly, it might miss company-wide opportunities or data sources that a centralized team would have the perspective to recognize.

TIP

A huge benefit is the ability to characterize the nature of the whole organization to the Board or CEO as well as each business unit or HR function. You get a "full view" of the organization; this is impossible for a distributed team to produce since they typically will not have access to all the data.

However, the downside of centralization is that it moves the people who generate the people analytics data further away from the people who make decisions based on the data. Among the groups that the people analytics team supports, this separation can create the sense that the people analytics team doesn't really understand their needs.

Many times, a business division or HR center of excellence creates its own people analytics team when it isn't receiving the support it needs from the company-wide centralized team. This team is sometimes called a *shadow team.* The term *shadow* may sound negative, and a shadow team is indeed widely believed to be an inefficient use of resources. On the other hand, it's hard to fault group members for investing their own resources to meet their own needs.

Centralizing the team also risks overwhelming your company's people analysts when multiple parts of the company come asking for support at the same time. Word spreads, and a centralized team can find a line of groups wanting their share of help. The centralized team has to prioritize the requests, which can create dissatisfied internal customers who feel that the centralized people analytics team is disconnected and bureaucratic and not doing enough to support them.

Distributed

A *distributed* structure is an inclusive model: Anyone and everyone in the company can potentially contribute to a people analytics project. Sometimes people call the distributed model *embedded* analytics because the tasks are embedded directly into each employee's job.

With the responsibility for people analytics distributed, there is no question that the people doing the work understand the problem they're working on, because it's their own problem. The team leaders are more likely to act on the information from the analysis because they completed the analysis themselves. They can understand and trust its insights.

This hyperfocus on your own problems can be a pitfall as well. For example, the Recruiting team might not know about or consider the data that the Compensation team uses, even if it's relevant to the problems of recruiting. The analysts on the Compensation team might not think about the benefit other teams can receive from the analysis, because they don't see themselves as supporting the other teams.

The most obvious potential problem with distributed people analytics is that the people with the skills you need might not have the time or willingness to take on another genre of tasks.

REMEMBER

Even with its drawbacks, the distributed approach is growing in popularity. Increasingly, even large companies are finding that a rigid, top-down centralized people analytics organization is not tenable. However, identifying and organizing a truly distributed network of expertise that is capable of advanced analytics can take years. If your company hasn't been hiring people all along into all areas of HR with analytical skill sets, it's facing an uphill battle.

A consensus is starting to form that the best architecture is one that blends centralized analysts with a heavier investment from distributed stakeholders. It's the we're-all-in-this-together approach. You can't expect everyone to be able to run advanced statistics, but you can expect them to be more conscious of the range of possibilities, be more analytical, and to use data when making important decisions.

MAKING YOUR OWN PATH

Too often, companies try to copy others' success and call it "best practices." Just because Acme Company did something and saw revenue increase doesn't mean that its strategy will work for you. Sometimes comparisons are compelling, but doing the same thing someone else did will never be a business differentiator.

(As a side note, I am waging a war against the concept of best practices. Implementing best practices is copying what someone else did because it worked for them, without consideration for the unique nature of your own business and situation. I'd rather we call them what they are: guess practices. Blindly copying is not a long-term strategy.)

Yes, you can learn from other companies. The most important thing to learn is that the successful ones defined what would make people analytics work by looking at their own goals, resources, and culture. Start small if you have to, and look for opportunities to adapt and grow. Your business will benefit from an analytical, data-driven approach to problem.

2

Elevating Your Perspective

Chapter **4**

Segmenting for Perspective

S egmentation is a fundamental and essential part of people analytics — or any analytics, for that matter. Segments are crucial when it comes to helping you understand and derive insight from your data.

A *segment* is a grouping of people who share common characteristics. A segment of people can be thought of as one whole unit or as a portion of another unit. For example, the people who work together in an industry form a segment of the total job market. The people who work together in a company form a segment of an industry, and the people in that particular company can be grouped into many much smaller segments.

Some simple examples of segments within a company are division, business unit, location, and job function (such as sales or engineering). People can also be segmented by characteristics that have nothing to do with the company and everything to do with the person — gender, ethnicity, socio-economic status, age, work experience, educational achievement and personality type, for example. People can be described by things that stay the same or things that change — some examples of things that change are years of work experience, company tenure, job tenure, pay, or attitude. There are nearly an infinite number of potential segments for any dataset about people because people can be described in so many different ways.

REMEMBER

Using data to observe a group of people with data is like looking at a diamond in the light: The brilliance of a diamond is determined by its number of cuts (or *facets*) and the clarity of the stone. Like diamonds, companies can be viewed in many different ways. The job of people analytics is to increase perspective and clarity.

In this chapter, I introduce you to segmentation, show you some of the ways it's used in people analytics, and point you toward the use of segmentation to improve the way you think about the people in your company.

Segmenting Based on Basic Employee Facts

As you explore your company's various systems, such as enterprise resource planning (ERP), human resource information system (HRIS), and applicant tracking system (ATS), you will find many hundreds of different facts about people stored in relational tables. In some cases, administrators input these facts. In other cases, individuals input the facts themselves — self-service, in other words. In other cases, the company actively seeks new facts by distributing surveys or forms. Finally, some facts are generated with no deliberate planning — data is just coincidentally collected by way of other activities or processes — for example email and meeting metadata.

Metadata is simply data that describes other data. Email or Meeting metadata refers to facts that can be observed from the use of company systems — facts that may be useful for analysis. For example, you could potentially learn a lot by analyzing the number of emails sent, number of words in emails, number of unique social connections, number of meetings, average meeting time, concentration of social connections by job function or location, and so on.

REMEMBER

In their primary form, the facts collected as data can seem useless; however, in informed hands, the facts can be transformed into useful information.

"Just the facts, ma'am"

What kind of people data are we talking about? Generally speaking, you can find facts from the following categories of information in one or more of your systems that contain employee data. (I list these facts first and then delve into how to make them more useful.)

Candidate facts

>> Name, or the name the candidate answers to

>> Candidate ID, which is a unique number representing the candidate

>> Source — recruiting method / channel (for example, LinkedIn, job board, referral, recruiter source, university recruiting, recruitment partner outsourcing)

>> Source — most recent employer

>> Source — most recent university

>> Education level, such as diploma/GED, some college, bachelor's degree, master's or MBA degree, or PhD

>> Requisition ID, or the unique number representing the job opening

>> Test score (For example, a technology company I worked for tested potential software engineer candidates for their level of acumen solving challenges with code. A pet retailer I worked for tested store customer service employees for their knowledge of pet topics following new hire training. A pharmaceutical company I worked for tested aspiring pharmaceutical sales representative for their product knowledge following new hire training.)

>> Application date, which is the date of first contact

>> Phone screen date, which is the date on which a recruiter first spoke to the candidate

>> Date of candidate's prescreen employment test, if applicable

>> Onsite interview date

>> Offer date

>> Offer acceptance or decline date

>> Hire date

Basic employee facts

>> Name

>> Employee ID

>> Company start date

>> Company tenure (how long the employee has been working at the company based on the company start date)

Job facts

>> Job title

>> Job code

>> Full-time or part-time

>> Contractor or employee

>> Salaried or hourly

>> Temporary or permanent

>> Job function, such as sales and marketing, manufacturing and operations, research and development, or general management and administration

>> Job management level, such as executive, director, manager, or individual contributor

>> Job compensation grade

>> Job start date

>> Job tenure, or how long the employee has been working in the current job based on the job start date

>> Annual pay

Managerial and financial structure facts

>> Manager — this is the name of the manager of the employee

>> Next-level manager — this is the name of the manager's manager (usually this is a director)

>> Executive — if you look at an organization chart, this is the name of the highest-level management officer under the CEO on the organization chart tree. (Usually this is a vice president)

>> Financial unit (usually the lowest level unit is called a *cost center.)*

>> Next-level financial unit, usually called an organization — there are multiple cost centers in each organization

>> Division, which is the highest-level financial unit before the company — there are multiple organizations within each division

A *hierarchy* is a relational classification system in which people or groups are ranked one above the other according to status or authority. The most obvious example is an organization chart built by employee-to-manager reporting relationships. Every company will have a different number of levels and different naming convention for their management hierarchy.

Location structure facts

>> Job location

>> City

>> Country

>> Country region, such as northeast, northwest, southeast, southwest

>> Global region, such as Asia Pacific, Europe, Middle East, Africa, North America, South America

Core demographic classifiers

>> Gender

>> Ethnicity

>> Disability status

>> Veteran status

>> Age

>> Generational cohort — Baby Boomers, Generation X, Millennials, and so on

>> Marital status

Demographics are important for evaluating the changing composition of the workforce, completing government-required Equal Employment Opportunity Commission (EEOC) reports, and analyzing your process for unconscious bias.

If your company is headquartered in the United States and has more than 100 employees and/or a U.S. government contract, you are required by law to file Employer Information Reports (EEO-1s) with the EEOC.

Though demographic information is useful for analyzing patterns, it is inappropriate to use non-job-related personal characteristics like gender, ethnicity, or age to directly make any employment decision, such as whom to hire, whom to promote, or how to pay. In the United States, there are laws that prohibit making employment related decisions on the basis of non-job related personal characteristics and specifically providing protection for gender, ethnicity, age and religion.

The brave new world of segmentation is psychographic and social

If you can get beyond the people data basics, you will someday understand that new insights about people are driven primarily by new and richer types of data about those people. People are cognitively advanced social animals who have minds of their own. To understand and predict their behavior, you have to "see" inside their minds — and in order to do this, you have to ask these animals some questions.

Here are a few examples of the many characteristics you can measure by using survey instruments or tests that can open up a whole new world of important insights to you:

>> **Personality types:** Some common personality instruments are the Big Five, the Myers-Briggs Type Indicator (MBTI), and StrengthsFinder.

>> **Attitudes:** Some common employee-survey measures are satisfaction, commitment, motivation, and engagement.

>> **Preferences:** A range of topics can be determined using basic questionnaires or advanced survey analysis tools.

>> **Technology adoption profile:** These factors include innovators, early adopters, early majority, late majority, and laggards.

>> **Opinions:** Survey questions might be designed to measure the likelihood to recommend the company to friends and colleagues or to exit the company for a better opportunity.

Look to survey instruments and tests to help you find important differences between people that help you understand, predict, and influence behavior. These types of instruments can help you develop segmentation that will unlock new insight.

Visualizing Headcount by Segment

In its most basic use, counting people by segment can help you see the company in new ways. For example, the numbers in the graphs shown in Figure 4-1 add up to a company's total head count of 3,100; however, each graph paints a different picture of the company based on the segmentation dimension. These are just six segmentations among hundreds of possibilities.

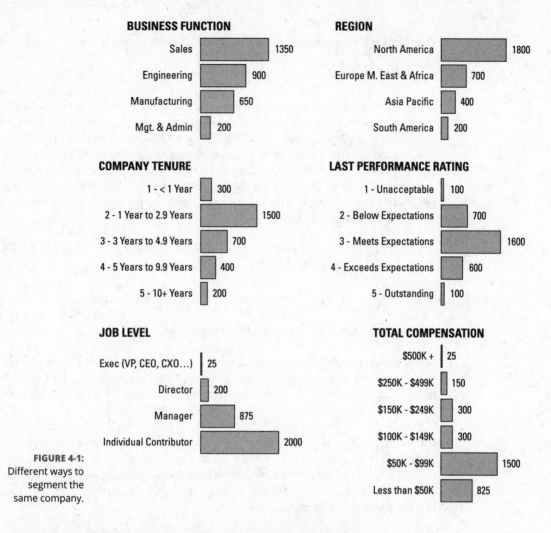

BUSINESS FUNCTION

Sales	1350
Engineering	900
Manufacturing	650
Mgt. & Admin	200

REGION

North America	1800
Europe M. East & Africa	700
Asia Pacific	400
South America	200

COMPANY TENURE

1 - < 1 Year	300
2 - 1 Year to 2.9 Years	1500
3 - 3 Years to 4.9 Years	700
4 - 5 Years to 9.9 Years	400
5 - 10+ Years	200

LAST PERFORMANCE RATING

1 - Unacceptable	100
2 - Below Expectations	700
3 - Meets Expectations	1600
4 - Exceeds Expectations	600
5 - Outstanding	100

JOB LEVEL

Exec (VP, CEO, CXO...)	25
Director	200
Manager	875
Individual Contributor	2000

TOTAL COMPENSATION

$500K +	25
$250K - $499K	150
$150K - $249K	300
$100K - $149K	300
$50K - $99K	1500
Less than $50K	825

FIGURE 4-1:
Different ways to segment the same company.

Analyzing Metrics by Segment

One of the main reasons to bother with segmentation is to provide a finer-grained (and thus more convincing) analysis of the data you're using to get to the root of a problem. Here's an example that illustrates the power of segmentation: *Exit Rate %* is a metric that measures the percentage of employees at your company who left to go work elsewhere over some specified period.

REMEMBER

Exit rate is synonymous with attrition rate, termination rate, and turnover rate.

The formula for Company Exit Rate % is calculated this way:

(Total # Company Exits ÷ Company Average Headcount) × 100

Company average headcount is calculated by counting the number of employees at the beginning and end of a period and averaging, or by counting the number of employees each day of a period and averaging, or by using any other consistent period sampling methodology. For example, you can average headcount over a year by weekly, monthly or quarterly snapshots. The reason to use an average headcount is that if the company is changing (either increasing or decreasing headcount) you will get a different answer depending on what day you count — average headcount standardizes.

If your company's Exit Rate % is 10 percent, it means that 10 percent of your employees left to go work elsewhere in the time frame of analysis.

When viewing Exit Rate % by segment, you calculate it this way:

= ((Segment # Exits ÷ Segment Average Headcount) × 100)

Segment average headcount is calculated by averaging the number of employees in the segment over the period. You are not dividing segment exits by the total number of employees. You are dividing segment exits by segment average headcount.

For example, if a segment called Segment A had an average head count of 100 people over a year and 20 people left in that year, then the Segment A Exit Rate % = 20%, or ((20 ÷ 100) × 100 = 20). In this example, Segment A has double the exit rate of the average, which is, as I mentioned, 10 percent. This tells you that something may be going on in Segment A.

Figure 4-2 shows quite clearly the explanatory power of moving beyond mere Company Exit Rate % and looking at specific segments within a company — Region, for example, or Business Function or Last Performance Rating. It lets you see the percentage of people within that particular segment who left the company during that period, not the percentage of the total population of exits.

REMEMBER

The reason for calculating segment exits as a percentage of segment headcount is that it allows a fair and consistent comparison between segments, regardless of the segment's size. If the calculation is not done as a percentage of segment average headcount, then the larger groups will always show a higher percentage of overall exits — which would tell you only that these were larger groups, not that there was something wrong with them.

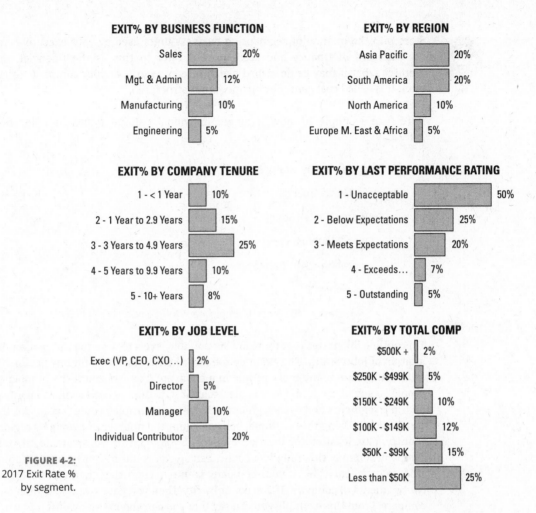

EXIT% BY BUSINESS FUNCTION

Sales	20%
Mgt. & Admin	12%
Manufacturing	10%
Engineering	5%

EXIT% BY REGION

Asia Pacific	20%
South America	20%
North America	10%
Europe M. East & Africa	5%

EXIT% BY COMPANY TENURE

1 - < 1 Year	10%
2 - 1 Year to 2.9 Years	15%
3 - 3 Years to 4.9 Years	25%
4 - 5 Years to 9.9 Years	10%
5 - 10+ Years	8%

EXIT% BY LAST PERFORMANCE RATING

1 - Unacceptable	50%
2 - Below Expectations	25%
3 - Meets Expectations	20%
4 - Exceeds…	7%
5 - Outstanding	5%

EXIT% BY JOB LEVEL

Exec (VP, CEO, CXO…)	2%
Director	5%
Manager	10%
Individual Contributor	20%

EXIT% BY TOTAL COMP

$500K +	2%
$250K - $499K	5%
$150K - $249K	10%
$100K - $149K	12%
$50K - $99K	15%
Less than $50K	25%

FIGURE 4-2:
2017 Exit Rate %
by segment.

When you report Exit Rate % per segment, you can see how much each segment's exit rate varies from the company average. Clearly, you want to know where each segment is in the range of values. You can use segmentation to identify the segments that require more attention, which helps you move the overall company average the most with the least amount of effort.

Understanding Segmentation Hierarchies

In people analytics, you can use many hierarchical dimensions to describe people, such as manager hierarchy, financial unit hierarchy (cost center hierarchy), location unit hierarchy, or job unit hierarchy. The details vary by company, based on what the units are called and the complexity of the unit relationship structure.

TIP

Start with the method of segmenting business units used by your executives for the purposes of finance and accounting. I refer to this as the financial unit hierarchy, but it may be described using different words at your company. (Most often it is called cost center or business unit structure.)

Here's an example of how a single individual can be found in a location hierarchy:

Location hierarchy example

Region = "North America"

   Country = "United States"

      City = "Mountain View"

         Location = "401 Castro Street"

            Floor = "3"

               Desk = "401-3-5901" Employee = "John Smith" ID = "11158"

This outline illustrates that there are six possible levels to describe the geographic location of John Smith. The example reflects a hierarchical tree for one person. Of course, there are many more people in a company. You can count the number of people by any of the levels in this hierarchical structure — each level will contain multiple segments and each segment will contain multiple people (except for the very bottom). Using this example, you can count the number of people by region, country, city, location, or location by floor if you want to. For example, at your company you may find only two countries you can count by but twenty different cities you can count by. If your company is in two countries, then you have only two segments to compare. If you count by city, then you have twenty segments to compare. From this example you can say that you can choose many different ways to count, even if we are only talking about location.

In Figure 4-3, you can see that the company has 2,000 employees in North America, 1,800 employees in the United States, 980 employees in Mountain View, 500 employees at the building at 401 Castro Street, 200 employees on the third floor, and one employee, at desk 401-3-5901, named John Smith.

As Figure 4-3 illustrates, each person exists only once; however, the same person can be described in many different hierarchical segment structures. Here are three other ways to describe where John Smith is in the company:

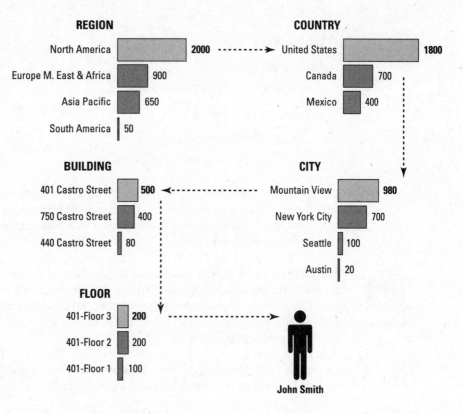

FIGURE 4-3:
You can keep
slicing the pie
until you get no
more pieces.

Financial unit hierarchy

Division = "Sales Division"

    Organization = "Enterprise Go-Team"

      Department = "Widgets"

        Cost Center Name = "Widgets – Southwest Territory"

          Employee = "John Smith", ID = "11158"

Manager hierarchy

CEO = "Sally Rodgers"

    VP = "Bob Woodward"

      Director = "Chris Henderson"

      Manager = "George Harris"

        Employee = "John Smith", ID = "11158"

Job hierarchy

Job Function = "Sales"

   Job Level = "Individual Contributor"

     Job Family = "Inside Sales"

       Job = "Inside Sales Rep 3"

         Employee = "John Smith", ID = "11158"

When conducting each analysis, you decide the right level of summarization that's useful for your analysis. For example, you can count by Division, Location or Job or any combination. All math and science begins with counting. What you count is determined by context and need.

REMEMBER

When you first begin reporting data, you will find lots of inconsistencies between data that's recorded in systems and what is in different people's minds. Without a place to store data, an agreed segmentation structure and regular reporting, what you and anyone else sees in their mind's eye is likely to be very different. Counting provides perspective.

In a certain light, the reconciliation between our mind, others' minds, and the data that is stored in systems is the point of analytics.

Creating Calculated Segments

Most of the segments I describe earlier in this chapter exist as a single entry in a database structure: for example, Division = "Sales" or Department = "Inside Sales". In the earlier examples, no calculation is involved in creating a segment — the segment is simply found in the system in the exact way it's described.

As you might have suspected, other types of segmentation are out there — more specifically, ones that require calculation. In the next few sections, I walk you through a few examples.

Company tenure

The graph showing company head count by tenure, as shown in Figure 4-4, looks like data that just comes out of a system the way it is. However, tenure is a calculated field that results in continuous data, which wouldn't look good on a graph the way it is. If tenure is calculated as the number of days since an employee started the graph would have as many bars as there are people because everyone would have a different tenure. It would therefore show nothing useful. However, if you take the tenure calculation and create a new variable that describes tenure as a category characterized by ranges of days (0 to 365 days, 366 to 730 days, and so on) then you can count people that fit within a range of days to produce a graph that has a more useful number of segments to produce insight.

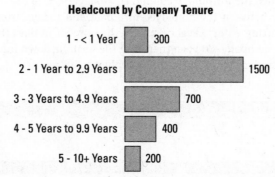

Headcount by Company Tenure

FIGURE 4-4:
Company head count, with all employees categorized into tenure group categories.

For example, you may want to count the number of people in their first year of employment. What you have in the HRIS is *start date*. Tenure can be calculated by counting the number of days between *start date* and *current date* and expressing it as the number of days or years or months. You might find people with 1.1 years, 1.5 years, 1.7 years, .89 years, .5 years, 20.7 years, and so on. Counting by data in this way wouldn't produce a good graph, because everyone's number would be unique. To graph by tenure, you need to count the number of people who fall within a range. Figure 4-4 uses the following five ranges:

Tenure =

< 1 Year

1 Year to 2.9 Years

3 Years to 4.9 Years

5 Years to 9.9 Years

10+ Years

Depending on whether you're working in Excel or SQL (a database querying language) or another data environment, the formula is different. You also always have more than one way to do anything with data. For example, to count all people in their first year of tenure, you could create a formula that first calculates tenure and then another formula that count those whose tenure is less than 1 year. The logic works like this: If tenure < 1.0 years, then assign a 1 or else assign a 0. Then sum.

To see how you'd do this calculation in Excel, check out Figures 4-5, 4-6, 4-7, and 4-8 below.

In Figure 4-5, you see a simplified employee roster that's been exported into Excel, where each row represents a unique currently active employee and each column represents a data fact about that employee. Column C is the employee hire date. I have added the formula in column D, =today()-C2, to calculate the number of days tenure between the employee hire date and today. After inputting this formula and hitting enter, Excel calculates the number of days the employee has worked for the company. You can then drag the formula down into the other rows or use other standard Excel functions to apply it to all rows.

FIGURE 4-5: Calculating employee tenure from Hire Date in Excel.

ID	Name	Hire Date	Tenure (days)	Location	Dept	Org	Grade	Title	Manager ID	Manager	Avg Perf
A6A000402	Destinee Hill	11/28/18	=today()-C2	Remote	Logistics	Operations	AO5	Director Of Logistics	A6A100291	Nick Esparza	4.50
A6A000525	Quinten Forbes	5/5/17		San Francisco	SW Infrastructure	Software Engineering	T4	Staff Software Engineer	A6A100424	Kaylynn Hanson	4.10
A6A000394	Sabrina Burns	10/19/16		San Francisco	CTO	CTO	T2	UX Researcher	A6A100002	Charlie Moon	3.50
A6A000386	Eden Medina	10/15/16		San Francisco	Health SW	Software Engineering	T4	Sr Systems Engineer	A6A000201	Alden Thomas	3.55
A6A000384	Nylah Bryan	6/10/17		San Francisco	Facilities	People Operations	A	Office Coordinator	A6A000468	Yusuf Riggs	3.90
A6A000372	Kieran Shaw	3/17/18		San Francisco	Health SW	Software Engineering	T3	Sr Software Engineer - Web	A6A000370	Izaiah Whitaker	3.60
A6A000378	Alec Warner	3/19/16		Sunnyvale	EPM	Hardware Engineering	T4	Engineering Program Manager	A6A000585	Marcos Yates	3.43
A6A100177	Draven Johnson	5/16/17		Pittsburgh	Clinical SW	Software Engineering	T4	Lead Software Developer	A6A100063	Drake Barry	3.20
A6A000382	Parker Gibson	10/7/16		San Francisco	Product Experience	Product Experience	E8	Exec Director Product Design	A6A100312	Shyla Phelps	4.80
A6A000965	Austin Pennington	7/7/17		Sunnyvale	Quality	Hardware Engineering	T4	Sr Quality Assurance Manager	A6A100001	Tony Melendez	3.20
A6A047830	Moses Oliver	12/30/16		EMEA	Sales EMEA	Sales	E6	Director Business Planning	A6A2705BN	Amaya Barton	4.20
A6A120320	Jessica Vaughn	1/12/18		Sunnyvale	Quality	Hardware Engineering	T3	Product Quality Engineer	A6A000595	Austin Pennington	3.45
A6A000228	Charlie Flores	1/29/15		San Francisco	HR	People Operations	AO2	Human Resources Coordinator	A6A000437	Jace Carney	3.20
A6A000900	Jonas Browning	7/28/17		San Francisco	Analytics	Product Management	B6	Director Analytics	A6A000171	Megan Valdez	3.10
A6A100258	Perla Payne	5/16/17		Remote	Sales US	Sales	B5	Director, Business Dev Lifestyle Pr	A6A100410	Javier Cisneros	3.30
A6A000965	Madelynn Wiley	8/6/16		Sunnyvale	Facilities	People Operations	A	Sr Facilities Coordinator	A6A100422	Alexis Montoya	3.80
A6A2895SN	Talon Wolfe	5/22/17		EMEA	Sales EMEA	Sales	S6	Head of Sales France Benelux	A6A58174N	Davin Hodge	2.85
A6A100249	Nyla Wilkerson	5/16/17		San Francisco	CTO	CTO	T53	Manager Adv Dev & Research Par	A6A100002	Charlie Moon	3.63
A6A42790N	Madden Cochran	12/4/15		China	Mfg Engineering	Hardware Engineering	T4	Operations Engineering Mgr	A6A001013	Madeline Tyler	3.55
A6A000198	Jaylin Harding	9/5/14		Sunnyvale	Software QA	Software Engineering	T56	Director Device Quality Assurance	A6A000148	Yurem Pruitt	3.17
A6A000413	Abigayle Cunningham	6/29/18		San Francisco	Health SW	Software Engineering	T52	Software QA Engineer	A6A000410	Kendal Kaufman	3.00
A6A100529	Rylee Olson	2/1/18		San Francisco	Procurement	Operations	B5	Global Supply Manager	A6A000997	Kristina Pierce	3.40
A6A000014	Salma Elliott	5/16/17		Pittsburgh	CTO	CTO	T6	Director HW Dev Mobile Lifestyle	A6A100002	Charlie Moon	4.40
A6A061566	Raphael Osborne	12/25/15		China	HR	People Operations	B3	Human Resources Generalist	A6A000287	Roland Ayers	3.40
A6A100248	Aurora Nixon	5/16/17		Pittsburgh	MIS	People Operations	T2	Ecommerce Developer	A6A100092	Damon Christian	3.57
A6A000463	Bailey Vaughn	1/28/17		San Francisco	Health SW	Software Engineering	T54	Sr Software Engineer In Test	A6A000410	Kendal Kaufman	3.45
A6A00327N	Jase Blankenship	10/7/16		China	Quality	Hardware Engineering	T3	Sr Supplier Quality Engineer	A6A29501N	Terrance Oneal	3.05
A6A000428	Alonzo Spencer	4/21/17		San Francisco	Product Experience	Product Experience	B3	Project Manager	A6A000472	Miracle Harris	3.80
A6A000012	Dayana Wang	12/10/16		Sunnyvale	HR	People Operations	AO4	Recruiter	A6A000477	Jace Carney	3.53
A6A000559	Gideon Lara	6/2/17		San Francisco	Sales US	Sales	B3	Execution Project Manager	A6A100410	Javier Cisneros	3.20
A6A001008	Davian Dalton	10/22/02		Sunnyvale	OSP	Software Engineering	T6	Media/DSP Architect	A6A000077	Ryder Carey	4.60
A6A000112	Leon Larsen	9/20/13		Sunnyvale	Systems Engr	Hardware Engineering	T4	Director Of Program Management	A6A000513	Leila Downs	2.85
	Judah Morse	5/26/17		San Francisco	Research	Product Management	B6	Director Customer Exp & Mkt Insig	A6A000171	Megan Valdez	3.35

With Figure 4-5, you can see employee tenure; however, this is not a perfect end state. In Figure 4-6 below, I add a formula to column E, which divides the number of days found in column D by 365 so you can see employee tenure converted into years.

Having employee tenure in years is useful, and yet you can see that almost every employee has a different tenure. If you were to count now by column E, you would not get a useful table or graph. In this example, what you want to do is count those employees with tenure less than 1 year. What I do in Figure 4-7 below is use the Formula Builder to add an if-then statement to column F. What the if-then statement does is add a 1 to column F if tenure (calculated in column E) is less than 1 or a 0 if tenure is equal to or greater than 1.

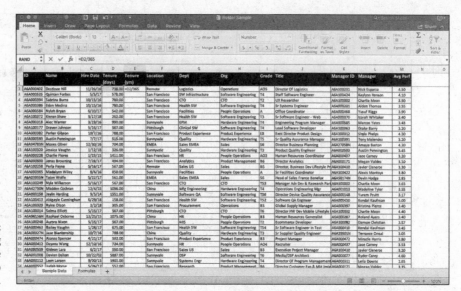

FIGURE 4-6:
Converting
employee tenure
from days into
years in Excel.

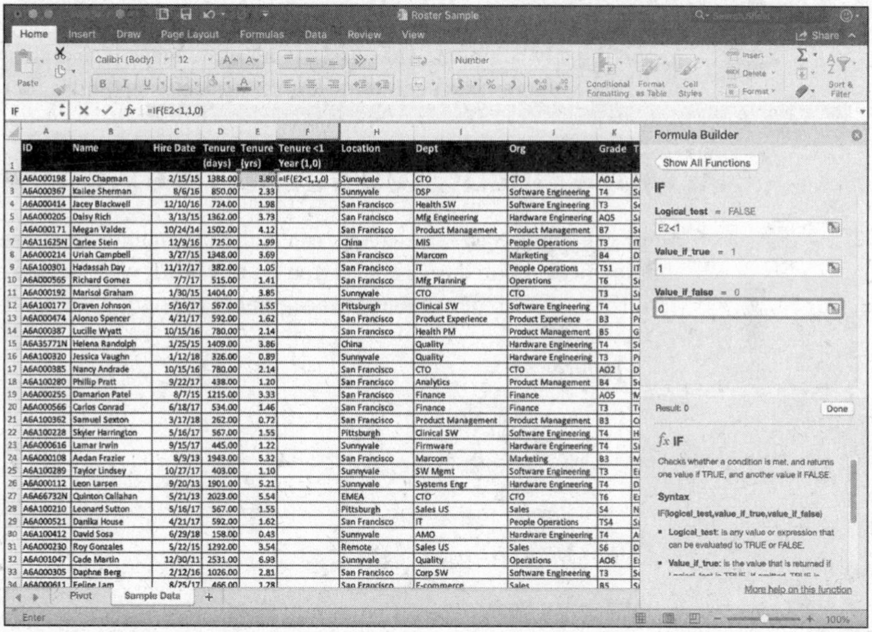

FIGURE 4-7:
Adding an
if-then
statement.

Continuing with this illustration, you can see in Figure 4-8 that I have extended the if-then statement to all rows in column F and highlighted some example rows for individuals that have less than 1-year tenure.

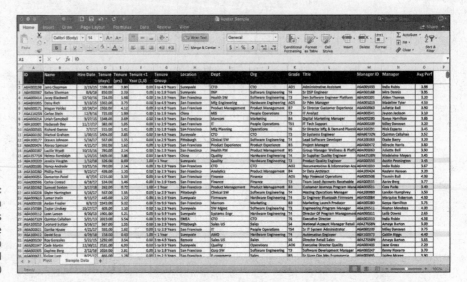

FIGURE 4-8:
Employees with
tenure less
than 1 year are
indicated with
a 1 and all
others a 0

TIP

Assigning a 1 or 0 to a data point changes continuous data into categorical data. A formula like this one may be embedded in the HRIS or in your analytics and reporting environments that assigns all employees into a classification segment and then changes this segmentation dynamically as tenure increases.

More calculated segment examples

Here are some fast-and-quick calculated segments that are useful for most employment-related analysis. If you do any work with people analytics, you will find that you use these calculated segments over and over again:

Tenure

> < 1 Year

> 1 Year to 2.9 Years

> 3 Years to 4.9 Years

> 5 Years to 9.9 Years

> 10+ Years

Total job experience

> < 5 Years

> 5 Years to 9.9 Years

> 10 Years to 14.9 Years

15 Years to 20 Years

20+ Years

Generation cohort

WWII and Silent Generation

Baby Boomer

Gen X

Gen Y — millennial

U.S. minority status (simple classification of ethnicity into two segments)

Minority

Non-Minority

Base Pay

>$100K

$76K to $100K

$51K to $75K

$25K to $50K

<$25K

Market pay group – variation A

>60th Percentile

40th to 60th Percentile

<40th Percentile

Market pay group – variation B

>75th Percentile

25th to 75th Percentile

<25th Percentile

Market pay group – variation C

>90th Percentile

10th to 90th Percentile

<10th Percentile

Cross-Tabbing for Insight

This section outlines how to get started working with data in segments. Cross tab-bing (also called cross-tabulation or cross-tab) is putting data together in a table in a particular way that allows you see if there is a relationship among variables. A basic cross tab puts one method of segmentation on the columns and one method of segmentation on the rows. You use a cross tab if you want to compare the similarities or differences of segments as divided by some other segment. For example, what proportion of employees in each division are men or women? Or do sales employees exit the company disproportionately to the size of their division when compared to the exit rate of other divisions? These and many other ques-tions can be answered without further complication by simply constructing cross-tab table and reviewing the numbers.

Setting up a dataset for cross-tabs

The key to working successfully with cross-tabs is to do the prep work correctly. This usually involves these two major steps:

1. Extract the data from wherever it is.

2. Organize the data in a way that is useful for reporting and analysis, using either a statistical application or a spreadsheet.

TIP

The majority of analysts extract data from a company's HRIS and work with data in Excel. Eventually, you should replace Excel with a more robust and permanent reporting solution; however, it's a great place to get started.

You may have fields where categorical descriptive information is contained that you need to change into numbers — location, for example. For each employee, you find 1 of 20 different locations. If you want to analyze U.S. versus non-U.S., you can create another field, named US–Reference, and make the value a 1 for any employee at a location in the U.S. and a 0 for any other location. Then you can count U.S. or use that variable in any other more advanced statistical procedure.

Table 4-1 shows you what I mean, by representing a few records from a simple dataset.

In the table, all U.S. locations were coded as 1 and those outside the U.S. were coded as 0. Also, I took the 0–10 Likelihood to Recommend the Company variable and added another variable (Likelihood to Recommend: High Reference (0,1), which indicates 1 when Likelihood to Recommend is greater than 7 and 0 if not.

A Simple Dataset

ID	Division	Location	US-Reference (0,1)	Likelihood to Recommend the Company (0–10)	Likelihood to Recommend: High Reference (0,1)
14568	Sales	Remote: Phoenix, AZ	1	9	1
21456	Engineering	Mountain View	1	2	0
11358	Operations	Dublin, Ireland	0	4	0

Getting started with cross-tabs

When a dataset is organized in a table, the next step is to count by "crossing" two or more variables against each other — known as creating a cross-tab. Cross-tabbing helps you see the interactions between two variables by explicitly revealing that some measured characteristics usually appear (or do not appear) in conjunction with other characteristics.

In the example in Table 4-2, you cross two columns from table 4-1 with each other into a two-dimensional table: Division by Likelihood to Recommend: High Reference.

Each cell in Table 4-2 contains the number of employees who fit the category listed as the row heading and the column heading. The 300 employees in Sales, for example, rated the company higher than 7 on Likelihood to Recommend, which was thus coded as a 1 in Likelihood to Recommend: High Reference.

TABLE 4-2 **Working with Two Variables**

	Likelihood to Recommend: High Reference = 1	Likelihood to Recommend: High Reference = 0	Row Total
Sales	300	150	450
Engineering	260	189	449
Operations	130	130	260
Column total	**690**	**469**	**1159**

The next step is to convert the numbers in Table 4-2 into percentages. You can calculate the percentage of rows or columns or the overall total, depending on what you want to know.

In Table 4-3, I calculated the percentage of each row, which tells you the percentage of each division segment that is likely to recommend the company. I used this formula:

Percentage of employees in cell = ((number of employees in cell) ÷ (number of employees in row total)) × 100

You can draw a lot of information from Table 4-3. For example, there appears to be some association between Division and Likelihood to Recommend the Company. Twice as many sales associates would recommend the company over those who would not, whereas the Engineering and Operations groups don't fare as well among their employees.

TABLE 4-3   **Percentage of Row Total**

	Likelihood to Recommend: High Reference = 1	Likelihood to Recommend: High Reference = 0	Row Total
Sales	67%	33%	**100%**
Engineering	58%	42%	**100%**
Operations	50%	50%	**100%**
Column Total	**60%**	**40%**	**100%**

USING SEGMENT DEFINITIONS TO DEFUSE DATA QUALITY CONCERNS

Very often, bad data is entered into systems, and there's nothing that the systems or the systems people can do about that. You have probably heard the term *garbage-in, garbage-out* get thrown around among systems people. It simply means that if you add bad data to a database when you report from that database, the data will still be bad.

At other times, the data in the system is technically accurate, but when it comes to reporting that data, the choices you make may make the data appear wrong to others. When people make different choices, they get different answers — it's as simple as that. When data won't perfectly compare, sometimes people assume that there's a data quality problem when the two reports may simply be using two different definitions.

Usually, disagreements about the data you're using come to the fore when you report to a group of executives. They may say, "We don't have 30 people in that group" or "Finance showed us a report with head count yesterday, and on their report it said 15 and yours says 10 — yours must be wrong." Often, the answer lies simply in the definition of *head count:* Finance may be counting contractors plus employees, whereas you may be counting only employees, for example.

There are many ways in which people can be included or excluded that could result in different numbers. Your dataset for head count can be affected by any of these factors:

- Employees and/or contractors
- Full-time and/or part-time
- U.S. and/or non-U.S.
- Exempt and/or non-exempt
- Regular and/or temporary workers

As if that weren't enough, here are even *more* ways to affect headcount:

- **Date:** Often, you get a different count, depending on the date the data was pulled. People are always coming and going, which means that one day may be different from the next. Do you count the number of people at the beginning of the period or at the end of the period, or do you use an average? Do you pull head count on the day you present? If all reports are run at exactly the same time, they have a better chance of matching — but they usually aren't run at the same time.

- **Fractions:** You can count part-time employees as partials based on the hours worked (.3) or count each one as (.5) or count them as a whole, just like a full-time employee (1), or you might not count them at all. As they add up on your report, you will end up with a different number.

- **Hierarchy choices:** If you're counting employees by a unit, you might count them by the financial structure definition of that unit (Example Sales), or you might count them as being anyone under the head of that financial structure unit (everyone that reports to managers that report to directors that report to the Vice President of Sales John Smith). You may think that these two methods should give you the same answer, but it may not — and it usually doesn't.

Work with others to create a standard definition or to make your own definition clear. You'll have valid reasons to count things in different ways.

Good Advice for Segmenting

Here are some additional tips you can use to create accurate and useful employee segmentation:

» **Tackle one task at a time.** Don't try to try to do everything at once. You'll become overwhelmed, as will the people you seek to share data with.

» **Focus your efforts.** Start with some research objectives, hypotheses, and questions to answer before you spend a lot of time on the data.

» **Be open-minded.** You may begin with a particular segmentation scheme, but it may evoke a new question, and you may need to add additional segments to your report to answer the new question.

» **Remember that segmentation can help you see things you might not have otherwise seen or thought to ask.** After collecting any data, most good researchers run reports by a bunch of fundamental segments, just to get a sense of what is going on in the data.

» **Expand your outlook.** By that, I mean that you shouldn't confine your segmentation design to only the data from a single data source. Many important people-related insights come from data found in transient sources like employee surveys. Assuming that you have collected and stored data the right way, there's no reason you shouldn't be able to combine data from multiple sources. Having data from multiple sources vastly increases the possibilities for segmentation and analysis.

» **If you're sharing data with others, pick out the most important segments to share based on what you have to communicate.** Leave out information that's interesting but that may, in the grand scheme, seem trivial or nonessential. Put segment data that you don't plan to present live in an appendix or another location that you can access quickly in case you need it to address questions.

There are a variety of ways you can segment employee data for the purposes of reporting and analysis. The options for segmentation are constrained only by the facts you collect (location, start date, and pay, for example) and your imagination. Imagination is important to help you figure out how you can use data to answer questions and how to get new data when necessary. If you don't have the data that you need in order to create a segment you want to create, you can use your imagination to find a way to get it. The options for segmentation are therefore infinite. What you do with segmentation should be determined by your purpose — the questions you want to answer — not by what has coincidentally been recorded in a system.

Chapter **5**

Finding Useful Insight in Differences

When I talk to leaders of human resources about unsuccessful early experiences with data in HR, most of the time I hear something like this: "We have lots of data, but we aren't getting any useful insights from it." They had been relying on the (mistaken) idea that having a lot of data at their fingertips would provide them with a lot of answers, and instead they found that the data they have simply doesn't speak to anyone, so no one is using it. For them, the big question is this: Does the lack of useful insight from the HR data stem from the quality of the analyst, the quality of the systems they are using, or the quality of the data itself?

I suggest another way of looking at the issue. The issue may not be any of those things — the issue may be an unclear problem focus. The goal of people analytics is to produce useful insight — to see a problem in a new and different way so that you can move past the problem toward new opportunities. Getting useful insights from data requires more than just the ability to perform a series of data tasks well — it also requires applying critical thinking to focus your effort on a worthwhile problem for the company. The real issue may not be the analyst, the quality of the systems, or the quality of the data itself — the real issue may be an absence of a specific problem focus.

REMEMBER

All data is useful for some purpose and yet, not for all purposes. Depending on what question you are trying to answer, some data is disproportionately useful, and some data is useless. Some data will help you and some data won't. Some data tasks will propel you forward, and some data tasks won't. There's no universal project plan to apply to determine what data is useful or what you should do with it — you have to determine what data you need and what you need to do with it based on which problem you're trying to solve. If you jump right into a bunch of tasks like system selection, system implementation, data collection, data cleanup, data governance, statistical methods, and/or visualization without first defining a clear focus, you are not likely to turn up anything useful at all.

So how do you define a clear focus? In this chapter you will learn how rummaging around a little in strategy first can help you find a focus to get more out of your data.

Defining Strategy

The word strategy is often used in vague and useless ways. Let me provide a definition. The word *strategy* originated in the military and has been most vividly illustrated in warfare. Here's the current U.S. military definition of strategy:

> *The art and science of developing and using political, economic, psychological, and military forces as necessary during peace and war, to afford the maximum support to policies in order to increase the probabilities and favorable consequences of victory and to lessen the chances of defeat.*

Companies compete with each other. Companies compete for customers. Companies compete for product and service superiority. Companies also compete for people; especially those they perceive to be the best people.

It should probably go without saying that winning would be easy if there were no competitor. When no competition exists, there's no need to strategize. Inversely, when competition does exist, you need strategy. Since in business there is competition, you need strategy.

Keniche Ohmae, the acclaimed Japanese business strategist and author of *The Mind of the Strategist,* has said that "the sole purpose of strategy is to enable a company to gain, as efficiently as possible, a sustainable edge over its competitors."

Clearly strategy entails creating differences that increase the odds of success or decrease the odds of failure.

Often in human resources, companies seek a universal set of people, programs, practices, or processes that they believe will lead to a business advantage. But if all companies pursue the same tactics then there is no advantage. Unfortunately, this means there is no universal set of best HR practices that will lead to a "permanent business advantage". As military history's greatest leaders have shown, there's no permanently best advantage, strategy, or set of tactics that will always lead to victory. The only certainty in competition is change. This is one big reason you need constant factual feedback (using data) that informs the actions you take and measures the results you get.

If HR strategy is one side of the coin, people analytics is the other. HR strategy is about carefully choosing a series of objectives that create advantages that tilt odds in your favor to achieve a primary objective: that is, helping your company be better than anyone else at something. People analytics provides a factual perspective to measure progress against your objective, whatever that objective may be. The advantage people analytics provides is in the ability to react with superior actions based on superior information. Superior information provides an advantage because it allows you to adapt your actions faster and more effectively than your opponents.

Here is my technical definition of people analytics that reflect a more complete picture of both the actions of people analytics and the purpose:

> The systematic application of science and statistics to people strategy to achieve probabilistic business advantages.

In chapter 1, I introduce people analytics as what exists at the intersection of behavior science, people technology systems, statistics and people strategy – I call these the *Four S People Analytics Framework*. (See Figure 5-1 for a representation of this framework.)

The premise of the Four S People Analytics Framework is that each of the areas of capability described — science, systems, statistics and strategy — make some valuable contribution to the application of people analytics to produce repeatable results. If you leave any of these Four S's out, you get some deficiency. Figure 5-2 represents the problem you find if you are attempting to do the work of people analytics without the appropriate context and HR domain expertise represented by the strategy component of the Four S framework.

In this context, strategy represents the domain expertise that is required to direct and absorb the efforts of the three remaining S's: science, statistics, and systems. The absence of a grounding in strategy results in a lot of work but produces a result that is not particularly useful to anyone. If you are doing a lot of work with data but nobody is using the end result, then it indicates you most likely missed the strategy part.

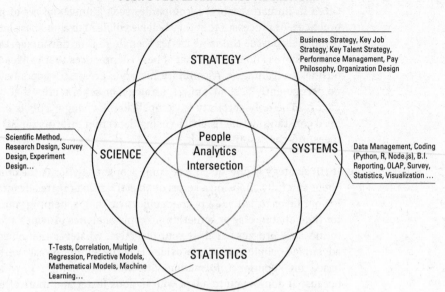

FOUR S PEOPLE ANALYTICS FRAMEWORK

STRATEGY

Business Strategy, Key Job Strategy, Key Talent Strategy, Performance Management, Pay Philosophy, Organization Design

Scientific Method, Research Design, Survey Design, Experiment Design…

SCIENCE

People Analytics Intersection

SYSTEMS

Data Management, Coding (Python, R, Node.js), B.I. Reporting, OLAP, Survey, Statistics, Visualization …

FIGURE 5-1: The Four S People Analytics Framework

T-Tests, Correlation, Multiple Regression, Predictive Models, Mathematical Models, Machine Learning…

STATISTICS

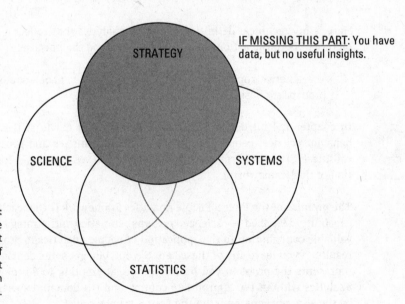

STRATEGY

IF MISSING THIS PART: You have data, but no useful insights.

SCIENCE

SYSTEMS

FIGURE 5-2: Missing the strategy part results in a lot of activity without a clear problem focus.

STATISTICS

REMEMBER

A common pitfall in any analytics project, including people analytics, is to get busy working on data because that sounds like the right thing to do but without knowing why you're doing what you are doing and in what context you will spend all your time shuffling data around from place to place and produce nothing of much use from it. Getting useful insights out of people analytics should begin by picking a problem focus that is useful to the company first, and only once that is settled get busy on data. The problem focus will inform the questions you have and the data you need to answer those questions. This workflow is very different from picking some data you happen to have on hand and getting busy on that data to see whether you can find something useful to share.

Focusing on product differentiators

If you have a specific business or people problem that is obvious or that someone has asked you to work on, by all means feel free to skip this chapter and start precisely on the work you have been asked to do. If nobody has provided you with a specific business or people problem focus to work on, then start here.

What is the product, service, or customer category your business wants to win? The answer to this question can become a focal point for your people strategy and your people analysis to provide the factual details as to how you are doing.

Differentiation is the heartbeat of strategy as well as the primary reason for business success or failure. Your company's area of product differentiation is how your company sets itself apart from all other companies that compete to sell a similar product. Continually winning the affection of your customers requires that you identify a specific intent to be different and create people advantages to carry out this intent.

Here are some examples:

>> You may have a *customer delight* difference, such as that practiced by Southwest Airlines. By hiring people who are fun and arming them with company values and policies that remind them to not take themselves too seriously, Southwest motivates employees to take pride in making travel fun, which translates to establishing a different experience for customers. Southwest may not be good at everything an airline can do, but they have deliberately chosen to be good at finding ways to make people who fly with them smile.

>> You may have an *innovation* difference, such as the one characterized by large successful technology companies like Google. Google knows that, as a technology company, its employees need to work to create the future — or someone else will steal their lunch. Google recognizes that creating the future's Next Great Product starts with great engineering talent — that's why the company makes extraordinary investments to acquire, engage, and retain people with extraordinary technical competence.

>> You may have a *product marketing* focus, such as the one practiced by Apple. Apple products are often markedly different from their competitors, based on the quality of the product design. To keep that streak going, Apple hires great design talent. Apple hires a lot of other people too, but it is more important to Apple's success to obtain the people who are best in the world at design. The result is that Apple may not lead the way in creating the fastest product or the most flexible product, but it is leading the way in design. This is a choice that Apple's leaders made that is reflected in where they focus their attention.

Maybe your intended company differentiator is one of the things I have stated above or maybe it is something else entirely. Maybe it is several things. Maybe it is something your company is trying to find again or change right now. From the outside looking in, it is sometimes hard to tell what the chosen differentiators are, but I believe all businesses that are successful over the long term have at least one thing they have decided they are going to be really good at. If it is not obvious to you already, you should get away from your desk to spend some with other people figuring this question out, and, if you can get their time, you should talk in particular to the executives.

Every company makes a series of decisions about how it wants to turn resources, raw materials, and the input of people into a product or service. This is what is sometimes called a *value chain*. Figure 5-3 spells out the series of simple questions you can use to try to get a picture of the way your company works.

BUSINESS VALUE CREATION MODEL

Clarify the chain of logic through which intangible assets will be transformed to tangible value.

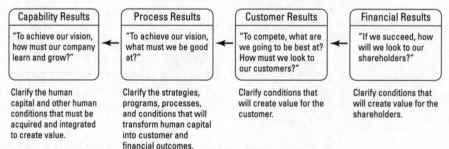

FIGURE 5-3: The chain of logic through which intangible assets will be transformed into tangible value.

Capability Results	Process Results	Customer Results	Financial Results
"To achieve our vision, how must our company learn and grow?"	"To achieve our vision, what must we be good at?"	"To compete, what are we going to be best at? How must we look to our customers?"	"If we succeed, how will we look to our shareholders?"
Clarify the human capital and other human conditions that must be acquired and integrated to create value.	Clarify the strategies, programs, processes, and conditions that will transform human capital into customer and financial outcomes.	Clarify conditions that will create value for the customer.	Clarify conditions that will create value for the shareholders.

Before your company can produce a product or service that is different than that of your competitors — and is superior in some way — you must acquire and engage the necessary capabilities in people that are required to produce a product or service that is different — and superior in some way — to that of your competitors. At some level, all business strategy rests on people. It starts and ends with people, but the question is, how do you create a real difference in people?

Sometimes just thinking about the value chain and mapping it out can help you figure out where your company seeks to be different in some way.

Identifying key jobs

When asked, most executives will say one of the main reasons the company they manage is better is because they have better people than everyone else. Well, if most executives say this, then it can't be true. Who is telling the truth, and who is lying? How do you know? How does your company produce better people than average? How do you keep them? Is there anything remarkably different about the way you approach people than anyone else? How do you define better? How do you measure it? Don't be discouraged; you can help your company answer these questions and more, but you need to help your company get a lot more specific first.

If you think you can be best at everything, then go for it — be best at everything. Unfortunately, if you try to be best at everything, usually you end up being not very good at anything. For this reason, *customer segmentation* is already an accepted and core concept in business strategy. Segmentation can also be a useful concept for human resources strategy. Segmentation can help you get a lot more focused. By finding observable differences, you can help your executives clarify the range of choices and determine where you are succeeding and where you are failing.

The answer to what is best will at a minimum vary by type of job. If you mix jobs together, you will not get a clear answer. What makes a good chef is probably not the same thing that makes a good host or waiter. What makes a good accountant is probably not what makes a good manager. These examples are arbitrary, but you get the point. People analytics is the tool you can use to see the ways that jobs are different, the ways people are different, and connect the two. If you have more information about a job and about how people with different characteristics perform in that job, you can encourage those characteristics that support success to create advantages as a company.

If you understand how jobs differ, you can get a better answer about what good and bad looks like for a particular job. The way you determine how jobs differ is through something called *job analysis*. If your company has not done job analysis before (or not recently) you should start there and head straight to Chapter 13. Job analysis will provide you with information about how jobs differ and allow you to create meaningful job segmentation breaks.

Assuming you have done some job analysis or have some other way of classifying all jobs at your company into categories, here is the next question you can answer to help you with focus. What jobs are most pivotal to your success as a company, given the current business strategy and intended nature of product superiority? What are the key jobs, in other words? For Southwest Airlines, a key job is the flight attendant because they represent Southwest's spirit to the customer. For Merck, a key job is a scientist because they find the scientific breakthroughs that lead to the next blockbuster drug. For PetSmart, a key job is dog trainer because they provide valued services that draw customers into stores. For Children's Health Dallas (a children's hospital), a key job is nurse because so much of the patient experience and care is delivered through the careful attention of nurses. For Google, a key job is the software engineer because they create the future. This doesn't mean that other jobs are not important in some way too. It's just a matter of emphasis and focus. You have to be really good at something, and you have to start somewhere.

After you have identified a job or set of jobs where amassing success will have a clear benefit to your company based on business strategy, then you can move on to looking for important questions you can answer with data to help your company win. This way of working with data will by definition produce useful insights.

TIP

I am not saying that you should only focus your analysis on one job permanently. It could be five important jobs, 20 important jobs or some other number. There is no set specific number. Maybe over time you can amass enough analysis to cover all jobs. I'm just saying it is helpful to begin with a focus — this being the case, you should start somewhere important first.

Identifying the characteristics of key talent

After you have identified the jobs where you want to focus your attention, the next question should be, "What would describe the ideal or perfect employee in these key jobs?" In other words, if someone who knew a lot about this job could pick one person from an ocean of talent, whom would they pick and most importantly, why? If no one can describe what is good and what is bad, you can't measure it. If you can't measure good and bad, you can't consistently create good.

REMEMBER

Jobs are not made the same, people are not made the same, and no one person would be good in all jobs — people and jobs have different characteristics. It is getting the combination right that opens up the door to success.

Imagine that all your competitors have suddenly decided to lay off all their employees. Now you alone are the only employer for people in your particular product or service niche. You cannot hire everyone, nor do you want to, but you have the pick. Whom would you pick, how would you select the people you pick, and what impact would it have on your future ability to win? How are these people different from others?

Would they be experienced employees of another company with some specific job title? Or would they be students from a particular university that you respect?

Would they have a proven track record of success? Is it something observable from a résumé, or would you have to ask questions to draw it out? Is it a particular personality type? Does it require a certain type of cognitive ability? Do they know certain things that other people don't know? Do they behave in ways that are different from others?

Now suppose that you have an answer to these questions. How did you arrive at the answer? Did you guess? Did you go with your gut? Did someone else give you the answer? My apologies for all the questions (you might think you're on a job interview), but the fact of the matter is that the questions are important because your answers determine the fate of the people who want to work for your company and the fate of your company. What I'm trying to get at here is that, yes, you use hard data to have better answers, but it starts with better questions. If you don't know the questions you don't have any chance of collecting the right data or knowing what to do with it once you have it.

WARNING

In marketing, they often use demographic variables like gender, ethnicity, age, socioeconomic status, and family characteristics in developing a target persona. In human resources, you can track these variables to measure and assess how you are doing with diversity, but you cannot use these variables for hiring. Instead, you should use reliable, validated job-related criteria. What you use to target hires has to relate to job success or you shouldn't be using it.

More often than not, the most important segmentation method for identifying, engaging, and retaining key talent may be the hardest to see from the outside. It is what is going on inside the mind that usually matters the most. People have unique personalities, knowledge, skills, abilities, experiences, and preferences that interact with a stimulus and an environment to influence the probability of success or failure. The patterns are recognizable, predictable, and influenceable, but with people you need a strategy to move information that is on the inside of the mind to the outside of the mind so that you can use it. For more on how you can achieve this feat, see Chapters 12, 13 and 14.

Measuring If Your Company is Concentrating Its Resources

Flowing naturally from a clarity about business differentiation and people differentiation is concentration. In the past, HR teams tried to please many different stakeholders, in the process spreading their resources thinly over too many areas and, as such, diluting the effectiveness of those resources to accomplish any single objective. In the past, many of the objectives of the HR leadership team were disconnected from —and, in some cases, in conflict with — one another, thus diminishing their overall effectiveness. The concept of concentration is an increasing part of modern people strategy because it is more effective.

Concentrating spending on key jobs

I recall, when I was working at a national pet retailer in a particularly difficult year, they faced a dilemma: If they distributed the entire annual pay increase budget among all retail employees evenly, the increase would amount to about 10 cents per hour, which was a whopping $2 per week for a part-time employee. That is less than the cost of a latte. Yet the cost for the pet retailer to provide everyone with that half-latte pay increase would be in the many millions of dollars. Unfortunately, the half-latte method of allocating the budget would have no positive impact on the company's success or employees' lives — spreading the money out this thinly would actually benefit no one.

The pet retailer as a whole benefited much more by investing its limited budget into creating more expensive but higher profit-producing service roles — like dog trainers, dog groomers, and doggie day care attendants — that were a differentiator for the pet retailer, brought more people into the store, and produced higher margins. When all was said and done, concentrating its spare budget on more important service roles first gave the pet retailer more money to spend on other employees over the long run.

REMEMBER

Concentrating resources on services was a good strategy for the pet retailer for reasons specific to their business strategy and situation but may not be the best approach for you. All companies have important differentiating jobs that do for their company what the service jobs do for the pet retailer; you just need to figure out what those important differentiating jobs are for your company.

A useful focus for people analytics insight is to use your compensation data, job analysis data, and decisions about job importance to analyze if the way the company is spending its money on people reflects the company's strategy and business change objectives or if it is off track.

Concentrating spending on highest performers

For the past 20 years, a significant modern people strategy has been the concept known as performance management. *Performance management* is the term used to refer to activities, tools, processes, and programs that companies apply to measure, manage and reward the performance of employees. The components of performance management are performance appraisal, generally coupled with a policy of allocating different pay and rewards based how well the employee performed relative to peers.

Performance management was popularized by Jack Welch, the longtime chairman and CEO of General Electric. Performance management is based on the idea that if you don't concentrate resources to reward your highest-level performers, the high performers will go to companies willing to pay them more, leaving behind only the low performers. For these reasons, left alone a company will tend to get worse over time, not better. Facing this dilemma, GE decided to measure all employee performance (providing a relative rating of each employee) and actively force out the lowest performing employees, while generously rewarding its highest performing employees from each team. GE applied this active process with hope to get better as a company over time.

WARNING

The criticism against performance management are many. The most important criticism is that, absent an objective job rubric for measuring performance, the performance evaluation is a subjective measure, which is too easily biased. Also, the performance management process is time consuming. Furthermore, performance management can be a frustrating experience for a vast majority of employees who are being told they are average or below average. This process is particularly disturbing for all parties if the manager cannot provide any specific information about how the employee can achieve the more lucrative top performer classification in the future. Finally, performance management may encourage employees to focus more attention on individual as opposed to collective objectives, withhold support for co-workers, deliberately cheat or sabotage others, or otherwise game the system to stand out.

The jury is still out on whether or not performance management works or what configuration of performance management works best. Most companies that implement performance management are not as aggressive about managing out the low performers as GE was; however, a large number of companies that apply performance management apply some pay differential based on performance.

While many companies go through this exercise of measuring performance and determining paying differently based on performance a useful insight you can generate with people analytics is to answer the question: are you doing enough? Alan Eustace, a Google vice president of engineering once said that one top-notch software engineer is worth "300 times or more than the average." He went on to provide examples that many of the most valuable Google services, such as Gmail and Google News were started by a single person. Nobody really knows the exact true value between the highest contributors from average but the general finding that there are order-of-magnitude differences has been confirmed by many studies. For this reason, Google instituted a philosophy to pay its top software engineers order-of-magnitude differences from average. We aren't talking about something like 10% more, we are talking about something more like 100% more. Alan Eustace explains, "it would be better for the company to lose an entire incoming class of engineering graduates than one exceptional technologist."

While paying people different amounts may not sound fair to everyone, companies implementing pay for performance will point out that paying the highest contributing employee more is actually a fair and legally defensible way of determining pay. Most people would agree that those who contribute more value should get paid more than those who contribute less. The problem is that often the way performance management is implemented it is a lot of work and the result is little differences.

There are a number of questions surrounding performance, value and pay you can look to answer with people analytics that answering can provide valuable insights. Are you really differentiating the pay between the best and worst doing enough to achieve the objective you were hoping to achieve? Are the pay differences noticed by the highest value producing employees? Do the best employees of other companies know you pay the highest value producing employees remarkably well? (an important targeted attraction tool if so, not so if not) Are pay decisions perceived as fair? Are the highest value producing employees happier with pay and more committed than average? In other words, are all your efforts actually producing differences or they just a waste of time and money? Believe me, executives want to know the answer.

TIP

There are a number of reasons why people in the same job get paid different amounts of money: pay in previous job, market pay at the time of hire, negotiation, tenure, pay differentials for geography, pay differentials for performance, pay differentials for special knowledge or skills or differences brought into pay through mergers, acquisitions or other circumstantial reasons. This observation is not to suggest a specific pay philosophy – it is simply to state the fact.

Pay is a sensitive topic – the context for pay differences is not clear to people who don't work with pay data such that they can't see the problem. For example, what would you do in the following scenario?

Five years ago you hired someone to do a job for $30 dollars per hour. As a result of annual pay raises, this employee now makes $35 per hour. In this time period, the economy has really taken off and today you can't find anyone qualified who is willing to leave their current employer to take this job for less than $55 per hour. Your offers for $35 per hour are failing to attract the level of talent you want. What should you do? Should you pay the new employee more than the current employee with 5 years tenure? Should you pay both employees the new rate, thus giving he tenured employee an overnight $20 per hour raise? How will co-workers working right next to that employee in other jobs feel when they don't get a comparable percentage increase at the same time? With only two people in the same job you could bite the bullet and pay them both the same. What if you have 1000 people in the same job who were hired at different times and therefore all making something different between $35 and $60 per hour? Now, what if incidentally women or minorities ended up making less on average than white males? Clearly, if this were discovered this would represent a major legal issue for your company whether you intended for this to happen or not. If you brought everyone to $55, today's going rate, the cost might be enormous — maybe even too much for the company to bear. Furthermore, is paying everyone $55 fair to the people who have many more years of experience then the new hire? Shouldn't the experienced employees make even more than the new hires? This nightmare scenario is not a far-fetched problem for large companies — this is a day in the life of an HR professional at any company with more than 100 employees.

REMEMBER

Traditionally, people known as compensation analysts or compensation professionals worked with executives to establish a coherent pay philosophy and then institute a series of process, analysis, and corrective procedures to try to bring alignment between philosophy and reality over time. Pay reality is never perfectly aligned with pay philosophy because of all of the complex moving parts and because (typically) there is not enough money to solve all the pay problems at once and remain profitable at the same time. Each year HR professionals, compensation professionals, and executives work together to try to move the pay reality closer to its ideal state based on the companies pay philosophy and business strategy.

A useful focus for people analytics is to use your compensation and performance data to analyze if the way the company is really spending its money on people reflects the company's pay philosophy and strategy or if it is off track. You can use data to determine if the actions the company is taking with pay are having the desired effect. For example, is the highest performer attrition rate lower than the average or lowest performers attrition rate? If the purpose of a performance-based pay differential is to make the highest performers difficult to poach, decreasing the rate of exit of highest performers relative to their peers, then by segmenting your attrition data per performance you can help your executives see if their money spent is actually achieving this objective.

REMEMBER

You can pour resources into any number of areas to try to make people happier that will have no impact on outcomes, or you can do other things for the same amount of money that will have an impact on the outcomes you're seeking. You want to apply resources to categories of change where the company scores can be improved and that result in a behavioral or business outcome you're seeking.

INTERPRETING DATA STRATEGICALLY

Often, it's difficult to interpret HR data without adding perspective. Consider Scenario A in the figure below. Is this Exit Rate% a good sign or a bad sign for the company? Exits appear to be increasing, which seems bad; however, there isn't much of a context here to come to a definite conclusion.

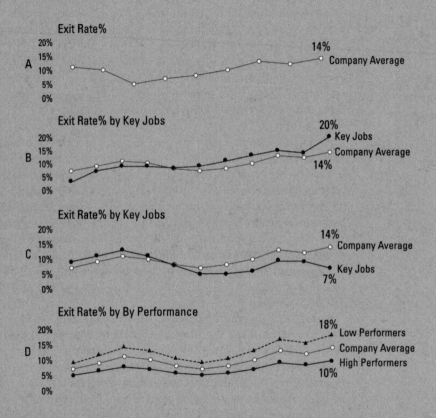

Now consider what happens when you add a key talent segment to this graph. In Scenario B, the company average is the same, but now you can see that the company is losing key talent at a faster rate than the company average. That is bad.

In Scenario C, the company is losing key talent at less than the rate of the company average. That is good, as is Scenario D, which focuses on Exit% By Performance. In Scenario D you see that the high-level performers leave at a lower overall rate than average and that low-level performers leave at a higher rate than average. That's a good thing!

In this manner, you can use people analytics to express your strategy of human resources and use data to understand whether the strategies you're taking are effective.

Finding Differences Worth Creating

Billions of dollars are spent on recruiting every year, aimed at convincing people to move from one company to another, and many companies are competing for the same people you want. The question is, how are you different?

Acquiring, engaging, and retaining people who are different from your competitors requires that you know what your kind of "different" looks like and also that you develop an environment and a job opportunity that looks good to that kind of person. Ideally, that environment is not just different; it also looks superior to them in comparison to wherever they are. If you want to consistently win and keep key talent, the offer can't just be good; it also has to stand apart from what this key talent can find anywhere else. In marketing, they call this a *unique value proposition*; in human resources terms, we call it a *unique employee value proposition*.

Many companies just try to match their competitors or try to be a standard-issue employer of choice, but this is difficult to achieve and may not be effective anyway. Continually winning the affection of the best people in the world at something requires that you identify a specific differentiating intent and be the best in the world at it. Your employee value proposition is where you set yourself apart from all other companies that compete to acquire the same employees.

How can you differentiate your employee value proposition in such a way that, as far as the people who would be most advantageous to your success are concerned, you're the only choice to work for in today's job market? If you can answer this question, it would enable you to be one of the most successful companies in your industry.

If people were machines, analytics would be a lot easier — in fact, managing would be a lot easier — but the truth is that people are not machines. That means you have to work a bit harder to get the information you need — more specifically, by developing methods to systematically collect, understand, and use data about your ideal talent's goals, wants, needs, motivations, hopes, dreams, and aspirations. It's also helpful to understand their work-related complaints, problems, fears, doubts, and worries that the opportunity you present to them will alleviate.

Many companies run surveys and use the information they gather to inform their plans for where they need to make additional enhancements to improve the work environment — all, of course, in order to attract, engage, and retain employees generally. You, too, will be doing a lot of work with surveys. Though high levels of satisfaction on items included in an employee survey is a good sign, it may not provide you with any real useful insight. When you cut this data by key job and performance segments to view how key talent segments are different, this will give you more useful insight than viewing the same data without this point of view. It is the differences between important segments that gives you the most important insights.

REMEMBER

You cannot develop a winning people strategy by trying to be everything to everyone, copying the choices of other companies, or working in the realm of anecdotes. You need data specific to your situation.

With people analytics, you can clearly and distinctly see the differences in people. With its help, you'll finally be able to:

>> Gather and analyze information about the preferences and opinions of your key talent in key jobs to shift the business advantage in your favor.

>> Test hiring and retention strategies with experiments.

>> Collect constant feedback so that your company can make the changes that are required in order to be the best in the world at what it does and also communicate how you are different to potential employees.

Chapter 6

Estimating Lifetime Value

Achieving sustained profitable business growth requires many things to go right at the same time. To name a few: differentiating products and services, the ability to profitably scale production, and the ability to attract, activate, and retain happy customers. To make matters more challenging, all this must be done in competition with other companies in a global market that never rests.

Many of these business outcomes can be measured and analyzed numerically: market share, revenue, profit, customer satisfaction, and customer retention, for example. These are the kinds of measures you find mentioned in annual reports, discussed in investor phone calls, and highlighted in balance sheets. These are the outcomes that, by definition, matter, but not all businesses are endowed with equal measure of these conditions. Given that fact, how do you cultivate these outcomes or change them?

Setting aside complicated financial manipulation for a moment, the answer is simple: Most successful executives agree that people are a company's largest and most important financial investment. People physically carry out the plans that differentiate the company from its competitors. People empathize with customers. People imagine products and services. People create business models and strategies. People are the beating heart and the eyes, ears, lips, and hands of your company. People hold the future of your company in their hands. People design, manage, and execute the actions of every productive enterprise.

We have all heard the statement that "people are a company's most important asset" — perhaps too many times. One question that comes to mind when such statements are made is this: "Are such statements sincere, or are they just lip service?" The next question is, "Can we determine the truth value of such statements in any measurable way?"

Though some might dismiss the ability to quantify something like this, the reality is that there are several ways to measure an employee's financial impact on a company. One of them is employee lifetime value (ELV).

In this chapter, you can see what ELV is, where it comes from, why it's important, how it can be used, and how to calculate it for yourself.

Introducing Employee Lifetime Value

Employee lifetime value, or just ELV, was inspired by customer lifetime value (CLV), a concept drawn from marketing.

So, what exactly is CLV?

CLV is the total profit estimated over the entire future relationship with a customer. As such, it's an important concept for marketing because it encourages a shift from a short-term transactional point of view of customer value to a long-term point of view of the customer, which is a much better context for cultivating healthy, ongoing customer relationships.

CLV was designed to put the cost of customer acquisition and retention into the proper context of the long-term profitability of each customer — on average, by segment, and in some cases by individual. CLV allows companies to compare the likely return on investment of spending for acquiring or retaining a customer with the total predicted value of the relationship.

The cost of acquisition and value of a customer will vary by segment. When you calculate CLV, you can calculate the CLV of the average customer, the CLV of the average customer of a particular customer segment, the CLV of an individual customer (provided you know what segments to classify them in), or the CLV of all members of a particular customer segment.

Importantly, the concept allows companies to compare the CLV of each segment on a relative basis. Why spend the entire finite marketing budget chasing customer segments that have less long-term value when those same dollars can provide a larger return if used on segments that have a higher long-term return on investment?

Turning now to employee lifetime value (ELV) proper, you can define it as an indicator or measurement of the estimated financial value (profit) that an average employee brings to an organization over their entire lifetime of working for the company. In this calculation, the *employee lifetime* is the period that starts when an employee first joins your business and ends on that person's last day. When you calculate ELV, you can calculate the ELV of the average employee, the ELV of the average employee of a particular employee segment, the ELV of an individual employee in the past (provided you maintain historical data and wait long enough), the forward-looking estimated ELV of each individual employee (provided you know what segments to classify them in), or the ELV of all members of a particular employee segment.

Understanding Why ELV Is Important

Much like CLV, ELV is important because it encourages management teams to shift from a short-term transactional point of view to a long-term point of view designed to cultivate a healthy ongoing employee relationship and to make better resource decisions. The ELV is also intimately linked to employee attraction, activation and attrition. (See Chapter 8 for an overview of these core concepts; for a detailed look at the analytics of each one, check out Chapters 9, 10, and 11).

Consider the situation in which one recruiter is filling niche jobs where the people who do that work are rare, and another recruiter is filling jobs where qualified people are common. To fill some jobs with high-quality talent that is rare, you might have to spend more time, you may have to spend more money, and you may need to hire more recruiters. If you evaluate the time and money required to recruit without taking these factors into account, you won't appreciate the higher difficulty level of finding rare talent and therefore won't take it into consideration when trying to make sense of the comparison results in context.

As a whole, you may achieve very different results considering the proportion of more difficult jobs you're attempting to fill or rare people you're attempting to hire. In particular, time and cost metrics are higher. This leads to difficulties when it comes to interpreting what is actually going on, raises questions of fairness in how you evaluate the performance of recruiters. and, more importantly, reduces incentives for recruiters to avoid working hard to find rare talent.

It isn't necessarily a bad thing to spend more time and money on recruiting if it's yielding more difficult-to-source and otherwise higher-quality hires. Even when you understand this, however you're still left with several problems:

>> How do you determine what *good* and *bad* mean in your talent acquisition measure?

>> How do you develop a working data-driven model to accurately predict how much time and money it will take to fill a workforce plan? Also, specifically, how many recruiters should you have?

>> How do you avoid creating the incentive for recruiters to look for more common talent and ignore the thankless pursuit of finding rarer and more difficult-to-convince talent?

>> How much money should you spend to attract, activate, and *retain* an employee of various types for your company?

>> How do understand and refine the return on investment (ROI) of the spending decisions you make?

>> How do you communicate the need for more resources to other people in a way that's convincing — and backed with data?

REMEMBER

The three A's, as I describe them, are the three big problems related to people that all companies must solve. Attraction represents the problem of getting talent into your company, activation represents the problem of getting that talent up to an optimum level of productivity (and keeping them there) and attrition represents the problem of keeping the highest value employees in the company well letting others go. (*Retention* fits in the category of attrition in that it is just the opposite of attrition: it is what you want to happen — when you *retain* an employee they stay at the company; when I talk about the good things that you want to have happen if you have it right, as opposed to when something is wrong, I use the word *retention* instead of attrition.)

The simplest use of ELV is to help put investments in employee attraction, activation, and attrition in the context of the total amount of money the company will spend on people over the lifetime working for the company. Most people would be shocked to know the large amount of money that will be spent on employees over their entire lifetime with a company.

If the average cost of a software engineer in San Francisco — including pay, benefits, equipment and space — is $200,000, with an average tenure of 5 years, the lifetime cost of each software engineer is roughly a million dollars. That is the cost *without* adding the return on investment of that spend. You wouldn't hire additional people if you were planning to just break-even — if this were the case you might as well just close up shop now.

REMEMBER

In Chapter 7 I suggest an additional assumption you can add for a return on investment — the value of that employee's effort above their cost. Cost represents a conservative starting point for calculating value, since it doesn't contain any assumption for the return on the dollars invested — a conservative assumption is that they must be worth at least what you pay them or the market would stop hiring them for this price.

In its simplest use, ELV can be helpful for making a business case for routine investments in human resources, which can sometimes sound like a lot to ask without context, but not a lot to ask in the context of the very large amount of money spent on employees overall and the value they produce. Almost everyone would consider a million-dollar piece of equipment depreciated over ten years to be significant. Most people would not question even a substantial setup or routine maintenance cost on such a large investment. Why not people? Looking at people in dollar terms allows you to compare people problems and opportunities in the context of dollars and long-term value — just like anything else the company considers to be important enough to invest money in.

If the average employee will earn over $1 million in their lifetime with the company, and if that employee's work is assumed to have at least an equivalent but probably much greater value to the company in profit, it seems almost frivolous to question some small additional expense to do a better job of attracting, activating, and retaining workers. For example, if you're going to hire ten software engineers, in whom you'll spend at least $10 million over 5 years ($1 million x ten engineers) and who might have a real value to the company anywhere from $20 million to $100 million (using 2x to 10x return on investment range) how much investment seems reasonable to tend to the needs of that talent? Probably a lot, right?

Applying ELV

You use ELV to calculate lifetime value to help prioritize where you need to focus your attention and how to allocate resources. ELV is applied to aid in the formulation of a sound people strategy that aligns with a business strategy that consists of more than just words on a page.

In Chapters 4 and 5, I discuss the importance of segmenting to people analytics and people strategy. One primary reason for the importance of segmentation is that not all employees are the same, which means that not all employees have the same type of relationship, cost, or long-term value for a company.

Employee segments vary in a number of important ways. Here are some examples:

>> Some job family segments have more value to a company based on the company's market position and business strategy, generating different value for the company over their lifetimes.

>> Some job family segments have wider variations in performance, generating different value for the company even within the same jobs.

>> Some employee segments tend to produce long-term employees who generate different value for the company over their lifetimes.

>> Some job family segments are very large in terms of head count but are paid very little on average.

>> Other job family segments are smaller in terms of headcount but are paid significantly more on average because they generate (on average) more value.

>> The higher-value job family segments are also generally scarcer, which means that they're more difficult to attract.

Segmentation plus ELV equals insight that provides for a more advanced people strategy. Here are some ELV-related questions that can stimulate new insight that can be applied to create a more advanced people strategy:

>> What is the difference in estimated ELV between each major job family segment at your company (average ELV per person and total dollar ELV per segment)?

>> What is the difference in estimated ELV in each job family by performance rating?

>> What is the difference in estimated ELV in each job family by varying prehire characteristics by source, knowledge, skills, abilities, or other?

>> What is the difference in estimated ELV increase from investing the same overall dollar spend on a people program intended to improve performance applied to different job families?

>> What is the difference in estimated ELV increase from investing the same overall dollar spend on different people programs for the same job family?

>> Within a segment, which is the best strategy to increase ELV? Is it by adding more employees in the segment, by increasing the value produced per employee in the segment, or by extending the expected lifetime tenure of employees in the segment?

Identifying the ELV of different segments enables you to balance the acquisition, activation, and retention efforts with expected long-term value by segment on an apple-to-apple basis using dollars. You also can use ELV to compare problems and opportunities by segment in the context of dollars.

If you allocated your budget for people-related programs equally per head, most of the dollars would go to the lowest-value-producing employee groups, which ironically are also the easiest to acquire, obtain consistent performance from, and replace. If you don't use ELV and you spread your money around, you decrease the likelihood of your actions being successful, and you spend your money in places where it will have less value.

Contrast this situation with an approach that allocates resources proportionally to the average ELV per job segment or to the total ELV per segment based on dollars, not on heads. By proportionally allocating resources to ELV, you can concentrate resources to obtain a better result and achieve higher return on investment in people.

Calculating Lifetime Value

The ELV metric is a foundational people analytics concept that can be calculated simply and can be improved with more complex math, should you want to go down a more advanced path.

REMEMBER

The more data you can gather about differences in employee performance and the value of additional productivity by segment, the more accurate your results will be. However, the simplest method I propose is quite easy, and you can get a good baseline ELV that you can use to get started.

Here are the four steps to calculate ELV the simple way:

1. Estimate average human capital ROI (HCROI). (Calculation provided below.)

2. Estimate average annual compensation cost per segment.

3. Estimate average tenure per segment.

4. Calculate the estimated ELV per individual or per segment by multiplying it out.

The next few sections look at each of these steps in greater detail.

Estimating human capital ROI

Human capital ROI (HCROI) can be defined as the pretax profit for each dollar invested in employee pay, including cash compensation, benefits, and equity compensation. This is the formula for calculating HCROI:

(Revenue – (Total Cost – (Regular Compensation Cost + Total Benefit Costs))) ÷ (Regular Compensation Cost + Total Benefit Costs)

TECHNICAL STUFF

If you prefer, you can use this alternate calculation instead of the calculation above:

(Profit ÷ Average Number of Employees) ÷ (Employee Cost ÷ Average Number of Employees)

HCROI compares operating profit to the total compensation dollars required to produce those profits. This measure answers the question, "How much profit are we earning for every dollar we've invested in the people?"

For example, a result of 1.0 means that the organization earns one dollar of operating profit for every one dollar invested in total compensation.

TECHNICAL STUFF

When it comes to the specific kinds of data you need in order to calculate HCROI, there are three different types of employee costs you may consider: cash compensation costs, benefits costs, and equity costs (stock options and grants). Some companies just use cash compensation in their HCROI calculation to keep it simple, others work out a more accurate estimate by applying assumptions for benefits, equity, and other less obvious costs. Annual cash compensation costs can usually be estimated well enough from the annualized pay field stored in your company's human resources information system (HRIS). For more accuracy, you can get actual historical pay tables from your payroll provider or located in your payroll system. Total revenue and costs can be found on the financial ledger. You should work with a member of your Finance team to estimate benefits cost based on information on the financial ledger. You also should work with someone in Finance if you want to estimate the value of equity (stock options and grants). Because benefits are purchased at a company level rather than at an individual level, it is difficult if not impossible to identify actual benefits costs by segment or individual. For this reason, most companies use a rule-of-thumb ratio to estimate benefit costs — for example, "for benefits assume an additional 30% of the cost of total cash compensation per individual or per segment."

Estimating average annual compensation cost per segment

Calculate how much money an average employee in each segment you want to analyze gets paid per year.

One way to do this is to calculate the total payroll (plus benefits and stock) from a segment of employees from the nearest time period, annualize, and then divide by the number of employees.

For example, the average annual salary plus benefits of an employee may be $110,000.

As was the case with HCROI, compensation can be calculated from the estimated annual compensation from the HRIS and adding benefits charges not available at the individual level from the financial ledger.

Estimating average lifetime tenure per segment

The actual average lifetime tenure will be different per employee segment, generally depending on what the job is, where in the world the job is, how much the employees are paid, how the job market is doing, and factors related to the employee experience.

For example, a software company in San Francisco, California, may find that the average software engineer tenure lifetime is three years, while the same company in Kansas City, Missouri, may find that the average software engineer lifetime tenure is five years. You will also find that the lifetime tenure varies significantly by industry and job. Retail store employees usually have an average lifetime tenure less than a year — maybe six months.

REMEMBER

You aren't calculating average employee tenure by taking all employees who are active and averaging tenure. That method doesn't work, because it assumes that everyone's first day with the company is as it was recorded in the HRIS and that everyone's last day with the company is the day you calculate it. Many of those employees will stay (hopefully!) much longer. You calculate average lifetime tenure using a sample of employees who have exited and averaging the tenures found at the time of exit.

For example, if in the history of the data, ten people have left the company, and at the time they left, their tenure in years was 7, 2, 3, 4, 5, 6, 2, 4, 3, and 4, the average tenure is 4 years, which is a straight average of those numbers.

TIP

Calculating average tenure per segment assumes that you have a large enough sample of people who have exited from a segment to abstract this measure to your total population in that segment. In some situations, you may need to estimate ELV using only an assumption of what you expect tenure to be in that segment because you don't have any historical data. Another reason for this may be that you want to model different ELV outcomes using different tenure assumption inputs. For example, you may want to model the theoretical value of increasing tenure by one year. Figuring out how to increase average tenure 1 year is another problem; for now, you just want to find out what it's worth.

Calculating the simple ELV per segment by multiplying

The simple method is to multiply estimated HCROI by the segment estimated annual cost by the segment estimated lifetime tenure (in years). Here's this formula, using other words:

Segment average ELV = (HCROI) × (annual cost) × (lifetime tenure)

For an example based on this formula, see Figure 6-1. In this example, the estimated HCROI was 1.5, with the average software engineer making $110,000 in total pay and benefits, with an average lifetime tenure of four years, which gives you $660,000.

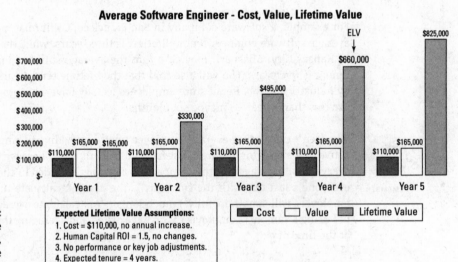

FIGURE 6-1: Average software engineer — cost, value, lifetime value, ELV.

If you have 50 software engineers, the total ELV for the software engineer job segment is $33,000,000 ($33 million).

If you plan to grow the company to 100 software engineers, the total ELV for the software engineer job segment is $66,000,000 — or $66 million. (See Figure 6-2.) That means the ELV for those extra 50 software engineers is $33 million.

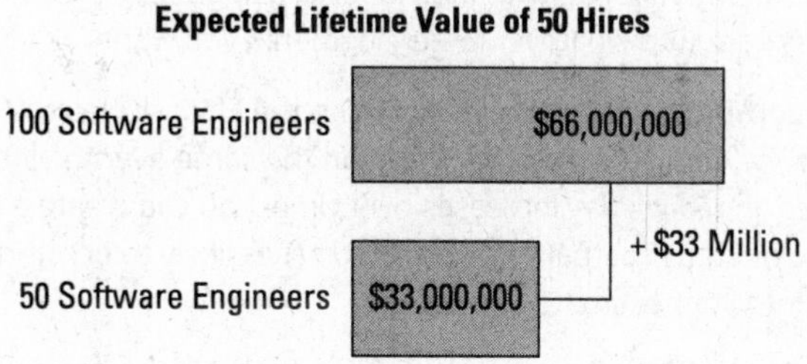

Expected Lifetime Value of 50 Hires

100 Software Engineers $66,000,000

FIGURE 6-2: The increase in ELV from 50 hires.

50 Software Engineers $33,000,000   + $33 Million

Figure 6-3 illustrates that there's more than one way to increase expected lifetime value (ELV). In the figure, the graph on the left shows an increase of $4.4 million by increasing the HCROI of the 50 software engineers from 1.5 to 1.7. The graph on the right shows an increase of $8.3 million by increasing the HCROI of the 50 software engineers from 1.5 to 1.7.

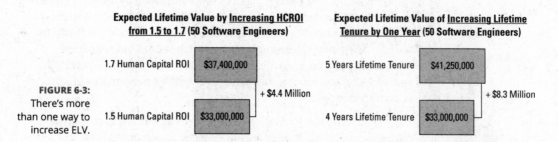

Expected Lifetime Value by <u>Increasing HCROI</u> <u>from 1.5 to 1.7</u> (50 Software Engineers)

1.7 Human Capital ROI $37,400,000

1.5 Human Capital ROI $33,000,000   + $4.4 Million

Expected Lifetime Value of <u>Increasing Lifetime</u> <u>Tenure by One Year</u> (50 Software Engineers)

5 Years Lifetime Tenure $41,250,000

4 Years Lifetime Tenure $33,000,000   + $8.3 Million

FIGURE 6-3: There's more than one way to increase ELV.

As you're considering where to focus your resources, ELV represents a tool to model and compare the theoretical value of the HR programs you plan to implement. Though ELV isn't an accounting measure and isn't intended to be a perfect representation of the value created by employees, it provides a relative point of comparison in dollars that allows you to make better decisions and test your results to see whether your assumptions were correct. With each subsequent test, you can refine those assumptions.

Refining the simple ELV calculation

The simple ELV calculation outlined in the preceding section can be refined in a number of ways. Here are a few of the elements that can be tweaked:

>> **Lifetime tenure:** A more accurate per segment lifetime tenure estimate can be made with a multivariate predictive model (a predictive model that considers many variables) per individual and aggregate the individual estimates back into whatever larger segments you want.

>> **Annual compensation increases:** So far, the ELV calculation I have provided assumes the compensation costs remain the same over the lifetime of the employee. In reality, pay increases over time. You can create a more accurate ELV calculation by estimating annual increases likely to occur in your tenure horizon into your estimate.

>> **Human Capital ROI:** Because companies generally operate and calculate profit as a whole unit, the most transparent method when it comes to calculating ELV is to apply the same ROI assumption to all job segments and people. However, you know not only that the actual productivity and ROI of people will vary based on their individual performance characteristics but also that it will vary across jobs based on their differing contributions to the company's economic engine.

For example, the best-performing sales representative may bring in $1 million in annual sales, and an average rep may bring in only $300,000. If you knew this, you could adjust the HCROI assumption by performance to illustrate that the high-performing sales representatives bring in three times what the average reps do. You could then more accurately shift your assumptions if you're looking at predicting, improving, or optimizing performance in whatever you're deciding.

REMEMBER

You should recognize, footnote, and reiterate to all who will listen that the calculations of HCROI and ELV are not intended as accounting measures — there is no widely agreed upon standard or certifying body. Such calculations are not intended to be perfect. They are intended to allow you to provide a point of reference using some internally consistent formula. I'm not saying that the value produced is of any extraordinary importance in itself; rather, it is useful as a thinking device and comparison point.

>> **Discount rate:** The discount rate is an economic idea that is used to calculate the present value of future revenues.

The basic idea of a discount rate is that "a bird in the hand is worth more than a bird in the bush." In financial assumptions, future dollars must be discounted because they are less certain. Would you rather have $100 today or 15 years in the future? The sample principle can apply to your assumptions about the return on human capital. Future profits are discounted.

If you are going to make a big presentation that asserts some large return on investment or recommends modifying some important business decision based on HCROI, then you should call on a Finance or Accounting professional to help you adjust your figures for this time value problem.

Identifying the highest-value-producing employee segments

Calculating ELV by different segments can help prioritize where you focus your attention and how to allocate resources. One primary reason that segmentation is important is that not all employees have the same type of relationship, cost, or long-term value for a company. Just like in marketing, not all investments in people will have the same return, so you should consider how you allocate spending among different options on some comparable relative basis. Putting segments into ELV dollars allows you to compare problems and opportunities by segment in the context of dollars and long-term value. Calculating the lifetime value of different employee segments enables you to look at the values of problems and opportunities among different segments in a different way than everything for everyone all the time.

For a concrete example of what I mean, check out Figure 6-4, which illustrates in graphic form the stark differences in ELV between segments. Segment 1 generates $30 million more in ELV than Segment 2, so it may make a lot of sense to spend proportionally more attention, time, and money on finding ways to make improvements to ELV in Segment 1.

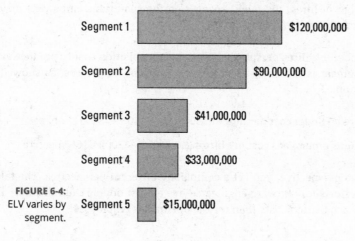

Expected Lifetime Value By Segment

Segment 1 — $120,000,000

Segment 2 — $90,000,000

Segment 3 — $41,000,000

Segment 4 — $33,000,000

Segment 5 — $15,000,000

FIGURE 6-4: ELV varies by segment.

Making Better Time-and-Resource Decisions with ELV

By looking back at the money spent for talent acquisition during a certain period in comparison to the lifetime value acquired for the company during that time, you can understand how much was spent per dollar of value produced, which helps you

>> See whether you're making good choices.

>> See how segments where difficulty-of-hire varies widely compare on the value produced.

>> See whether you're improving how you spend your money on talent acquisition as time goes on.

The following equation represents return on investment (ROI) for talent acquisition efforts:

Segment talent acquisition ROI = ((segment ELV – segment talent acquisition cost) ÷ (segment talent acquisition cost))

For example, the software company spends $300,000 on talent acquisition for 100 software engineers that returned $10 million in ELV. The same company spends $200,000 on talent acquisition of 300 operations employees that returned $5 million in ELV.

If you're considering the difference in talent acquisition productivity based purely on the number of hires, the talent acquisition for operations employees may be considered much more efficient.

Using a number-of-hires perspective, the talent acquisition cost to produce every software engineer is 4.5 times as much as operations employees, as showed by this calculation:

Software engineer cost per hire = (($300,000) ÷ (100)) = $3000 per hire

Operations employees cost per hire = (($200,000) ÷ (300)) = $667 per hire

Using a value perspective, you get a completely different perspective. The talent acquisition efforts for software engineers have almost double the value over that of the talent acquisition costs than for the operations employees:

Software engineering added ELV = ($10,000,000 – $300,000) = $9,700,000

Operations added ELV = ($5,000,000 – $200,000) = $4,800,000

If you distribute that ELV per hire it works out to the following:

Software engineering: $9,700,000 ÷ 100 hires = $97,000 ELV per hire

Operations: $4,800,000 ÷ 300 hires = $16,000 ELV per hire

Based on the calculations from this example, even though the software engineering recruiting costs is much more per hire, a successful recruitment generates almost 6 times as much value. If you are only using a cost perspective, your report or analysis might conclude the engineering recruiting cost-per-hire is not as good as the operations cost-per-hire, but from a value standpoint you could take the opposite conclusion. It is important to look at both cost and value before making a conclusion.

Drawing Some Bottom Lines

Expected lifetime value is a thinking tool for relative comparisons and prioritization in human resources. There are a number of ways you can improve the assumption in ELV over the basic techniques I have illustrated, but remember that ELV isn't intended to be used as a precise accounting system. The most appropriate use of ELV comes as an aid in enhancing critical thought.

One important way that ELV varies from customer lifetime value (CLV) is that, in customer lifetime value, every dollar spent is collected as value, whereas in ELV not every dollar spent is collected as value. For most jobs, money will be spent regardless of whether the employee produces any real value for the company. There are many potential reasons that an employee's effort can produce more or less value. Chapter 7 proposes a framework that can be applied to employee value that makes a more realistic assessment of the range of potential value produced by employees and a useful tool for helping the company see where its human resource efforts will have the most financial impact.

Chapter **7**

Activating Value

We know that acquiring uniquely talented people is important to helping any company create a high-performing workforce. We also know that retaining people — specifically, uniquely talented people — is important. A topic that doesn't get nearly enough attention is what happens to those employees day-to-day after they're inside the company. Some call this *culture,* or *engagement;* what I want to introduce you to is a simple concept I call *activation.*

If each employee in the company were a component from which the company derived some value, activation would simply indicate whether the switch is on or off. Imagine, if you will, that every employee's forehead sports an On–Off switch. (I know it sounds like something out of *The Twilight Zone,* but bear with me.)

In a simple real-life example of activation, you have hired a software engineer who is at work but cannot really start working for two weeks because they are waiting for their computer to arrive. In those two weeks, the engineer is unable to deliver the value from work that you hired her to do, so if she had an On–Off switch, it would be in the Off position. Of course, more things matter than having a computer, but if that's the one thing that she was missing, the switch would move to the On position whenever the computer arrived.

Not all activation problems are this simple to fix. In another example, after the engineer was hired, team members never completely agreed about the best way to solve a problem, so the engineer ended up working for six months on code that would never be used because of conflicting perspectives among the broader team. You paid her during this period, but the company was unable to materialize value from her work. Again, in this scenario the engineer is working but her activation switch is in the Off position.

REMEMBER

When you're paying employees but they aren't activated, you aren't deriving value; when they are activated, you are deriving value. The challenge of correlating HR activities to business outcomes is that there's more to it than just knowing you have the "best" or "right" set of people or HR programs; what you really need to know is how many individual value switches are On or Off.

When you think about a company from the standpoint of producing optimum results from employees' efforts, you need a data-informed perspective on the three A's (attraction, activation, and attrition) if you really want to see what is going on as a whole with employees at your company. Let's see what happens when you have two of the three nailed down, but not all three:

>> **Attraction and activation (without retention):** When your business can attract uniquely talented employees but you're not retaining them (not retaining means they are leaving), you're expending a lot of energy but simply going in circles.

>> **Activation and retention (without attraction):** When you're activating employees and retaining them, but you're unable to attract uniquely talented employees, you face the danger of simply being beaten out by those of your competitors who have more talented employees working on whatever it is you want your product focus to be.

>> **Attraction and attrition (without activation):** Finally, when you're attracting uniquely talented employees and are able to retain them, but you don't know how to activate them to a high level of performance, you aren't getting the most out of the money you're spending on those employees. You have the right people, and you are going to pay them regardless of the value they produce, but you are not obtaining optimum value from them.

For an illustration of the points I make earlier, check out Figure 7-1.

Now that you know in broad terms what activation is and where it fits into a people analytics HR strategy, I can break activation down into greater detail in the following section.

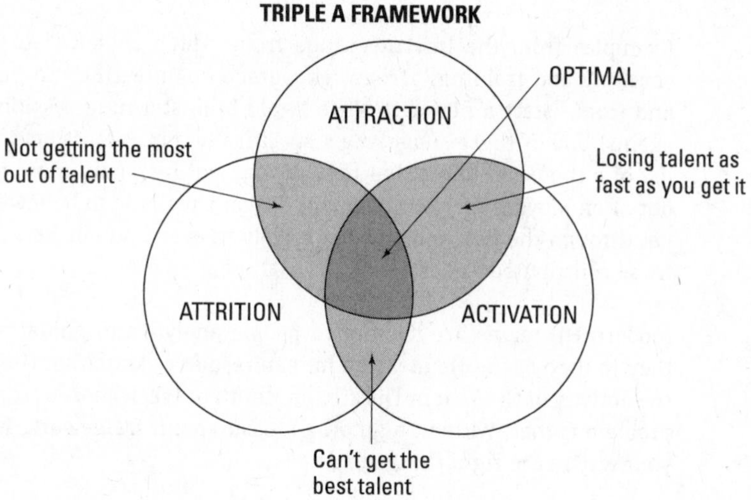

TRIPLE A FRAMEWORK

OPTIMAL

ATTRACTION

Not getting the most
out of talent

Losing talent as
fast as you get it

FIGURE 7-1:
The pitfalls posed
if there are
problems in
attraction,
activation, and
attrition.

ATTRITION

ACTIVATION

Can't get the
best talent

Introducing Activated Value

The influence of human resource management on organizational performance is a central research question capturing the interest of academics and practitioners for decades. My own literature review turned up more than a hundred articles on the topic of the impact of human resource practices on firm performance that were published in peer-reviewed scientific journals between 1990 and 2018.

Researchers have repeatedly demonstrated that implementing a bundle of people management practices centered on creating strong employee involvement and morale can have a relevant and important influence on company performance.

A 2013 Gallup meta-analysis accumulated data representing well over 1.3 million employees from 263 research studies to study the relationship between employee engagement and business outcomes. Of the nine outcomes studied — customer loyalty and engagement, profitability, productivity, turnover, safety incidents, shrinkage, absenteeism, patient safety incidents, and quality — all proved to be related to employee engagement. According to Gallup, the difference between falling in the top quartile and the bottom quartile of their engagement index could mean a 22 percent difference in profitability, 21 percent in productivity, and 37 percent in absenteeism, to name just a few of the advantages.

The fact that what you do with people impacts company performance shouldn't be a surprise or be that difficult to understand. What isn't clear is how to get repeatable results in different contexts. Instead, what you find is an array of disconnected measurement ideas and a dizzying list of suggestions that total in the hundreds, if not thousands, of activities.

Examples from the Internet range from "ditch cubicles" to "provide ongoing coaching and training," from "encourage volunteering" to "incentivize goals," and from "start a newsletter" to "hold brainstorming session." I have nothing against any of these suggestions specifically, but it isn't helpful to begin with a list of a thousand items that may or may not help gain more performance value out of employees for your company. It isn't realistic to believe that you will ever get through the list, and you're unlikely to ever find out how much value any of these contributed or destroyed.

Modern HR teams are looking to people analytics to guide their focus because they're tired of the old idea of a human resources team that tirelessly implements the Activity of the Year or Quarter or Month or Week chosen from a magic hat. The problem is that, without a guiding measurement framework, it's difficult to find your way to the right things to do.

In the hope of providing just such a framework, I have come up with something I call *activated value,* a concept designed to focus attention where it will produce the most business value.

The Origin and Purpose of Activated Value

Activated value is a concept I developed after giving up employment at large companies like Google to start consulting for smaller companies that have less time and fewer people and resources, yet are still trying to repeat Google's success.

One of my first clients was a 500-person start-up that at one point had been a San Francisco start-up darling blessed with a venture capital valuation of over a billion dollars and loved by employees, customers, and investors alike. Much of the company's initial growth was from its first product, which was a smash hit among its customers. However, this product was not enough to achieve profitability and, before long, competitors copied its design. For a period of years, employees tried to figure out who they wanted to be as a company as they tried to get other products launched. Unfortunately, their best efforts weren't so successful, because their second and third products didn't "wow" customers as much as the first. By the time I started working with them, it was clear that the company was having financial problems but had a proud history of achievement and that employees were still confident they could turn this company around.

The imitation trap

The first thing I observed while working with the small, troubled company was that I could see much more clearly when smaller companies try to buy the

affection and loyalty of employees by imitating the HR practices of larger companies, it can make them look good on the surface for a time but if large scale success
is not found quickly, these can undermine the company's success in the long term.

For this company, imitating the expensive real-estate, open floor plan layout,
bean bags, ping pong tables, micro kitchens, free lunches, and other liberal benefits and perks of neighbors like Google, Apple, and Facebook made the startup
look like a great place to work, but beneath the vibrant surface and upbeat
demeanor important problems were hiding. Attempting to look like the much
larger, better capitalized and profitable companies in compensation, benefits,
perks, and expensive office space undermined the startup's success by increasing
the startup's per-unit cost of production over that of the competitors that had
much bigger war chests. At the same time, the company had to face competitors in
other countries, where workers have lower expectations and cost less, resulting in
a much lower unit cost of production. This put the startup in a difficult position of
not being particularly competitive on price. The ongoing higher cost of production
undermined profitability and this required executives to continually go back to
investors to put in more money. Each time they went back to investors for more
funds, the employees' share of the equity pie kept shrinking to the point where it
became clear that the employee stock options may eventually be worth nothing.
This undermined the reason the most talented employees took the risk on the
start-up rather than work at an established company — they wanted their work to
matter and they wanted a piece of the company for their contribution. As the real-
ization that the company might fail became clear and the stock options that were
holding people in place had less value, critical employees began to leave, which in
turn helped make the self-fulfilling prophecy for company failure more likely.

The most important thing I observed in working with a smaller company is that
implementing all the little things the large companies do simply is not possible at
a smaller company. It could bankrupt them, and it was doing just that. Aside from
the problem of the money to buy the coolest toys, the smaller company just didn't
have enough people on the HR team to implement everything larger companies
were doing even if they wanted to — there wasn't enough time in the day for that
small team. The smaller company had to figure out what of the many things the
larger companies do matter most, or they had to find their own way forward, or
else they would be unable to beat larger, more profitable competitors that had a
lot more money to spend on human resources. A smaller company can compete
with a larger competitor, but not by playing by the rules of the larger competitor's
self-serving game.

REMEMBER

With no standardized, reliable way to measure the deep things that matter (like
goals, motivation, capability and support), neither HR nor managers can be held
accountable for actually achieving a great culture — so their attentions go to what
is happening on the surface (bean bags, ping pong tables, and food). More specifically, managers' attention goes to wherever they're being held accountable, and

HR's attention goes to activities that are pursued until complete, regardless of whether anyone has a way of knowing whether those activities matter. This missed opportunity to get the deep cultural things that matter right while focusing on the Fashion of Corporate Success undermines the company's real success over the long term by first increasing the costs over that of competitors and then increasing the company's need to continue acquiring people to replace those who are leaving. As the old saying goes, "what gets measured gets managed." If nothing deep and important is measured, then nothing deep and important is managed.

The need to streamline your efforts

All companies can benefit from measures of how effectively they are managing people and, as I have been pointing out all along, many of those measures can be found within the emerging practices of people analytics. The problem is that whereas some large companies doing innovative work in the people analytics sphere have hired 20 or more people to exclusively work on people analytics and many other companies experimenting in people analytics have teams of 5 more people working exclusively on people analytics, many smaller companies may not even have that many people working in all of HR.

Given how necessary people analytics is to the effective management of people, small growing companies need people analytics as much (or more) than large companies, but they just don't have the same resources to apply, so they need it to approach it in a different way. A large-company approach to people analytics requires large, upfront investments in systems as well as large teams full of people who can do advanced systems, behavioral science, and mathematics work — usually, people holding highly specialized training, including full PhDs. The large-company approach to people analytics simply wasn't possible at the startup I was working with and wouldn't be possible at any other small or medium sized company, either.

TECHNICAL STUFF

My definition of a small company is any company with less than 250 employees, while my definition of medium-sized company is 250 to 2000 employees, and my definition of large is above 2000. Others may have a different definition. The point remains that companies of different sizes have different challenges and have to address the problems of human resources in different ways.

Initially, I thought that I could meet the HR measurement needs of the smaller company by introducing a basic set of HR metrics and a comprehensive annual survey on employee culture. While my own extraordinary efforts were generating useful insights for the small company, my methods weren't accessible to operators to take over from me — the everyday people who work in HR and manage people as opposed to the data scientists. It became clear that even the basics required too much work and expertise to safely hand off to a group of already overworked people. It just is not going to happen if someone isn't responsible, but one person can't do it all — especially not one that isn't well versed in all four S's: strategy, science, statistics and systems. I could do many things myself because of my previous experiences, but not everything, and it is difficult to find someone with experience to hand the whole people analytics thing off to, and clearly the small company couldn't truly create a complete team just for people analytics.

THE SPECIAL PROBLEM OF HUMAN RESOURCES FOR RAPIDLY GROWING SMALL- AND MEDIUM-SIZED COMPANIES

The problem of a successful and therefore rapidly growing small- or medium-sized company is that, relative to their size, they are much busier in HR than the HR people at a larger company. Just imagine — HR at a small- or medium-sized growing company may be supporting a company that is doubling in size every year, which represents a substantial volume of recruiting and other important HR work.

The extraordinary efforts of HR at the small- or medium-sized growing company really matters for that business to succeed, where the HR employees at a larger company may just need to keep the lights on. In a small company, every hire matters a lot, whereas in a larger company the impact of a single employee, single HR decisions, or single hires is diluted so you can survive more mistakes.

Furthermore, the small- and medium-sized company HR team must design, implement, and iteratively refine a dizzying array of systems, processes, policies, and practices at the same time, whereas the larger company just needs to build on an existing body of work that came before. The larger company doesn't have to build, implement, or refine the entire HR gamut in one year — the HR team at the smaller company may need to do just that.

Often small companies hire someone to lead their HR department from the HR department at a larger company, hoping to replicate the success of the HR department at the larger company. However, because responsibilities are distributed at the larger company, the HR person taken from the larger company may not have participated in the design and implementation of all of the varied HR systems, processes, policies, and practices at the larger company. They may not have even completely understood all the HR systems, processes, policies, and practices at the larger company. The conundrum for the smaller company is how to design and implement everything it needs to with a much smaller team and budget. The skill required to do this is very different than the skill required to serve as a representative of HR team in some specific capacity at the larger company. Furthermore, the complete package of institutional knowledge that created the success of the larger company team doesn't transfer easily, if at all, through a single individual.

Because I wouldn't be able to effectively find a way to collect, report, and find insights for hundreds of metrics and survey questions, I set out with a goal to find a smaller number of people–measures that could be related to business results that connects employee value with business value and that can be administered anywhere by people without a PhD in calculus or industrial organizational psychology. With that goal in mind, I set out to design a key performance indicator (KPI) that I envisioned would be a composite measure (or index) of a few items that can be collected through a survey instrument, but this measurement system wouldn't require hundreds of questions, hundreds of HR metrics, or advanced data science to still be highly useful. It would necessarily miss a lot of things, but it would measure the most critical things.

I was looking to implement a system of measurement that can be boiled down into a single indexable key performance indicator (KPI) that could

- Be practical to implement
- Be easily grasped by front-line managers
- Correlate to employee performance and contribute to the understanding of employee performance
- Correlate to business performance and contribute to the understanding of the relative performance of different business units or of the company when compared to competitors in an industry
- Simplify the production of the measure and clarify the possible range of options in the response
- Be used by managers and HR to track their performance regularly: quarter-by-quarter or (preferably) month-by-month
- Be used in conjunction with other people and business data to make better business decisions

After I worked through what was required, the single indexable measure I came up with that satisfied all requirements is what I call *activated value*.

Measuring Activation

Anyone who has studied the research literature of human performance improvement knows that a frustratingly complex body of research that's out there examines behavior influences of individual performance. Though it's safe to say that many factors can drive or affect performance, what I sought to do was come up with a way of measuring just the bare-minimum conditions required for ideal performance to occur that anyone can agree with. Activated value is a way of simplifying the process by focusing on those factors that are important contingencies of a "system of interrelated factors" that produce performance. More importantly, the concept of activated value would be especially easy to understand for managers and nontechnical people.

Determining the minimum conditions necessary for successful performance

The theory of activation proposes that, taken down to its essence, four conditions must exist for an employee or a team to consistently produce at or above performance expectations. The employee or team must

>> Be *capable* of performing the actions required

>> Be *aligned* on what a good result looks like

>> Be *motivated* to perform the actions

>> Have all the tools and *support* that are required for successful performance of those actions

If any of these four conditions is missing, it's difficult, if not impossible, for the employee or team to perform reliably.

REMEMBER

To say that four conditions are absolute requirements to achieve performance isn't to say that other aspects don't matter at all. Many things can matter — the purpose of activation is to simplify your understanding of performance to the bare minimum. At the point at which you fully understand the presence or absence of these four conditions, you can control these four in analysis to more reliably identify other factors that matter to performance.

The following list summarizes each of the four conditions of activation:

>> **Capability (knowledge, skills, and abilities):** In its most basic sense, an individual who is capable has the knowledge, skills, ability, and other characteristics necessary to perform the job. Capabilities are what people bring to the company — personal qualities such as technical knowledge, learning agility, social skills / emotional quotient (EQ), and grit, for example.

The company can increase capability in two ways: recruiting and training — keeping in mind that some characteristics aren't possible to create through training and others are but would cost too much time and money.

The primary channel that the company has to increase capability is the optimal selection of people for jobs based on selection criteria related to job performance as determined by strategic planning and job analysis.

Sometimes when all the other factors of activation have been handled well, some of the characteristics thought to be critical to performance aren't actually critical in practice. Inversely, even an extraordinarily capable person put into a situation without appropriate supports will fail.

REMEMBER

It doesn't matter whether people are aligned, motivated, and supported if they aren't capable of performing the job with a high level of ability.

>> **Alignment:** Employees who are aligned know what they're expected to accomplish, under what conditions, and how they're performing in relation to those expectations.

The company can increase alignment by way of goal setting, performance appraisal, and regular executive, manager, and employee communication.

REMEMBER

It doesn't matter whether people are capable, motivated, and supported if individuals, teams, managers, and leaders don't understand and agree on expectations.

>> **Motivation (preferences, commitment, engagement):** Motivation is the general desire or willingness of someone to do something.

Motivation reflects the interaction of personal preferences with the job, working environment, company culture, leadership, managers, peers, rewards, and incentives, which result in motivation or demotivation to perform the tasks at hand.

When the company adequately addresses the other factors, motivation often takes care of itself. Regardless, the company can take many actions to create an environment conducive to high levels of motivation. The most important action is to find and select people who are excited about the company's mission and products. The second most important way the company can maintain high levels of motivation is to listen to employees when they specify the tools and support they need to perform at their best.

TIP

Attempts to "pump up" motivation without managing the other factors generally doesn't produce the desired outcome.

It doesn't matter whether people are aligned, capable, and supported if they aren't motivated to perform the job.

REMEMBER

>> **Support:** This category covers not only the particular technical tools used to perform work but also any other support that's necessary, such as access to documentation, access to manager and teammates to help solve problems, resources designed to produce skills and knowledge in the individual, technical support, and camaraderie.

TIP

In assessing support, it's also important to assess negative consequences built into the work environment and work process, such as the failure by other departments to fulfill orders or conflicting or competing objectives between teams or peers that punish or fail to reward individuals for doing the right thing for the company. Investing in common supports, such as training, can be unproductive if done without ensuring that influences are aligned.

It doesn't matter whether people are aligned, capable, and motivated if they aren't provided with the supports they need to perform the job.

REMEMBER

Now that you know what activation is, it's time to step it up a level. When you think about a company from the standpoint of producing results through people, you need a data-informed perspective on capability, alignment, motivation, and support of people if you truly want to perform individual and group diagnostics that a) provide useful information about what is preventing performance or b) allow you to use data to make predictions.

Now that you know in broad terms what activation is and where it fits into a people analytics HR strategy, I can break activation down into greater detail in the following sections.

The calculation nitty-gritty

You can infer all four model variables — capability (C), alignment (A), motivation (M), and support (S) — with a short, 8-item survey using a 0–10 agreement scale. Here are the survey questions:

Survey design

For scale, let's use an agreement scale from 0 to 10.

TIP

Pay careful attention when dealing with a 0–10 agreement scale; 11 responses are possible on such a scale (0,1,2,3,4,5,6,7,8,9,10).

Survey items are described in the table below:

TIP

On the actual survey, you would just list the statements in the survey tool along with the suggested 0-10 agreement scale. While the categorical classification of each item should not be shown on the survey, for the sake of background see the sub-categories or dimensions noted in the first two columns of Table 7-1. You maintain the categories in the background so that you so you can calculate and report by any of the four major categories on the survey in addition to calculating an overall index as a whole using all eight items. Others do not need to be distracted or burdened by the details of how you categorize each item, and in particular these distractions should not be on the survey itself.

TABLE 7-1 **Setting up a CAMS survey**

CAMS Component	Format of Item	Survey Item Statement
Alignment	Team	There is a clear objective around which myself and the people I work with rally.
Alignment	Individual	I have a clear understanding of the difference between an average contribution and a great contribution for my role.
Capability	Team	My primary work group has all the capabilities it needs right now to achieve top performance as a team.
Capability	Individual	I have the capabilities I need right now to achieve top performance in my current role right now.
Motivation	Team	The people I work with are willing to help even if it means doing something outside of their usual activities.
Motivation	Individual	I am motivated to do more than minimum expectations.
Support	Team	I have the cooperation and support from others at *<Company>* I need in order to be successful.
Support	Individual	I have the resources and tools I need to be successful.

Note that all of the statements used are positive, so the 0–10 scale response can be interpreted consistently, such that a 0 would be the worst response and a 10 would be the best response for all items. This allows a simple calculation of the index.

The index calculations proposed in this chapter assumes 8 positively worded items on a 0–10 agreement scale. If, for various reasons, you want to use a different agreement scale, for example 1 to 5 or 1 to 7, or add or remove an item you may do so; however, you would have to take this into consideration in the index calculation and other uses of this data described below. If you change the structure of the survey, then you will have to adjust the index and your interpretation of the index accordingly.

TECHNICAL STUFF

Note that the items in each category are intentionally similar — one, however, is asked from the perspective of the team and one is asked from the perspective of the individual. Asking about the same concept in more than one way creates a better performing index. Each survey item is framed in a particular way, which is subject to a particular bias. Asking the question in more than one way is intended to provide balance to minimize the impact of various types of bias. The overall index will be more reliable than the response to a single item or subset of items.

Calculating the CAMS index

Sum the total counts (0–10) from the individual response to the eight items. This should produce a score ranging from 0 to 80 per individual, known as the *CAMS index*.

Calculating Net Activated

Net Activated is a metric that is a count of the number of people who have responded positively enough to the eight questions to be considered sufficiently activated for purposes of reporting and other calculations.

To calculate Net Activated, assign a categorical description for all individual survey respondents using the following rules:

>> **Activated** = *CAMS index* equal to or greater than 70

>> **At-Risk** = *CAMS index* less than 60

Count the number of individual survey respondents that are Activated and At-Risk.

Calculate Net Activated Percent

Net Activated Percent is a metric that calculates the percentage of the workforce that is activated. Use the following formula to calculate the *Net Activated Percent*.

Calculate Net Activated Percent = (# in workforce – # at-risk in workforce) ÷ (total headcount of company)

Additional reporting

While it is nice to see the average CAMS Index and the Net Activated Percent for the company, it will be much more useful to calculate these by segment so you can see what is going on in different parts of the company and compare segments of the company to each other.

Follow these steps:

1. **Calculate the average CAMS index per segment.**

TIP

A segment can be any number of different layers or dimensions of the company. For examples you can segment by division, by department, by director, by manager, by job family, by job, by job level, by location, by performance, by key jobs or key talent, by gender and so on and so forth. For more on segmentation see Chapters see chapters 4 and 5.

2. **Cross-tab the average CAMS index by segment. (For more on cross-tabs, see Chapter 4.)**

3. **After completing more than one survey, trend each segment over time.**

   This will show you if each segment is getting better or getting worse over time.

4. **Cross-tab each of the four sub categories (Capability, Alignment, Motivation & Support) as well as each of the seven individual items in order to provide more specific feedback about what is going well or going poorly.**

   I'd concentrate specifically on where the greatest opportunity to improve the CAMS index is. Is there is a problem in capability, alignment, motivation, support or some combination?

5. **Follow steps 1-4 above for Net Activated Percent as well.**

Survey administration

This 8-item inventory is short enough that it can be distributed monthly or quarterly as a regular management ritual and key operational tool that can be associated with other outcomes without degrading response rate or presenting difficulty when it comes to producing and distributing reports.

This survey should be conducted confidentially by a third-party agent so that individual responses can be joined with other data and reported by segment while protecting the integrity of the process and the safety of individual responses.

REMEMBER

It can sometimes take a few survey cycles for certain employees to feel comfortable that they can trust you with their honest replies. If you have never taken a survey, look at it from their perspective. How all this works and what you're going to do after they give you their responses is still a little fuzzy to them. After you have successfully completed a few survey cycles, more people will feel more comfortable that they understand the process and have increasing confidence that they won't be singled out for retribution. (Don't laugh: Some people are convinced that it will happen.)

Though we protect the individual responses for the integrity of the process and the accuracy of the data, you can and should have follow-up group or one-on-one meetings where people who feel safe doing so have the opportunity to talk about the four factors (capability, alignment, motivation and support) and contribute inputs for solutions. These meetings should be facilitated so as to be voluntary, positive, constructive, and safe for everyone involved.

KEEPING THINGS CONFIDENTIAL — OR IS IT ANONYMOUS?

All survey invitations should provide a clear definition to the survey taker of who is collecting the data, for whom, for what purpose, and how the data will be stored and used.

In survey parlance, "anonymous" means that survey results cannot be associated to individuals at all. Imagine, you have a giant cauldron and all employees walked by and dropped in their response. You would never know who put in what. The responses are just in the cauldron and you can't count them as a whole — that's all you get. This being the case, you can't join any other data to report by segment.

Still speaking in survey parlance, "confidential" means that survey results can be associated to individuals for purposes of data management and analysis; however, the caretaker of the survey (either internal or external to the company) have agreed to not share individual responses with anyone. The agreement of the caretaker is to only report survey results in aggregate. The best practice is to use a third-party — a firm that is not part of your company, in other words — to administer your survey. The company will only receive data back in aggregate from the third-party, not the individual detail, so it is impossible for anyone at the company to look at the individual detail.

The third-party caretaker can join data, perform analysis, and report the data by any meaningful segment of your workforce; however, they have agreed to only share data back with the company in segment sizes that achieve a minimum threshold to protect individual confidentiality. A minimum segment size of three is large enough to make it impossible to figure out specifically who responded in a particular way; however, most companies use segment sizes of five just to be safe. In any case, the guidelines are designed so that no manager, rogue HR person, or whomever can pin a negative response on a specific individual. You apply and communicate the guidelines to help people taking the survey feel comfortable about sharing honest feedback without the fear that the company will use what they say against them.

The best approach for surveys is to use a third-party external agent to run your survey confidentially to completely remove the conflict of interest of the person holding the data so people feel safer to share their honest feedback and to project professionalism. I call this a "Third Party Confidentiality Assurance."

Survey Analysis

With the same 8-item inventory, you can

» Identify which of the four factors, if any, can be categorized as a weakness for the company as a whole or for a particular segment.

» Provide executives a perspective across the entire business to enable them to see strengths, weaknesses, risks, and opportunities among divisions and teams so that they can work with managers to solve problems and hold managers accountable.

» Measure the performance of managers at facilitating activation among the teams they manage and provide individual advice based on the profile of the groups they manage.

» Identify whether the specific issues blocking activation vary among groups or if the issue is relatively consistent across many groups.

» Correlate activation to other survey, performance, or business outcome data, if such data is available.

Combining Lifetime Value and Activation with Net Activated Value (NAV)

In Chapter 6, I introduce employee lifetime value (ELV) as the people analytics version of customer analytics customer lifetime value (CLV). There I talk about how CLV is the total profit estimated over the entire future relationship with a customer. CLV was designed to put the cost of customer acquisition and retention into the proper context of the long-term profitability of each customer — on average, by segment, and in some cases by individual. CLV allows companies to compare the likely return on investment of spending for acquiring or retaining a customer with the total predicted value of the relationship. With ELV, companies now have an important method of putting employee-related issues on a financial basis for the purposes of relative prioritization that is similar to CLV.

Remember the important difference between customer lifetime value (CLV) and employee lifetime value (ELV): Whenever a customer spends money, that value is immediately captured; when you spend money on an employee, the value of that spending may or may not be captured by the company, depending on what the employee does. It's entirely possible for employees to show up and collect their paychecks but exert no effort to create value for the company — or they can make the effort and still miss the mark. Because ELV is contingent and therefore less predictable, you have to look at ELV a little differently from CLV.

Net Activated Percent (NA%) is a metric described earlier in this chapter that represents the percentage of employees that are activated. Net Activated Value (NAV) combines the concepts of NA% with ELV into one measure. NAV helps you navigate the winding path of employee lifetime value on the employee journey. In this section, I show how you can build on this measure to obtain more insight.

You can obtain a clear focus on where to spend your time and money if you compare the estimated value represented in a particular segment if 100 percent of that segment's employees are activated versus the estimated value of that segment at the current Net Activated Percent (NA%). If you multiply the ELV of the segment times the current Net Activated Percent (NA%), you have a new measure called Net Activated Value (NAV). This new measure, NAV, represents roughly the value of the efforts of the people in the segment that are activated. NAV discounts the expected value of segment, taking into consideration that because not all employees are activated, the segment can't possibly deliver full value.

Here's the formula for calculating Net Activated Value (NAV):

Segment NAV = (Segment NA%) × (Segment ELV)

As shown in Table 7-2, you can compare the dollar value of the opportunity by group to figure out where to focus your attention to have the largest business impact.

TABLE 7-2   ## Net Activated Value

Job Segment	Segment NA%	Segment Total ELV	Segment NAV	Opportunity (ELV – NAV)
Segment 1	95%	$120,000,000	$114,000,000	$6,000,000
Segment 2	**85%**	**$90,000,000**	**$76,500,000**	**$13,500,000**
Segment 3	80%	$41,000,000	$32,800,000	$8,200,000

In the example shown in Table 7-1, going to work on increasing NAV in Segment 2 is the best investment of your time and resources, based on the information you have that combines Net Activated Percent with employee lifetime value.

TIP

NAV (like ELV) is not intended to be used as a rigorous financial accounting exercise. Rather, these are tools to put concepts like employee attraction, activation and attrition into a relative dollar context, recognizing that not all jobs or people have the same value and the value that is produced may be different than the value expected as a result of some missing contingency as represented by CAMS. The conversion of headcount to ELV helps to get the magnitude of values you are dealing with right and then Net Activated Value shows how efforts to improve value from different segments (based on the information you have at the time) compare on a relative basis for prioritization. Do not confuse this with asserting that the fix is worth $X million dollars from a Finance standpoint. I think it is safe to say that if a group of employees is being paid and they can't perform optimally (a fact backed up by survey results), then some value is lost. NAV just helps you prioritize your focus among the various options and use the same consistent measure to track changes over time.

Using Activation for Business Impact

You can use the activation measurement framework in a number of ways to improve the bottom line. I list the most effective ways here first and then delve a little deeper into each approach over the course of this section. First off, you can

>> Gain business buy-in on the people analytics research plan

>> Analyze organization problems and design solutions

>> Support managers

>> Support organization change

The following sections spell out the details.

Gaining business buy-in on the people analytics research plan

Often when I work with companies, I have to quickly gain consensus among the various influencers and decision makers (from different departments or functions within the organization) about the specific business goals and job outputs (accomplishments) we are trying to understand and improve with people analytics.

People often see "part of the elephant" when it comes to concepts that they believe influence attainment of business unit performance goals — that's to say they see the parts that interest them or are familiar with, but not the other parts. Some people may be focused on compensation issues, others look at company climate and culture, others emphasize employee selection, and still others may be focused on learning and development. Though it can be frustrating to mediate between so many different points of view, this diversity of perspective is helpful for people analytics.

When you work with a large group, you can draw the 4-factor activation model on a whiteboard (you know — the capability-alignment-motivation-support concept), begin jotting down each person's interests or concerns in the appropriate columns, and drive the discussion toward an understanding of how it all fits together as a whole to influence behavior and its performance products. When you explain that these same four factors of influence will be used to define your approach for analysis, it should soon become clear how many parties will need to work together to ensure a successful analysis and eventual solution to any underlying problems. (As you might expect, not just one stakeholder or team can be expected to tackle the task)

REMEMBER

By using the activation model to explain how all four factors fit together, looking for examples of misalignment (expectations and incentives in conflict), and expanding all participant's views to include the entire four factors, you will be able to gain increased alignment on objectives and how to proceed.

Analyzing problems and designing solutions

Phase 1 of most analysis should be the 4-factor activation survey outlined earlier in this chapter. The findings from this survey can be used in the design of data measurements collected from systems, additional surveys (as needed), interviews, and other sources.

In addition, the four factors provide a useful way of organizing information to guide discussion. When a stakeholder has a specific "best practice" solution in mind, I have found that one of the most powerful applications of the model is to use it to explain that investments in one factor will not pay off if it's not the problem or if other needed factors are missing or in conflict. You can use a discussion like this one to manage the risk that the stakeholder may implement a solution without making other equally important changes — and then expressing frustration at not seeing the expected results. Introducing the 4-factor model early on in the engagement can sometimes provide a transition from a tactical focus to a focus on business impact.

When you make a recommendation for a solution — even a simple one — you can use the 4-factor framework to assess relevant information in each of the factors and to suggest a comprehensive solution that includes all four. The model can be used to create checklists to ensure that the items to be considered when preparing to roll out an intervention are not missed.

Supporting managers

Front-line managers like the simplicity and practical language of the activation model. It takes about five minutes to introduce in a minimal way. In a few hours, it's possible to provide a systematic introduction to how managers can use these factors for assessing the main factors that affect the performance of the groups and individuals they manage.

Performance-appraisal discussions between managers and employees can benefit from the 4-factor activation model as well. Once managers agree with their people on goals or targets, they can use the four elements of activation to collaborate with employees to find the pieces' missing supports that might help make a difference.

Supporting organizational change

An important function of a model is to establish a common language. A common language can be a huge advantage, especially when you have to obtain consensus among many stakeholders. The 4-factor model proposes a fundamental language for how to support performance, moving the company beyond fixation on the result to a focus on the conditions that are required to gain a better result.

Taking Stock

In Chapter 4, I specify that you can break your workforce down into many different types of segments and that each segment may offer a different perspective. In Chapter 5, I explain that the way you segment the workforce and where you should put your dollars to achieve the biggest return on investment on people will not be the same as in any other company. In Chapter 6, I describe how to put all segments into a comparable financial basis — in dollars — for a long-term perspective using employee lifetime value (ELV). In this chapter (Chapter 7), I tell you how to adjust ELV for activation, a concept that reflects the minimum conditions for value to be produced and then measured by NAV. With NAV, you can evaluate where to spend time and money on people to gain the highest return on investment.

Part 2 of this book establishes a flexible, lean measurement framework for people analytics. Part 3 gives you the fundamental measurement and analysis tools for the employee journey.

3

Quantifying the Employee Journey

IN THIS PART . . .

Measure how good your company is at attracting talent (Attraction), activating talent (Activation) and controlling the rate of talent exit (Attrition)

Get in front of productivity problems by using data to proactively evaluate the four minimal conditions for performance — capability, alignment, motivation and support

Meet the five models of people analytics

Clarify, improve, and communicate your analytics journey and post-analysis action plan with the help of models

IN THIS CHAPTER

» Understanding the employee
experience from the perspective
of the employee journey

» Measuring the influence of key touch
points on the employee experience

» Creating a measurement framework
to produce insight and continuous
improvement in the employee
experience

Chapter **8**

Mapping the Employee Journey

f you were to conduct a careful review of the options available for measuring the performance of Human Resources, you would come up with a list of more than 200 potential metrics and just as many survey questions. (I know, because I've done both.) Starting a people analytics journey that includes all these metrics and survey questions in its scope would be daunting — and a lot of work to complete. If you ever completed the task, it would still be a confusing result: Among all these measures, how would you know the good or the bad of it, and where would you focus? Rather than attempt to measure all things that are possible, or arbitrarily choose a focus, it's better to align the measures to a broader objective or problem focus area. To guide this effort, I propose the "triple-A framework" — *attraction, activation,* and *attrition* — as shown in Figure 8-1.

The triple-A framework provides some clarity by narrowing the range of possible areas of focus to three broad opportunities or problems:

» **Attraction** represents a set of metrics and analyses intended to measure the attractive force of the company to acquire the quality of talent it wants. In other words, how are you doing on getting talent into the company?

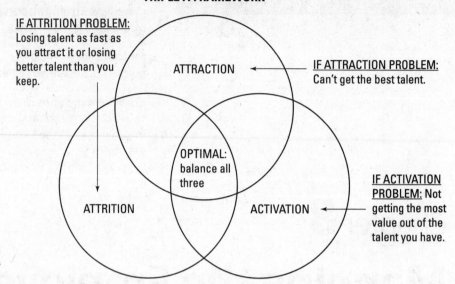

TRIPLE A FRAMEWORK

IF ATTRITION PROBLEM:
Losing talent as fast as
you attract it or losing
better talent than you
keep.

ATTRACTION

IF ATTRACTION PROBLEM:
Can't get the best talent.

OPTIMAL:
balance all
three

ATTRITION

ACTIVATION

IF ACTIVATION
PROBLEM: Not
getting the most
value out of the
talent you have.

FIGURE 8-1:
The triple-A
framework.

>> **Activation** represents a set of metrics and analysis intended to measure the proportion of people and teams who have all the basic requirements to produce high performance. In other words, how are we doing at creating the conditions that make for productive employees?

>> **Attrition** represents a set of metrics and analysis intended to measure the degree of control the company has over the quality of the talent it's able to retain versus the quality of talent it allows or encourages to exit. In other words, how are you doing keeping your highest performers, while letting others go on to the next stop in their career?

In Chapters 9, 10 and 11, I give each component of the triple-A framework (attraction, activation and attrition) their chapter to provide a deeper exploration of the topic and to provide a sampling of measures you can use to get started analyzing them.

For the time being I elevate the triple-A framework to your attention because of its foundational role in refining your focus from among many measures and connecting the many measures together. The three A's — attraction, activation, and attrition — describe the three primary talent management problems each company must solve collectively and also describe the main phases of each individual's journey as well. All employees go through a period of attraction, activation, and attrition on their journey with the company. This chapter is about what you can learn about how the company is doing from the standpoint of the employee journey, as opposed to from the standpoint of areas of HR specialty or from the standpoint of HR systems and processes.

The survey-based measurement system I propose in this chapter provides a way to measure how well you're doing at different stages of the employee journey from the standpoint of candidates and employees.

Standing on the Shoulders of Customer Journey Maps

An *employee journey map* is a visualization of the major stages and touch points that employees experience from the time they become aware of an opportunity at the company, during interviews, throughout their first day of employment, into their first year and into later tenures, and then ending when they leave the company.

The idea of an employee journey map has roots in the *customer journey map* — a visual document that charts the customer experience as it progresses through the stages of a company's sales-and-marketing funnel into a buyer/seller relationship to achieve goals for the customers.

The customer journey map for service design was first introduced by the (then up-and-coming) international design-and-marketing firm IDEO, back in 1999. (The company had come up with the idea and applied it to the Acela high-speed rail project, where it was used to visualize the customer experience for interactions with — and feelings for — the rail system.) The customer journey map, now widely used in marketing, is particularly useful as a tool for visualizing, analyzing, communicating, and improving intangible services.

The goal of the customer journey map is first to define the path that key customer types take to the product or service and then break down the elements of that path in order to better understand how these types find their way to (and experience) the product or service. This map brings together major interactions, known as *touch points,* that the customer has with the company and documents the changing feelings, motivations, and questions that key customer groups have at the touch points. The customer journey map is used to compare customers' perceived interactions with the company's vision of the experience. Understanding the customer's point of view throughout the journey makes it possible to solve problems and design a better experience that meets or exceeds the expectations to produce advantages versus competitors.

The success of the customer journey map led many to ask whether its principles can be applied to the employee experience. I'm happy to say that the answer to this question is emphatically yes. Below I show you how to create an employee journey map for yourself.

When completed, the map visually shows the stages that employees go through, details specific company touch points, specifies feedback tools that are used to quantify the candidate or employee experience at each stage, and even includes a summary of what the data shows all in one view.

We will build this map together. Figure 8-2 below shows three different ways of categorizing the stages that all employees go through in their relationship with a company.

EMPLOYEE JOURNEY MAP

TRIPLE-A FRAMEWORK	ATTRACTION					ACTIVATION			ATTRITION
CUSTOMER JOURNEY STAGES	AWARENESS	OPINION	CONSIDER	PREFERENCE	DECISION	ACTIVATION			DECLINE
EMPLOYEE JOURNEY STAGES	LABOR POOL	INVITE OR APPLY	PHONE SCREEN	ON-SITE INTERVIEW	OFFER	0–90 DAYS	90 DAYS–1 YEAR	ANNUAL ANNIVERSARY	EXIT
TIME	→

FIGURE 8-2:
Employee journey map: the first step is to identify the stages.

In Figure 8-2, the first row is included so you can see how the detailed employee journey stages found below fit into the over-arching triple-A framework. The second row expresses the cognitive stages that an employee goes through, borrowing from how a marketer thinks about a customer moving from no awareness of a product to having a relationship with the product, until eventual decline. The third row lines it all up with the activities that occur in the recruiting process. The arrow below shows that the map works left to right, showing how a person moves from no awareness of the company to becoming a productive member of the company to eventual decline.

As Figure 8-2 illustrates, the employee journey map should accommodate the entire journey that people make as employees — from their first contact with the company during the recruiting process to new-hire orientation to onboarding to the first 30, 90, and 180 days to the first anniversary and on to future anniversaries until the point of exit.

REMEMBER

Your recruiting process or way of framing the employee experience in stages may be a little different from mine and that is fine. You can draw your map how you want to — the one I have included is just a generic example.

Figure 8-3 builds on the foundation we've started by citing the important company touchpoints that align to each stage.

As I have sampled in Figure 8-3, your next step is to brainstorm all of the points of contact between the company and the person to clarify the opportunities you have to influence the opinion of the candidate or employee about the company.

By connecting touch points to the employee journey map, you can figure out where your best opportunities are to apply resources to make the most impact on opinion at any given phase of the employee journey.

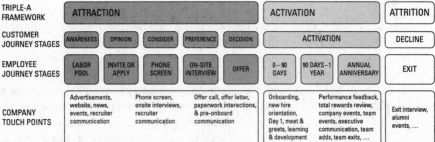

EMPLOYEE JOURNEY MAP

FIGURE 8-3: Employee journey map: the second step is to add the company touchpoints.

The next step is to indicate how you are going to measure company performance at each stage. Surveys help you see the journey map beyond merely aspiration and anecdote. With survey data, you can measure each stage of the employee journey in such a way that you can see the average, the range, and trend over time, compared by segment and by stage. Survey data allows you to record incidents and attitudes along the way to see how incidents and attitudes that you find at prior stages correlate to what you find at later stages. With this information, you can focus on improving the experiences at earlier stages that you know are important because of the long-term consequences for the company. Well-designed surveys, when used together with other data, can help you see many things that you otherwise would be unable to see.

Figure 8-4 adds the names of the surveys you can use to obtain a quantitative measure of the attitude or opinion of people at each stage.

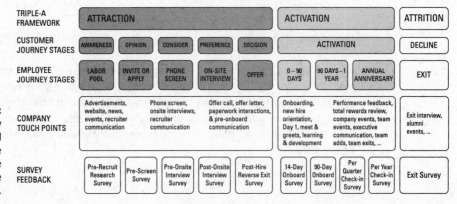

EMPLOYEE JOURNEY MAP

FIGURE 8-4: Employee journey map: the third step is to decide how you are going to measure each stage.

Figure 8-4 provides a generic title for a series of surveys you can use to obtain feedback on each stage. I provide some sample surveys later in this chapter. but keep in mind that you can name your surveys whatever you like and modify your surveys as you like — again, what you find here is merely an example to show how it all fits together.

The data you can use in conjunction with your employee journey map is not limited to survey data only. The data blueprint shown in Figure 8-5 is a conceptual diagram of what's happening in the employee journey which, with a little work, can be expressed as metrics using data that you can obtain from systems. Unlike the data described above that is collected through surveys, this type of data is obtained from the applicant tracking system (ATS) or human resource information system (HRIS). After detailed data has been extracted from these systems, you can express the counts of the number of people at each stage, the number of people entering and exiting each stage, and the movement of people between stages in many different useful ways.

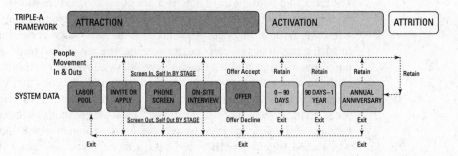

FIGURE 8-5:
Employee journey map: you can also use data from systems.

Figure 8-5 illustrates diagrammatically how people move from one stage to the next (or exit out entirely) and provides the names of the base measures that can be used to count and measure the volume of movement. You may use these base measures alone or together with other data to paint a picture of what is happening overall — a picture which cannot be gained by relying on personal experience or anecdotal evidence.

Figure 8-6 brings everything we have done so far together in one place.

As you can see in Figure 8-6, the employee journey map allows you to see in one place how a lot of different concepts fit together as one — this is in fact the entire point! The example I have included works left to right and has rows that allow you to see how the triple-A framework, customer journey stages, employee journey stages, company touchpoints, survey feedback tools, and system feedback tools all fit together.

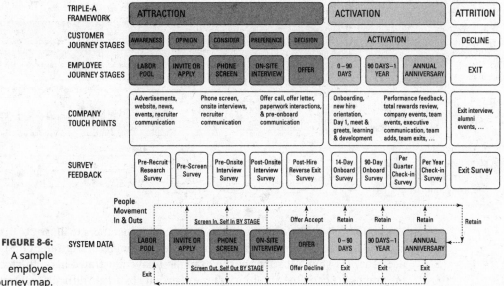

TRIPLE-A FRAMEWORK	ATTRACTION					ACTIVATION			ATTRITION
CUSTOMER JOURNEY STAGES	AWARENESS	OPINION	CONSIDER	PREFERENCE	DECISION	ACTIVATION			DECLINE
EMPLOYEE JOURNEY STAGES	LABOR POOL	INVITE OR APPLY	PHONE SCREEN	ON-SITE INTERVIEW	OFFER	0–90 DAYS	90 DAYS–1 YEAR	ANNUAL ANNIVERSARY	EXIT
COMPANY TOUCH POINTS	Advertisements, website, news, events, recruiter communication	Phone screen, onsite interviews, recruiter communication		Offer call, offer letter, paperwork interactions, & pre-onboard communication		Onboarding, new hire orientation, Day 1, meet & greets, learning & development	Performance feedback, total rewards review, company events, team events, executive communication, team adds, team exits, ...		Exit interview, alumni events, ...
SURVEY FEEDBACK	Pre-Recruit Research Survey	Pre-Screen Survey	Pre-Onsite Interview Survey	Post-Onsite Interview Survey	Post-Hire Reverse Exit Survey	14-Day Onboard Survey	90-Day Onboard Survey	Per Quarter Check-in Survey / Per Year Check-in Survey	Exit Survey

FIGURE 8-6: A sample employee journey map.

TIP

A detailed employee journey map like the one in Figure 8-6 should definitely be available for use by anyone on the HR team and should be collectively reviewed from time to time, but I'll admit it is a tad overwhelming to look at if you were not the one involved in creating it. This does not mean you should not do an employee journey map — don't throw out the baby with the bath water — but you can put the detail away for use by those people who need it when they need it and just provide a summary to the casual audience.

Figure 8-7 is an example of what the employee journey map could look like with less detail on its inner operations while still including summary data that can be obtained from survey and system sources.

Check out what's been added in Figure 8-7. On the Survey Data Summary row, you can review the height of any bar all the way across to compare stages to each other. There are four bars for each stage, which represent a quarterly view so you can also see if you are getting better over time. Because this is just illustrative, my labelling is not specific (Q1, Q2, Q3, Q4), but in your case you could be more specific: for example: Q1-2018, Q2-2018, Q3-2018, Q4-2018. You also could report it by intervals other than quarters — bi-annually or annually, for example. The point of the design I have suggested here is that you can compare stages to each other and also see how each stage is changing over time in a single glance.

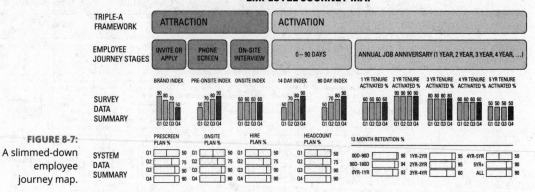

FIGURE 8-7:
A slimmed-down
employee
journey map.

The bottom row, labelled System Data Summary, is just there to illustrate that you can also include system data facts and/or leverage graphs of a different design, as necessary for your situation. In the example I have illustrated here, the focus of the graphs is not on the absolute volume of activity by stage (difficult to interpret), but rather on a metric that compares the volume of activity to what was planned in advance — the metric expressed is essentially the percentage of plan achieved for key stages. These bars can range between 0 and 100 (with 100 being perfect) and the line indicates how close the company got to plan. Again, I have added bars labelled by quarter so you if this were real data you could see how the company is improving over time — or not. You could also see how missing the plan in earlier stages can quickly add up to a situation where you miss plan in later stages. This design allows you to quickly trace the problem back to where it started.

The graphs on the far right of the bottom row are different than the ones to the left. The graphs to the far right represent the percentage of employees retained (the ones that didn't leave the company) over a 12-month period by job tenure group. If this were real data, these graphs would show you at what point or points in the employee's job tenure you begin to see high percentages of employees exit the company. Seeing retention in 1-year job tenure intervals allows you to find the right time frames to move employees into new jobs, address whatever the problems are common among each tenure interval which may be different than exits among other tenure intervals, and plan for inevitable exits.

The intent of the graphs included in this chapter is not to convey a real data insight or to explain how to create them. These are sketchy examples with fake data. My goal here is to show you that, with a handful of graphs, you can create a powerful dashboard that can be easily understood in the context of the employee journey with a quick glance — this does not occur by accident, this occurs by design.

Why an Employee Journey Map?

The goal of recruiting people into a company isn't to produce a hire and then simply congratulate yourself on a job well done — the point is to have that hire become a productive, contributing member of the company for as long as possible. It isn't a one-time or sporadic relationship — it's a high-cost, high-value relationship that must be renewed by employees and employers every working day.

TIP

Consider the entire journey that the employee makes with the company and how the actions (or inactions) taken by the company affect the motivation and productivity of employees over time.

The goal of an employee journey map is to identify those areas or transition points where people tend to encounter problems — whether those problems occur at the initial interview stage or while working for your company — and identify opportunities for improvement.

A closer look at the various metrics available to Human Resources departments not only reveals a bewildering array of options but also shows that some options have different ways of measuring progress. It also shows that some of those ways come in conflict with one another because they highlight different priorities.

An employee journey map can also help unify often disparate and competing efforts within the same company by providing everyone with a single framework that maps the activities of Human Resources with the employee experience.

Everyone has blind spots. Everyone has a lot to do, and — left unchecked — everyone gets caught up in what they're trying to accomplish individually, sometimes at the expense of people who do other jobs or at the expense of the company as a whole. The employee journey map allows you to take a bird's-eye view of actions by different stakeholders who work together to impact the employee experience.

REMEMBER

Unless you work in a very small company, Human Resources isn't a single person, single knowledge area, or single job. The contribution to the company from people who work under the umbrella of HR fits into multiple categories. HR *Centers of Excellence (COEs)* are centralized units within the function of Human Resources that have a specialized expertise and job focus. Examples of HR COEs are Talent Acquisition, Compensation, Benefits, Employee Relations, Learning and Development, and Organization Design (OD). Someone who works in Compensation doesn't do Recruiting's job, and someone in Recruiting doesn't do Compensation's job, and so on. Sometimes, the policies, programs, processes, and other efforts of people in different COEs pull in different directions. What you want to do with data is help these specialized members of HR connect what they do to an overarching objective.

AVOIDING THAT "STUFF HAPPENS" MOMENT

Stuff happens, right? Not necessarily. One advantage of a detailed employee journey map is that it can help you avoid typical speed bumps in the hiring-and-retention process. The two examples in this sidebar show you how things can go wrong in that process — and how an employee journey map might help you catch the warning signs.

Recruiters

The natural incentive for a recruiter is to produce a hire quickly and move on to the next one, recruiters are measured by their number of hires — an incentive that results in behaviors that produce hires without regard to quality or care for the experiences of candidates and sometimes the future teams where the candidates will work. You need for recruiters to produce not only hires but also the best-quality hires possible while accurately representing the job — and to do so without leaving a trail of dead bodies. If you aren't measuring the contribution of the recruiters in light of the entire employee journey, you may have recruiters doing what is best for themselves while operating against what is best for the candidates or the company in the long run.

Managers

The natural incentive for managers is to hold on to their best-performing employees as long as possible – they are measured by the performance of their team. If they let their best employee shuttle to another team or get promoted, then they have to take a risk and start over. Though this tendency is convenient for managers, eventually employees may want to progress their careers into the next step for *them*. When the entire responsibility for managing the careers of employees remains only in the hands of managers and employees, employees will find it best to exit the company to achieve their next career moves. This unfortunate and unnecessary loss for the company can be prevented by having processes that continuously evaluate the tenure of employees and proactively present new internal opportunities at the right times. Absent an entire employee journey perspective and a company-wide system of measurement, managers who are left to their own devices won't make decisions that are best for the company or its employees — and then everyone loses in the end when employees exit the company.

The benefit of considering the employee experience at different signposts in the employee journey is that it provides a longer-term perspective from which to evaluate and prioritize actions. If you were to consider the employee journey only from the standpoint of the employee experience all mixed together all at one time, you can miss signposts and get off track.

Creating Your Own Employee Journey Map

Creating a customer journey map can sound like its own ambiguous and arduous journey, but it need not be. Though it's important to align your map to data, it doesn't have to be overly complicated. It only needs to contain the necessary detail to communicate the stages, touch points, influences, and emotional reactions to help you understand what is going on and drive action.

Mapping your map

The initial spadework for mapping isn't that onerous. Here's what you need to do first:

1. Pick a key job group or another employee segment at your company.

2. Define stages or steps of your recruiting process for candidates in this job group.

   For example: outreach, resume review, phone screen, on-site interview 1, onsite interview 2, offer, hire, onboard, and so on.

3. Define the key touch points for candidates in this job group.

   For example: recruiter's first email to candidate, recruiters first phone conversation, recruiters follow-up phone conversation, greeting at the company, interview, employee orientation, greeting on first day, greeting with the team, and so on.

4. Identify the key information needs and questions that a typical person experiences at each touch point. Also consider the information needs that the company has at each touch point.

5. Define measurement instruments and metrics for each stage.

6. Collect quantitative and qualitative data.

7. Identify the problems and opportunities. In the *Offer* stage, for example, it may be of concern that candidates can't differentiate the job opportunity except by level of pay.

8. Identify who is accountable to act for each problem or opportunity identified. Many efforts can be combined, but one person must be accountable to direct those efforts.

9. Monitor continuously to see whether the actions that are taken address the problems and opportunities in the manner expected and to uncover new problems and opportunities.

10. Repeat the process for each important employee segment at your company.

That's the framework. The success (or failure) of your employee journey map depends on how you fill in that framework. And the most important element you'll use to fill in that framework is, of course, data. So it's time to tackle the data question, and that means reading the next section.

Getting data

The employee journey map should be based on data that describes the reality of candidates and employees, not on your idea of what that reality should be. Here are some ways you can get reliable information to fill in the gaps on the employee journey map:

>> **Leave your office behind:** An important first step to increasing your perspective about the employee experience is to walk away from your desk and observe people working where the work is being done. You can often spot issues that nobody else would have thought to tell you about or that you wouldn't have noticed in data you already have. Evaluate what actually is happening rather than what people say or what arbitrary information has incidentally accumulated in systems or in previous surveys.

>> **Walk in someone else's shoes:** In some companies, you can shadow someone, do a ride-along, or work in a role for a day. Though this process may be anecdotal and produce too much detail for a journey map, it can stimulate your understanding of, and empathy with, the type of people you employ. It can also help you understand what good work looks like and the types of people who do it.

Getting close to the action produces the opportunity to ask questions in a face-to-face environment in a context where people are already comfortable — and where you can understand the things you're being told.

>> **Conduct stakeholder interviews:** Interview employees in the key job families for which you want to create a journey map. Interview managers, recruiters, and other support staff. Interview candidates — not for jobs but rather to ask them questions regarding their experience in applying for a job at your company. Interview former employees — many people will take your phone call and will be happy to talk to you about what went right and what went wrong.

When you do as I suggest in this list — leave your office behind, walk in someone's shoes, and do stakeholder interviews — go ahead and capture anecdotes; do not, however, rely totally on them as a final source of information. (I realize that it can be tempting to get caught up in a good story and run with it.) Eventually, it's important to validate anecdotal inspirations with data collected from a larger sample; the three tasks I just mentioned can be useful creative thinking devices to help you express those patterns to other people in a way that is compelling after you have confirmed these observations. Look first to confirm that the stories do exist as consistent patterns in systematically collected data; and then, only when this is confirmed, use anecdotes to help you express those patterns to other people.

» **Conduct surveys:** In my career, I have designed a lot of employee surveys. In my experience, focusing on a collective perspective of people through surveys always a) makes a profound contribution to whatever question I am trying to answer b) helps to identify compelling stories and c) is less complicated to deploy and explain than most other analytical methods.

» **Looking at data in systems:** You can use lots of data on your employee journey map in the operational data systems — like the applicant tracking system (ATS), human resources information system (HRIS), enterprise resource planning system (ERP), or any other systems that contain information about candidates and employees.

Using Surveys to Get a Handle on the Employee Journey

Since the employee journey map is centered around the experiences of living, breathing people, a key part is collecting feedback from living breathing people with surveys. In this section, I provide you with some sample surveys you can use to put real data to your employee journey map.

REMEMBER

When you use the survey items I outline in the following sections, simply replace *<Company Name>* with your company's name and replace *<Insert Industry Example>* with relevant talent competitors.

Pre-Recruiting Market Research Survey

On a scale of 0 to 10, how likely are you to seriously consider a new job opportunity in the next year? (0= not at all, 10 = very likely)

If it applies, please describe a moment when you have felt genuine happiness at work.

If it applies, please describe anything that is preventing you from being as successful as you would like to be in your current role.

"Which top three employers would you consider for your next career move?" Choose three.

>   *<Insert here your own custom list here>*

>   *<Insert Industry Example>*

>   *<Insert Industry Example>*

>   *<Company Name>*

>   *<Insert Industry Example>*

>   *<Insert Industry Example>*

>   *<Insert Non-Industry Example>*

>   *<Insert Non-Industry Example>*

>   *<Insert Non-Industry Example>*

>   Other: _____

>   Other: _____

>   Other: _____

On a scale of 0 to 10, how likely are you to consider a job opportunity at *<Company>*? (0= not at all, 10 = very likely)

When you think of *<Company>* brand and culture what words, if any, come to mind? (List as many as you can)

When you think of *<Company>* brand and culture what words, if any, come to mind? (Selected all that apply)

<Insert here your own custom list here>

Examples:

>   Arrogant

>   Conservative

>   Creative

>   Diverse

>   Ethical

>   Friendly

>   Fun

Innovative

Intelligent

Intimidating

Performance

Professional

Quality

Successful

Snobby

Traditional

Trustworthy

Unethical

Brand Exposure

Have you ever used the products and services of *<Company>*? (Yes/No) (If yes, detail: _____)

On a scale of 0 to 10, how familiar with *<Company>* are you? (0= not at all, 10 = very familiar)

Have you ever been to an event sponsored by *<Company>*? (Yes/No) (If yes, detail: _____)

Do you know anyone who works at *<Company>*? (Yes/No) (If yes, detail: _____)

» Have you ever been approached before by a recruiter at *<Company>*? (Yes/No) (If yes, detail: _____)

Have you ever applied for a job at *<Company>*? (Yes/No) (If yes, detail: _____)

Sourcing Channels

How did you find out about your current job?

What professional websites or blogs do you follow?

What periodicals and magazines do you read on a regular basis?

What professional associations or meetup groups do you regularly participate in?

What websites do you use to learn about or look for job opportunities?

Pre-Onsite-Interview survey

On a scale from 1 to 5, please indicate your level of agreement with the following statements: 1) Strongly disagree. 2) Disagree. 3) Neither agree nor disagree. 4) Agree. 5) Strongly agree.

The recruiter has clearly defined what the job is.

The recruiter has expressed a unique selling point for the job.

The opportunity that is described to me is compelling.

I know everything I need to know about the job opportunity for now.

I have a clear understanding of <Company Name>'s brand identity and products.

<Company Name> seems like it's in a position to succeed.

<Company Name> compares favorably with competitors as an attractive place to work.

I think that my long-term career goals can be met at <Company Name>.

I'd be proud to work for <Company Name>.

On a scale from 0 to 10, how likely are you to consider a job opportunity at <Company Name>?

When you think of <Company Name>'s brand and culture, which words, if any, come to mind? (List as many as you can.)

Post-Onsite-Interview survey

On a scale from 1 to 5, please indicate your level of agreement with the following statements: 1) Strongly disagree. 2) Disagree. 3) Neither agree nor disagree. 4) Agree. 5) Strongly Agree.

The recruiter gave me the information I needed to prepare for the interview.

The interviewers showed up on time.

The interviewers made me feel welcome and as comfortable as I could be at an interview.

The interviewers were well prepared to speak with me

The interviewers were knowledgeable about the line of work I do.

The interviewers were interested and curious about me.

The interviewers explained and applied an interview method designed to reduce bias.

The interviewers have realistic expectations about the job.

In the interviews, I was given the opportunity to fully describe what is unique about me.

The hiring process at <Company Name> is much better than my experience with other companies.

How can we improve our recruiting process?

What aspects of the opportunity are most compelling to you?

What aspects of the opportunity are a concern to you?

When you think of <Company Name>'s brand and culture, which words, if any, come to mind? (List as many as you can.)

Post-Hire Reverse Exit Interview survey

Immediately before joining us at <Company Name>, did you work for another company? (Yes, No)

If no, were you (select one):

Personal: Caring for children or significant others

Personal: Going to school

Personal: Pursuing nonpaid interests

Personal: Other

If yes:

Was your last employer in the same industry? (Yes, No)

What was the name of your last employer?

At <Company Name>, do you expect to gain or lose in the following areas? 1) Lose a lot. 2) Lose a little. 3) Neither lose nor gain. 4) Gain a little. 5) Gain a lot.

Overall company quality

Leadership team quality

Manager quality

Peer quality

Work quality

Learning and development opportunities

Current offered job level

Long-term career opportunities

Expected 1-year value of total compensation package (base, bonus, stock)

Expected 3- to 5-year value of total compensation package (base, bonus, stock)

Benefits (health and retirement, for example)

Perks (meals, on-site services, and fitness, for example)

On balance, how would you characterize your decision to leave your last employer? (Select one.)

Mostly for work-related reasons within your prior employer's ability to address.

Mostly for personal reasons outside of your prior employer's ability to address.

Personal: Other

If it applies, please describe a moment when you have felt genuine happiness at work.

If it applies, please describe anything that prevented you from being as successful as you wanted in your former role at *<Company Name>*.

Please tell us about the events leading up to your decision to leave *<Company Name>*.

Is there anything your prior employer could have done differently to keep you longer? (Yes, No)

Please tell us what your prior employer could have done differently to keep you longer?

14-Day On-Board survey

On a scale from 1 to 5, please indicate your level of agreement with the following statements: 1) Strongly disagree. 2) Disagree. 3) Neither agree nor disagree. 4) Agree. 5) Strongly agree.

I feel welcomed by the people I will work with here at *<Company Name>*.

I received all the information and learning resources I needed to get up to speed quickly.

I have received the time I need with others to get up to speed quickly.

This onboarding process at *<Company Name>* is well thought out and well designed.

I was given accurate information during the interview process.

<Company Name> compares favorably with competitors as an attractive place to work.

How can *<Company Name>* improve the onboarding process?

How can *<Company Name>* make first few days of working at better?

When you think of our company brand and culture what words, if any, come to mind? (List as many as you can.)

90-Day On-Board Survey

On a scale from 1 to 5, please indicate your level of agreement with the following statements: 1) Strongly disagree. 2) Disagree. 3) Neither agree nor disagree. 4) Agree. 5) Strongly agree.

I feel welcomed by the people I will work with here at *<Company Name>*.

I received all the information & learning resources I needed to get up to speed quickly.

I have received the time I need with others to get up to speed quickly.

This onboarding process at *<Company Name>* is well thought out and designed.

I was given accurate information during the interview process.

<Company Name> compares favorably with competitors as an attractive place to work.

The work I have do in the next 12 months is compelling.

I have everything I need to perform at my best.

My manager is working with me to adapt myself to the team and role.

My manager is working with me to adapt the role to my strengths.

I have a clear understanding of the difference between an average and great contribution for my role.

I have a clear understanding of what I need to do to make a great contribution in my role.

I have the capabilities I need to make a great contribution in my current role at this time.

The actions I need to take to be successful in this job are achievable and within my control.

I really care about achieving great work here.

I am willing to put in a great deal of effort beyond that of the average person in order to be successful here.

I have the cooperation and support I need to be successful.

I have the resources and tools I need to be successful.

How can <Company Name> improve the onboarding process?

How can <Company Name> improve the first 90 days of working at <Company Name>?

When you think of our company brand and culture, which words, if any, come to mind? (List as many as you can.)

Once-Per-Quarter Check-In survey

On a scale from 1 to 5, please indicate your level of agreement with the following statements: 1) Strongly disagree. 2) Disagree. 3) Neither agree nor disagree. 4) Agree. 5) Strongly agree.

I have a clear understanding of the difference between an average and great contribution for my role.

I have a clear understanding of what I need to do to make a great contribution in my role.

I have the capabilities I need to make a great contribution in my current role at this time.

The actions I need to take to be successful in this job are achievable and within my control.

I really care about achieving great work here.

I am willing to put in a great deal of effort beyond that of the average person in order to be successful here.

I have the cooperation and support I need to be successful.

I have the resources and tools I need to be successful.

My manager is helping me develop in my career.

My manager communicates clear goals for the team.

My manager regularly gives me actionable feedback.

My manager avoids micromanaging me.

My manager consistently shows consideration for me as a person.

My manager keeps the team focused on priorities, even when it means declining interesting projects or putting less important projects on the back burner.

My manager regularly shares relevant information from senior leadership.

My manager has had a meaningful discussion with me about my career development in the past six months.

My manager has the functional expertise required to manage me effectively.

My manager makes tough decisions effectively.

My manager effectively collaborates across the organization.

My manager values my perspective, even when she doesn't agree with it.

I would recommend my manager to others.

I can recommend <Company Name> as a great place to work.

I can recall a moment in the past three months when I felt genuine happiness at work.

If it applies, please describe a moment in the past three months when you have felt genuine happiness at work.

If it applies, please describe anything that is preventing you from being as successful as you wanted at <Company Name>.

Once-Per-Year Check-In survey

On a scale from 1 to 5, please indicate your level of agreement with the following statements: 1) Strongly disagree. 2) Disagree. 3) Neither agree nor disagree. 4) Agree. 5) Strongly agree.

I have a clear understanding of the difference between an average and great contribution for my role.

I have a clear understanding of what I need to do to make a great contribution in my role.

I have the capabilities I need to make a great contribution in my current role at this time.

The actions I need to take to be successful in this job are achievable and within my control.

I really care about achieving great work here.

I am willing to put in a great deal of effort beyond that of the average person in order to be successful here.

I have the cooperation and support I need to be successful.

I have the resources and tools I need to be successful.

My manager is helping me develop in my career.

My manager communicates clear goals for the team.

My manager regularly gives me actionable feedback.

My manager avoids micromanaging me.

My manager consistently shows consideration for me as a person.

My manager keeps the team focused on priorities, even when it means declining interesting projects or putting less important projects on the back burner.

My manager regularly shares relevant information from senior leadership.

My manager has had a meaningful discussion with me about my career development in the past six months.

My manager has the functional expertise required to manage me effectively.

My manager makes tough decisions effectively.

My manager effectively collaborates across the organization.

My manager values my perspective, even when she doesn't agree with it.

I would recommend my manager to others.

I would like to pursue career advancement at <Company Name>, in the next 12 to 24 months.

I would be thrilled to be working in the same job 12 months from now.

Overall, I think that I can meet my career goals at <Company Name>.

I can recommend <Company Name> as a great place to work.

I can recall a moment in the past three months when I felt genuine happiness at work.

I am proud to work for <Company Name>.

I fit in well in the <Company Name> employee culture.

I am inspired by the people I work with at <Company Name>.

I find personal meaning in the work I do at <Company Name>.

I have the opportunity to do what I do best at <Company Name>.

I am motivated to do more than expected to help those I work with succeed.

I have no desire to leave <Company Name> right now.

If it applies, please describe a moment in the past three months when you have felt genuine happiness at work.

If it applies, please describe anything that is preventing you from being as successful as you wanted to be at <Company Name>.

Key Talent Exit Survey

After you leave <Company Name>, will you be working for another employer? (Yes, No)

If no, will you (select one):

Personal: Care for children or significant others

Personal: Go to school

Personal: Pursue nonpaid interests

Personal: Other

If yes:

Is your new job in the same industry? (Yes, No)

What is the name of your new employer?

For your new employer, do you expect to gain or lose in the following areas? Scale: 1) Lose a lot. 2) Lose a little. 3) Neither lose nor gain. 4) Gain a little. 5) Gain a lot.

Overall company quality

Leadership team quality

Manager quality

Peer quality

Work quality

Learning and development opportunity

Current offered job level

Long-term career opportunity

Expected 1-year value of total compensation package (base, bonus, stock)

Expected 3-to 5-year value of total compensation package (base, bonus, stock)

Benefits (health and retirement, for example)

Perks (meals, on-site services, and fitness, for example)

On balance, how would you characterize your decision to leave <Company Name>? (Select one.)

It's mostly for work-related reasons within <Company Name>'s ability to address.

It's mostly for personal reasons outside of <Company Name>'s ability to address.

If it applies, please describe a moment when you have felt genuine happiness working at <Company Name>.

If it applies, please describe anything that prevented you from being as successful as you wanted to be at <Company Name>.

Did any recent actions or events affect your decision to leave <Company Name>? Choose all that apply:

Work related: Action/inaction by your manager

Work related: Action/inaction by leadership team

Work related: Action/inaction by peers in your work group

Work related: Action/inaction by peers not in your work group

Personal: Personal health, health of others, or birth of child

Personal: Career opportunity for significant other is making you move

Personal: You or a significant other reached retirement eligibility age

Work related: Other

Personal: Other

Please tell us about the events leading up to your decision to leave <Company Name>.

Is there anything <Company Name> could have done differently to keep you longer? (Yes, No)

Please tell us what <Company Name> could have done differently to keep you longer.

Is there anything <Company Name> can do now or in the future to get you back? (Yes, No)

What can <Company Name> do to get you back?

REMEMBER

The survey items above are examples that I have selected to get you started for purposes of gaining a summary perspective on the employee journey. In addition to this, *People Analytics For Dummies* includes a comprehensive survey guide ("Appendix B: Great Employee Survey Questions") as an online resource at the web site associated with this book. This resource includes many other categories of items that you can use to explore specific problem or opportunity areas in more depth.

Making the Employee Journey Map More Useful

You may use my journeyman example if you like, but you need not be confined by my example. I encourage you to find your own way for making your employee journey map come alive for your company. Below are some suggestions for you as you do so:

TIP

>> **Apply creativity to make the employee journey map relevant and interesting.** You don't have to use a boring flowchart or copy the artistic design of another company's journey map. Take inspiration from the world around you, but make it your own. For example, if you're at a transportation company, consider making it transportation-themed. If you're at a manufacturing company, consider making it manufacturing-themed. The possibilities are endless.

The uptake of the employee journey map may well depend on the degree to which it captures the imagination of the leaders, managers, and employees of your company, so it's worth taking a little time to think about it.

>> **Make it simpler, but not simple.** As you add more steps or layers of insight, you make the employee journey map more complex. Try to get it just right, but if you have extra data, you can create versions that summarize that data, followed by versions that contain the additional data or places where you can drill down into detail as necessary.

>> **Make the employee journey map interactive.** Consider having a hyperlinked version of your employee journey map that allows navigation between different journey maps for different job families and also allows you to drill down, as needed, into more graphs and data details if you have a lot of data.

>> **Capture problems and opportunities and assign an owner.** The employee journey map is a pointless exercise if you don't identify problems and opportunities and assign someone to take ownership over investigating and correcting them.

Using the Feedback You Get to Increase Employee Lifetime Value

In Chapter 6, I spend some time discussing the purpose and calculation of employee lifetime value (ELV). As a refresher, ELV is the estimated value that an individual employee will generate for your business over his lifetime.

You are mapping the employee journey to improve the employee experience, not just to make people happy for its own sake, but also in order to increase ELV.

ELV can be increased in one of these three ways:

>> Extend the tenure of an employee (individually or on average by segment) by addressing employee goals and needs. In the Triple-A framework this is addressed by focusing on the attrition problem.

>> Increase the value that an employee (individual or on average by segment) produces by increasing performance or increasing the nature of key talent's job contributions over time. In the Triple-A framework, this is addressed by focusing on the activation problem.

>> Retain higher-value producing employees while replacing lower-value-producing employees with higher-value producing employees over time. In the Triple-A framework, this is addressed by focusing on the attrition problem.

All these objectives can be enhanced by learning from the employee journey and then applying focused effort where it will have the most impact. Given that different segments of employees will have different experiences as well as different employee lifetime value (ELV) potential than others, start working on the employee journey map from the perspective of key job and key talent segments, and then work to others as time permits.

Chapter **9**

Attraction: Quantifying the Talent Acquisition Phase

Any company that competes on a product-and-service level needs, at minimum, to attract talent, coax good work out of those people, and hold on to its most productive people. If the company cannot attract the quantity and quality of talent it needs, it's reflected in diminished productivity relative to competitors.

Attraction represents the force of the organization to draw in or attract talent for its purposes, whatever that purpose may be. Attraction's principal importance to company performance is straightforward: In order to grow, a company must acquire new people to perform work for the company. The company's current and future success is determined by the company's ability to acquire a sufficient quantity and quality of talent to design, produce, and sell more products. If the company cannot attract the people it needs in order to operate, none of your other management strategies or systems matter.

Introducing Talent Acquisition

When a company is just starting out, the work of talent acquisition often is performed by a key founder or ends up being shared by everyone on the team. As a company grows, the demands of talent acquisition become more complex. Eventually, the company must hire people to take responsibility for the work of acquiring more people. Historically, this highly specialized role within an organization has been called either Staffing or Recruiting — increasingly, it's being called Talent Acquisition.

Whatever you call it, it isn't unusual for a growing company to have dozens (if not hundreds) of people doing this work. I have worked in some companies — Merck and Google are two prominent examples — that have over 300 recruiters. Talent acquisition is like a business within a business. And, with its high volume of activity, the inputs, activity, and outputs can seem difficult to see, manage, and control.

The operative word here is *seem*. The fact of the matter is that talent acquisition, like sales or supply chain management, is a production-oriented function for which there are straightforward ways to measure success — there are, in other words, clear inputs (applicants) and clear outputs (hires) and start and end time stamps. In this respect, you're dealing with a classic *throughput funnel* (see Figure 9-1), where a large initial pool is whittled down to a relatively small final result.

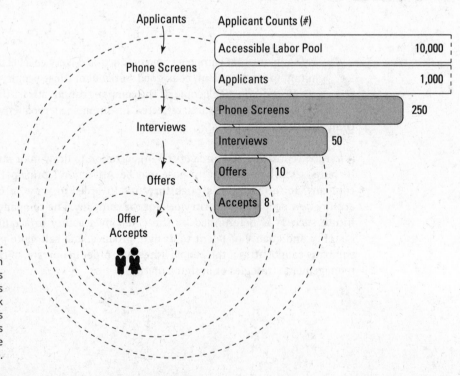

FIGURE 9-1: Talent acquisition professionals find candidates and then work those candidates through stages until a hire is made.

As Figure 9-1 illustrates, first you have a lot of activity and eventually a hire is made — and it's this activity that needs to be managed correctly. Talent acquisition measurement isn't limited to the number of hires that come out the other side of a funnel. You can use a variety of metrics and analysis to wrangle better control over what is going on *in* that funnel. Important measurement categories include volume, efficiency, speed, cost, quality, and the experience of candidates and hiring managers.

REMEMBER

Measurement helps you see what is working well, what isn't (and why), and how to make it work better. In some cases, you'll have to use measurements to justify making the best decision possible under the circumstances.

Making the case for talent acquisition analytics

The design and day-to-day running of a company involves a lot of decisions — not just decisions made by the CEO but also those countless decisions made every day throughout the command structure of an organization. The aggregate quality of these decisions determines success or failure. Talent acquisition is a job function that facilitates decisions that have great consequences for companies.

Making the right decisions means asking the right questions. For example: How do you attract to your company the best candidates in each field or discipline? How do you determine what "best" even looks like? Where do you find these stars? How do you get them to agree to leave where they are and come to you? How much should you offer? Should you pay for quality and let the pros do their thing, or should you hire upstarts for less and bring them into a system that makes them high quality over time? When you need to defend your hiring decisions, how can you convince others that you made the best choices?

Answering these questions correctly determines whether your company consists of the best band of people out there who are committed to excellence or is a mismatched collection of mediocrities just trying to muddle through the best way they can. Measurement and analysis are designed to help you systematically improve your chances of getting the right answers and thus improving your decision-making process. And what is it that can actually be measured and analyzed when it comes to talent acquisition? I thought you'd never ask.

Seeing what can be measured

Analytics can be applied to an array of decisions from within the talent acquisition function. The following examples show the types of decisions that can be made better with data:

» **Priorities:** Which jobs and candidates should you focus resources on, in what order should you focus on them, and how much of your resources should be directed to each one?

» **Goals:** Should you optimize the talent acquisition process for speed of hire, cost of hire, quality of hire, candidate experience, or a balance?

» **Candidate characteristics:** Which candidate characteristics should you favor in the talent acquisition process (generally and per job) in order to produce higher-quality hires, stimulate a more efficient process, support company culture, or help a hiring manager solve a specific problem on a team?

» **Screening and selection instruments:** Which screening and selection instruments (methods of thinning applicant pools and rating candidates) should you apply?

These are some examples of frequently used selection instruments:

Unstructured interviews: In an unstructured interview, the format and the questions asked are left to the direction of the interviewers.

Structured interviews: A structured interview uses a predetermined list of questions that are asked of every person who applies for a particular job. For example, a situational interview focuses not on personal characteristics or work experience, but rather on the behaviors needed for successful job performance.

Sample job tasks: These tasks can include performance tests, simulations, work samples, and realistic job previews that assess performance and aptitude on particular tasks.

Personality tests and integrity tests: These assess the degree to which a person has certain traits or dispositions (dependability, cooperativeness, and safety awareness, for example) or aim to predict the likelihood that a person will engage in certain conduct (theft or absenteeism, for example).

Cognitive tests: These assess reasoning, memory, perceptual speed and accuracy, skills in arithmetic and reading comprehension, as well as knowledge of a particular function or job.

Criminal background checks: These provide information on arrest and conviction history.

Credit checks: These provide information on credit and financial history.

Physical ability tests: These measure the physical ability to perform a particular task or the strength of specific muscle groups, as well as strength and stamina in general.

Medical inquiries and physical examinations: Such exams could include psychological tests designed to assess current mental health.

>> **Resources:** There are substantial options for applying resources (money, time, materials) to talent acquisition strategy and tactics.

Where and when should you invest resources (and which ones) in talent acquisition channels, staff, technology, training, incentives, new selection techniques, and other supports?

REMEMBER

All these "people decisions" add up and over time impact the long-term success or failure of every company. Superior talent acquisition can lead to competitive advantages. If your company had an attrition rate of 25 percent per year and its talent acquisition efforts produce below industry average hires, it will take only two years for 50 percent or more of employees at your company to be below industry average. 25% turnover may be an extreme example, but even with a 10% turnover rate any company can go from great to below industry average in 5 to 10 years if they don't have hiring quality figured out. Conversely, in the same scenario, if the talent acquisition function produced exceptional hires, it could quickly change the talent profile and trajectory of the company in a short time as well.

Getting Things Moving with Process Metrics

Talent acquisition, as I mention earlier in this chapter, is best thought of as a process of inputs and outputs. The job of talent acquisition is to take inputs (applicants) and produce outputs (high-quality hires). (Refer to Figure 9-1.)

Talent acquisition can be measured, managed, and improved by targeting four distinct areas: speed, cost, quality, and experience.

In this section, I walk you through the major measures of talent acquisition from a process standpoint. I start with the output of the process in mind first and work my way backward from there.

Answering the volume question

The goal of talent acquisition is to produce hires. As you might expect, you have an easy way to gauge success here — just count the number of hires made. Of course, one guy standing there next to the water cooler doesn't fully represent all the work that occurred to hire that guy. Behind the scenes, you need to measure a lot more to have a complete appreciation for what it takes to hire another guy like this one. (Here's a quick peek at the important numbers here: number of initial candidates, number of phone screens, number of onsite interviews, and number of offers.)

REMEMBER

Most executives don't care how many phone screens you make as long as the company gets the number of hires they expected. Yet counting these activities is essential for the purpose of analysis; just remember that the goal of talent acquisition is to produce more hires, not to perform more activity. The volume of activity at each phase of the talent acquisition funnel is data you need, though it may not be the data you show to executives. Talent acquisition funnel data is more useful behind the scenes for purposes of evaluating activity and isolating where the company can be more efficient.

To evaluate how successful you are at talent acquisition, you should understand that companies have different head count growth needs and targets and that your own company's growth needs and targets will change over time. Successfully hiring 100 people sounds good, but if you needed to hire 200 people to achieve the company's objective, 100 isn't so good. Conversely, if you needed only 100 and you hired 200, that would also be bad.

The way to address this problem is to compare volume to a need or plan. Did your talent acquisition team produce enough hires to meet the company's head count objectives? This cannot be measured by simply measuring the number of hires made — it requires understanding hires in the context of head count and head count plans.

In this section, I spell out some of the basic metrics necessary to measure talent acquisition output as it relates to head count and head count plans by segment.

Head count measures

Let's get some basic terminology out of the way. First and foremost, you have three ways to express what I've been calling head count:

>> Use the head count value at the beginning of a period.

>> Use the head count value at the end of a period.

>> Take an average of the beginning and ending head count values.

REMEMBER

Situationally, you need all three numbers for different reasons and different calculations, some of which I describe later in this chapter.

In the HR data world, you can find a variety of rather strange terms, such as the ones defined in this list:

>> **Active:** An active person has a record in the database and is working with the company in some way in the time period of the report focus.

>> **Terminated:** A terminated person has a record in the database and is no longer working with the company after the date provided. (You should be excited to hear that *Terminated* doesn't mean the company hired an android that looks like Arnold Schwarzenegger to go back in time to destroy that person. Though the person's future self may or may not be in actual trouble, the historic self should be just fine.)

>> **Employee:** An employee is someone who works for the company with a specific wage or salary and has an employment contract (written or implied) with the company; the company controls what will be done and how it will be done.

If you had to evaluate all these criteria each time you attempted to count the number of people employed by the company, the exercise would become tedious and riddled with error. Fortunately, all mature companies have a database, known as a human resources information system (HRIS), in which each person who is an employee is recorded as an employee with other personal details as well as any employment-related transactions that occurred. For this reason, HRIS is often referred to as the *system of record:* By definition, a person is not an employee if the system of employee record doesn't have a record of her as an employee. This definition sounds redundant but is in fact accurate.

REMEMBER

When it comes to identifying who is an employee for people analytics, the HRIS is the primary source of truth — the judge and jury. It is the system of record.

>> **Non-employee:** A non-employee is a person working for your company who isn't an employee — that is, the relationship between the two parties is between two businesses, one of which is providing a service to the other. The non-employee may be self-employed or may be the employee of another company that has the contract with your company. I tend to call these folks *contractors,* though your HRIS may have many worker classification types. Contingent worker and board member are two examples of non-employees. Though the distinction may seem petty, the detailed distinction is truly important because of the legal and tax implications (which are *not* petty). To further complicate the matter, a single individual can move between different worker types over time. Fortunately, the HRIS records these changes by design.

To keep things simple, I discuss just two types of workers here, employees and non-employees, because I'm primarily interested in who is an employee on a given day or range of days. Because many terms can be used to designate a non-employee, you should establish a filter to include only employees on a given date, which excludes anyone with any other classification on this date.

Extracting information from a specific database to determine the answer to a question can be complex, and hinge on a number of important details, even if the question is as basic as "How many employees did we have on this day?" I'm not in a position to give a detailed step list for carrying out a database query on your database, not knowing what you have done with it, so I keep my descriptions general (yet still helpful, I hope). For the purpose of this discussion, assume that everything you do with head count is filtering for employees and excluding non-employees. Therefore, what you find here is a blueprint you can abstract from for the purpose of general design principle, not as a legal document.

End-of-Period Headcount (Headcount.EOP)

Let's look at how you arrive at end-of-period head count (Headcount.EOP). If you define Headcount.EOP as a count of active employees in a particular segment on the last date of a particular period, you can write this shorthand expression this way:

{Headcount.EOP} = Count of [Active].[Employee].[Segment].[Period].[Last Date of Period].[plus any other necessary qualifier].

For simplicity's sake, I refer to it as

{Headcount.EOP} = Count of [Segment].[Period].[Last Date of Period]

You should take [Segment] to include any qualifiers you add to get to the segment of the overall population you want to count, even if those qualifiers are numerous. I put [Segment] in the formula to represent where that logic will occur so that you can move forward without endless distracting detail.

I calculate this shorthand expression using source data, extracted from the HRIS. (Table 9-1 provides a tongue-in-cheek version of such source data, using a company that seemingly hires only former presidents of the United States.) I use curly brackets {} to denote that the result is a record set or a list of values. The use of square brackets [] refers to a filter or dimension of the data. The underlying data and values within the filters determine the form of the output. After computing the Headcount.EOP expression, you could end up with no result, a single value, or multiple values.

TABLE 9-1 **Headcount.EOP Detailed Active Employee List: Report Dates: 9/30/2017, 10/31/2017**

Date	Period	Worker ID	Name	Worker Type	Status	Region	Other Detail
9/30/2017	2017-09	10006	George Bush	Employee	Active	East	...
9/30/2017	2017-09	10007	Ronald Reagan	Employee	Active	West	...
9/30/2017	2017-09	10008	Barack Obama	Employee	Active	East	...
10/31/2017	2017-10	10006	George Bush	Employee	Active	East	...
10/31/2017	2017-10	10008	Barack Obama	Employee	Active	East	...
10/31/2017	2017-10	10009	Bill Clinton	Employee	Active	North	...

For purposes of the example, here's the shorthand expression of the {Headcount.EOP} definition restated to filter to a set of records that represent all employees in the East region on the last day of the month of October 2017:

{Headcount.EOP} = Count of [Segment:Region=East].[Period=2017-10].
[Last Date of Period =10/31/2017].

In this example, I have provided a distinct instruction for each filter that, when combined, will result in all records that exist that match the filter criteria.

TIP

To identify head count on a specific date, you have to account for the changing status and the associated dates. Without adding extensive complexity, one way of doing this is to extract separate reports for each date you want to look at. You can extract reports for every day, for just the end of each week, or for the end of each month, for example. Other segmentation details regarding each individual can be added in columns to the right of Region, such as Division, Manager, Pay, Job Function Category, Job, or Survey Responses.

Now let me walk you through the shorthand expression:

{Headcount.EOP} = Count of [Segment:Region='East'].[Period=2017-10].
[Last Date=10/31/2017]

It turns out that, given the source data as specified in Table 9-1, only George Bush and Barack Obama meet the filter criteria. The result of the shorthand expression is a value of 2:

Count of [Segment:Region='East'].[Period=2017-10].[Last Date=10/31/2017] is 2

Because the result could be multiple outputs, if you were to formulate the segment categories and segment value filters differently, you typically show the output in a format that works no matter what the definition is. Described in table form, it would look like Table 9-2.

TABLE 9-2   Headcount.EOP: Output Table (with Filter for East)

Metric	Segment Dimension	Segment Value	Period	Date	Headcount Value
Headcount.EOP	Region	East	2017-10	10/31/2017	2

Start-of-Period Headcount (Headcount.SOP)

Whatever you do for End-of-Period Headcount, you can also do for Start-of-Period Headcount. Because the periods in the example are months, you would run reports and extract a list of employees as of the first day of the month rather than the last day of each month. However, feel free to base the period of analysis on quarters, which means that Start-of-Period is the first day of each quarter. (If you want to live dangerously, you can use years as the period of analysis; then Start-of-Period would be the first day of the year.)

The shorthand expression for Start-of-Period Headcount (Headcount.SOP) will look like this:

{Headcount.SOP} = Count of [Segment:Region].[Period].[First Date in Period]

Average-Headcount

I have shown you how to calculate head count at the start of a period and at the end of a period. Sometimes, however, you might need the average head count. In fact, Average Headcount is used in the denominator of many of the HR metrics that you'll actually care about. (Two examples that come to mind that use average head count are exit rate and hire rate.)

There's more than one way to calculate average head count — ways that have varying degrees of precision and varying degrees of practicality. A basic method is to add together the Start-of-Period head count and the End-of-Period head count and divide the sum by 2. A more precise method is to calculate head count by segment for every day and then take the average of all days in the period. Constructing a daily average increases the amount of computing that's necessary and so is less practical. For a compromise, calculate head count by equal intervals in the period. For example, if you're calculating average head count for a year, you might calculate head count by segment at the end of each week, the end of each month, or the end of each quarter over one year and average this by segment.

Average-Headcount-Basic

Here's the shorthand expression representing the way you calculate the average number of employees in each segment employed during the selected period, calculated with beginning and end divided by 2:

> **Average-Headcount-Basic:** [Segment].[Period].Headcount.SOP **+** [Segment].[Period].Headcount.EOP ÷ 2

Average-Headcount-Daily

Here's the shorthand expression representing the way you calculate the average number of people employed in each segment during the selected period using daily values:

> **Average-Headcount-Daily:** [Segment].Headcount.Day1 + [Segment].Headcount.Day2 + [Segment].Headcount.Day3 + [Segment].Headcount.Day4 + [Segment].Headcount.DayX . . . (until last day of period or sample) ÷ Number of days in period.

Whichever way you go, you end up with an employee list for each day in the period you want to use, which you then combine into a single combined data extract.

You will add a variable to the extract for counting — labeled, appropriately enough, the counting variable. When conditions are met for what you want to count, the counting variable contains a value of 1; when conditions are not met, the field contains a value of 0. In the example. if the individual is an active employee on the date specified, a 1 is applied in the counting variable; if the individual is not active and/or is not an employee on that date, the variable contains a 0. This allows you to apply a simple repeatable methodology of summing the counting variable across all dates in the dataset and simply dividing by the number of distinct dates found.

TECHNICAL STUFF

In statistics, a one/zero counting variable is called a *dummy variable*.

If you examine the calculation to produce average head count using the start-of-period head count and the end-of-period head count, you're creating an average by summing the segment head count using records from the first day of the month and records from the last day of the month. Because two distinct dates are found for each monthly period, producing two records per individual, you're summing the head count for each segment in each period and dividing by 2. If you had a record for each day of the month, you would be dividing by 28, 30, or 31, depending on the number of distinct days in each monthly period. Because you have only beginning and end days in the example, you're dividing by 2.

Hires

A *hire* is, by definition, someone who was not an employee that became an employee. To calculate the number of hires, you extract a list of all active and terminated employees and count the employees within a given segment with a start date squarely within the period you're interested in.

The shorthand hire expression looks like this:

Hires: Count [Segment].[Period].Hires

Hire-Rate

The *hire rate* is the number of hires during a period, expressed as a percentage of average head count in that period. To calculate the hire rate, you divide the number of hires within a given segment within a given period by the average head count of the same segment for the same period:

Hire-Rate: Count [Segment].[Period].Hires ÷ [Segment].[Period].Average-Headcount

Figure 9-2 illustrates a hire rate example.

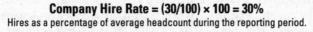

Company Hire Rate = (30/100) × 100 = 30%
Hires as a percentage of average headcount during the reporting period.

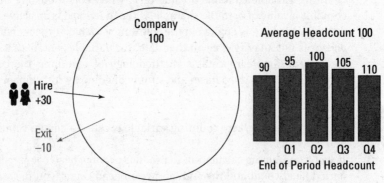

FIGURE 9-2: Calculating hire rate.

Headcount-Growth

Headcount growth is the increase in the number of employees from the start of the period to the end of the period. To calculate head count growth, you subtract start-of-period head count for a given segment in a given period from the end-of-period head count for the same segment in the same period:

Headcount-Growth: [Segment].[Period].Headcount.EOP – [Segment].[Period]. Headcount.SOP

Headcount-Growth-Rate

Headcount growth-rate is the increase in the number of employees from the start of the period to the end of the period as a percentage of head count at the start of the period. To calculate Headcount-Growth-Rate, you divide the head count growth within a given segment within a given period by the start-of-period head count of the same segment for the same period:

Headcount-Growth-Rate: [Segment].[Period].Headcount-Growth ÷ [Segment]. [Period].Headcount.SOP

Figure 9-3 shows a (rather unimpressive) growth rate calculation.

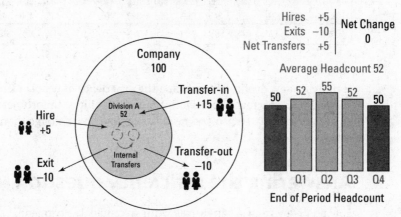

"Division A" Growth Rate = (0/50) × 100 = 0%
Net Change during the reporting period as a percentage of headcount at start of period
(start of period is the same as previous period headcount end.)

FIGURE 9-3: Calculating growth rate.

Headcount-Plan-Achievement-Percent

Most company leaders have plans for how many people they want to have as a whole and in different segments by a future date — I call this a *head count plan*. Headcount-Plan-Achievement-Percent is a particular segment's head count on a particular date expressed as a percentage of that segment's head count plan on the same date:

Headcount-Plan-Achievement-Percent: [Segment].[Period].Headcount-EOP ÷ [Segment].[Period].Headcount-EOP-Plan

Figure 9-4 graphically illustrates actual achievement versus the head count plan.

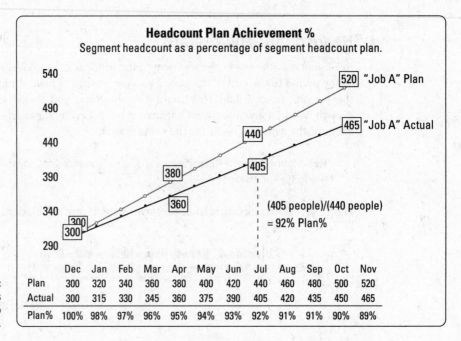

Headcount Plan Achievement %
Segment headcount as a percentage of segment headcount plan.

(405 people)/(440 people)
= 92% Plan%

	Dec	Jan	Feb	Mar	Apr	May	Jun	Jul	Aug	Sep	Oct	Nov
Plan	300	320	340	360	380	400	420	440	460	480	500	520
Actual	300	315	330	345	360	375	390	405	420	435	450	465
Plan%	100%	98%	97%	96%	95%	94%	93%	92%	91%	91%	90%	89%

FIGURE 9-4: Somebody needs to step up their game.

REMEMBER

If time, money, quality of hires, and the experience of people were no object, you could stop all this math homework at number of hires. Unfortunately, speed, cost, and quality all matter, so you need to measure more things than just volume of activity.

Answering the efficiency question

You don't go from a single call with a candidate to making an offer in one step. You talk to lots of people, and you use many steps to refine the list of people you're talking to until you arrive at the end with the hire.

The movement from one important step to the next can be measured by talent acquisition funnel metrics. The rest of this section looks at the metrics you can use.

Requisitions

A *requisition* is a request for applicants to fill an open job. To calculate the measure I call requisitions, you count the number of requisitions in a selected segment in a selected period:

Requisitions: Count [Segment].[Period].Requisitions

TECHNICAL STUFF

Requisition is the technical term for an open job request — these terms are used interchangeably. What name you use depends on either what you prefer or what people in your company have used in the past. If nobody at your company has heard of the word requisition before you, might prefer to tell other people you are counting the number of open job requests, rather than tell them you are counting the number of requisitions.

Candidates

Candidates are people who are considered for open jobs. Here's the shorthand expression:

Candidates: Count [Segment].[Period].Candidates

Applications

An application is a formal request by a candidate to be considered for an open job (a job requisition). To calculate applications, you count the number of applications in a selected segment in a selected period:

Applications: Count [Segment].[Period].Applications

TECHNICAL STUFF

While the words "applicant" and "candidate" may often be used as synonyms there is an actual technical distinction reflected in the databases that are used to track talent acquisition activity. Anyone who has been considered for any job has a candidate record. If you are using a unique identifier, all candidates should have just one record in the talent acquisition database regardless of how many different jobs they have applied for at your company. This is to be contrasted with the word applicant. A candidate may have applied to multiple job openings, and so a candidate may have multiple application incidents, each of which would have a unique identifier, known as the applicant ID.

Interviews

An interview takes place when the people who will participate in the hiring decision formally assess a candidate for decision either by phone or in person:

Interviews: Count [Segment].[Period] Interviews

Offers

An offer takes place when a candidate has been selected and a formal invitation has been given to the candidate to join the company:

Offers: Count [Segment].[Period].Offers

Offer-Accepts

Offer-Accepts is the number of candidates with offers who have accepted those offers:

Offer-Accepts: Count [Segment].[Period].Offer-Accepts

Funnel-Stage-Pass-Percent [Pass%]

Here's the percentage of applicants that pass from one stage to the next stage, by segment, by period:

Pass-Percent: [Segment].[Period].[Stage X+1 Applicants] ÷ [Segment].[Period]. [Stage X Applicants] ×100

Funnel-Stage-Fail-Percent [Fail%]

Here's the percentage of applicants that do not pass from one stage to the next stage by stage, by segment, and so on:

Fail-Percent: [Segment].[Period].[Stage X+1 Applicants] ÷ [Segment].[Period]. [Stage X Applicants] × 100

Funnel-Yield-Percent [Yield%]

Here's the percentage of applicants who make it all the way to offer-accept, by segment and so on:

Yield-Percent: [Segment].[Period].Offer-Accepts ÷ [Segment].[Period]. Applicants × 100

Figure 9-5 shows what a yield-percent calculation would look like.

REMEMBER

Talent acquisition funnel metrics contain important insights about how successful you are at effectively thinning the pool of applicants as you work through the selection process. The less you thin at one stage, the more thinning you have to do at the next stage. However, if you thin too much at the top of the funnel, the applicant pool may get too small to produce someone to pass to the next stage to produce a hire.

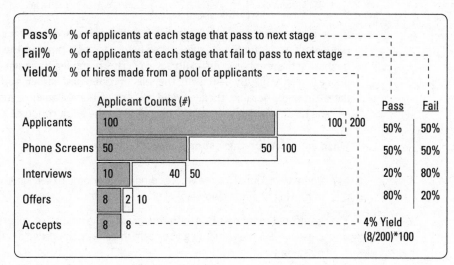

	Applicant Counts (#)			Pass	Fail
	Pass%	% of applicants at each stage that pass to next stage			
	Fail%	% of applicants at each stage that fail to pass to next stage			
	Yield%	% of hires made from a pool of applicants			

Pass%   % of applicants at each stage that pass to next stage
Fail%   % of applicants at each stage that fail to pass to next stage
Yield% % of hires made from a pool of applicants

Applicant Counts (#)				Pass	Fail
Applicants	100	100	200	50%	50%
Phone Screens	50	50	100	50%	50%
Interviews	10	40	50	20%	80%
Offers	8	2	10	80%	20%
Accepts	8	8		4% Yield (8/200)*100	

FIGURE 9-5:
Getting to 8.

Figure 9-6 shows two funnels: B takes twice as much effort to produce the same number of hires as A, so in this comparison, A is far better than B based on volume.

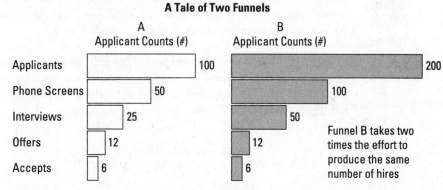

A Tale of Two Funnels

	A Applicant Counts (#)	B Applicant Counts (#)
Applicants	100	200
Phone Screens	50	100
Interviews	25	50
Offers	12	12
Accepts	6	6

Funnel B takes two times the effort to produce the same number of hires

FIGURE 9-6:
A tale of two funnels.

In scenario A, you get 6 hires from 100 applications, 50 phone screens, and 25 interviews. In Scenario B, you also get 6 hires, but you had to screen 50 more applicants by phone and have an interview round with 25 more people. If each interview is 1 hour long and each applicant in the interview round must have interviews with five people, you have spent 125 additional hours (25 x 5 x 1 hour) interviewing. If the average pay of the interviewers is $50 per hour, the inefficiency of scenario B cost the company at least $6,250 more. Also, time was lost unnecessarily.

Producing more candidates gives you more options to choose from, but having more isn't a good thing if it just requires you to do more work to produce the same number of hires. If, however, having more candidates can produce more hires and/or higher-quality hires, the increased volume can be justified.

If you suspect that you're in Scenario B or if you can see that your funnel is taking more work or taking longer than it had before to get a hire out the funnel, consider increasing the number or difficulty level of criteria applied to screen candidates at the phone screen stage. By increasing the selection standard earlier, you let fewer candidates through; because those candidates are of higher quality, more of them will become hires, which increases the hire yield on the work conducted at each stage.

When you calculate these funnel metrics, you can

>> Compare a funnel for the whole company over time to see whether you're improving or getting worse.

>> Compare the funnels from different divisions, locations, recruiters, or other creative ways of segmenting your data to derive perspective or answer a question.

>> Derive how much activity needs to occur in order to produce a set number of hires in a set time frame and/or forecast how many hires the current funnel will produce over the next quarter based on what you have achieved in the past.

REMEMBER

Understanding what's going on in the talent acquisition funnel can help you work toward correctly balancing the volume, time, cost, and quality that you want to achieve in talent acquisition as a company. Results vary.

In addition to measuring the shape and overall yield of the funnel, you can use the funnel metrics to measure how many recruiters, how many applicants, and how much action are required in order to produce a hire in a given time frame. (See Figure 9-7.)

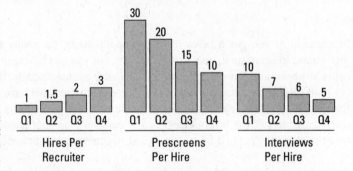

FIGURE 9-7:
Looking at talent acquisition efficiency.

Average-Hires-per-Recruiter

You can calculate the average number of hires made per recruiter in a given period using the following approach:

Average-Hires-Per-Recruiter: [Segment].[Period].Hires ÷ [Segment].[Period].[Recruiter].[Average-Headcount]

Average-Phone-Screens-per-Hire

Here's the shorthand formula for calculating the average number of phone screens it took to make a hire in a given period:

Average-Phone-Screens-Per-Hire: [Segment].[Period].Phone-Screens ÷ [Segment].[Period].Hires

Average-Interviews-per-Hire

The shorthand for getting the average number of interviews it took to make a hire in a given period looks like this:

Average-Interviews-Per-Hire: [Segment].[Period].Interviews ÷ [Segment].[Period].Hires

Interview-Offer-Percentage

To calculate the number of offers extended as a percentage of distinct candidates interviewed during the selected period, use the following:

Interview-Offer-Percentage Formula: [Segment].[Period].Offers ÷ [Segment].[Period].Interviews

Knowing on average how many recruiters and how much activity are required in order to produce a certain number of hires is important so that you know how to scale resources up or down to meet a changing hiring plan over time. It's also helpful to know how long it will take.

Answering the speed question

Another way of looking at the funnel is to measure the difference in time between the day each job was first opened for applications and when they were filled (time-to-fill) or measuring the difference of time between when each candidate started in the process and when they start as an employee (time-to-start).

Hiring speed is important because it

» **Helps your company develop an advantage over slower talent competitors (usually larger companies) by moving much faster than they do to get to an offer-accept**

   Every day that a candidate waits in the process increases the chance that she will have a conversation about an opportunity with another company that you then will have to compete with at the offer stage. If you move faster, the candidate is less likely to receive an invitation to interview with other companies before receiving your offer. The worst-case scenario is that, by the time you get around to making an offer, the candidate has two other offers to choose from. In this scenario, your overall probability of getting the candidate to accept has dropped to 33 percent. You may also enter a bidding war, which means that you'll have to pay more money to the candidate. If you offer this candidate more than you pay your existing employees, you will have to increase their pay, too, at the next annual pay review to stay out of trouble.

» **Communicates to the candidate that when you reached out, you were serious — you mean business!**

   Compare a crisp process to a process where the candidate has a conversation with a recruiter, ends the call, and then waits weeks to hear from anyone. Someone who doesn't hear from you for a long time may conclude that the company isn't interested in hiring her or may believe that she isn't the company's first choice. Speed is part of the experience. There's something exhilarating about getting something you want quickly.

» **Adds value to the company**

   The less time it takes for you to fill a position, the less time jobs remain vacant. Vacant positions reduce productivity and put strain on co-workers, increasing their likelihood to leave as well. Finally, if you can move faster to fill positions, you will be able to do more things in a given quarter or year, regardless of whether you use that time to produce more hires or do something else with it.

As I mention earlier, you can use two major metrics to measure time in recruiting: time-to-fill and time-to-start. Though I haven't called attention to it as a metric, the average time between each stage can also be measured. Examples of *stages* are Application, Pre-Screen, Onsite Interview, and Offer. Understanding the time between each stage can help you diagnose where you're losing time to reduce the overall time.

Time-to-fill

The average time it takes to find and hire a new candidate, measured by the number of days between publishing a job opening and the candidate's acceptance of a job offer, is the *time-to-fill*, or the time it takes to fill a job for the company. If you were to open a job today, how long is it likely to take to fill that job? How does this vary by job function or level? You should be able to answer these questions. If you can't, measure time-to-fill:

Time-to-fill: Sum of [Segment].[Period].Days between job post date and offer accept÷ [Segment].[Period].Offer-Accepts

Figure 9-8 illustrates a time-to-fill calculation.

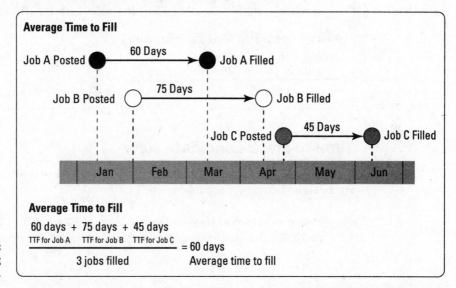

Time-to-start

Time-to-start measures the average number of days between the moment a candidate joins the process and the moment the candidate starts the job. In other words, it measures the time it takes for a candidate to move through the hiring process after they've applied.

To calculate the average number of calendar days from the date a job requisition is approved to the date a new hire begins work, follow this shorthand formula:

Time-to-start: Sum of [Segment].[Period].Days between job post date and employee start date ÷ [Segment].[Period].Hires

Figure 9-9 illustrates a time-to-start calculation.

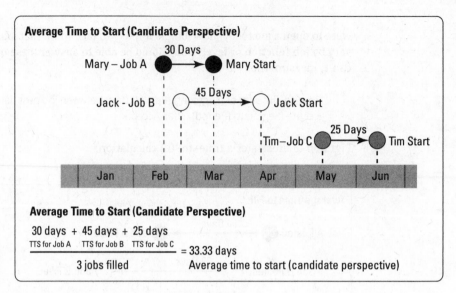

Average Time to Start (Candidate Perspective)

Mary – Job A → Mary Start (30 Days)

Jack - Job B → Jack Start (45 Days)

Tim – Job C → Tim Start (25 Days)

Jan | Feb | Mar | Apr | May | Jun

Average Time to Start (Candidate Perspective)

$$\underbrace{\underset{\text{TTS for Job A}}{30 \text{ days}} + \underset{\text{TTS for Job B}}{45 \text{ days}} + \underset{\text{TTS for Job C}}{25 \text{ days}}}_{\text{3 jobs filled}} = \underset{\text{Average time to start (candidate perspective)}}{33.33 \text{ days}}$$

FIGURE 9-9: Calculating time-to-start.

Time-to-start: Candidate view

This formula calculates the average number of days elapsed between application start date and employee start date.

Time-to-start (candidate view): Sum of [Segment].[Period].Days between application start date and employee start date ÷ [Segment].[Period].Hires

MAKING SENSE OF METRICS

By themselves, metrics do not convey insight. The only way to interpret whether 50 hires is good or bad is in context. Depending on the goal, 50 means very different things. Were you planning on hiring 10 people, 50 people, or 100 people?

Here are several ways you can turn neutral data into insight:

- **Compare segments to each other:** Seeing how different segments compare to each other can help you determine what is normal and abnormal, what is good and bad performance, and what changes make a difference.

  Suppose that you're measuring time-to-hire and one division consistently has a time-to-hire of 30 days while other divisions have a time-to-hire of 55. You may not know the reason for the discrepancy, but at least you know that 30 days isn't outside the realm of possibility. With this information, you can set the bar higher for other segments until you can get them to 30 days as well.

- **Correlate the metric to another measure that matters to you**: For example, if you're in a retail business, you might run a statistical analysis of store performance to correlate Quality-of-Hire with Customer-Satisfaction. If what you really care about is customer satisfaction, correlating time-to-start may help you determine whether time-to-start is in fact a good thing, a bad thing, or a neutral thing as it relates to customer satisfaction.

- **Trend the metric over time:** See how the metric is changing over time to provide perspective on what is normal and what is abnormal. If you see that you have never really had any major problems and this metric is hovering around the same place as before, you probably have nothing to worry about now, either. If the metric is increasing or decreasing, you can evaluate whether that's a good thing or bad thing for you in the context of what you're trying to achieve. If you have no clear insight about it, just ignore the metric — don't try to use a metric you don't understand just for the sake of using one.

- **Compare with other companies using HR Metric benchmarking sources:** You can turn to a number of credible paid sources when you want to make use of HR Metric benchmark data. Here are some better-known options:

  PWC: www.pwc.com/us/en/services/hr-management/people-analytics/benchmarking.html

  SHRM: www.shrm.org/resourcesandtools/business-solutions/pages/benchmarking-service.aspx

  CEB: www.cebglobal.com/professional-services-technology-provider/benchmark-data-diagnostics.html

  The Hackett Group: www.thehackettgroup.com/hr-metrics

  Benchmarking can provide you with a perspective about where your numbers are relative to other companies, but it doesn't tell you where your metrics should be.

  The companies you're comparing to may be different in ways that cause their numbers to be different. Here are some ways that comparison companies can be different:

  - They may be a different size.

  - They may have a different growth rate.

  - They may have a different employee job distribution.

  - They may have a different employee tenure and age distribution.

  Because all these options can affect metrics, these other companies may not be an apples-to-apples comparison for you and so what anyone else is achieving may not actually represent an appropriate goal for you.

Answering the cost question

Counting how much money you spend is always a useful exercise in self-reflection that can lead to productive restraint. Cost is a particularly important measure in business.

It's useful to understand your overall hiring costs to monitor whether you're getting increasing productivity from the spend or whether your costs are increasing with each hire. It's also useful to make sure you're getting an adequate return on your investment.

The first and most traditional measure of recruiting cost is cost-per-hire, as I explain next.

Cost-per-hire

Cost-per-hire measures the economic cost of the effort taken to fill an open job. Given that filling an open job is in no way, shape, or form a uniform task, you can imagine that a multitude of factors come into play when determining the real costs of each new hire. Generally speaking, you can divide them into these two types of costs:

» **Internal**

Additional management costs (the time necessary for additional management involvement in recruitment marketing events, interview, and selection meetings)

Employee referral incentive

Nonstaff costs (office costs, for example)

Other, internal staff cost overhead for government compliance

Talent acquisition staff costs (salaries, benefits, and training, for example)

Relocation and immigration fees

Sourcing staff costs

» **External**

Advertising and marketing

Background check, eligibility to work, drug tests, and health screens

Campus talent acquisition activities

Career site development and maintenance (costs related to building and maintaining the site and keeping it populated with fresh, relevant content)

Consulting services (including EEO consulting)

Contingent fees

Immigration expenses

Job fairs and talent acquisition events

Recruitment process outsourcing (RPO) fees (for prescreening and assessing candidates)

Relocation

Sign-on bonus

Social media (the time involved in planning and creating social content and engagement with prospects along with the cost of any sponsored content)

Technology costs such as LinkedIn Recruiter licenses, applicant tracking systems (ATSs), background-check software subscriptions, onboarding applications, and any other technology costs to support talent acquisition such as some of the new sourcing tools, like Entello

Third-party hiring agency fees

Travel costs

Most of these costs are accumulated and recorded by Accounting in the aggregate, not specific to each hire. To calculate cost-per-hire, you add up all of these costs and divide by the number of hires. The level of aggregation of financial data restricts the range of options you have for segmenting cost-per-hire data, which in turn restricts the level of insight you can produce — for this reason, financial measures are not a very precise tool. Cost-per-hire is sort of like putting your finger out to feel the direction of the wind — you get a sense of the force and direction of the wind, but it is not very precise.

TIP

For all the painful details on calculating cost-per-hire, check out the Society for Human Resource Management's cost-per-hire standard at

> www.shrm.org/ResourcesAndTools/business-solutions/Documents/
> shrm_ansi_cph_standard.pdf

REMEMBER

Cost-per-hire doesn't account for the value produced from making investments to increase hiring volume or quality; it only focuses on the expense.

Hiring ROI

As I mention earlier in this chapter, cost-per-hire is the most traditional and frequently encountered measure for looking at talent acquisition spending.

Cost-per-hire is nice to know and trend; however, the problem is that it doesn't take into consideration the difficulty of filling different types of jobs or the value produced by those jobs. When these perspectives are lacking, it would be impossible to interpret increasing or decreasing cost-per-hire. It may be that costs are increasing, but that more difficult and higher-value-producing hires are being made.

A new measure that puts the cost of hiring into the context of value is hiring ROI. Hiring ROI requires that you first estimate the total Employee Lifetime Value (ELV) of the hires the costs are associated to.

When you calculate cost-per-hire, you divide all talent acquisition costs in a period by the number of hires made in that period. When you calculate hiring ROI, you divide the ELV of all hires in a period by all talent acquisition costs in the period. When using the hiring-ROI metric, you're measuring the dollar output of each dollar input into the recruiting process. When using the cost-per-hire metric, you're measuring the number of hires produced for every dollar input into the recruiting process. They're both measures of efficiency, but hiring ROI has some advantages.

Hiring ROI is a new concept that allows you to evaluate your spend for talent acquisition relative to the value the hires are producing for the company. This is important because the difficulties involved in producing the output the company needs will vary over time and will vary between companies. If you're evaluating performance based on cost-per-hire and not considering the generated value, you may find your resources unnecessarily constrained when you are chasing after unusually valuable talent, which reduces your ability to effectively produce high-quality candidates in a provided time frame. In the past, evaluated costs were based on the number of hires produced; however, the difficulty of sourcing, selecting, and hiring isn't equal by job or the quality of candidates, so reporting costs by number of hires is misleading and fraught with peril. For example, it costs much more money to source and hire an executive-level job than a lower-level job, and it can cost more to source and hire for a technical job than for a general job, like cashier. It's much better to align resources with value and focus on where you want to spend your time and money to produce higher quality.

Answering the quality question

When you hire people for your company, you like to believe that they will prove to be the best hires you've ever made, but in reality, you won't be right as often as you might think.

To find out whether you got it right, you have to follow your choices through to the future to see what happens. True, you can't see the future, but if you go back in time you can see how well the company has done in the past. If you do this, you will find some successes and many failures. Each situation by itself seems entirely unique, but if you put them together in aggregate form, you can see overall rates of success and failure that can be used to measure the quality of hires produced by the selection decision process.

If measuring hiring quality is important to you, here are some of the foundational principles you need to use when measuring hiring quality:

>> Measure the percentage of success and failure of the decision process over a large number of selection decisions over a long period. Do *not* be satisfied with short-range assessments.

>> Implement a method of measuring success and failure that is separate from the methods used in making the selection decision itself.

>> Come up with clear definitions of success and failure as they relate to on-the-job performance.

>> Develop a rubric to classify strong success (above-average performance), moderate success (average performance), and failure (below-average performance) for each job family and level. A rubric is important to increase objectivity and to detach the quality evaluation from a typical process of performance evaluation that is subjective and may use a scale that, unfortunately, isn't useful when measuring hiring quality.

REMEMBER

A *rubric* is a scoring guide. Scoring rubrics are used to delineate consistent criteria for measuring performance. A scoring rubric allows managers, employees, and recruiters to communicate and evaluate performance criteria, which otherwise can be elusive, complex, and subjective. A scoring rubric isn't intended for only one task — it can provide a basis for self-evaluation, manager review, peer review, hiring decisions, and documentation of job requirements. The goal is to produce as much of an accurate and fair assessment as possible while also fostering a common understanding. This integration of performance measurement and feedback by way of rubrics is called *ongoing assessment* or *formative assessment*.

Using critical-incident technique

The critical-incident technique is an investigative tool for capturing *critical incidents* — stories of past events that involve highly effective and highly ineffective job performance in a job for purposes of developing a rubric for evaluation. The goal of carefully scrutinizing critical incidents is to examine past experiences in order to identify the knowledge, skills, abilities and other characteristics that are necessary to produce successful job performance in the present or future. In particular, you should be most interested in identifying the knowledge, skills, and abilities that truly differentiate good from poor performance.

REMEMBER

Because the repetition of *knowledge, skills, abilities and other characteristics* is tedious I will refer to them as KSAOs or collectively as competency. Competency represents the characteristics necessary to perform some job function successfully. Competency is a catch-all phrase that doesn't care whether the necessary characteristics are knowledge, skill, or ability or whether the characteristic is developed over time or innate.

In the current context, I am suggesting you use the critical-incident technique to develop a scoring rubric you can use to measure hiring quality through the performance evaluations of employees in their first 90 days. If you apply the rubric consistently, then you can measure changes in hiring quality over time.

The rubric can also be used to develop valid pre-hire assessment tools for screening candidates, for measuring ongoing performance on the job, and to facilitate ongoing conversations about performance. The rubric should be continuously evaluated and improved over time by correlating previous quality scores using the rubric with other job performance measures, peer feedback, and objective productivity measures.

Figure 9-10 illustrates a performance rubric for the Listening skill in the form of a behaviorally anchored rating scale.

Figure 9-10 is an example of a behaviorally anchored rating scale (BARS) for a skill we refer to as "Listening". This particular BARS example provides a scale from 1 to 7. By definition, a BARS rating scale provides statements that can be used in juxtaposition to other statements to determine where someone may fall. Imagine if you were asked to rate someone on listening using a scale of 1 to 7. How would you know what a 1 is versus a 3, versus a 7? You may guess, but your guess would be different than mine. The statement provided in BARS are used to generate a greater degree of reliability in the measure. The BARS rubric for listening allows the rater to look for the statement that best describes the relative complexity level of listening (either described or directly observed). This measurement of listening will be better than one made without a behavioral anchor.

Example 9-10 is an example rubric of one factor you may be looking for in either candidates or employees. The first purpose of critical incidents technique is to identify the factors that differentiate between the best and worst performance in each job — which of course will vary. The second purpose of the critical incident's technique is to develop the rank order list of behavioral anchors you will use to measure each factor. The total rubric will include several factors, each of which will have their own BARS.

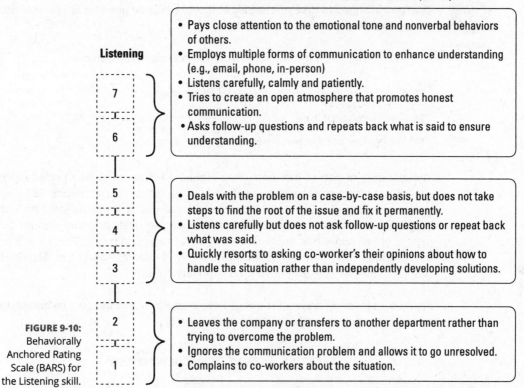

BEHAVIOR ANCHORED RATING SCALE (BARS)

Listening

7 / 6
- Pays close attention to the emotional tone and nonverbal behaviors of others.
- Employs multiple forms of communication to enhance understanding (e.g., email, phone, in-person)
- Listens carefully, calmly and patiently.
- Tries to create an open atmosphere that promotes honest communication.
- Asks follow-up questions and repeats back what is said to ensure understanding.

5 / 4 / 3
- Deals with the problem on a case-by-case basis, but does not take steps to find the root of the issue and fix it permanently.
- Listens carefully but does not ask follow-up questions or repeat back what was said.
- Quickly resorts to asking co-worker's their opinions about how to handle the situation rather than independently developing solutions.

2 / 1
- Leaves the company or transfers to another department rather than trying to overcome the problem.
- Ignores the communication problem and allows it to go unresolved.
- Complains to co-workers about the situation.

FIGURE 9-10: Behaviorally Anchored Rating Scale (BARS) for the Listening skill.

Kell, H. J., Martin-Raugh, M. P., Carney, L. M., Inglese, P. A., Chen, L., & Feng, G. (2017). Exploring Methods for Developing Behaviorally Anchored Rating Scales for Evaluating Structured Interview Performance. ETS Research Report Series, 2017(1), 1-26

You can use a variety of ways to capture critical incidents, including interviews, surveys, written reports, and facilitated group discussions. The people involved in developing the critical incident material should be chosen from a pool made up of people who do the work, managers of those people, and others who know the job — customers, vendors, consultants, and subordinates. The information captured when the critical-incident technique is applied isn't intended to evaluate current performance or to assign individual credit or blame for past performance — it's used to develop criteria for evaluating good and bad so you can identify the knowledge, skills, abilities, and other characteristics (KSAOs) used to produce exceptional performance so those KSAOs can be searched for in the talent acquisition process. Because the rubric is based on the critical incidents of good performance in contrast to critical incidents of poor performance, everyone can agree the KSAOs measured by the rubric are useful to the company.

REMEMBER

The conversations to develop the rubric should never be punitive or else you will not receive accurate information.

At a high level, the critical-incident technique captures three items:

» The circumstances in which the job behavior occurred

» The job behavior itself

» The positive or negative consequences of behavior

These reports of critical incidents often highlight instances of poor performance and outstanding performance as well the personal characteristics (KSAOs) perceived to be related to the behaviors and outcomes. A single incident isn't of much value, but dozens or hundreds of them can effectively help you identify the pattern of behaviors that are most likely to lead to a good result. The list will be made into a rubric that can be used to critically evaluate observed or described actions and behaviors to assign a level of quality.

Figure 9-11 is an overview of the workflow to apply critical incident technique to develop behaviorally anchored rating scales (BARS).

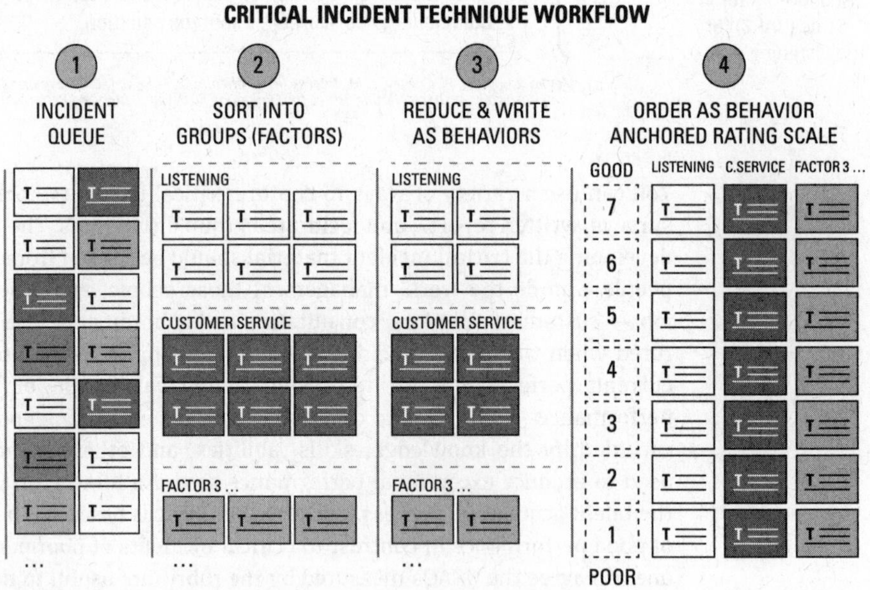

CRITICAL INCIDENT TECHNIQUE WORKFLOW

1	2	3	4
INCIDENT QUEUE	SORT INTO GROUPS (FACTORS)	REDUCE & WRITE AS BEHAVIORS	ORDER AS BEHAVIOR ANCHORED RATING SCALE

FIGURE 9-11: Critical Incident Technique Workflow Overview

The four-steps depicted in Figure 9-11 is just an overview. Below is a more detailed outline of how to perform the critical-incident technique in order to identify job success factors and create an associated behavior anchored rating scale:

1. **Create a group of subject matter experts.**

   Identify, invite, and gather subject matter experts in a group setting.

2. **Record critical incidents.**

   After making introductions and providing an ice-breaker, have the subject matter experts individually document specific positive and negative job performance incidents on a form or on index cards. Somewhere on the form or card, have the participants write the individuals' behaviors or attributes that are perceived to be the key to producing the unusually positive or negative experience. The first write-up may be rough. Have a facilitator read each scenario described on a card, and as a group, confirm understanding of the incident and the associated behaviors or KSAOs; edit and condense as needed.

3. **Sort similar cards into groups.**

   Have the subject matter experts move the index cards into groups of similar concepts. You can call these groups of statements *factors* — either success factors or failure factors. Have the subject matter experts refine how you're organizing the index cards until you arrive at what you believe are the core factors related to extraordinary job performance and the best organizing framework in which to place each statement. At the end of the exercise, you should have some factor headers, and the detailed examples supporting those concepts will be on index cards pinned or taped below.

4. **Order the incident index cards.**

   Sort cards containing the examples into positive and negative categories within each group. Then further arrange the cards on a scale from 1 to 7, with the examples related to the highest level of performance at 7 and the examples of the worst performance at 1. A moderate example should be put in the middle.

TIP

You can modify the scale smaller or larger, depending on how much material you have: 1 to 3, 1 to 5, 1 to 7, or 1 to 10.

You can accomplish this sorting task in different ways, either individually or together as a group. However, I suggest that you have each subject matter expert assign his own score and then average across all participants. If there is wide disagreement on the position of an index card, you can have a discussion as a group to find out what the reason was and come to a consensus on where to place this card.

TIP

If you can't come to consensus on an example, it's best to exclude it.

5. **Fill in the gaps**.

   After all the cards have been placed under a factor and sorted on the scale you've chosen, look for the gaps and request additional incident examples that can be placed into any gaps. Having some of the puzzle pieces in place will aid recall of situations that fit above, below, or between the categories. With the whole in place, you can go back to ask now whether anything is still missing.

6. **Review the factor scales**.

   You should use subject matter experts to review the completed scales and weigh in on the scale's relevancy and accuracy for the job you want to apply it to.

7. **Save the work of the meeting.**

   You can take pictures or have someone in the meeting type up each factor and each card and then record the relative position of the cards electronically. Eventually, you'll have a clean electronic copy of the factor scales, with crisp examples you can use to get the opinions of others who were unable to participate in the group exercise. Reconcile feedback until you can reconcile no further. Again, if there is broad disagreement among a sample of stakeholders, it may be best to remove whatever the stakeholders can't agree on and go with what they can.

8. **Finalize into a behaviorally anchored rating scale (BARS), apply, and analyze.**

   After you have fully vetted the scale, you have a completed assessment framework that represents a theory of how behaviors are associated to job performance. As a result of the preceding steps, you'll have a series of factors and a 1-to-7 scale with an example for each rung on the scale to help an assessor decide what number to choose when evaluating someone for that factor.

   The scores from the various factors should be combined into a final combined index. For example, if there were three factors, each rated on a 7-point scale, each person can be evaluated to receive points between 0 and 21.

REMEMBER

   You can assess performance using BARS in a variety of different time frames for a variety of different purposes. For example, you can assign each candidate a score using BARS following a structured behavioral job interview. You can also use BARS to measure job performance after a hire has been made. In the context of the interview, the interviewer must evaluate the interviewee based on the interviewee's own description of their past behaviors in situations that relate to the interviewer's question. In the context of using BARS to measure job performance after an employee is hired, the rater (managers or peers) is evaluating the employee based on their actual observations of job behavior.

The best way to measure hiring quality is to apply BARS to the observation of actual on-the-job performance following the hire. You can create a preliminary measure of hiring quality based on the application of BARS in the interview process but this will always be inferior to the measurement of observations of actual job performance. If you hold onto your pre-hire assessment and correlate it to ongoing performance assessment, then you can continuously evaluate the overall predictive power of the rubric you use in the interview process and at the same time scrutinize each component of the rubric you use.

REMEMBER

If you are measuring something in the interview process that is not correlated to job performance, you should stop measuring it. Conversely, if you are not measuring something in the interview process that is correlated to job performance, then it should be added.

The choice of where to put people on the BARS scale will always be subjective, but the critical-incident technique can at least help you develop scale anchors that provide a consistent point of reference rooted in objective experiences.

The scales you have developed through the critical-incident technique facilitate a transfer of qualitative information into a numerical measurement framework, which allows it to be combined with other data to be analyzed as a model. The scales will never be perfect, but they are better than having no anchor, and through repeated use and analysis, the scales can be improved.

REMEMBER

A talent acquisition process measures how well decisions about the talent acquisition process design and about whom to hire are made. All the techniques covered in this chapter should be judged in light of that main goal. Make the techniques work for you.

Chapter **10**

Activation: Identifying the ABCs of a Productive Worker

I f people were robots, you would simply hire them and they'd do whatever it is they were designed to do for you. The robots would be productive whenever they were turned on, so you'd know that you'd get a certain value return on every robot dollar spent. You can't assume the same about people, however. People can show up and do nothing or do the bare minimum or enthusiastically find ways to make your company run better. People can help you outsmart the competition, or they can keep their mouths shut. The analysis of activation is about whether you're getting the most out of your people and how you can manage people better.

If you're analyzing machines, you simply need to understand the basic parameters of those machines, and then you can have near perfect ability to understand, predict, and control the machine's behavior. Unfortunately, or fortunately, controlling the behavior of people isn't as easy. People make their own, independent choices about their own behavior; therefore, the behavior of people is more difficult to understand and predict. That is not to say that people's behavior is completely random and cannot be analyzed or predicted. Discernible patterns can help you understand the behavior of people and make predictions; you just have to understand the ways that the behavior of people is influenced.

REMEMBER

The models that predict the behaviors of humans are fundamentally probabilistic, not deterministic. They postulate what is likely to happen, not what by necessity will happen.

If you want to understand, predict, and influence the actions of people, you need to make the less-visible influences of people's behavior more visible with data.

Analyzing Antecedents, Behaviors, and Consequences

The goal of people analytics is to understand cause-and-effect relationships so that when you carry out an action, you can produce a better outcome for companies and the people who work for them. Just as the alphabet is the starting point for all human communication, you need a starting point for people analytics. The ABC Behavior Change framework shown in Figure 10-1 is this starting point.

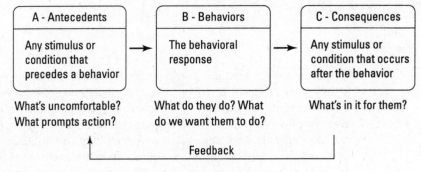

FIGURE 10-1:
The ABC
Behavior Change
framework.

The ABC framework has these three parts:

>> **Antecedent:** Those measurable factors that precede an observed behavior and/or consequence. Antecedents can refer to measurable company conditions, such as employee culture or climate, and/or it can refer to specific program or policy actions intended to stimulate some behavior or consequence.

>> **Behaviors:** Measurements of the ways in which a person or group of people act in response to a particular antecedent situation or stimulus or absence thereof.

>> **Consequences:** Results that directly follow from that behavior. The goal of the ABC framework is to come up with theories about behavior that you can test with data, which drives a specific measurement and analysis plan that you can act on.

REMEMBER

Each behavior has both individual and company consequences and these consequences have different impacts on individual and collective behavior. Company consequences are dispersed among many people, so company consequences have less impact on individual behavior than individual consequences. Individual consequences can reinforce or discourage individual behavior. Effective management works to bring company and individual consequences into alignment.

You can't manage what you don't see, and data is useful for seeing things that otherwise are difficult to see. The ABC framework is a heuristic tool used to organize theories about behavior, which is the starting place for developing scientific methods to test your theory and (eventually) improve how you manage people using data. To test theories with data, you have to codify the behavior, the circumstances that lead to the behavior, and the outcomes that are associated with the behavior in ways that are measurable. After you have all three elements of the ABC framework described as measurements, you can apply mathematics to find out whether your theories hold true. In this way, the ABC framework is a jumping-off point for a data-informed way to identify the best course of action to take in order to influence behavior to achieve the outcomes you want.

Looking at the ABC framework in action

Say that you're in a busy grocery store checkout lane and an angry customer accuses the cashier of mispricing an item. The customer asks the cashier to check the price of the item, but the cashier insists that the price is correct. The customer presses the issue, and the cashier follows up by getting angry at the customer in return. Everyone in line is held up while the cashier phones the office for a clerk to go check the price. The price is found to be correct, though the item had been picked up in the wrong place. Now an even angrier customer leaves his groceries with the cashier and storms out of the store. The rest of the people waiting in line are exasperated at the delay.

Let's examine this situation with the ABC framework. First, the customer, using an angry tone, asked the employee to do a price check. That was a critical antecedent, though there were many others. For example, the item was in the wrong place. (Clearly, other antecedents are not described in the preceding paragraph, but I'll come back to them.) Next, the employee reacts with recalcitrance and anger — a wrong behavior, especially in a retail environment. The ideal behavior would be to acknowledge the misunderstanding but offer the product to the customer for the lower price anyway or offer the customer some type of reward for pointing out the problem. If nothing else, a caring response may have deescalated the situation. In any case, the consequences of the wrong behavior are that the store has lost this particular sale, has potentially lost this customer for life, and has diminished the experience of other customers. It wasn't a pleasant experience for anyone. Some would say, "That's work" or "That's retail." However, not all store experiences and cashiers are the same — some handle these situations more adeptly than others. How do they do it?

This situation is anecdotal, but if I were to analyze this problem, I would want to step back and think about other, less obvious antecedents. Has the store been staffed properly? Is there a general culture and expectation that cashiers will be happy and responsive to customers? Is this an enthusiastic employee, or does this employee consider the relationship between cashiers and management to be contentious? Is there is a policy in which the cashiers can make their own decisions under a certain price limit? How frequently is that policy evoked? Have cashiers been selected for unflappable personalities? What is the range of variability and percentage of different types in the store? Is there an expectation that cashiers will behave in a certain way or be sent home? Are lots of other people modeling good behavior? Have employees been trained in how to deal with difficult customers? Do other employees exhibit the expected behaviors? Is this a fun place to go to work every day, or is this workplace total hell?

TECHNICAL STUFF

Total hell is a technical term referring to a place to work that is much like the total hell described in Dante Alighieri's *Inferno.* If you can imagine suffering where you're subjected to burning, fiery coals, you're on the right path to understanding total hell.

In some ways the store and the employee consequences can be aligned. Are there social or disciplinary consequences for poor behavior? Are there rewards for good behavior? Is there an aggressive career opportunity program at the store, or are cashiers treated as temporary expendable help? Is there employee profit sharing? Does the company, and do the managers, work with employees to create a compelling mission and vision for their work, thus creating a connection between the actions that individuals take and the greater impact on other lives or society? You can picture in your mind a store that has the antecedents and behaviors that would lead to a much better outcome for everyone. Maybe you have experienced one. It's a remarkable difference, isn't it?

Extrapolating from observed behavior

There are all kinds of antecedents, behaviors, and consequences going on all around us all the time. Antecedents drive consequences, and consequences in turn create new antecedents, like billiard balls bumping into each other. Much of what is driving behaviors is unseen because each encounter seems independent and random. This is just a flaw in perspective, however. One major goal of people analytics is to increase the breadth and depth of awareness collectively and individually.

A Johari window (see Figure 10-2) is a heuristic illustration that helps people think about how information can vary between the self and others to see the implications. The Johari window is used in corporate settings as a heuristic tool to explain why getting feedback is essential for the success of the enterprise.

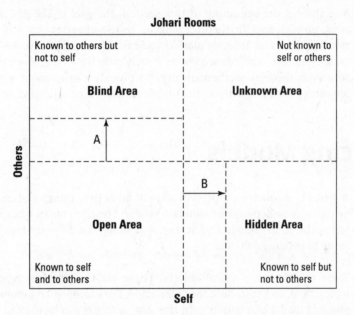

FIGURE 10-2:
A Johari window.

The philosopher Charles Handy came up with a twist on the Johari window that he calls the *Johari house.* Essentially, he reconfigures the four panes of the Johari window into a house with four rooms. Room 1 is the part of yourself that you and others see. Room 2 contains aspects that others see but you are unaware of. Room 3 is the private space that you know but hide from others. Room 4 is the unconscious part of you that neither you nor others see. The idea of the Johari house is that although your understanding of yourself and the world around you will always be imperfect, there is some advantage to improving it. The factors that you measure and report in people analytics primarily offer value by providing feedback about things that are otherwise outside of your field of awareness — increasing the size of those rooms, in other words. You're architecting a different house.

TIP

Sometimes, you will already have access to regularly collected data that you can use to create collective and individual feedback. In other situations, you don't have the measurements and you will have to develop new measurement methods. In my experience, the best-performing people analytics teams and analysts do a lot more of the latter. The best analysts produce an advantage by coming up with creative methods to measure things, not by applying the same methods everyone else is using, but with fewer mistakes. The difficult mathematical tasks are performed by software, so you're not making a lot of mistakes in mathematics. You're making more mistakes in what you put into the software and in interpreting what you get out of the software.

As I state at the beginning of this section, the goal of the ABC framework is to come up with specific theories you can test — theories that will drive a specific measurement and analysis plan. If you can express your theories about antecedents, behaviors, and consequences clearly, you have created a blueprint to measure your theories mathematically. To provide clarity about your theories and organize them, you will use the tool described in the following section.

Introducing Models

A *model* is an abstract representation of an object (thing) and its components to help people understand or simulate reality. The term *model* has a number of uses, so I spend some time in this section describing the different types of models that apply to people analytics.

Some models are physical objects. These are the simplest types of models to understand, so I start here for illustration. For example, an architect may create a physical model of a building. In this way, a model can be used to convey the idea of the building and test this idea before the building is constructed in the real world. Everyone can look at the model and decide whether they like it. If they don't like it, the architect can ask why not. The model removes non-essential detail and material. Material is added when the decision is made to proceed.

Conceptual models are abstractions that connect or organize ideas. These are often illustrated diagrammatically or with mathematical notation. Though more abstract than physical models, conceptual models serve the same purpose as physical models — but for items you can't hold in your hand. The model serves a useful purpose by helping you see in your mind this thing you can't touch or feel. All of what you work with in business strategy and applied behavioral science is conceptual. Figure 10-3 shows an example of a conceptual model.

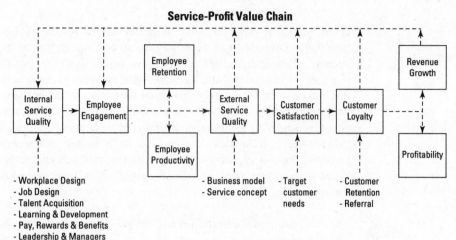

FIGURE 10-3:
The Service-Profit
Value Chain
model.

The Service–Profit Chain model illustrates the researchers' point of view about the important antecedents, behaviors, and consequences of a retail company at a high level. It's a way to communicate abstract notions of what matters in order to first elicit reactions by others and then form a plan for analysis and testing. Though this model may be useful for a retail company as a starting place, each company creates value and profit differently — sometimes by adopting the strategies of other companies and sometimes in some rather unique ways.

REMEMBER

The conceptual model illustrated by the Service–Profit Chain is not the only way people use the word *model* or that you will use the word *model.* As I mention at the beginning of this section, the term *model* has many forms, which can be confusing. The following sections categorically describe the most important forms of conceptual models in business.

Business models

Business models are frameworks that describe how a business creates value or, as management theorist Peter Drucker has said, business models are simply "a theory of a business."

A *business* model is a conceptual model that describes and represents the elemental structure of how a business will earn profit that can be contrasted to the ways that other businesses earn profit. These conceptual models describe the elements of a business that include: problem focus, target customer focus (market), unique value proposition, channels, methods of generating revenue, total addressable market (projected target customer market estimates), projected costs, projected revenues, and any believed or real business differentiation advantages.

Often, unusually large business successes are the results of the application of a new business model that nobody else saw coming. Examples include the initial success of companies like Ford (mass production), McDonald's (fast food), Amazon (e-commerce), and Netflix (digital streaming). Each new business model has antecedents and consequences that stem from or affect the way the company works with people — the way that companies harness people to produce profits — which you refer to as human resources. In a historical context, what companies like Ford and McDonalds decided to do with human resources was remarkable for their time. It is only over time that the methods they deployed faded into a common experience to such an extent that their innovations now seem unremarkable.

REMEMBER

The business model determines the unique characteristics of what, how, where, and why people matter. The work of people analytics is to develop a unique model of how people deliver value to customers and to keep refining that model to increase the number of happy customers before running out of time and resources. You come up with theories, you test them, and if you learn something, you improve your model.

Scientific models

A *scientific* model is the conceptual model that describes and represents the component structure, relationship, behavior, and other views of a scientific theory for a physical object or process. A scientific model is a simplified abstract view of a complex reality. Sometimes these are expressed as mathematical equations, and at other times they're expressed as diagrams to make them more accessible.

The well-known $e=mc^2$ is a mathematical expression of a scientific theory of how the universe works. It was developed from theory, refined with mathematics, and tested by experiments. It's abstract, but it has been applied to do some concrete tasks like travel into space, create large explosions, and develop ways to harness the energy that is all around us.

The quality of a scientific field can be assessed by how well the mathematical models developed on the theoretical side agree with the mathematical results of repeatable experiments. Lack of agreement between theoretical mathematical models and experimental measurements often leads to important advances as better theories are developed based on the nuances of the findings.

Mathematical/statistical models

A *mathematical* model is a conceptual model that describes and represents the mathematical structure, relationships, behaviors, and other views of real-world situations, represented as equations, diagrams, graphs, scatterplots, tree diagrams, and other elements. A mathematical model is a simplified abstract view of a more complex real-world phenomenon. Mathematical models can take many forms, including dynamical systems, statistical models, differential equations, or game theoretic models.

With mathematical/statistical models, we are at the very heart of how data can be used to impact business decisions. Take, for example, a rocket manufacturer. It goes without saying that, when designing a new engine, the manufacturer starts by designing a mathematical model and conducting simulations on a computer rather than incur the costs of building physical million-dollar rockets and blowing them up just for testing purposes. If the only way you could learn was by blowing them up, things might get pretty expensive. Eventually, you have to test your rockets in the real world, but hopefully you can do this only after you worked out most of the bugs through a mathematical model. This isn't where it ends, though. Eventually, even as you launch real rockets, you will also collect data to see whether the rocket performs as predicted and to adapt your model based on real-life data.

Similar to the rocket example, before you implement some new way of hiring employees, some new training program, some new way of paying people, or some new benefit, you should do some rudimentary mathematical testing to make sure you aren't going to blow up your company. Companies can and do frequently go bankrupt as a result of the inadequate modeling of people-related decisions or an inability to understand how to control the motivations of the workforce, which determines success or failure in the marketplace.

Data models

A *data* model is the conceptual diagram or other technical language that describes and represents the component structure, relationships, behaviors, and other views of data elements in an information system that in turn represent objects or processes of the real world. It's a simplified, abstract view of complex data relationships.

You truly bore down into the nuts-and-bolts when you get to data models. Data models assist software engineers, testers, technical writers, IT workers, analysts, business users, and other stakeholders to understand and use a common data definition of the concepts represented by data and their relationships with one another. With that common definition, you're now in a position to facilitate

>> The design of systems

>> Efficient data management in databases and data warehouses (also known as data repositories) and reporting applications

>> Multiple stakeholders in analyzing data in a consistent way

>> The integration of multiple information systems that contain common elements

The first phase of a data model is conceptual. The data requirements are initially recorded as a set of technology-independent conceptual specifications. For instance, a data model may specify that the data element represent a primary object, which is composed of data elements and relatable to other objects. See Figure 10-4 for an example.

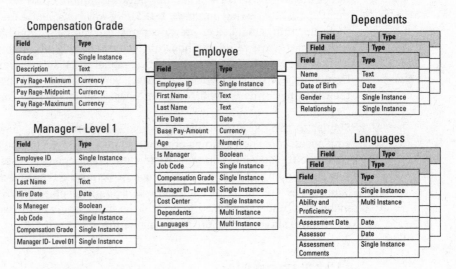

Compensation Grade

Field	Type
Grade	Single Instance
Description	Text
Pay Rage-Minimum	Currency
Pay Rage-Midpoint	Currency
Pay Rage-Maximum	Currency

Manager – Level 1

Field	Type
Employee ID	Single Instance
First Name	Text
Last Name	Text
Hire Date	Date
Is Maneger	Boolean
Job Code	Single Instance
Compensation Grade	Single Instance
Manager ID- Level 01	Single Instance

Employee

Field	Type
Employee ID	Single Instance
First Name	Text
Last Name	Text
Hire Date	Date
Base Pay-Amount	Currency
Age	Numeric
Is Manager	Boolean
Job Code	Single Instance
Compensation Grade	Single Instance
Manager ID–Level 01	Single Instance
Cost Center	Single Instance
Dependents	Multi Instance
Languages	Multi Instance

Dependents

Field	Type
Name	Text
Date of Birth	Date
Gender	Single Instance
Relationship	Single Instance

Languages

Field	Type
Language	Single Instance
Ability and Proficiency	Multi Instance
Assessment Date	Date
Assessor	Date
Assessment Comments	Single Instance

FIGURE 10-4: A tiny part of an HR data model.

In the example, an employee object consists of related data elements such as job title, location, start date, and manager. The employee data elements can be related to elements in other systems, such as customers, products, and orders, which are recorded in a sales system.

The conceptual model of what data elements you have, their nature, and how they are associated can then be translated into a logical data model, which documents structures of the data that can be implemented in databases — entities, attributes, relations, or tables, for example. The logical data model describes the semantics of the database, as represented by a particular data manipulation technology, whether they are tables and columns, object-oriented classes, XML tags, or other items. Implementation of one logical model may require multiple submodels.

The last step in data modeling is transforming the logical data model to a physical data model that organizes the data into physical assets that accommodate access, speed, and other situational needs. The physical data model describes the physical means by which data are stored in the servers, partitions, CPUs, tablespaces, and the like.

System models

Systems modeling is the use of models to conceptualize and construct business information systems in business.

In business information systems and IT development, the term *systems modeling* has multiple meanings. It can relate to

» The use of a model to conceptualize and design systems

» The interdisciplinary study of the use of these systems

» The systems simulation, such as system dynamics

» Any specific systems modeling language

Check out Figure 10-5 for a rudimentary example of all the systems and databases that may be connected in an operating people analytics environment in a large company. It functions as a simplified conceptual diagram of the systems a company may already have in place (and thus need to fully understand) when embarking to establish an automated people analytics data workflow through these systems.

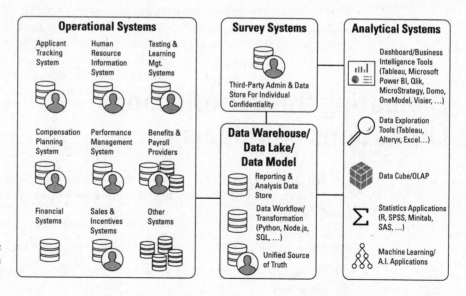

FIGURE 10-5:
A sample system diagram.

TECHNICAL STUFF

A common type of systems modeling is *function* modeling, with specific techniques such as the Functional Flow Block diagram. These diagrammatic models can be linked to requirements and extended in breadth or depth. As an alternative to functional modeling, another type of systems modeling is *architectural* modeling, which uses the systems architecture to conceptually model the structure, behavior, and other views of a system. The Business Process Modeling Notation (BPMN) is a graphical representation for specifying an entire business process in a workflow. (In that sense, BPMN can also be considered a system modeling language.)

Evaluating the Benefits and Limitations of Models

A model's primary objective is to convey the fundamental relationship and functions of the system of elements that it represents without unnecessary detail. Models can

>> Enhance understanding of the system of parts through their organization.

>> Facilitate efficient communication between stakeholders using a common language.

>> Document the system of objects for future reference and provide a means for collaboration.

>> Study the effects of different components, make predictions about behavior, and test ideas.

>> Provide an outline for analysts to perform their work while also offering a tool for practitioners to formulate ideas on how to solve problems and see the impact.

Though the use of models offers many benefits, it also has some limitations.

>> A model is not a perfect representation of reality, and so by definition will omit some things.

>> A model can be obtuse to others if they aren't yet familiar with the pieces.

>> A model regarding dynamic systems (people, for example) can and will change over time. Your work is never done.

>> A model may not apply well between different situations, industries, companies, and locations.

REMEMBER

The most important insight that can be gleaned from the limitations of models is that they need to be created, validated, and rebuilt for each situation.

To take just one example, imagine owning a pet retail company that has discovered the high probability that a candidate who has five or more pets at home will make a great employee. With this information in hand, you might put the question "How many pets do you have?" into your pre-hire screening process with the intent to measure whether it matters in the performance prediction model. The point here is that this same question doesn't predict success for other companies — an electronics retail store, for example. At most, other companies relying on this information to make hiring decisions would be wrong. Furthermore, collecting such information would be a waste of everyone's time and would prevent you from collecting something else that would be much more useful.

You won't be able to derive a unique model from a common dataset. You need a way to know which data to collect. Which data you collect is determined by a theoretical model. Without this model, the amount of data you could apply approaches the entire possible universe of data — infinity, in other words — which clearly won't work. This means you have to create different datasets for different businesses. Of course, you will use some common data ingredients at all companies (employee roster lists, exit lists, and hire lists, for example), but these won't provide you with the answers to important questions about your business without other data as determined by scientific theory. This part of people analytics is a creative activity rather than a routine activity.

Obtaining unique insight requires defining a unique scientific model for a unique business, which requires collecting unique data. After you have the correct data, the analysis is routine and therefore easy. The problem of identifying what of all possible new data to add to the model to produce new insight cannot be solved with a system because all of data you need doesn't reside in the existing systems yet. This understanding moves the priority of work from system and statistics to the design of scientific models and data collection instruments to fill those models. The design of the scientific model must precede all other system and data efforts, or else those efforts will fail. This understanding moves the initial priority of work from systems and data governance to the conversations and actions required to develop a thoughtful scientific model for each business, which informs you on what data you need, what the shape of that data should be, and what analysis is necessary.

Using Models Effectively

Just like an architectural blueprint does for a construction site, a model is a design blueprint for a series of activities that is intended to come together into a finished product. The blueprint allows the people working on the different parts to know what to do and where to do it while also providing a basis for communication between each other.

Imagine building a house. You cannot begin certain activities until other activities have already occurred. You can begin work on framing only if the foundation is in place. You cannot begin working on the electrical system until the framing is in place. You cannot finish the walls until the electrical system is in place and approved by inspectors. Each part has to be built, and then they all must eventually fit together, or else the house won't work. The blueprint provides the structure, and the project plans provide the order. Models provide the same guidance in people analytics.

When you pay careful attention to how HR professionals talk about their difficulties with people analytics, you will hear a lot of if-only statements:

>> "If only we had all our data in one place, then we could do people analytics."

>> "If only we had better data governance, then we would have better data and then people analytics would (finally) work."

>> "If only we could hire someone who can tell a story with our data in a compelling way, then people here would use data more successfully."

>> "If only executives wouldn't rush ahead to make decisions without data."

If you have undertaken this long journey to implement systems and do all this work with data and you are then confronted at the end by one or more of these if-only statements, you will stop dead in your tracks and find that you have wasted money and time. Then you will have to start over.

In a system-oriented people analytics workflow, success is achieved if you

>> Have implemented systems with relevant data.

>> Have data quality governance to produce good, clean data.

>> Have extracted all the relevant data and joined it.

>> Have structured the dataset correctly for your analysis.

>> Can fit an insight from the data to your unique business situation.

and

>> Can, after all that, fit that insight to the needs of someone who can act on it.

Each if-only statement contains a contingency that can cause overall failure. The sheer number of contingencies suggests that the system of work will have a very low probability of success. This is especially true when you consider that, at your company, you're solving a problem that nobody has ever solved and that may be unlike the problem at any other company.

Using a method of people analytics that I developed called lean people analytics, you reduce risk and waste by working in a different order — one which postpones the more expensive risks to later in the process. You only move to the next step after you have completed the last, which increases the expected value of the overall system of work.

Figure 10-6 illustrates how the order of activity in lean people analytics is the opposite of a system-oriented analytics order of activity.

As Figure 10-6 shows, in the system-oriented analytics development workflow you start with the system first and you work to the right toward deducing an insight that has relevance to a particular business. You then try to find people to listen. The assumption is that if you can make the system workflow more efficient or if you can visualize the data marginally better at the end, you will get a better result. The entire premise is flawed if you don't have the correct data to derive a valuable insight in your systems from the beginning. You can't add by analysis what you left out to begin with. Consequently, a system-oriented analytics development workflow is better at helping you more efficiently produce the metrics you are already producing from the data you already have, as opposed to developing new insights.

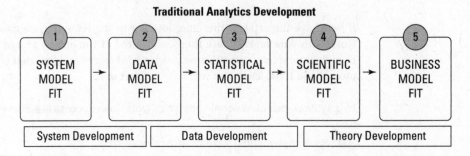

Traditional Analytics Development

1	2	3	4	5
SYSTEM MODEL FIT	DATA MODEL FIT	STATISTICAL MODEL FIT	SCIENTIFIC MODEL FIT	BUSINESS MODEL FIT

System Development	Data Development	Theory Development

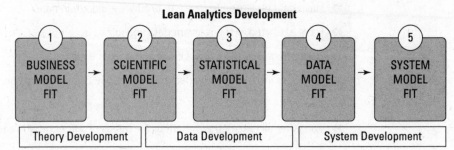

Lean Analytics Development

1	2	3	4	5
BUSINESS MODEL FIT	SCIENTIFIC MODEL FIT	STATISTICAL MODEL FIT	DATA MODEL FIT	SYSTEM MODEL FIT

Theory Development	Data Development	System Development

FIGURE 10-6: Contrasting people analytics workflows.

In the insight-oriented analytics development workflow, you go in a different order. Here is the order of the insight-oriented analytics development workflow I propose:

1. Define your company's business model.

2. Add to this definition a scientific model that illustrates how you think people connect to your business model.

3. Collect the relevant data.

4. Create a statistical model.

5. Build a permanent system model to systematize this information for routine ongoing use.

REMEMBER

The first crucial step is that you must learn the company's unique business model. Only then can you work out theories of how people connect to this business model.

After you have a theory of how the antecedents and behaviors of people relate to how your company produces happy customers, you can then test your theory with data to see whether it is correct. As you learn what is useful and what isn't useful, you can change the model. When you start out, you want to collect new measurements and conduct new analyses in a manner as nimble and inexpensive as possible. Survey tools are inexpensive and are therefore an optimum tool for this phase of development.

After you have come up with a report or an analysis that provides feedback that others have found useful, you can make it more efficient by systematizing ongoing data collection, processing, and delivery in a permanent data model represented by permanent systems. A system model begins as a conceptual model that you can use to communicate the flow of data to technical partners. Eventually, this conceptual model will be used to codify a physical data workflow and database or system structure.

Getting Started with General People Models

The idea that every company is different and every person is a snowflake may be true, but it's about as useful as saying that you can reach the North Pole from any direction you want. You need to know where you are, and you need a generalizable navigation system to put (and keep) you on the right path, or else you're just going to go around in circles.

The general navigation system I suggest for dealing with people is called net activated value (NAV). (For more on NAV, check out Chapter 7.) If you're looking for nirvana, I have no idea what will bring that to you, but if you're looking for business results, value will always point you in the right direction.

The concept behind NAV is a simple one: You get business value from employees when they're activated, and you get no value from employees when they aren't activated. Imagine if all employees were like money machines with a light on the front and you could see which ones were functioning and which ones weren't. Then, if you wanted more money, you would go to work on the ones with the lights off. Seems obvious, doesn't it? What isn't obvious is seeing why the ones that aren't working aren't working, and if there is any consistent pattern to the failure. For this, you need to take some measurements.

Activating employee performance

Carrying forward this idea that the value creation motors of folks are either on (activated) or off (not activated), your job as technician is to figure out how to get as many of them running as possible.

What you want to understand is whether there's a pattern. Are the machines broken at a particular location? Is it a particular model? Within the machine, what part of the machine is broken? How long does the machine run before breaking? What happened immediately before the machine stopped? To complicate this matter, there are different scenarios: Just because one machine needs oil doesn't mean that all machines aren't working because they need oil.

If you can see inside the machine, you can see which parts are broken and replace them. You want to do the same thing for your employees. If you were to rip open these humans and see what was broken, you would have a chance to fix it like you would a machine, but that wouldn't be humane. Instead, one way you can measure which elements of the human equation are broken is by way of scientific inference — specifically, you infer what is broken by using survey instruments. After this is done, you apply creative solutions, and later you survey again to see whether the theory was correct. Did the behaviors or consequences you were concerned about change as a result of your creative solutions?

REMEMBER

Though you will never know everything that makes a particular human tick, fortunately, that isn't your goal. Your goal is to understand the minimum conditions necessary for employees to consistently produce value for your business. Though many things could be beneficial to humans — free lunch and back massages, for example — you need to know what is absolutely essential for this human to produce value and get a handle on that first. You can work on lunches and massages *after* the essential factors that produce value are working properly.

Whatever creative solutions you come up with, they will have to come to terms with the four minimum conditions necessary for this human machine to produce value: *c*apability, goal *a*lignment, *m*otivation, and *s*upport (CAMS). If each of these conditions is turned on, the value that your employees produce is either what you pay them or some multiple of this value.

Figure 10-7 shows one way of expressing capability, alignment, motivation, and support (CAMS) in a framework of antecedents, behaviors, and consequences.

In Figure 10-7, CAMS is in the second Antecedents column, meaning it is believed to influence behaviors and consequences that are represented in columns to the right. For example, the model is suggesting the CAMS antecedent should be correlated to measures of work quality and work intensity behavior and these should in turn correlate to the other downstream consequences such as measures of job performance and productivity.

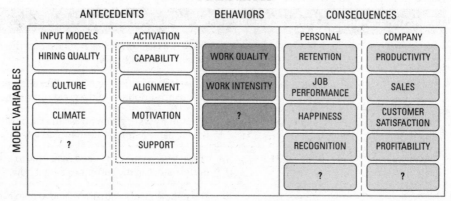

CAMS MODEL

ANTECEDENTS		BEHAVIORS	CONSEQUENCES	
INPUT MODELS	ACTIVATION		PERSONAL	COMPANY
HIRING QUALITY	CAPABILITY	WORK QUALITY	RETENTION	PRODUCTIVITY
CULTURE	ALIGNMENT	WORK INTENSITY	JOB PERFORMANCE	SALES
CLIMATE	MOTIVATION	?	HAPPINESS	CUSTOMER SATISFACTION
?	SUPPORT		RECOGNITION	PROFITABILITY
			?	?

FIGURE 10-7: One possible CAMS model.

You can infer a measure of all four CAMS variables — capability (C), alignment (A), motivation (M), and support (S) — with a short, 8-item survey using a 0–10 agreement scale. Implicit in all 8 of these survey statements is the theory that individual success requires, at minimum, four conditions:

>> Agreement on goal

>> Capability to perform the goal

>> Motivation to perform the goal

>> Support

The absence of any of these four conditions results in something less than great performance.

Survey design

Come up with statements where you can get a disagree or agree reaction for evaluating if the four minimum necessary conditions for success are likely present or not present — statements that touch on the four model variables of capability (C), alignment (A), motivation (M), and support (S) — using a 0–10 agreement scale.

TIP

Pay careful attention when dealing with a 0–10 agreement scale; 11 responses are possible on such a scale (0,1,2,3,4,5,6,7,8,9,10).

All of the statements I use are all positive, so the 0–10 scale response can be interpreted consistently such that a 0 would be the worst response and a 10 would be the best response for all items.

Survey items are described in Table 10-1 below.

TABLE 10-1 **Elements of a CAMS survey**

CAMS Component	Format of Item	Survey Item Statement
Alignment	Team	There is a clear objective around which myself and the people I work with rally.
Alignment	Individual	I have a clear understanding of the difference between an average contribution and a great contribution for my role.
Capability	Team	My primary work group has all the capabilities it needs right now to achieve top performance as a team.
Capability	Individual	I have the capabilities I need right now to achieve top performance in my current role right now.
Motivation	Team	The people I work with are willing to help even if it means doing something outside of their usual activities.
Motivation	Individual	I am motivated to do more than minimum expectations.
Support	Team	I have the cooperation and support from others at <company> I need to be successful.
Support	Individual	I have the resources and tools I need to be successful.

TIP

On the actual survey, you would just list the statements in the survey tool along with the suggested 0–10 agreement scale. I have included some categorizations of each item in the first two columns of the table below for your sake, but no one other than you need worry about the how you categorize each item.

The index calculations proposed later in this chapter assumes 8 positively worded items on a 0–10 agreement scale. If, for various reasons, you want to use a different agreement scale (going with 1 to 5 or 1 to 7, for example) or add or remove an item, feel free to do so; however, you would have to take this into consideration in the index calculation and other uses of this data described below. If you change the construction of the survey, then you will have to adjust the index and your interpretation of the index accordingly.

TECHNICAL STUFF

Notice that the items in each category are intentionally similar; it's just that one is asked from the perspective of the team and one is asked from the perspective of the individual. Asking about the same concept in more than one way creates a better performing index. Each survey item is framed in a particular way, which is subject to a particular bias. Asking the question in more than one way is intended to provide balance to minimize the impact of various types of bias. The overall index will be more reliable than the response to a single item or subset of items.

Calculating the CAMS index

Sum the total counts (0–10) from the individual response to the eight items. This should produce a score ranging from 0 to 80 per individual, known as the *CAMS index*.

Calculating the net activated

The CAMS Index can be used by itself to get a detailed look at activation levels, but sometimes you just want to count the number of people who meet a minimum threshold of activation. Start of by setting your threshold. Here's one I came up with:

>> **Activated** = *CAMS index* equal to or greater than 70

>> **At-Risk** = *CAMS index* less than 60

Then all you need to do is count the number of individual survey respondents who qualify as Activated. Given the criterion you set, these respondents make up the *net activated* pool.

Calculate Activated Percent

Activated Percent is a metric that calculates a count of the number of activated respondents divided by the total number of survey responses.

Activated Percent = (# activated) ÷ (total survey responses)

Although such a company-wide metric can be useful, as with all surveys it is possible to narrow the focus to one particular segment of the company. The formula for that approach would be as follows:

Activated Percent = (# activated in segment) ÷ (total survey responses in the segment)

The beauty of a segment approach to a CAMS diagnostic is that you can identify whether there's a consistent pattern among segments of your work population and by process of elimination determine what, among the four CAMS conditions, is the problem. After you have identified where the problem is in your population and which specific CAMS condition is missing, you can contrast the activated and non-activated employees to try to isolate which antecedents matter. You compare activated employees to non-activated employees and try a treatment method on some portion to see, after applying the antecedent change, whether the condition that had concerned you has been resolved for the treated individuals. If the condition has been resolved, you have your answer.

Survey administration

The 8-item inventory described above is short enough that it can be distributed monthly or quarterly as a regular management ritual and key operational tool that can be associated with other outcomes without degrading response rate or presenting difficulty when it comes to producing and distributing reports.

This survey should be conducted confidentially by a third-party agent so that individual responses can be joined with other data and reported by segment while protecting the integrity of the process and the safety of individual responses.

While the questions are necessarily directed to obtain the opinion of individuals, for purposes of reporting you will group responses by units (similar jobs, teams, division, company, and so on) to evaluate conditions by team and make corrections by team.

Figure 10-8 uses a slice of items from the Activation survey to show how a simple index can be created by assigning points based on the level of agreement with a series of statements. (The slice in Figure 10-8 concentrates on Alignment and Capability.) The responses from survey participants are scored and combined into an index per concept.

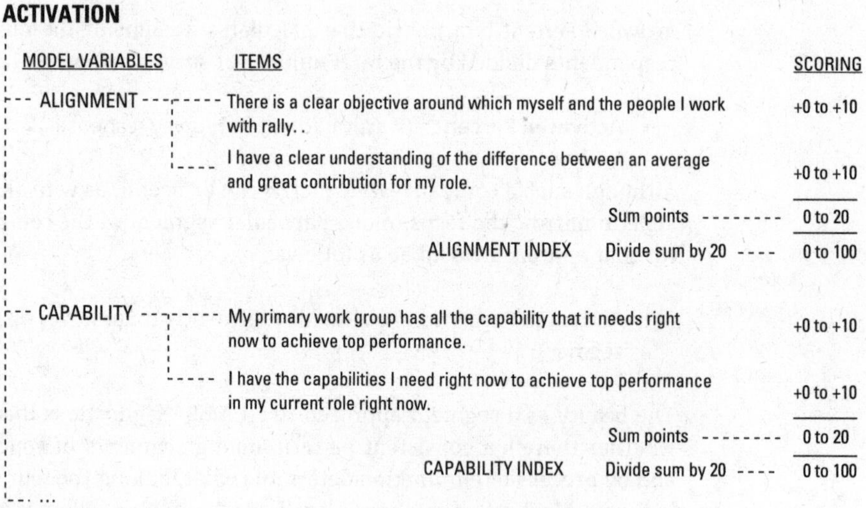

ACTIVATION

MODEL VARIABLES	ITEMS		SCORING
ALIGNMENT	There is a clear objective around which myself and the people I work with rally. .		+0 to +10
	I have a clear understanding of the difference between an average and great contribution for my role.		+0 to +10
		Sum points	0 to 20
	ALIGNMENT INDEX	Divide sum by 20	0 to 100
CAPABILITY	My primary work group has all the capability that it needs right now to achieve top performance.		+0 to +10
	I have the capabilities I need right now to achieve top performance in my current role right now.		+0 to +10
		Sum points	0 to 20
	CAPABILITY INDEX	Divide sum by 20	0 to 100

FIGURE 10-8: An example of activation subindex scoring.

In Figure 10-8, each selection on the 0–10 scale determines the points assigned to the item, which are then combined for each of the variable concepts. Here, there are two statements for each of the two CAMS items. You add the scores for the two statements together then divide the points by the total number of points possible — in this case by 20. After you divide the points achieved by the points possible, you end up with a percent between 0 and 1. Multiple this by 100 to get an index value between 0 and 100. Using this method, each individual in the survey database will have an index score between 0–100 for each CAMS variable you've measured.

REMEMBER

The steps are different depending on what your analysis uncovers. If you were solving a capability problem, the follow-up analysis I suggest is totally different from when you're solving a motivation problem, a support problem, or a goal alignment problem.

The idea of models is to organize all the concepts so that you aren't adding questions to surveys either indiscriminately or based on what someone else is doing. The idea is to add those survey questions that help you learn something specific related to the problem you're trying to solve. Without a conceptual model to keep things organized, you will start off with a lot of fuzzy ideas about people, collect a lot of data, and end up in a situation where you won't know what the data really means for you or what to do with it. You have managed to ask a ton of questions, but it's not quite clear how the answers to those questions connect to the behaviors and consequences you care about. It also isn't clear whether you have asked the appropriate questions among the infinite number of possible questions.

In the next section, I take a stab at firming up some of the more common "fuzzy ideas" found in business these days by presenting models that allow you to move from vague notions to quantifiable measurements. The conceptual models I describe are intended to be illustrative. You can find or create many more.

Using models to clarify fuzzy ideas about people

One of the fuzziest ideas out there is the notion of *organizational culture* (usually defined as a "corporate personality"), consisting of the shared values, beliefs, and unstated rules that influence the behavior of people as members of an organization. Now, *culture* is a concept borrowed from anthropology, where it's defined as those unique characteristics — knowledge, beliefs, art, morals, law, customs — held in common among a group of humans that are transmitted via social learning. Members of a company are, first and foremost, part of a broader social cultural context (continent, religion, country, ethnicity, community) and also the specific social culture context of where they work.

REMEMBER

Contrary to how the term is frequently thrown around, *company culture* is not good or bad or wrong or right in any universal sense. On the other hand, a company culture may or may not be the right fit for a certain place, market, or time or may or not be what you expect it to be. It's the difference between the current state of affairs and people's expectations that matters.

Culture may not be good or bad universally, but it can be strong or weak, and this can have implications. A *strong* culture is one that people clearly understand and can articulate. A *weak* culture is one that people have difficulty defining, understanding, or explaining. The benefit of a strong culture is that people behave and make decisions consistently because they agree on a common set of expectations and values. Companies with strong cultures operate like well-oiled machines. Hardly a word needs to be said, and everyone knows exactly what to do. Conversely, in a weak culture, there is little common understanding and agreement about expectations and values, which means that control must be exercised by way of extensive instruction, rules, and bureaucracy.

Some of the benefits derived from cultivating a strong culture are that it

>> Gives similar-minded people a reason to embrace this company.

>> Better aligns the company toward achieving its vision, mission, and goals.

>> Achieves higher intrinsic employee motivation and loyalty.

>> Increases team cohesiveness among the company's various departments and divisions.

>> Promotes consistency and coordinated effort among the company.

>> Shapes employee behavior at work with less bureaucratic controls, enabling the company to operate more efficiently.

TIP

You can quantify organization culture through field observation, interviews, or surveys; however, surveys are much more efficient and useful for your use in people analytics.

The Culture Congruence model

A lot of public peer-reviewed research on organization culture is available, and the methods of measuring culture proposed by these researchers have been defined in many different ways. Though I share just one way with you — the Culture Congruence model — I want to know that you can do it in other ways, if that serves your purpose.

Figure 10-9 illustrates the high-level concepts that are measured as variables in the organizational culture assessment instrument (OCAI), a well-respected tool for assessing current and preferred organizational culture that was developed by professors Robert Quinn and Kim Cameron of the University of Michigan. The main OCAI variables shown on the left side of the figure — dominant characteristics, leadership style, strategic emphasis, management style, and so on — are represented as antecedents to a series of attitudes, behaviors, and consequences. (There's tons more information about the OCAI at www.ocai-online.com.)

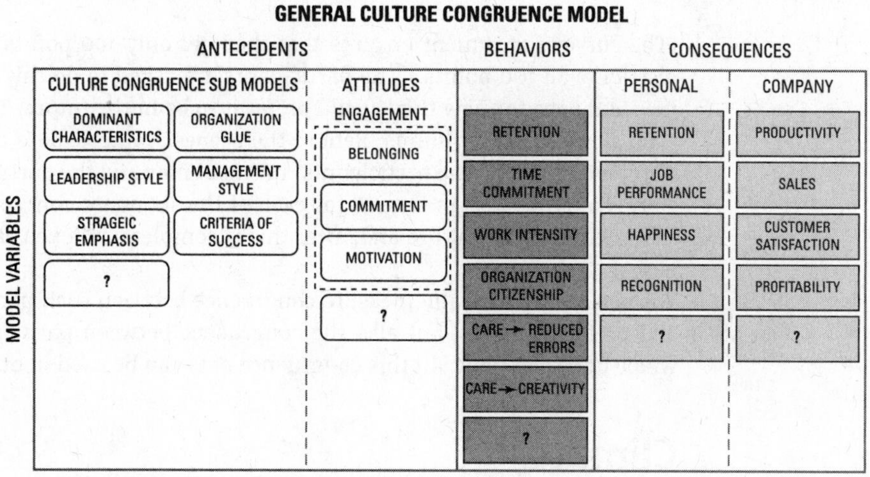

GENERAL CULTURE CONGRUENCE MODEL

FIGURE 10-9: The OCAI Culture Congruence model.

Culture is measured a little differently in the OCAI survey instrument from most other types of instruments. Because culture is presumed to be neither universally good nor bad, the way the OCAI uses culture data is by measuring the differences between the current and expected states, a concept I refer to as *congruence*. Figure 10-10 shows one way to measure congruence for dominant characteristics, one of the six concepts included in the OCAI instrument.

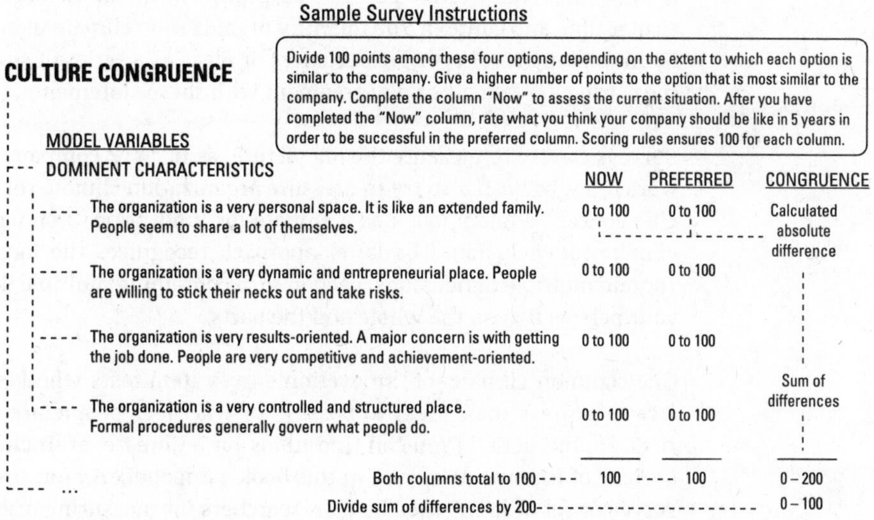

FIGURE 10-10: Sample scoring of OCAI for dominant characteristics.

In the OCAI, participants are asked to divide 100 points between four options, depending on the extent to which they find that each option lines up with what they see at their company. The participants are instructed to give a higher number of points to the option that jibes closest with their experience of the company.

(The survey instrument ensures that they get only 100 points and they have to distribute all 100 points.) The participants are asked to do this twice — once for now and once for how they would prefer it to be in the future. These are in separate, side-by-side columns. Behind the scenes, you calculate congruence as the difference between the participants' rating of now and the participants' preferred state. Congruence is measured for each of the six major concepts included in the OCAI definition of culture and, after this is complete, indexed as a whole.

TIP

You can mathematically measure congruence between each participant's current and preferred states, but also the congruence between participants, either as a whole or by segment. All this congruence data can be used in other models.

Climate

Organization culture and organization climate are similar ideas often used interchangeably, but the two have marked differences. Yes, both culture and climate describe a company and influence behavior, but culture defines those aspects of the company that are ubiquitous, deep, and stable, whereas climate arises more from perceptions that are less agreed on and change more frequently. In other words, climate is influenced by culture; culture is not influenced by climate.

Organization climate is a measurement of the patterns of opinion, attitudes, and feelings that characterize people's perception of life in the organization at a particular time and context. You quantify organization climate using surveys, usually by first listing a variety of experiences or ideas as a series of statements and then measuring agreement or disagreement with these statements.

Surveys can try to measure the big picture, as in "XYZ company is a great place to work," but you can also try to measure organization climate relative to some specific concept domain, such as a climate for innovation, a climate for safety, or a climate for inclusion. The latter approach recognizes the fact that climate can contain multiple dimensions, each in turn containing multiple items, which shape your perspective on the whole and the parts.

One common climate-of-innovation survey item tests whether "employees feel free to express their ideas to bosses" or whether "people are not afraid to take risks around here." (You can find items for a Climate-of-Inclusion survey and a Climate of Innovation survey in this book's Appendix B.) But there is no universal survey or set of items used by all researchers for measuring organization climate. Though some items find their way onto most surveys, you will see items drift on or off surveys based on the particular interests of researchers or consultants.

Figure 10-11 is one take on a climate survey, illustrating the high-level concepts that are measured as variables of an organizational climate instrument (OCI) based on the work of Bedell Hunter and M.D. Mumford. The climate concept variables — mission clarity, autonomy, organization integration, and so on — are on the left side of the figure and are represented as antecedents to a series of attitudes, behaviors, and consequences that are theorized to be influenced, at least in part, by climate.

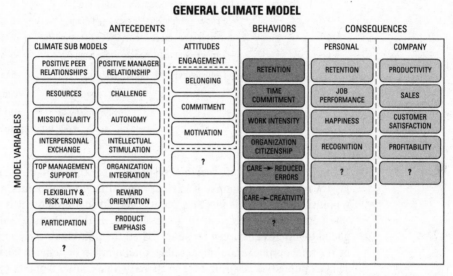

FIGURE 10-11: An organizational climate instrument (OCI) model.

The climate model survey instrument is a little easier to score than the culture survey instrument because it's designed around agreement or disagreement with a series of positive statements. Figure 10-12 takes a small slice of items from the climate survey and shows how a simple index can be created by assigning a point system to the Likert scale. The responses from survey participants are scored and combined into an index.

TECHNICAL STUFF

A Likert agreement scale is a survey research question response scale design named after its inventor, psychologist Rensis Likert. When responding to a Likert Agreement item, respondents specify their level of agreement on a symmetric Agree-Disagree rating scale for a series of statements. That scale is as follows:

» Strongly Disagree

» Disagree

» Neither Disagree or Agree

» Agree

» Strongly Agree

Strongly Disagree	Disagree	Neutral	Agree	Strongly Agree
Points 0	0	2	4	6

CLIMATE

MODEL VARIABLES	ITEMS	SCORING
ROLE CLARITY	I have clear goals and objectives for my job.	+0 to +6
	I am clear about my priorities at work.	+0 to +6
	I know what my responsibilities are.	+0 to +6
	I know exactly what is expected of me.	+0 to +6
	I know what most people in the company do.	+0 to +6
	I know what most people around me do.	+0 to +6
	I know what most departments do.	+0 to +6
	Sum points	0 to 42
	Divide sum by 42	0 to 100
		ROLE CLARITY INDEX

FIGURE 10-12:
An example of climate model scoring.

Using the method of scoring responses to the climate survey shown in Figure 10-12, any response less than neutral is worth 0 points, neutral is worth 2 points, agreement is worth 4 points, and strong agreement is worth 6 points. The points from each item in a variable — in this example, role clarity — are added together per survey response. Then the points per recipient can be divided by the total number of points possible: total number of items in the variable times 6. This example has seven items, so there is a possible 42 points (7×6). After you divide the points achieved by the points possible, you end up with a percent between 0 and 1. Multiple this by 100 to get an index value between 0 and 100. Using this method, each individual in the survey database gets an index score between 0–100 for each variable measured in the survey.

TIP

As you score surveys, you will obtain a response to each item, an index of each variable, and a combined index of all questions for each person who takes the survey. All this data can be correlated to each other or to other antecedent, behavior, and consequence data by joining datasets using a unique employee identifier. Examples of unique identifiers are employee ID and email.

REMEMBER

The idea here is to only view, analyze, and report the data in aggregate, not at the individual employee level of detail. If individuals suspect that their individual answers are being scrutinized by management, they might come up with answers that they believe management wants to hear rather than come up with the truth. Nevertheless, for purposes of data management and analysis, you must retain this individual level of detail and unique identifier so that you can join the data to correlate to other datasets containing relevant antecedents, behaviors, and consequences not contained in the survey dataset itself. Because of the sensitivity of the individual level of data being collected, you should work with a third party (someone who isn't a member of your company) to perform this work so that you can collect sensitive survey data while providing assurances of confidentiality or pseudoanonymity to employees.

If it's a truly anonymous survey, you cannot connect the results to an individual; however, this means you can't use the data within an antecedent, behavior, and consequence model joining to any other data sources outside the survey. From my perspective, a strictly anonymous survey is not worth doing, for this very reason.

Engagement

Employee engagement is a fundamental concept in the effort to understand and describe quantitatively the nature of the relationship between a company and its employees. While the definition of engagement can vary somewhat depending on who you ask, my definition of an "engaged employee" is one who is committed to the company, enthusiastic about their work, and willing to take positive action to further the company's interests. The distinction between employee engagement and the older concept of employee satisfaction is that engagement measures more than just how satisfied employees feel — it is about whether or not employees have the motivation to make efforts on behalf of the company, too. You can imagine a well-paid employee that is committed to stay at a company as long as the company will let them stay, but that is not motivated to make any effort on behalf of the company more than the bare minimum to keep their job. Because engagement implies some motivation to apply additional personal discretionary effort on behalf of company interests, you might imagine therefore that companies with "high" employee engagement should be expected to outperform those with "low" employee engagement.

Figure 10-13 illustrates the high-level concepts that are measured as variables of an engagement model. The engagement concept variables — belonging, motivation, commitment, and so on — are in the second column, with some additional antecedents like culture and climate to the left because these are believed to influence engagement. Further to the right are a series of attitudes, behaviors, and consequences that are theorized to be mediated by engagement. (You can find sample engagement survey item variations in this book's Appendix B.)

When you compare Figures 10-14 and 10-15, you can see that there's more than one way to operationally measure engagement.

The engagement model illustrated in Figure 10-14 measures three concepts — belonging, commitment, and motivation — and brings them together into a composite measure referred to as *engagement*. Other researchers prefer to keep concepts such as belonging, commitment and motivation as separate measures and to measure each component by itself. (See Figure 10-15.)

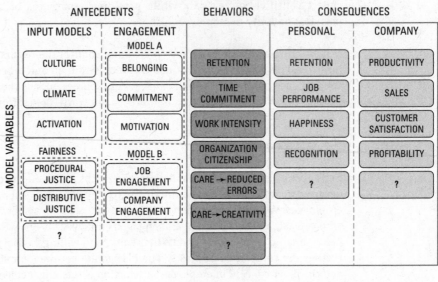

GENERAL ENGAGEMENT MODEL

ANTECEDENTS		BEHAVIORS	CONSEQUENCES	
INPUT MODELS	**ENGAGEMENT** **MODEL A**		**PERSONAL**	**COMPANY**
CULTURE	BELONGING	RETENTION	RETENTION	PRODUCTIVITY
CLIMATE	COMMITMENT	TIME COMMITMENT	JOB PERFORMANCE	SALES
ACTIVATION	MOTIVATION	WORK INTENSITY	HAPPINESS	CUSTOMER SATISFACTION
FAIRNESS	**MODEL B**	ORGANIZATION CITIZENSHIP	RECOGNITION	PROFITABILITY
PROCEDURAL JUSTICE	JOB ENGAGEMENT	CARE → REDUCED ERRORS	?	?
DISTRIBUTIVE JUSTICE	COMPANY ENGAGEMENT	CARE→CREATIVITY		
?		?		

MODEL VARIABLES (vertical label on left)

FIGURE 10-13: An engagement model.

	Strongly Disagree	Disagree	Neutral	Agree	Strongly Agree
Points	0	0	2	4	6

ENGAGEMENT (A)

MODEL VARIABLES	ITEMS	SCORING
BELONGING	I am proud to tell others that I am part of (Insert Company).	+0 to +6
	(Insert Company) has a great deal of personal meaning for me.	+0 to +6
COMMITMENT	I do not have an intention to change to another company at this time.	+0 to +6
	I would be happy to spend the rest of my career with (Insert Company).	+0 to +6
MOTIVATION	I am willing to give extra effort to help (Insert Company) meet its goals.	+0 to +6
	I feel motivated to go beyond my formal job responsibilities to get the job done.	+0 to +6
	Sum points	0 to 36
	Divide sum by 36	0 to 100
		ENGAGEMENT INDEX

FIGURE 10-14: Putting engagement model A through its paces.

Figures 10-14 and 10-15 show you that different researchers make very different choices about how they measure concepts and express them as variables. This is true of all inferential science, not just engagement. I raise this point to illustrate that an important part of the work of people analytics is deciding what method you want to use to measure a variable and testing your choices to determine whether the method of defining the measure you picked is reliable and valid. (*Valid* here means that it's measuring what you intended it to measure.)

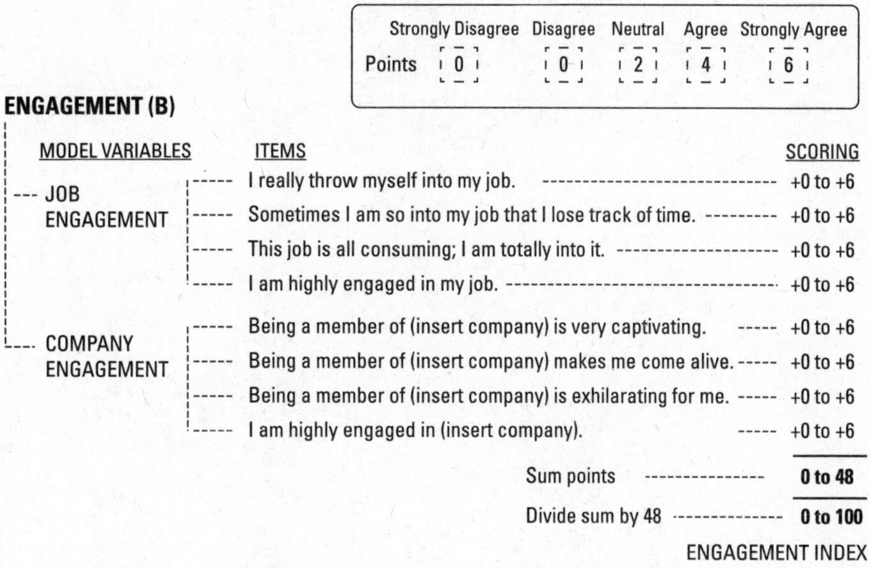

	Strongly Disagree	Disagree	Neutral	Agree	Strongly Agree
Points	0	0	2	4	6

ENGAGEMENT (B)

MODEL VARIABLES	ITEMS	SCORING
JOB ENGAGEMENT	I really throw myself into my job.	+0 to +6
	Sometimes I am so into my job that I lose track of time.	+0 to +6
	This job is all consuming; I am totally into it.	+0 to +6
	I am highly engaged in my job.	+0 to +6
COMPANY ENGAGEMENT	Being a member of (insert company) is very captivating.	+0 to +6
	Being a member of (insert company) makes me come alive.	+0 to +6
	Being a member of (insert company) is exhilarating for me.	+0 to +6
	I am highly engaged in (insert company).	+0 to +6

Sum points ------------- **0 to 48**

Divide sum by 48 ------------- **0 to 100**

ENGAGEMENT INDEX

FIGURE 10-15: Putting engagement model B through its paces.

The great thing about analytics is that you get to experiment with measures to decide for yourself what works best for your purposes. Measure everything in pieces, put them together, take something out, or put something else in. You do so until you find the combination that works best for the question you are trying to answer. After you know what works best, you can share that information with the world if you want or keep it secret if you want. You wouldn't be the first. It is all up to you!

» Measuring employee commitment

» Carefully examining the reasons why people leave

» Example exit survey

Chapter **11**

Attrition: Analyzing Employee Commitment and Attrition

Attrition refers to the number or percentage of employees who are leaving a company to work for other companies or who have decided to pursue other opportunities. *Attrition rate* is the measurement you'd use to determine the percentage of employees who have left a company in a given period. (Some might use other terms to refer to attrition rate — *termination rate* and *exit rate* come to mind — but they all mean the same thing.)

If you're convinced that, in the grand scheme of things, attrition is out of your control, you're in for a rude awakening. To create an above-average company, you have to do three things well: a) hire employees capable of high performance b) activate those employees to a level of high performance and c) keep in the fold more employees with above-average performance than those with average or low performance. This chapter is about your ability to control the last option (c).

The effort required in order to find, select, and get employees to a high level of performance can be substantial. As a result, the cost of replacing each employee, all factors considered, can exceed an entire year of employee pay. The cost of losing an above-average employee in a key position may be two to three times the person's annual pay. That fact may explain why there is no more frequently discussed topic among HR professionals as employee attrition and why employee retention (the inverse of attrition) is the most frequently cited justification for HR programs and projects. And, if you need even more proof of the importance of managing employee attrition for an enterprise, it turns out that it's the most often used HR key performance indicator (KPI) — *the* standard for measuring how successful an organization is in meeting its business objectives.

Despite the importance of controlling the employee attrition rate to both HR professionals and executives, most strategies meant to reduce attrition are based on vague theories built on anecdotal evidence rather than on measurable data. Many HR departments exert a great deal of effort in the hope of influencing their organization's attrition rate measure, only to see that it tenaciously remains the same or erratically moves up and down with little explanation. In such a world, executives keep doing what they're doing and HR keeps reporting the attrition rate as a KPI, but everyone's actions end up having little influence on the attrition rate.

Fortunately, there's a wealth of easily collectable data you can use to better understand and control employee attrition. Rather than rely on anecdotes and generalities, you can test your assumptions about attrition through analysis. Armed with that new information, the actions that are doing nothing to reduce attrition can be run out of town, making room for actions that will actually help you reduce attrition.

In this chapter, I point out common misconceptions about employee attrition, show you a better way to think about attrition, and give you the playbook for how to measure and control attrition using data analysis rather than whatever someone said around the water cooler.

Getting Beyond the Common Misconceptions about Attrition

A lack of evidence-based information causes a company's senior leaders to build retention strategies on misconceptions. The most common misconceptions about attrition can be summarized in this simple list:

>> Attrition rate is only related to what you do or don't do well as a manager or company.

>> People leave for only a single reason.

>> All employee attrition is the same.

>> All attrition should be prevented.

>> You can compare the attrition count of one group directly to another.

>> You can control employee attrition with general, one-size-fits-all efforts.

Basing retention strategies on misconceptions can be both costly and ineffective. The purpose of people analytics is to provide evidence-based recommendations by determining the statistically significant relationships between antecedents, employee behavior, and outcomes. Let me walk you through how evidence-based approaches can put to rest misconceptions about attrition.

Misconception 1

Attrition rate is only a result of what you do or don't do well as a manager or company.

Evidence-Based Perspective

- What other companies do or don't do matters as much as what you do.

- The number of job- and person-specific external opportunities that are available matters.

- The economy and job market matters.

Misconception 2

People leave for only one reason.

Evidence-Based Perspective

- The decision to leave a company is *multivariate:* There is no single cause. As with lifespan, there are many reasons that contribute to or protect against attrition. Some factors push and pull in different directions. Saying that there is a range of different things that matter is not to dismiss analysis with "stuff happens." My point is exactly the opposite of this — you can determine the precise balance of each variables' contribution to attrition using a multivariate regression model that includes all of the variables you want to test to see how much each variable proportionally contributes to attrition.

- Some of the factors that influence attrition aren't a part of the conscious decision to leave, making the face-value answer to "Why?" problematic. If you're given a single answer by an existing employee, it may or may not be the real reason, but it certainly isn't the only reason. Some variables mathematically increase the probability of employee attrition but are never a part of the employees' actual conscious awareness. If an important variable is not in their awareness, they cannot possibly mention it in an exit survey.

Misconception 3

All employee attrition is the same.

Evidence-Based Perspective

- Attrition of job types at a higher responsibility level has more impact on company performance than attrition at lower-level job types.

- Attrition of people from jobs of more strategic value — determined by the company's unique product or service value proposition — has more impact on company performance than attrition of more general job types.

- Attrition of employees with above-average performance has more impact than with employees who have average or below-average performance.

Misconception 4

All attrition should be prevented.

- Some level of attrition is good to bring in new talent with fresh energy and create opportunities for job movement within an organization.

- Most companies have pay-for-performance compensation practices and potential-based leadership succession planning programs. The intent of these programs is to decrease the likelihood of high-performing employees leaving while letting the attrition rate of lower-performing employees increase. It's antithetical to these resource-intensive practices to try to reduce all employee attrition with other, resource-intensive programs. These programs would be working against each other.

- What is more important than overall reduction in attrition is control of attrition so that there's a lower-than-average attrition in the segments where you want to retain high-performing employees and higher-than-average attrition in the segments where that attrition is acceptable or desirable.

Misconception 5

You can compare the attrition rate of one group directly to another.

- Some job types will always have higher attrition rates than other types. For example, highly interchangeable roles like cashier, customer service rep, or sales rep have higher average attrition rates than more specialized or technical roles.

- People in different tenure horizons (0–1 year, 1–3, 3–5, 5+, and so on) and people at different locations have very different annual attrition rates.

- It's unfair to compare the attrition rate of groups that have different team composition by job type, location, or tenure, because these factors influence the overall probability of attrition as much or more than controllable factors.

Misconception 6

You can control employee attrition with general, one-size fits all efforts.

- Targeted intervention is most effective.

- For one person, a well-timed promotion within the company is an effective retention tool; for another, an above-market pay offer is the only strategy that would work; and for another, it's correcting bad manager behaviors or providing necessary support at the team level — by making interventions proportional to the most likely need per segment, you can more effectively reduce attrition.

- Targeted intervention permits a greater concentration of resources to achieve better results than general solutions do.

What happens if you ask one hundred different people what they think spurs people to leave their jobs? You'll probably hear some of the most common explanations repeated over and over — pay dissatisfaction, job dissatisfaction, lack of promotion opportunities, burnout, or the ever popular "People leave managers, not companies." Certainly, it is easy to imagine how someone subjected to one of these conditions would be more likely to pursue another job opportunity.

Some recent research has also illustrated how critical workplace events or life shocks play a role in the decision to leave the job — sometimes a shock may increase a person's likelihood to exit who may not have otherwise been influenced by any of the conditions expressed by the popular opinions above prior to the shock. Examples of shocks are being passed over for an expected promotion, the announcement of a merger, a spouse being offered a job out of town, the birth of a child, or stock options vesting at a greater-than-expected value. If you were not to include the measurement of relevant shocks in your analysis, then your analysis will overemphasize some things and may miss other things that matter altogether.

REMEMBER

Though none of the many possible explanations I mention is totally and always wrong, it isn't helpful to have so many opinions. People analytics involves using data to understand the situational attrition risks that different companies, groups, and individuals experience and to help determine with more certainty what actions will reduce attrition, as opposed to relying on lists of dozens of possibilities based on generalities or anecdotes.

Measuring Employee Attrition

If you're going to analyze employee attrition, first you have to quantify it into a measurement. Right off the bat, you'll want to calculate your organization's exit rate. Read on to find out how.

Every measurement begins with a working definition and a mathematical operator. Here's how to operationally define exits, the base component of exit rate. An *exit* is someone who was an employee that is no longer an employee. To calculate the number of exits, you extract a list of all current and former employees and count the employees within a given segment with an exit date squarely within the period you're interested in.

TIP

Most human resources information system (HRIS) have a preconfigured exit list that can provide a list of all employees who have exited in a given period, along with some basic facts about the employee, like worker ID, start date, job, manager, business unit, division, location, base pay, and gender. If you do not know how to get this list, you can ask someone from IT or HRIT to help you get a list like this.

The shorthand formula for exits looks like this:

Exits Formula: Count [Segment].[Period].Exits

Say that you want to know how many statisticians exited in 2017. In words more humans are likely to understand, you count exits in the following way:

> If employee exit date is equal to or greater than January 1, 2017 and less than January 1, 2018 AND job equals ["Statistician"] then count it; if not, then don't.

You may achieve this count using an If-Then statement in Excel or any programing language:

> January 1, 2017 to January 1, 2018 represents the period. Period = [2017].

> "Statistician" is the job, which represents the segment. Segment = [Statistician].

Using the shorthand method I just mentioned, you're applying the following operation:

> Count [Statistician].[2017].Exits

In practice, you would apply this operation for all relevant segments and time periods to prepare a dataset for your graph output or visual dashboard.

You might also prepare this dataset as a base input for other, more complicated compound measures that combine two or more measures with more operators — for example, exit rate. The next section deals with that concept.

Calculating the exit rate

If you think about exits simplistically, you may take the position that a segment or time period with more exits is worse than a segment or time period with fewer exits. The problem with this position is that, because there are a different number of employees in each segment, you can't compare the number of exits to each other directly to make a meaningful comparison.

Let's compare Group A to Group B in the same period. Group A in Period 1 has 100 people. Group B in Period 1 has 50 people. If 10 people leave from both Group A and Group B in Period 1, that represents 10 percent of Group A and 20 percent of Group B. Although we're talking about the same number of exits, employees are exiting Group B at two times the rate of Group A.

You'll encounter the same problem if you're comparing Group A to itself over time. Let's say that Group A has 100 people in Period 1 and has 200 people in Period 2. If 10 people leave in Period 1 and 20 people leave in Period 2, you may assume that exits are two times larger in Period 2 — but this assumption isn't true. Exits are 10 percent of head count in both cases, even though Period 2 had more exits on an absolute basis. (The math here is simple: 10÷100 = 10%, and 20÷200 = 10%.)

In most situations, exit rate is a far more useful figure to calculate than exit count.

It's important to understand what exits mean in some relative context so that you can compare different segment sizes to each other. For this reason, you report segment exits as a percentage of segment average head count — this is the best way to calculate exit rate. To calculate the exit rate, you divide the number of segment exits within a given segment within a given period by the average head count of the same segment for the same period:

Exit-Rate Formula: Count [Segment].[Period].Exits ÷ [Segment].[Period].Average-Headcount

Figure 11-1 illustrates an exit rate example.

Statistician Exit Rate = (62/526.38) × 100 = 11.8%
Exits as a percentage of average headcount during the reporting period.

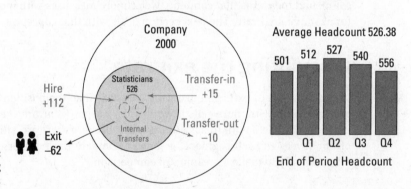

FIGURE 11-1: Calculating exit rate.

For this calculation, you need to count the total number of exits from a segment for the period of analysis. Then you divide the exits by the average number of employees in that segment.

Calculating the annualized exit rate

If you know the number of exits for part of a year, you can extrapolate this information for the rest of the year — the *annualized* exit rate, in other words — using the following formula:

Annualized Exit Rate = ({YTD Exit Rate} × (12 ÷ #-of-Months))

Annualization satisfies the basic problem that you cannot compare a partial year to a full year and therefore it's difficult to make sense of partial year data without putting it on a more commonly understood annual basis. Annualization allows you to view the partial year, if what occurred in the months that elapsed happened over 12 months.

REMEMBER

Annualization is a basic forecast. Annualizing based on a portion of the year may miss regular seasonal variations that may skew the results. Annualization will also miss any acceleration or deacceleration that may be occurring. Annualization isn't intended to provide a perfect forecast — it can help you compare the data you have to historical annual data or other benchmark data expressed on an annual basis. There are other, more rigorous methods for forecasting and prediction if that is your intent.

Refining exit rate by type classification

Not all exits are the same. When an employee's exit is recorded in a HRIS, the administrator will be asked to input some classifications of the exit. I call these *exit types*. More than one classification type framework is possible, and these can be used alone or used together for various ends. The classification type framework will vary by company and the desired level of analytical precision.

In this list, I describe some of the most commonly used exit classification types:

>> **Voluntary:** An exit is *voluntary* if the employee voluntarily exits the company of their own choice and free will.

>> **Involuntary:** An exit is *involuntary* if the employee exits the company and it isn't their choice — it's the company's decision. Involuntary may be as a result of the employee being fired or being laid off in restructuring or reduction in force. All exits are either voluntary or involuntary.

REMEMBER

If you want to understand changes in head count for the purpose of accounting or projection, you would include in your exit rate all exits. If you want to understand whether employees are "voting with their feet," you need to look specifically at exits coded as voluntary, excluding all involuntary exits, which aren't the employee's choice. Combining voluntary and involuntary confounds the conclusion.

» **Avoidable Voluntary:** Admittedly, all exits are either voluntary or involuntary, but it's possible to break down the voluntary exits a bit further. You can call an exit an *Avoidable* Voluntary if the employee voluntarily exits the company of their own choice and free will and there was something the company could have done to prevent the employee from exiting.

» **Unavoidable Voluntary:** An exit is *unavoidable* if the employee exits the company and it was completely unrelated to anything the company can control. For example, if an employee exits the company because a spouse is taking a job in another city and your employee is moving with them, this is an unavoidable exit. Other unavoidable reasons include exits to go to school, care for a sick relative, or raise a child, for example.

To make this Avoidable/Unavoidable distinction, you need some interaction with the employee regarding his reason of exit at the time he submits his resignation. For purposes of the avoidable or unavoidable classification, you don't necessarily need all the details, but you do need to know whether the person is leaving for some reason that is obviously completely outside the influence of the company.

» **Nonregretted Voluntary:** An exit is *nonregretted* if the employee voluntarily exits the company and at the time of exit the employee has a below-average performance rating. You might not regret losing this person because you could replace them with someone that will likely have better performance than the person leaving – meaning you are getting a performance upgrade out of this transaction. (If the employee has no performance rating at the time of exit, it's probably best to default to regretted.)

» **Regretted Voluntary:** Another way to break down voluntary exits basically involves your attitude to the exit. An exit is *regretted* if the employee voluntarily exits the company and at the time of exit has an average or above-average performance rating.

The Regretted/Nonregretted distinction isn't intended to be rooted in cruelty. The distinction is made to formulate a Voluntary Exit KPI that takes into consideration that there is a fitting process. What is best for the company and employees is that the company retains a high percentage of the employees who perform best in its environment over time and allows or even prompts other employees to go to environments where they can achieve better performance. The company wants to have a lower regretted exit rate than nonregretted so that it knows it's getting better, not worse, over time. Without the distinction, there's no way of knowing which way the company is heading.

OKAY, BUT WHAT REALLY IS UNAVOIDABLE?

The person charged with making the Avoidable/Unavoidable type classification must have some information about the exit and must make a judgment call on which type to pick. Because other people providing the classification may not fully understand your definition or purposes for making this type of decision, I suggest that you apply specific criteria to determine the Unavoidable classification. The simplified rule framework I use is this:

> Is the person leaving for another job or to do something else? (Job, No Job). If No Job, then the exit is Unavoidable. If Job, then continue.
>
> If Job, is the person moving? (Moving, Not Moving)
>
> If Moving, which scenario applies better:
>
> > A.) The person is moving to a new city for reasons other than the job.
> >
> > B.) The person is moving to a new city because she took a new job.
>
> If it's A, then it's unavoidable. If it's B, then it's avoidable.

Avoidable or unavoidable seems like an arcane detail; however, it's relevant if you plan to use Voluntary-Exit-Rate as a key performance indicator (KPI) or if you plan to design a predictive model. For example, if I were to compare two managers with ten employees and each had two people exit, they would both have a 20% voluntary exit rate, but one of them had two unavoidable exits and the other had two avoidable exits, which have two very different meanings. One manager has a 20% voluntary avoidable exit rate and the other has a 0% voluntary avoidable exit rate. The distinction may seem trivial to you, but it wouldn't be trivial to the manager, particularly if you assess the managers performance on the basis of employee exits. The avoidable and unavoidable distinction can also improve the accuracy of predictive models. It works better if you design one model to predict avoidable voluntary exits and another model to predict unavoidable voluntary exits and then put the two models back together to a single overall exit model than it is to smash all types of exits together from the start.

In either of these scenarios, you want to model unavoidable exits separately. The cleanest measure of "people who vote with their feet" is Avoidable-Voluntary-Exit-Rate. This careful distinction will improve your KPIs and reduce error in your predictive models.

Calculating exit rate by any exit type

In practice, when calculating by any exit type or even a combination of exit types, you calculate exit rate the same way, while filtering for the type you want to report. Use the following formula to calculate [Exit-Type]-Exit-Rate:

[Period].[Segment].[Exit-Type].Exits ÷ [Period].[Segment].Average-Headcount × 100

If you work with the example shown in Figure 11-1 — the statistician exit rate — you would use the following numbers:

[2017].[Statistician].[Voluntary].Exits ÷
[2017].[Statistician].Average-Headcount × 100

In this example, if only 35 of the 62 Statistician 2017 exits are Exit Type = Voluntary, then the Statistician 2017 Voluntary Exit-Rate is

$35 \div 526.38 = 0.0665 \times 100 =$ **6.7%**

The 6.7% figure means that, in 2017, 6.7 percent of the statisticians left the company for voluntary reasons.

Segmenting for Insight

Segmentation is the practice of categorizing employees into different groups based on certain common characteristics. This process takes on great significance when it comes to the quality of your people analytics. If you have too many segments, you end up with thousands of ways of looking at the same metric. That, of course, leads to long reports, dashboards that require a lot of user filtration, and/or alert-fatigue. If you have too few segments, you can fail to see any meaningful insight.

Rightly segmenting the dataset is what can make the difference between the success and failure of your people analytics to engage your audience and demonstrate useful insight. You can segment employee exit rate into different types of business units, job families, jobs, job tenures, locations, demographic segments, behavioral segments, attitudinal segments, or any other meaningful segment.

Figure 11-2 illustrates some of the common categories of segmentation in people analytics.

EMPLOYEE SEGMENTATION

FINANCIAL STRUCTURE	GEOGRAPHY STRUCTURE	LEADERSHIP STRUCTURE	JOB STRUCTURE	DEMOGRAPHIC STRUCTURE	PSYCHOGRAPHIC STRUCTURE	OTHER
Division	REGION	VICE PRESIDENT	JOB FUNCTION	GENERATION COHORT	ATTITUDES	TENURE
DEPARTMENT	COUNTRY	SR. DIRECTOR	JOB FAMILY	GENDER	OPINIONS	PERFORMANCE
ORGANIZATION	CITY	DIRECTOR	JOB LEVEL	ETHNICITY	PERSONALITY	PAY
COST CENTER	BUILDING	MANAGER	GRADE	DISABILITY	KNOWLEDGE	COMPENSATION MARKET RATIO
			JOB TYPE	SIMILARITY TO MANAGER	SKILLS	COMMUTE DISTANCE
			JOB		ABILITIES	

FIGURE 11-2: Segmentation categories.

REMEMBER

Without segmentation, the target group is lost in the population. Rather than focus on the entire company at once, segmentation allows you to break down the company to see what's going on in specific niches. But segmentation brings with it other advantages. Here are the most significant ones:

>> **Tailor-made dashboards:** Through segmentation, you get to personalize your reporting to different audiences instead of having a generic, watered-down dashboard for everyone. And when you focus on specific groups, traits, and characteristics, you're more likely able to bring to the foreground what executives should focus on, what matters, and what to do about it.

>> **Identifying evidence-based learning opportunities:** An analyst can study the exit rate by segment and then compare it to the company average or forecast benchmarks to understand how unusual (either high or low) the segment is. Segments with big statistical differences from average (either high or low) represent excellent research opportunities!

>> **More effective retention efforts:** Simply put, segmentation helps you better understand your employees' needs so that you can do a better job of solving problems, because segmentation refrains from treating all people as the same.

>> **Optimum use of productive resources:** Because you aren't wasting resources trying to influence the behavior of everyone, segmentation helps to reduce costs *and* increase the effectiveness of your resources. It allows you to concentrate your resources, money, time, and effort on the segments and problems that have the most value. Rather than apply watered-down efforts across all people, you can apply more concentrated resources to a targeted need.

So, what kinds of things might you discover by segmenting employee voluntary exit rate? With segmentation, you might learn that women and men are equally likely to exit — which would call for one type of retention strategy — or you might learn that women are more likely than men to exit or vice versa (which would call for very different strategies). If there are differences, you may decide to look further to determine what is the cause of those differences.

With segmentation, you might learn that on average employees have a 10 percent voluntary exit rate in their first year, 5 percent in their second year, 20 percent in their third year, and 5 percent each subsequent year. With this information, you may decide that by the end of the second year, someone should communicate with all employees about their next career opportunity at the company.

With segmentation you might learn that sales reps are, on average, twice as likely as statisticians to voluntarily exit — 20 percent versus 10 percent, regardless of manager — and that this has remained true over time regardless of the overall company exit rate. With that information, you might not want to compare the exit rate of managers in charge of sales reps with managers of statisticians.

With clever segmentation, you might learn that people who agree with the statement, "I know my next career move at the company" are one-third less likely to exit in the next 12 months as someone who disagrees with the statement.

With segmentation, you might learn that there's no major difference in exit rate between people in a similar job who are being paid widely different amounts of money.

Measuring Retention Rate

Employee retention rate is the opposite of exit rate — the other side of the coin, in other words. The *retention rate* is the percentage of employees who start a period and then make it to the end. To truly understand, predict, and control employee attrition, you have to have a theory of not only why people are leaving but also why people are staying. One thing you can be sure of is that if you can increase employee retention, you will reduce employee attrition. Though retention and attrition are quite similar, in some contexts, retention rate is a better metric than exit rate.

As with most metrics, there's more than one method to calculate retention rate. The easiest method to grasp is built using several other metrics that you already know how to calculate:

[Segment].[Period].{Headcount-SOP} = the count of employees in a defined segment on the first day of a defined period

[Segment].[Period].{Headcount-EOP} = the count of employees in a defined segment on the last day of a defined period

[Segment].[Period].{Hires} = the count of employees hired in the segment in the period

(Generally speaking it's best to exclude transfers in and out of from the entire analysis, because these could add unnecessary complexity to the measure.)

The shorthand Retention Rate formula looks like this:

(([Segment].[Period].{Headcount-EOP} - ([Segment].[Period].{Hires}) ÷ [Segment].[Period].{Headcount-SOP}) × 100.

To calculate the segment retention rate, you first count the number of people with a defined segment classification at the end of a defined period. Then you count and subtract the number of new hires with a defined segment classification in the defined period and then divide the result by the number of employees classified with the defined segment at the start of the defined period. Finally, you multiply that result by 100 to get the segment retention rate.

Measuring Commitment

Fortunately, you don't have to wait until people actually exit the company if you want to find out where you stand and in what segments you can work to improve employee commitment to reduce attrition.

Commitment is a measure of psychological attachment to the company. Broadly speaking, employees who are committed feel a connection to the company, feel that they fit in, and feel that they share the goals of the company. As a result, employees who are committed are more loyal to a company and less likely to leave it. In short, commitment is a measurement of the bond between an individual and a company.

Organizational scientists have developed many nuanced definitions of commitment, as well as numerous survey scale options to measure it. The scientists have also demonstrated that these survey-based measures of commitment predict actual work behaviors such as attrition, organizational citizenship behavior, and job performance.

In this section are ten questions selected to help you calculate a composite index of commitment, which you should offer as statements with a Likert agreement scale. (For more on the Likert scale, check out Chapter 12.) These questions can be used together, in a smaller batch, or as independent items. That said, indexes that consist of a larger number of items tend to perform better than single items — the composite index covers a broader range of issues and is a more reliable predictor of future behavior.

First, here's the scale you should be using:

Likert agreement scale:

(1) Strongly Disagree

(2) Disagree

(3) Neither Agree nor Disagree

(4) Agree

(5) Strongly Agree

And here are the statements:

For each statement, respondents indicate how much they agree with the statement by choosing a value from the Likert scale, just described:

- I am very happy being a member of *<Company>*.

- *<Company>* has a mission that I believe in and am committed to.

- *<Company>* has a great deal of personal meaning for me.

- I would be very happy to spend the rest of my career with *<Company>*.

- I enjoy discussing *<Company>* with people outside it.

- I feel like I'm "part of the family" at *<Company>*.

- I feel a strong sense of belonging to *<Company>*.

- It would be very hard for me to leave *<Company>* right now, even if I wanted to.

- I feel that I owe this organization quite a bit because of what it has done for me.

- *<Company>* deserves my loyalty because of its treatment toward me.

Commitment Index scoring

Each item can either be reported independently by each Likert selection choice or combined into an indexed scale. For example, if you used all ten items, you can define the Commitment Index as the cumulative response total over the ten items, where 1 point is assigned for Strongly Disagree, 2 points for Disagree, 3 points for Neither Agree nor Disagree, 4 points for Agree, and 5 points for Strongly Agree. Applying this method, those who take the survey can achieve a possible commitment score between 10 and 50 points.

Commitment types

You may take the Commitment Index one step further and categorize all survey responses as one of three commitment types:

>> **High:** Scored 40 to 50

>> **Uncertain:** Scored 30 to 39

>> **Low:** Scored less than 30

Calculating intent to stay

Though the method is less robust than the 10-Item Commitment Index, you can also simply ask employees whether they intend to stay. This item also uses a Likert agreement scale.

> If I have my own way, I will be working for this organization one year from now.

I have identified a strong correlation between the response on this Intent to Stay item and an exit over the next 12 months. Admittedly, the intent to stay is not a perfect individual predictor, but it is a great predictor of exits by segment (for example, by business unit). By this I mean that the lower the average response to this item in a business unit, the more exits you see in that unit. It provides a signal indicating where you should go to work.

WARNING

The Intent to Stay item does have a few built-in flaws. Most employees have no idea what will happen in the next year — they may have no plans at the moment to leave, but this may change later. For those who plan to leave, you're getting a fairly accurate predictor of their future behavior if presented with an opportunity; however, if no desirable opportunity presents itself, such individuals are still employed at the end of the period you're reviewing.

These flaws tell you as much about how to analyze the problem as the accurate predictions. We now know that the problem is, at minimum, one part intention and one part external opportunity. What you need to understand is both what the employee wants and how likely a recruiter is to call them. This is an illustration of how error cases can help you refine your understanding of the problem and how you collect and model your data in the future.

CALCULATING THE BENEFITS OF MEASURING COMMITMENT AND INTENT TO STAY

I want to stress that the Commitment Index and the Intent to Stay item are both helpful when it comes to comparing segments with each other in order to identify which segments are more likely to experience high attrition in the future, before it happens. Both the Commitment Index and the Intent to Stay item can be trended over time to see whether the attrition risk is increasing or decreasing.

Though not all high commitment employees will be retained and not all low-commitment types will exit, if you hold on to the survey data and one year later report exit rate segmented by the recorded commitment type you recorded one year before, you will probably find that low-commitment employees are at least two to three times more likely to exit than employees on average, and that high-commitment employees are two to three times less likely to exit. If your average exit rate is 10 percent, this could mean that low-commitment employees could have an exit rate of 30 percent or more, though high-commitment employees could have an exit rate of 5 percent or less. I encourage you to collect commitment data on surveys and try this analysis yourself. In any case, my research and the research of many other professionals have validated the fact that measures like Commitment Index and Intent to Stay is useful in predicting employee exit. It may not be the only factor predicting the likelihood to leave, but it is still useful.

Finally, if you have included the Commitment Index and the Intent to Stay item in a larger annual survey requesting opinions about a range of other topics (managers, pay, leaders, company prospects, and so on) you can correlate the responses to all topics with a commitment to see which items best explain commitment. What you're looking for are the items where you see the greatest difference between high-commitment and low-commitment employees. Though correlation doesn't imply causation, those items that correlate with the Commitment Index and the Intent to Stay item can help you identify the key drivers of employee exit and retention. (To find out more about how to conduct key driver analysis, see Chapter 14 in this book.)

TIP

You may question whether employees will respond honestly to any direct questions you pose. The degree to which employees will provide you with accurate information on employee surveys is influenced by the decisions you make. The most important decision here is to have your survey professionally administered by a third party who can help you work with the sensitive information that employees provide confidentially and can assure your employees that such confidentiality will be strictly enforced.

Understanding Why People Leave

The Streetlight effect (also known as the Drunkard's Search principle) is a type of observational bias that occurs whenever people search for something only where it's easiest to look. Both names refer to a well-known joke circulated among data professionals. The story goes like this:

> A policeman sees a drunk man searching for something under a streetlight and asks what the drunk has lost. He says he lost his keys and they both look under the streetlight together. After a few minutes the policeman asks the man if he is sure that he lost them here, and the drunk replies no — he lost them in the park. The policeman asks why he is searching here, and the drunk replies, "This is where the light is."

The drunkard looking under the light is a metaphor for how employee attrition is typically analyzed by new analysts. Often analysts will be asked to analyze employee attrition to tell their superiors whether the data shows that anything is broken, what is causing it, and what to do about it. Unfortunately, unless careful forethought was put into collecting the relevant data beforehand, this is much like the drunk hopelessly looking for the keys just under the place where there is light.

In the next section, I share the ways that things go wrong with exit surveys, talk about what information you need to collect in an exit survey, and then provide an example of what a good exit survey would look like.

Creating a better exit survey

An exit survey represents the last opportunity you have to ask questions before the employee moves on. Exit surveys can help you classify exits, identify talent competitor threats, understand how talent competitors are winning your people, and learn what you can do better to keep people. If you're serious about wanting to gain control over attrition, you need to do exit surveys. Unfortunately, a lot of bad exit surveys are out there, and not many companies are getting much use from them. In this section, I explain what can go wrong and then provide you with an example of a more effective exit survey instrument. Table 11-1 spells out the problems posed by many exit surveys.

TABLE 11-1 **Dealing with the Problems of Exit Surveys**

Problem	Detail
Problem 1: You have a low response rate.	Most companies achieve less than a 30 percent response rate on their exit surveys. In this scenario, the largest categorial reason (70 percent) that employees leave should be reported as "Unknown."
	You suffer from poor execution: The survey isn't requested in time before the employee leaves and there isn't appropriate follow-up.
	The survey is clearly run by Amateur Hour. The lack of a professional third-party administration for execution and confidentiality telegraphs a disqualifying lack of seriousness.
Problem 2: Your company lacks confidentiality.	A lack of professional third-party administration to provide assurance of confidentiality is a deal-breaker.
	Employees have little to gain by digging deep to provide their best answers. They may think, "Why burn bridges?" and "I had an answer, but it's water under the bridge for me, so it's not worth the effort."
	If you have a third-party agent collect the data for you and provide assurances that they will only share data back with the company in aggregate, then people will feel safer to speak their mind.
Problem 3: Poor design: You have errors in question logic that bias responses.	Many exit surveys aren't designed by survey professionals, and so they have errors in logic that bias response and confound interpretation. A common example is asking "Why did you leave?" — and then providing a list of options to choose from, where several of the options on this list are duplicate or overlapping and other important options are omitted. Furthermore, the question implies that there's only one reason when in fact there may be several. Also, sometimes the biggest influencers of behavior are actually unknown or inaccessible cognitively.
Problem 4: Poor design: You aren't asking the questions necessary to get the most important information you need at the time of exit.	More important than the details of the complex "Why are you leaving?" questions are other questions that are often missed.
	For example, "Where are you going?," "When did you decide to leave?" and "Did any critical incidents influence your decision?" would be equally important questions to ask.
	What you don't ask is often the larger design mistake because it is irreparable.
Problem 5: You've muddied the waters by a) including together data from regretted and nonregretted exits.	You have employees that you want to attract and employees whose exit you wouldn't mind at all. If you don't distinguish between the two, the data you collect will pull you in either no direction or the wrong direction. For an ill-fit or otherwise low-performing employee (nonregretted exits), you *want* the company experience, pay, or manager relationship to be uncomfortable. If you lump these together with regretted exits, then you will have made the reasons regretted exits leave blurry, particularly if you have more nonregretted exits than regretted.
	If you collect data for both regretted and nonregretted exits it is OK, but you should use a separate survey or designator so you can separate these very different exit types at the time you report the data.

TABLE 11-1 *(continued)*

Problem	Detail
Problem 6: You have errors in analysis and interpretation.	A common mistake is interpreting the reason for exit from only exit survey data, without a point of reference. There is a severe logical flaw if you review exit data without a point of reference and use it to interpret the reason why people are exiting. A better analysis is to compare the response to the same survey questions between stayers and leavers.

Example exit survey

Enough of the problems! On to a more effective exit survey instrument. The exit survey example below was carefully constructed, taking into consideration the problems described in the table above. The design of the example exit survey cannot solve some of the problems described in the table — for example, it cannot solve Problem 6. The design of the example exit survey included below is intended to take advantage of the opportunity you have to collect some data at the time employees leave while attempting to steer clear of the most obvious logical flaws noted above. In any case, take the information you obtain from any exit survey with a grain of salt. It is a single data point from a broader range of data you have the opportunity to collect and analyze to validate a hypothesis. The logic of your analysis is just as important (or more important) than the calculation. If you begin with a good model, use all of opportunities you have to collect data together and be careful with the logic of your analysis, you will arrive at a better answer then if you view each data source independently.

REMEMBER

As always, replace *<Company>* with your company's name.

Here's the kind of survey designed to get you the information you need:

Sample Exit Survey

After you leave *<Company>*, will you be working for another employer? *(Yes, No)*

If no, will you be *(select one)*:

- **Personal:** Caring for children or significant others
- **Personal:** Going to school
- **Personal:** Pursuing nonpaid interests
- **Personal:** Other

If yes, then . . .

- Is your new job in the same industry? *(Yes, No)*
- What is the name of your new employer?

For your new employer, do you expect to gain or lose in the following areas?

Scale: *[1. Lose a lot. 2. Lose a little. 3. Neither lose nor gain. 4. Gain a little. 5. Gain a lot.]*

- Overall company quality
- Leadership team quality
- Manager quality
- Peer quality
- Work quality
- Learning and development opportunity
- Current job level
- Long-term career opportunity
- Expected 1-year value of total compensation package (base, bonus, stock)
- Expected 3- to 5-year value of total compensation package (base, bonus, stock)
- Benefits (health, retirement, and so on)
- Perks (food, onsite services, and fitness, for example)

On balance, how would you characterize your decision to leave *<Company>* *(select one)*?

- Mostly for work-related reasons within *<Company>*'s ability to address.
- Mostly for personal reasons outside of *<Company>*'s ability to address.

If it applies, please describe a moment when you have felt genuine happiness working at *<Company>*.

If it applies, please describe anything that prevented you from being as successful as you would have liked to have been at *<Company>*.

Did any recent actions or events affect your decision to leave *<Company>*? *(Choose all that apply)*

- **Work related:** Action/inaction by your manager
- **Work related:** Action/inaction by the leadership team

- **Work related:** Action/inaction by peers in your work group
- **Work related:** Action/inaction by peers not in your work group
- **Personal:** Personal health, health of others, or birth of child
- **Personal:** Career opportunity for significant other is making you move
- **Personal:** You or a significant other reached retirement eligibility age
- **Work related:** Other
- **Personal:** Other

Please tell us about the events leading up to your decision to leave <Company>.

Is there anything <Company> could have done differently to keep you longer? (Yes, No)

If yes, please tell us what <Company> could have done differently to keep you longer?

Is there anything <Company> can do now or in the future to get you back? (Yes, No)

If yes, what can <Company> do to get you back?

4

Improving Your Game Plan with Science and Statistics

Chapter 12

Measuring Your Fuzzy Ideas with Surveys

When you come right down to it, a *survey* is just a question, or group of questions, designed to make things that are hidden inside the human mind knowable as data. Survey research, therefore, provides access to attitudes, beliefs, values, opinions, preferences, and other cognitive descriptors that, without the help of survey tools, remain anecdotal or entirely indescribable and therefore not useful to math, science, or people analytics. In other words, surveys help you convert nebulous concepts into hard numbers so that you can analyze them. Other things might be going on, but the main benefit from surveys is that they allow you to relate fuzzy concepts to more concrete and observable things, like individual and group behaviors and outcomes. To this end, surveys have been a fundamental tool in fields like psychology, sociology and political science for hundreds of years — and in newer fields, like marketing, for decades. It should come as no surprise, then, that surveys are important to people analytics, too.

Employee surveys and related feedback instruments, when managed well, are great tools to diagnose what employees think — *and* they can help you determine the relationship among these views and important outcomes at scale. Extending from these observations, it's possible to obtain the nuanced details you need in order to take the right actions to influence collective behavior and to predict future outcomes. A good survey can uncover great insights about things going on inside folks' minds — insights that have the potential to guide meaningful actions that drive collective success outside their minds. When surveys are designed and executed poorly, though, the impact can range from producing survey fatigue to exactly the opposite of what you're looking to achieve — eroding employee trust and commitment.

Discovering the Wisdom of Crowds through Surveys

James Surowiecki's *The Wisdom of Crowds: Why the Many Are Smarter Than the Few and How Collective Wisdom Shapes Business, Economies, Societies and Nations*, as the title implies, is all about how the aggregation of information in groups can result in decisions that are better than decisions made by any single member of the group.

The premise of the wisdom of crowds is that, under the right conditions, groups can be remarkably intelligent — that is to say that the estimate of the whole can often be smarter than the smartest person within them. The simplest example of this is asking a group of people to do something like guess how many jelly beans are in a jar.

So, if I had a jar of jelly beans and asked a bunch of people how many jelly beans were in that jar, the collective guess represented by the average would be remarkably good — accurate to between 3 percent to 5 percent of the actual number of beans in the jar, as a matter of fact. Moreover, the average of the guesses would likely be better than 95 percent of all individual guesses. One or two people may appear to be brilliant jelly bean guessers for a time, but for the most part the group's guess would be better than just about all individual guesses, particularly over repeated tries.

Though counting jelly beans doesn't sound practical, what is fascinating is that you can see this phenomenon at work in more complicated and more useful situations. For example, if you look at the odds placed on horses at a racetrack, they predict almost perfectly how likely a horse is to win. In a sense, the group of bettors at a racetrack is forecasting the future.

Think about something like Google, which relies on the collective intelligence of the web to seek out those sites that have the most valuable information. Google can do a good job of this because, collectively, the individualized efforts of this disorganized thing we call the World Wide Web, when understood through mathematics, can be incredibly useful when it comes to finding order in all the chaos.

Wisdom-of-crowds research routinely attributes the superiority of crowd averages over individual judgments to the elimination of individual noise, an explanation that assumes independence of the individual judgments from each other. In other words, for the wisdom of crowds to work, you have to be able to capture and combine individual predictions while avoiding group discussion that creates groupthink. The crowd also tends to make better decisions when it's made up of diverse opinions and ideologies and when predictions are captured in a way that can be combined and evaluated mathematically. That sounds a whole lot like a survey to me.

The wisdom-of-crowds concept suggests that even subjective flawed information can have great predictive value if the chaotic thoughts of people can be organized in a way that they can be analyzed together. Pay attention carefully — what I propose doing is working to harness more successfully the wisdom of crowds for your company using the careful application of survey design and implementation.

O, the Things We Can Measure Together

You may think of a survey as a single-use, company satisfaction poll; however, survey data can be used in many more ways than this.

At a high level, surveys can be used to either quantify what was previously a qualitative idea, identify that idea's frequency in a population, compare a part of a population to the whole, compare one population to another, or look for changes over time. After a qualitative idea has been quantified as a survey measurement, these measurements can then be mathematically correlated with each other and with other outcomes. Though the subjective opinion may be true or false, accurate or inaccurate, precise or imprecise, it's true to itself and as data it is inarguably a new data point. The degree to which the new data point is useful in analysis for explaining or in predicting phenomenon will have to stand on its own two feet. The proof is in the pudding.

REMEMBER

The range of possibilities for what concepts you can describe using a survey, how you use the data the survey produces, and why you use the data the survey produces are nearly endless. And, when it comes to all the varied ways you can apply surveys to learn about people, the possibilities there are endless as well. That said, I'll highlight some key survey types and uses as a way to fire up your imagination for the work ahead of you.

Surveying the many types of survey measures

Employee surveys can be designed to capture many different types or categories of information stemming from or influenced by psychology. In the following list, I describe nine categories and provide an example of what a survey item would look like using a Likert agreement rating scale design:

>> **Awareness:** An awareness is a knowledge or perception of a situation or fact. For example:

- I have a clear understanding of the priorities of <Company> this quarter.
- I have a clear understanding of what others expect of me in this job over the next quarter.

>> **Attitudes:** An attitude is a psychological tendency or predisposition that is expressed by evaluating a particular object with some degree of favor or disfavor. It could be about a person, a group of people, an idea, or a physical object. Attitude is formed by a complex interaction of cognitive factors, like ideas, values, beliefs, and perception of prior experiences. The attitude can characterize the individual and can influence the individual's thought and action, and the results in turn can either change or reinforce the existing attitude. For example:

- I am inspired by the people I work with at <Company>.
- I feel motivated to go beyond my formal job responsibilities to get the job done.

>> **Beliefs:** Beliefs are ideas about the world — subjective certainty that an object has a particular attribute or that an action will lead to a particular outcome. Beliefs can be tenaciously resistant to change, even in the face of strong evidence to the contrary. For example:

- Overall, I think I can meet my career goals at <Company>.
- I have the opportunity to do what I do best in my work at <Company>.

>> **Intentions:** An intent is something a person is resolved or determined to do. For example:

- I intend to be working at <Company> one year from now.
- If I have my own way, I will be working for <Company> three years from now.

>> **Behaviors:** Behaviors are the ways in which a person acts or conducts herself, especially toward others. For example:

- My manager gives me actionable feedback on a regular basis.

- My manager has had a meaningful discussion with me about my career development in the past six months.

>> **Values:** Values are ideals, guiding principles, or overarching goals that people strive to obtain. For example:

- The values and objectives of *<Company>* are consistent with my personal values and objectives.

- I find personal meaning in the work I do at *<Company>*.

>> **Sentiments:** In its purest sense, a sentiment is a feeling or an emotion. (Some definitions of *sentiment* overlap with *opinion* or *attitude*.) For example:

- I am proud to tell others I work for *<Company>*.

- I can recall a moment in the past three months when I felt genuine happiness at work.

>> **Opinions:** An opinion is a subjective view or judgment formed about something, not necessarily based on fact or knowledge. A person's opinion is kind of like an image — the picture the person carries in his mind of the object, in other words. A picture may be blurred or sharp. It may be a close-up, or it may be a panorama. It may be accurate, or it may be distorted. It may be complete, or it may be just a portion. Each person tends to see things a little differently from others. When people lack information — and we all do — we tend to fill in a picture for ourselves. For example:

- *<Company>* seems like it's in a position to succeed over the next 3 to 5 years.

- I have the resources and tools I need to be successful.

>> **Preferences:** A greater liking for one alternative over another or others. Though there are exceptions, you'd generally measure preferences by asking a series of contrasting trade-off questions and then inferring from the responses you get to the whole set how employees rank-order each option. Here are a few simple item examples (you would have a lot more):

- I prefer that *<Company>* put more future investment in the 401k *<Company>* match over increasing the *<Company>* contribution to health-care premiums.

- I prefer that *<Company>* put more future investment in employee technical learning-and-development programs over the big annual *<Company>* event.

Though these simple examples are enlightening, it doesn't get you very far. You have to decide what you're trying to learn, what items you want to use to learn it and why — and then you have to put it all together. The next several sections show you how.

Looking at survey instruments

Aside from the range of categories of psychological or social information that can be obtained from a survey, you have a number of people-related focus areas you can choose from when it comes to designing a survey. It's a self-limiting trap to think of that annual employee survey and assume that this is the only type of survey instrument you have to collect data about employees. If you're a skier, this would be like tying one leg behind your back and then setting out to ski down the highest and most difficult route down the mountain.

Here are some of the many types of surveys you can use to measure the employee journey and people operations — and the employee experience.

I have provided sample questions for all of these in Appendix B.

Employee journey: Time-context deep dives

- Pre-recruiting market research
- Pre-onsite-interview candidate survey
- Post-onsite-interview candidate survey
- Post-hire "reverse exit" survey
- 14-day onboard survey
- 90-day onboard survey
- Annual check-up
- Quarterly pulse check-in
- Exit survey

People operations feedback: Subject-focused deep dives

- Recruiter feedback
- Interview team feedback
- Talent acquisition process feedback
- Company career page feedback

- New hire orientation feedback

- First day feedback

- Manager feedback

- Onboarding process feedback

- Company employee intranet portal feedback

- Career advancement process feedback

- Learning and development feedback

- Talent management process feedback

- Diversity facilitation feedback

- Facilities feedback

Getting Started with Survey Research

In the last decade, there has been an explosion of new feedback tools powered by new technology and services partners. Nowadays, it's virtually impossible *not* to give and get feedback. There are surveys, polls, reviews, and open channels galore, and the workplace is no different. Inside companies, inexpensive online tools like Survey Monkey make it possible for anyone in your company to ask questions of anybody else in the company at any time, and, unfortunately, all too frequently they do.

Aside from increasing access to structured survey tools, members of today's workforce aren't shy when it comes to the many other outlets for unstructured feedback available for use. They contribute to anonymous employer-rating web-sites like Glassdoor or industry blogs like ValleyWag (although this specific one is now defunct). Twitter, LinkedIn, and Facebook are all outlets through which people's real opinions about working for your company go bump in the night. Even tools designed without feedback in mind at all — your run-of-the-mill collaboration-and-productivity tools — can become yet another place for "always on" feedback from individual to individual or from individual to company — grist for the analytical mill.

That makes for exciting times in this industry and for people analytics every-where, but *more* does not always equal *better*. Feedback without structure is noise, and noise with no purpose is the worst form of noise. Though a gentle white noise may at times be accepted to drown out the outside world so that you can lull yourself to sleep, there's nothing like an unpleasant shrill tone to evoke a swift search and removal of the offending speaker.

All this is not to dismiss the increasing predominance and interest in unstructured feedback devices. However, before you go chasing dragons disguised as windmills, you might consider learning the fundamentals first. That's what this chapter provides. Although options for feedback are abundant and diverse, the key principles of how you determine good from bad, useful from useless, and music from noise is about the same. Learn the fundamentals; then innovate.

Designing Surveys

Defining and communicating the purpose of a survey and its learning objectives are critical first steps of a successful survey strategy. Start with defining the desired objective and specifying how the information needed for that objective will be used when acquired. If you don't have a clear picture of these elements from the get-go, your survey effort will drift aimlessly — or even turn into a total waste of everyone's time. All design begins with defining what you're trying to change and why. When that is determined, it's simply a process of working backward and defining assumptions carefully, which you either accept, reject, or modify with the evidence you collect.

The whole of people analytics — all data science, for that matter — boils down to the following sequence of meta-research activity that you (or your hired-gun analyst) is responsible for facilitating. As you can see, you can sum up the process as your attempt to find the right answers to the following questions:

>> What do you want to change?

>> Can you measure this thing you want to change? How?

>> What other things influence this thing? How can we measure those things as well?

>> Upon measuring the outcome that concerns you and the things you think may matter, can you relate them and infer a direction for, and the strength of, this relationship?

>> Can you predict one measure from another measure?

>> Can you infer a causal relationship so as to obtain the information you need to control the outcome you care about?

>> Can you influence the outcome you care about by changing one or more of the antecedents?

These questions make it clear that it isn't enough to just survey the thoughts of people on a concept you think you care about — say, employee happiness, employee engagement, or employee culture — and then measure their responses. Sure, you can define your research objective as simply the effort to measure these things and then label the completion of the survey process a success; however, these measures collected by themselves leave many of the important questions unanswered. Even the surmountable achievement of making a fuzzy, previously unknowable concept measurable is a wasted effort if you don't learn anything about a) how these measures connect to other important company outcomes and b) how to control those outcomes.

REMEMBER

What you get out of a survey effort, or any analytical project, is predestined in the design phase. A poor research design amounts to taking a very-low-odds shot at learning anything of value; a high-quality design means a greater chance at gaining insights that will move your company forward.

Working with models

Observing and trying to interpret what you observe is a native human activity. It's the foundation for all survival. In your everyday life, however, you're often blissfully unaware of the nature of your observations and interpretations, with the result that you make errors in both. People analytics makes both observations about employees and the interpretation of those observations conscious, deliberate acts.

People analytics examines the "people side" of companies as it is, as opposed to how folks with their less-than-reliable "sixth sense" believe it should be. People analytics is superior to the vagaries of individual bias and delusion because its goal is to observe and explain repeating patterns among groups of people, as opposed to attempting to explain the motives of particular individuals. In this, people analytics focuses on the variables that differentiate people into group segments — based on years of prior work experience, for example, or educational background, personality, attitude, intelligence, pay, type of work, tenure, gender, ethnicity, age and many more — in hopes of discovering patterns among these variables.

The understanding and interpretation of those things you measure in people analytics is the reason for using a *model*: an integrated conceptual mapping representing the relationships of variables, displayed either as a picture, a mathematical formula, or a series of statements containing a verifiable theory. Such models can be extremely detailed and complex, or they can start out as a simple hypothesis: "Producing happier employees produces more productive employees," for example.

Implied in such a conceptual mapping of variables is a verifiable theory, one that is operationalized into measures, collected from either systems or surveys, and then tested mathematically. If you're going to measure the hypothesis statement, you must first define what you mean by *happy, productive,* and *employee.* After you have defined the necessary terms, you need to figure out how to measure them — but take pleasure in the fact that you're halfway there to designing a successful survey just by defining the terms carefully and specifying the measurement tools. These steps act as the foundation of your research design, which then shapes everything that comes afterward.

Conceptualizing fuzzy ideas

Conceptualization refers to the process of identifying and clarifying concepts: ideas that you and other people have about the nature of things. For example, think of the common words used in management and human resources — *satisfaction, commitment, engagement, happiness, diversity,* and *inclusion.* What do these words mean? When talking about diversity, are you talking about measuring the composition of your workforce by gender and ethnicity, the presence of stereotypical beliefs, any specific acts of discrimination, feelings that reflect prejudice, relational associations that reflect inclusion or exclusion, or all of the above? Is your focus on understanding how these matters apply (or don't apply) when looked at through the lens of gender, ethnicity, age, disability, socioeconomic status, economic background, personality, philosophical bent, or another factor? You need to be specific if you want to create a research plan and measurement framework that works. Otherwise, you're just talking about fuzzy ideas that nobody understands or agrees on. You can't analyze that.

Operationalizing concepts into measurements

Though conceptualization represents the clarification of concepts you will measure, operationalization is the construction of actual concrete measurement techniques. By *operationalization,* I mean the literal creation of all operations necessary for achieving the desired measurement of the concept. The whole of all people analytics rests on the operationalization of abstract concepts for the purposes of analysis. The creativity and skill that are applied to this operationalization effort is indicative of the quality of the analysts — which might explain why results vary so widely.

For example, one operationalization of employee commitment is to record the level of agreement of the employee to the survey item ("I am likely to be working for this company three years from now") using the standard 5-point agreement rating scale. Another operationalization of employee commitment is to ask the same question with a 7-point agreement rating scale. Yet another operationalization of employee commitment is to provide several statements representing commitment, have the subject record the level of employee agreement for each, and then combine the response to all these statements into an index.

Though any single statement may miss the mark, the idea of an index is that, by using a combination of statements, you're better able to grasp the whole.

Though you have a number of different ways to ask survey questions, constructing surveys so that all survey items are using the same agreement response scale format has several important advantages:

>> First and foremost, it's difficult if not entirely perilous to mathematically evaluate responses to items when different response scales are used.

>> It's much easier and less error prone for the person taking the survey if they're asked to use just one scale for the entire survey.

>> Last but not least, once you get into the groove of it, you'll see that you can measure a wide range of topics by simply coming up with a statement that expresses the essence of an idea and then asking the person taking the survey whether she agrees or disagrees with that statement.

Designing indexes (scales)

An important tool for operationalizing complex ideas is an index, also referred to as a scale. An *index* measures a respondent's attitude by using a series of related statements together in equal (or, in some cases, varied) weights. By measuring attitude with multiple measures, defined together as an index, you can gauge the sentiment of respondents with greater accuracy. The combined measure helps to determine not only how a respondent feels but also how *strongly* he feels that way within a broader range of values.

You'll find a ton of examples of statements in the Survey Question Bank in Appendix B.

Let's say you want to measure levels of employee commitment at your company. Using an index to evaluate commitment as a whole would entail using several (carefully chosen) survey items — perhaps items like these:

>> I believe strongly in the goals and objectives of *<Company>*.

>> I fit well into the culture of *<Company>*.

>> I am proud to tell others I work for *<Company>*.

>> If I were offered a comparable position with similar pay and benefits at another company, I would stay at *<Company>*.

>> At the present time I am not seriously considering leaving *<Company>*.

>> I expect to be working at *<Company>* one year from now.

>> I expect to be working at *<Company>* five years from now

>> I would be very happy to spend the rest of my career at *<Company>*.

If you go with the Likert scale, where each question has a possible value from 1 to 5, the range of the overall index spans from 8 to 40.

REMEMBER

Though indexes at first glance may seem to be asking the same old question in several different ways, they have several important advantages over single items:

>> Well-constructed indexes are more accurate measurement tools than single measures. Though good survey question design insists that you measure only one thing at a time, frequently concepts that you want to measure have no clear unambiguous single indicator. If considering a single data item gives only a rough indication of a given variable, working with several data items can provide a more comprehensive, accurate, and reliable picture.

>> Often, you want or need to analyze the relationship between several distinct concepts, but measures with only a handful of response categories may not provide the range of variation necessary for the math to isolate a clear correlation. In that case, an index formed from several items may be able to provide you with the variation you need. A single question with 5 responses has a range restricted by 5 possible values, but 10 questions with 5 responses has a range of 40 possible values. It's much better to correlate to 40 than to 5, especially if your other variables have a wider range as well.

TIP

Feel free to weight each statement more or less based on its independent correlation to some validating outcome measure — or any other sound logic you want to use. This would mean that, with the same 10 questions, you can achieve a range of values even greater than 40.

>> Indexes that gauge sentiment by including employee satisfaction, commitment, or engagement in the mix have proven to be more useful for predicting things like employee exit than any single item alone.

>> Indexes produce important summarizations for analysis and reporting: several items are summarized by a single numerical score while preserving the specific details of all individual items for further analysis or explanation

only if and when that detail is necessary. This means that instead of reporting all items from the index, you can begin by just reporting the index as a single measure – you may refer to it as a key performance indicator (KPI). Reporting one measure broadly is much easier for everyone to grasp and work with than is reporting the response to all the items that are contained in the index.

When it comes to creating an index, just follow these four simple steps:

1. Identify a research question that focuses on a single concept.

2. Generate a series of agree-disagree statements that relate to the concept in varying aspects or intensity.

   The intent is not to create your final index but rather come up with items you want to test for possible inclusion of an index.

REMEMBER

3. Establish a test group to test your possible index items in order to obtain a survey response to all test items together and to get subjective feedback on each item from test subjects.

   You should use a combination of subjective feedback and mathematical analysis to choose the best items to include in the final index. When testing survey items for the first time, you should sit down with at least 10 people and ask them if they find any ambiguity or confusion in the new items. You should also proactively ask the test subjects to explain how they interpret the items on the survey. These conversations, while subjective, will help you see problems you may not have otherwise seen.

4. After finalizing your list of statements and combining them into an index, decide whether you want to leave each statement at the same weight in the index or if you want to assign each statement a different weight based on some mathematically defensible logic.

Testing validity and reliability

After you have initially operationalized a measure, your work is far from done. You still need to stack up each specific measure against other concrete measures that either support or contradict the theory you're trying to prove. For example, if you're measuring commitment, it makes sense to evaluate your commitment measure against actual employee retention/exit over time or referrals of candidates to open jobs. Stacking measures against other measures (particularly, objective measures) allows you to test, validate, and improve the accuracy of your survey measures over time. If it turns out that your measure of commitment is an unreliable predictor of other, more objective measures that you think should be related, you will need to make changes to improve the measure. If your tweaks don't work, it's time to abandon the measure.

IMPROVING SURVEY DESIGN

Here's a handy list of do's and don'ts when it comes to survey design:

- **Avoid hearsay.** Ask mostly first-person questions, or in some cases ask about observable behaviors of other specific people. Don't ask respondents to speculate about "the company" or "the culture" or about unidentified people's thoughts and motives. Don't worry — you can still measure abstract ideas like "the company" and "the culture," but you need to frame each item in ways each person can respond using first hand observation or experience and then group these responses up to describe the larger abstract collective, as opposed to asking individuals to speculate about the abstract collective.

- **Avoid compound sentences or "double-barreled questions."** In other words, avoid questions that merge two or more topics into one question.

- **Avoid loaded and leading questions.** That means you shouldn't use terms that have strong positive or negative associations. If your language implies that you expect the respondent to realize that she had better choose the answer you want, then there is a chance she'll choose the answer you want — no matter whether this answer correctly depicts her opinion.

- **Avoid unnecessary distractions.** Be careful of unusual question groupings and page breaks, which studies have shown can change the way people respond. Be spartan, deliberate, and consistent.

- **Avoid questions or scales that pose problems.** Use one response scale throughout the entire survey and make sure that the scale has regularly spaced labels of similar length, if at all possible.

  It also helps to use a scale with an odd number of choices (3,5,7,11 . . .). Odd scales allow respondents to naturally choose between an option that is on either end of the scale or neutral. While some survey designs are attempts at forcing difficult choices, research indicates this may frustrate the survey respondent and introduce error in situations where the respondent genuinely has a neutral opinion.

  Questions designed to require ranking of multiple items in a list can be useful for some purposes, but this technique should be used sparingly because it is more difficult for the respondent to complete and more exposed to errors than question designs. If your objective is to find the relative positions of a series of statements, there are other ways to infer an order mathematically from the inputs of survey respondents — using a Likert scale, for example — without requiring survey respondents to rank multiple items at once.

- **Maintain balance and adhere to healthy design constraints.** As much as possible, design survey sections so that they contain a similar number of items, make sure items have a similar word count, and create indexes that have a similar number of items.

- **Assess each question for focus, brevity, and clarity.** Is the question expressed as briefly, clearly, and simply as it can be? Eliminate overgeneralization, overspecificity, and overemphasis.

- **Assess each question for importance.** Cull survey questions so that only the concepts that have previously been linked to important company outcomes remain. If questions haven't previously been measured, at least choose items that have a clear theoretical relationship to an outcome you intend to drive.

- **Assess vocabulary.** Use the words and phrases that people would use in casual speech. Limit vocabulary so that the least sophisticated survey-taker would be familiar with what she's reading. Eliminate ambiguous words.

- **Test for problems.** If you can, try to include some items that can be independently verified for purposes of validation.

- **Watch the clock.** Test to make sure the survey can be completed in 20 minutes or less.

- **Plan to report survey results using the smallest unit of analysis possible within the parameters of the confidential sample-size restrictions.** Of course, you can and should also report at higher-level aggregations and by chosen segments (diversity, location, manager, and so on). Specificity and breadth of reporting combined with creativity can help you achieve the level of impact from survey you are hoping for.

TIP

Sooner or later, you will learn two important ideas:

>> There's no single way to measure anything.

>> Not all measures are equal to all tasks.

TECHNICAL STUFF

I often hear people provide the advice that you should reduce the number of questions on your employee surveys to increase your survey response rate. My own research and personal experience find this advice to be false — in controlled studies, response rate is virtually unaffected by the number of questions on the survey or previous surveys completed. Once people begin the survey, they are more likely to complete the survey, regardless of the number of questions (within reasonable limits) than those who never enter the survey. Research demonstrates that a list of other factors, notably executive attitude and communication factors, are more important to response rate.

Managing the Survey Process

Large companies with abundant resources (time, people, and money, in other words) might have the option to build their own survey and analytics technology (and support team). Most, however, will likely research the market for options and buy a subscription to one of the many services available. There's a plethora of service providers for employee surveys that range from the high-touch consulting outfits to self-service software. Besides providing the latest technology, survey vendors can also provide industry-validated measures, thought partnership, benchmarks, robust reports for a large number of segments, in-depth data analysis, and other support such as communication templates, training, and advice. The most important element to address before getting excited about all the bells and whistles is ensuring that your chosen partner has the appropriate infrastructure, documentation, and internal experts to provide employee confidentiality and keep your data secure.

Getting confidential: Third-party confidentiality

Confidential means that personal identity information is attached to individual survey answers but is agreed to be kept private and expressed only outside of the survey database at group levels. It's a common practice to outsource collection and analytics of survey data to external vendors to facilitate administration of the survey while providing confidentiality. This convention allows the third party to link other employee data that helps with turning results into insights while protecting individual identity and employee trust.

To keep individual confidentiality, responses are expressed at a group level. The best practice is to enforce that results are only expressed for segment sizes of five people or more people. In most cases the criterion is that there must be five or more survey responses to produce a report for a segment.

Some companies, looking to stretch reporting to a broader audience of managers, apply the rule of five to the size of the actual segment population, not to the number of surveys returned, while applying a second criterion for response rate. For example, when I ran the survey program at Google, we applied a dual criterion: a) the segment must contain five or more employees AND b) the segment must have three or more survey responses. We also used these same criteria when I was working with Jawbone. In both cases, we established these criteria because we wanted to get more manager reports and the dual criteria created equivalent confidentiality. Under more simplistic guidelines, the majority of managers could not get a report since a manager of 5 would require a 100% response rate to get a report.

When it comes to confidentiality, however, you have options:

>> **Confidentiality with explicit exceptions:** Companies with a dedicated internal people analytics team are more and more likely to collect confidential data as described above, while only providing access to the personal details of respondents to specific trusted members of the team for the purposes of data management and analysis. (This option would need to be clearly defined in the employee survey FAQ and would not apply if the people responsible for people analytics "wear many hats" — meaning that they serve in other official HR or management capacities; in this situation, you'd be asking for trouble if you gave such individuals access to individual survey results.)

>> **Total anonymity:** Anonymity means what you think it means — the personal identity of a respondent is kept hidden. The intent of anonymity is to make it impossible to trace back to a specific individual something someone said so that they feel safer to speak their minds. As admirable as the intent may be, this particular practice greatly limits your ability to turn the feedback you receive into deeper insight by connecting it to other employee data. In certain fringe situations, anonymity may be called for, but in my opinion, anonymity isn't a good choice for people analytics, particularly when it's possible to use a third party.

REMEMBER

Anonymity can produce more problems than it solves. A common example is that a single employee may hack the anonymous process to provide repeated responses in order to game the overall results or try to get a manager fired. In other situations, employees may just mistakenly assign themselves to groups they don't belong to. (Trust me — this happens.) Then, when the manager gets the survey results, she discovers that there are a total of 15 responses for a team of 12 people. Such mistakes undermine the integrity of the survey process, leading many to doubt its efficacy. There's no way to undo the damage here, so the effort — months of work and everyone's time to take the survey — is totally wasted.

TIP

If you have real concerns about how your employees feel about sharing their thoughts, I strongly recommend taking the advice I give at the beginning of this section: Hire a third-party professional service that can provide services to connect individuals' responses with data confidentially.

Ensuring a good response rate

The *response rate* is the percentage of people who have responded to the survey. If you sent the survey to 1,000 people and 700 responded, your overall response rate is 70 percent.

Without getting into the nitty-gritty math of the situation, you don't require a 95 percent response rate to have a 95 percent certainty that you know what you need to know. The fundamental basis of polling (and, in fact, all of modern science) is that you can mathematically predict the response of a larger body of people with the response of a much smaller sample if you have selected people randomly. Generally, you need many fewer survey responses than you think you do.

REMEMBER

Keep one important assumption in mind: the random part. If there is some pattern to when and why people respond — if who responds is not totally "random", in other words — then all bets are off. Often, it's hard to recognize patterns in a smaller dataset, so for this reason you try to get as high a response rate as you can, to cover more ground.

Determining a good response rate

A U.S. senator once made this comment: "This is regarded as a relatively high response rate for a survey of this type" regarding a poll of constituents that achieved a 4 percent return rate. Though a customer satisfaction survey with a response rate greater than 15 percent might be considered a stunning success over in Marketing, those same response rates will get you fired fast in the People Analytics department.

Like most important things, the answer to "What is a good response rate?" is "It depends." If I had to come up with some answers here, I'd say that a 60 percent response rate is adequate for analysis and reporting, while a response rate above 70 percent is good, and a response rate above 80 percent is very good. Keep in mind that these are rough guides and that demonstrating the absence of a systematic response bias is more important than a high response rate.

REMEMBER

I'm convinced that there's way too much fuss and frantic guessing about what drives the employee response rate for surveys. If I have learned any generalizable truth working with employee surveys at many different companies, it is this: Employees are dying to provide feedback. You don't have to plead for feedback; just make an effort and get out of their way. If you want an especially high response rate, make the effort as comfortable as you can, given the circumstances.

Examining factors that contribute most to high response rates

If you want to achieve Olympic-medal levels of survey response rates, make sure you have the following down pat:

>> **High-quality communication:** Everything about the survey needs to communicate a sense of purpose, professionalism, and integrity. Throw in some charm and/or winks to unique aspects of company culture and you have the recipe for a huge success.

>> **Third-party confidentiality:** Use a professional third-party survey partner to provide confidence in individual confidentiality. State the rules clearly. This isn't a survey among parents for your child's birthday party. This is a whole lot of working people sticking their necks out for their company — at a minimum, they should be certain that their boss or someone in HR isn't looking at it and saying, "Well, that one can go if they feel that way." The employee must have confidence that his response will be reviewed with discretion *and* that he won't be singled out.

>> **A sincere interest in the results:** Response rates for employee surveys improve dramatically when a range of important people known to the employee stand up and say, "I want to hear your feedback; it's important to me." Communications from SurveyRobot.com (fictitious example) and/or HR are standard triggers for eye rolls when what you really want is a high response rate. Depending on your communication design, you may have a message from the head of HR or automated survey reminders in your bag of tricks; however, these should be preceded and followed by messages from other people: key founders, the CEO, the heads of divisions, managers, and even analysts! People want to know that a real person is responsible for this survey and that they (and the people behind them) care.

If you use a survey provider, they can work with your IT department to send out invites and reminders from specific people at you company (with their permission). It is also helpful if leaders at your company are willing to send out personal messages before the survey period, during the survey period, and after the survey period. You should have a communication plan in place so each message is unique, personal, and covers the important points that need to be covered.

>> **Repeated reminders:** One survey invitation is not enough. You might think people are ignoring your emails on purpose, when in reality they're just busy. They think that they'll return to the message, but the onslaught of other ones pushes it down their inboxes until your message is entirely out of their minds. Little reminders are an important way to regain attention.

Aside from the obvious email reminders, it's useful to put up posters, set out table cards in the cafeteria, use the lobby and elevator video screens, put "stickies" on desks, schedule time on work calendars, and so on. Be creative!

>> **High-quality survey design:** There's nothing worse than a poorly designed survey administered in an unprofessional manner and run by people who clearly don't know anything about what they're doing. Opportunity squandered. It is awful, it shows, and people are tired of it. Don't wing it. Get help.

>> **Make it competitive and fun:** One of the tried-and-true observations I have is that the mere public reporting of the response rate by executives will drive response rate among the teams of all executives. Aside from creating transparency and an indirect spirit of competition, upping the fun factor shows that corporate communication doesn't need to be boring. I admire executives who inspire their people by competing with other executives. And, by all means, come up with prizes: parties, dunk tanks, swag, bragging rights, and trophies may be just the ticket.

WARNING

It's good to encourage competition over participation, but never sanction a competition between executives in the survey results themselves. By this I mean that employees should never be cajoled, harassed, or threatened for particular response to a particular item. By this I mean, none of that "Hey guys, please rate me a five" stuff. First of all, it's tacky, and second, it defeats the entire point. I know some companies that actually go as far as to fire managers for trying to influence survey results in that manner. Hopefully, you never have to take that step but, in any case, make it clear to everyone that the survey is not a popularity contest. Just get out the vote! Let the crowd do the rest.

>> **Establish a track record of running good surveys, doing the right thing, and taking action:** The first employee survey at Google achieved a 55 percent response rate, the second was a 65 percent response rate, the third was 75 percent, and then the rate moved up from there. It takes a few years to earn employee trust in the survey effort, but trust can be won. Just be patient — and remember to do the right thing

REMEMBER

Yes, you do want to use communication to the best of your ability so that you can achieve a sufficient response rate for analysis. Despite all that, keep a cool head about your real objective, which is to learn something useful for the good of the enterprise, not to achieve responses.

Planning for effective survey communications

Loads of bad surveys are out there. Toss a stone and you'll hit a bad survey. And, because folks have had it up to *here* with bad surveys, getting participation requires catching people's attention and convincing them that this particular survey is worth their time and effort. A comprehensive, thoughtful, and engaging communications plan can help. All the prep work you did to set objectives will come in handy now: who, what, when, and why. Now you only need to interpret that from the perspective of the survey takers.

Never met the acronym WIIFM? Well, say hello to good old "What's In It For Me?" That's the key question you have to answer for everyone but yourself. Why should people fill out your survey? If you did a good job of identifying action owners and engaging them in the creation process, it's easier to develop an enticing value proposition and to enlist other people who are both recognized and respected to deliver "the ask." No, HR emails and notifications from the survey tool are not enough to do it. You need to enlist the big guns. Remember to make it personal and enlist the support of the village.

The stakes involved should be made clear at the beginning, which means right there in the survey invitation. Here are the questions you need to address:

>> What is this survey about?

>> Who wants to know this information?

>> Why do they want this?

>> Why was I picked? (if this is a sample)

>> How important is this?

>> Will this be difficult?

>> How long will this take?

>> Is this anonymous, confidential, or what? Will I be identified?

>> Is it safe for me to share my opinion? How?

>> How will this be used?

>> What is in it for me?

>> When is it due?

Here's what a survey invite might look like:

Hi, Mike.

I'd like to invite you to participate in the *XYZ Survey* to help us understand more about your experience as an employee at *XYZ Company*. We do this survey each year to get a sense of how happy you are, where we're improving, and where we can get better. *XYZ Company* is a truly special place, and we want to make sure we preserve that uniqueness as we grow. Your feedback will help guide our decisions as we think about where we stand and where to focus our efforts so that we can advance together as a company.

To participate, please follow this *(Hyperlink: Link)*.

The survey should take about 5 to 10 minutes to complete.

Please be assured that your responses are completely confidential. We have commissioned an independent employee research agency, People Analytics, to conduct this survey on our behalf. Their work is being conducted in accordance with our *(Hyperlink: People Analytics Code of Conduct).*

If you have any questions about the survey, please email: *(Email: survey @ xyz.com)* or visit the *(Hyperlink: FAQ page).*

I very much value your feedback, and I hope you will take the time to participate.

Sincerely,

XYZ

Comparing Survey Data

To compare your survey data, you need something to compare it to. One logical point of comparison is to look at how companies in the same field are faring. That's where *benchmarks* come in — a set of averages of the responses to the same or similar question collected from other enterprises. Survey vendors and other consulting firms are quite happy to provide (sell, in other words) such benchmarks. They can then be used to understand how your company compares to other companies. Is an Engagement Index score of 70 out 100 good or bad? The answer may not be clear; however, if you can determine that 70 is in fact a statistically significant difference and 33 percent better than that achieved by similar companies, then you can say with some degree of certainty that an Engagement Index score of 70 out 100 is pretty darn good.

Understanding where your employees stand relative to the employees of your competitors or relative to high-performing companies can produce vital feedback, especially regarding crucial concepts, like compensation and benefits. Obviously, most people like to have more of the good stuff and less of the bad stuff — what is more useful to know is the degree to which your population varies from others in your industry, either due to your best efforts or despite them.

External benchmarks can be quite useful; however, you should consider these limitations:

>> **Imperfect comparison error:** Gone are the days when giant consulting firms could retain their customers indefinitely because they had the best brand-name clients. Nowadays it's hard to find one firm that holds data from all the top companies in a certain industry. And, if they claim that they do, ask probing questions and you'll find the holes. For example, some use 5-year rolling averages, which allow them to market old data as new. An aspiration to

grow a unique culture coupled with investment and advances in technology and analytics have increased companies' capability to generate and gather intelligence on their own. Therefore, top brand companies that used to keep decade-long contracts with the Deloittes and PWCs of the world are now quitting consulting firms and mining (keeping) their own data.

» **Benchmark target error:** There is no single target for all. In today's world, companies have not only moving targets but also personalized targets. In other words, what makes Google great will not necessarily work for Facebook. It's okay, and even smart, to check external reference points —and the more, the better. However, do not make those external benchmarks your company's goal. If you do, you may reach the target but in so doing miss focusing on those items that are important for you.

A better way to win is by looking to improve the key measures that correlate to the outcomes you're trying to achieve as a company, regardless of whether you're already ahead of the pack. Let's say that scores for innovation at your company match external benchmarks, but work-life balance is significantly below the norm. Where would you recommend taking action? I hope you answer "It depends." If a culture of innovation is a necessary differentiator for your company and the key motivator for the type of people you want to attract, but work-life balance isn't even in their vocabulary, then focusing on improving satisfaction with work-life balance could be a bad investment for your company.

» **Vanity measure error:** Even if your company is ahead of all benchmarks, you can't rest on your laurels. Outperforming against peers can make you complacent, and that is a dangerous thing in today's fast-changing world. Always be looking to improve, and use external benchmarks for what they are: comparative information at a specific time.

Here's an arrogance-breaker. Through all of my years of working with employee surveys at different companies, I have noticed an important pattern: New employees nearly always respond more enthusiastically to survey questions than do the same employees a few years later. This may seem to be a natural phenomenon — it fits the pattern of all intimate human relationships — so you may not think much of it. However, if you're comparing your company to other companies or comparing units to each other within your company, those with newer employees have a distinct advantage hidden in their average. They will seem to have it all together and everything they do is golden; however, as growth slows and tenure increases, the average survey score will tenaciously decline. The natural temptation is to jump to the opposite conclusion: Something is entirely wrong, and these old managers must be driving the company into the ground. These attribution problems are dangerous. The manager may not be either as good or as bad as you think she is. Comparisons without control should be suspect. The question you should always ask is this: Are we comparing apples to apples? The fact is, when it comes to employee surveys, you cannot compare a group that has 50 percent new employees with a group that has 10 percent new employees. If you do, go ahead and crown as "best manager" the manager of the group with the new employees, without even looking at data.

So, yes, you do need a relative point of reference to interpret any point of data (especially surveys), but this point of reference need not be an external benchmark. Other point of reference options include:

» **Current segment score versus previous segment score (Trend):** Did the segment measure improve, stay the same, or get worse?

» **Segment versus company average (Average):** How does the segment measure compare to the company average? Is the segment above, the same, or worse than the company average?

» **Segment versus all segments range (Range):** How does the segment measure compare to the range of scores for segments of a like size? Is the segment in the high range, in the middle, or at the bottom?

» **Segment versus target (Target):** How does the segment measure compare to a segment target determined either by executive prerogative or by a number mathematically representing good derived from multivariate analysis of previous survey responses?

Chapter **13**

Prioritizing Where to Focus

n this book, you find lots of measures — metrics as well as survey questions — all designed to unearth information you wouldn't otherwise see. The thing is, you may start out with just a couple measures, but then, like a feral cat, before you know it you have hundreds of kittens. Yes, kittens are cute, but it's possible to have too much of a good thing. The same rule applies to the real world. There may come a time when you wonder, "After we get all this data, what will we do with it?" or "How can we possibly keep all these balls in the air and be good at everything we set out to do in the way we approach employee brand and culture?" The good news is that you don't need to be good at everything: What you need to be good at are those things you've decided to prioritize.

Key driver analysis (KDA) is one data tool you can use to determine what you need to prioritize. It helps you identify which changes will have the biggest impact on the outcome you desire. In addition to being one of the more powerful techniques that you can use to help understand the data you have found in surveys, it's a powerful technique to help your company prioritize what they are working on in people analytics and human resources in general.

REMEMBER

You don't need an endless list of things you need to do to improve as a company — what you need is to find a short list of things you can change that are important. When it comes to survey data, KDA is useful for exploring a lot of issues and quickly getting to the few that matter.

In this chapter, I show you an example of what the results of a KDA might look like, and then I walk you through the steps it takes to create one on your own.

Dealing with the Data Firehose

Definitions of analytics vary, but I think it is safe to say that everyone can agree that the goal of analytics is to use data to produce something of greater value than the data itself. The "something of greater value" differs from situation to situation. At times, it may be a new way to make decisions, a new insight that would not otherwise be possible, a new solution to a problem, or some other new advantage. Whatever "it" is, we can further say that the goal of people analytics is to produce new business value from our people analytics activities (just like any other version of analytics). The main difference here is that people analytics produces new value through people (the original source of all business value) using people data. The people data we use to generate value can take various shapes:

>> In Appendix A of this book, you will find the technical definitions of over a hundred different metrics that you can use to measure different aspects of companies that have to do with people — metrics to measure the flow of people in, within, and out of the company, metrics to measure the shape of the organization of people, metrics to measure compensation, benefits, diversity, learning, performance distributions, and more.

>> In Appendix B of this book, you will find examples of over a hundred different items you can measure on surveys. The survey items can be viewed as standalone measures or applied as segments to the aforementioned metrics in Appendix A.

>> In Chapter 4 of this book, I introduce some of the options for segmenting HR data, although I did not comprehensively cover all options. In any case, with a little brainstorming you could easily identify over a hundred different ways to segment the metrics or survey items described above. Each method of segmentation may have anywhere from two segments to hundreds of segments in it.

>> In addition to the base elements I have described in the first three bullets (metrics, surveys, and segments) there are many ways to analyze data — people data or data of any other stripe. From a reductionist point of view there are five

basic types of analysis you can do with any measure: A) observe a single measure alone at single moment in time, B) observe a single measurement over time to see change, C) observe a single measure by segment to examine differences, D) observe relationship (correlation) between two measures x(y), and E) observe the way that differences or changes in an outcome measure (y) are explained by many other measures (x1, x2, x3, . . .)

Other than to provide a summary, the point of all of this is to show you the number of permutations of activity that can be created by combining the basic elements and assumptions I have provided. First, if you just combine the metrics and survey measures together, you get 200 (100 + 100 = 200). Second, if you multiply the number of measures times the five types of analysis you get 1,000 things (200 x 5 = 1000). Third, using an online permutation calculator (Example: www. mathsisfun.com/combinatorics/combinations-permutations-calculator. html) if you calculate the number of possible analysis outputs you could create if you did these 1000 things applied to 500 segments you get . . .

Drum roll. The answer is that you get 2.7028824094e+299 options for output. That's the short answer. Typing this out the long way, the complete number of analysis outputs you can produce is: 27028824094543656951561469362597527549615200844654828700739287510662542870552219389861248392450237016536260608502154610480220975005067991754989421969951847542366548426375173335616246407973788734436457416111949760457104498575628788051460099421942675236691585660313686260248442810929690586379982121632O.

That's a lot of output! Making output tell a better story with better visualization techniques is a good idea, but dang, you're going to have a lot of different stories to sort through. If the goal of people analytics is not more activity, but instead more value per unit of activity, it begs the question, "How do you know which of the many possible activities and outputs will offer the most value?"

Because the goal of people analytics is to extract value from data before the end of your lifetime, or at least just before running out of time and resources at your current company, then speed, learning, and focus are going to be essential. You know that speed is important — the time clock is always ticking. You also know that learning — specifically, learning about people with data — is important. It's kind of the point. But something that doesn't get nearly enough attention is *focus*.

Here's where key driver analysis (KDA) can be of help, since its sole purpose is to use employee survey data to investigate the relationship between a number of measured items (drivers) and some specific attitudes, behaviors, or other consequence (intended outcome). A specific attitude, behavior or other consequence can be a *key performance indicator*, or KPI for short. To keep our terminology straight, in the section below I explain a two-pronged approach to survey design and analysis that acknowledges the role KPI's play in KDA.

Introducing a Two-Pronged Approach to Survey Design and Analysis

There are really two very different types of surveys: key performance indicator (KPI) surveys and key driver analysis (KDA) surveys. You should use both types of surveys or, at the very least, know which one you are doing when, how and why.

Going with KPIs

The primary purpose of a KPI survey is to evaluate ongoing success at achieving some pre-defined objective. You do this by asking respondents to express their level of agreement with a statement or series of statements. (If you want to use a series of statements as a KPI, they should be combined as an index.) To ensure wide respondent participation, a KPI survey should have a specific and narrow focus. That means a KPI survey should be constrained to only a handful of questions — 10 items or less, for example. By definition, a KPI survey should be suitable for rapid, repeated, ongoing administration with little cost.

The primary method of analysis of a KPI survey is to report the ongoing trend (as a whole and by company segment), compare segments to each other, and provide a basis to correlate a regularly collected survey-based employee KPI with other operating and business measures captured in the same segment frame and time frame.

REMEMBER

A KPI can be measured regularly in a survey devoted entirely to just capturing this one KPI or it can be added to a bigger, less frequent survey. The reasons for conducting an independent KPI survey as opposed to making it part of a larger survey are different. I will talk about the purpose of a larger survey in the next section.

Taking the KDA route

In a key driver analysis (KDA) survey, the primary goal of the survey is to understand which of many different survey items best explain or predict a chosen consequence the company cares about — a chosen KPI. Although a KPI serves as the focal objective of key driver analysis (KDA) survey, do not confuse the purpose, design, and analysis of the KPI survey with the KDA survey – the two are used together but are totally different animals.

Contrary to many believe, the purpose of including so many items on an employee survey is not to evaluate opinion on many items relative to each other — instead it is to evaluate the relative strength of the item variance to explain or predict the variance in some behavior or consequence. You ask so many questions so you can evaluate key drivers of a KPI, not because you believe all the questions on the survey should be treated as their own KPI.

The primary method of analysis in KDA is correlation; at least the important part. The KPI is used as the dependent measure (y variable) and all other survey items are the independent measures (x variables). The KPI may be pulled into the KDA dataset from outside the survey effort (attrition, performance, customer satisfaction, sales, on time departures, and so on) or it may be measured on the survey itself at the same time.(Engagement Index, Commitment Index, Intent to Stay, Team Effectiveness, or Employee Net Promoter Score, for example. are common survey-derived KPIs, often collected along with a lot of other items thrown in "just for good measure".)

After the items from the KDA have been analyzed to determine which ones are most and least important in explaining (or predicting) the KPI, the next KDA survey should be modified to remove those items that have little value in understanding the KPI. The removal of items frees up room to test new items which may prove to be more valuable than the old items you've discarded.

In contrast to KDA, KPI measures should remain consistent over time. KPI surveys are for measuring things you *already know* matter; KDA surveys are for learning new things you *don't know already*. Learning new things requires deliberate experimentation. The introduction of new KDA measures should be guided by the advancement of a theory, as represented by a model you've settled on. (For more on models, see Chapter 10.)

KDA surveys occurs less frequently than KPI surveys, but they contain more items so you can identify which actions would have the highest probability of influencing the KPI measure. After a series of high priority actions have been identified, the actions can then be tested for impact on the KPI using control and experimental groups. If after applying the action there is no change in the KPI, then the theory was incorrect, and you must go back to your KDA data or conduct a new KDA survey with new items. If the related issues identified by the KDA are dealt with successfully, you should then see a change in the KPI measure, which indicates you should systematically expand the successful action across the company.

Evaluating Survey Data with Key Driver Analysis (KDA)

KDA is important because it combines two perspectives into one analysis: the percent of responses to the item that were unfavorable and the correlation of the item to a KPI. Rather than jump right to the end of the story, I want to show you these two perspectives separately, just as they are found in their natural habitat. See Figure 13-1 for a view of typical employee survey data output sorted from least favorable to most favorable.

Factor	Survey item	Percent Favorable	Percent Unfavorable
Company	<Company> makes operational decisions based on its mission and values.	31%	69%
Company	There is a clear intent around which all of <Company> rallies.	32%	68%
Leadership	<Company>'s leadership team makes sound decisions on the basis of intellectual rigor and data.	34%	66%
Leadership	<Company>'s leadership team has provided clear information that is useful for making decisions.	35%	65%
Leadership	<Company>'s leadership team creates an environment that is conducive to 'speaking up'.	39%	61%
Comp & Benefits	<Company>'s pay is as good as or better than the pay in other companies.	42%	58%
Leadership	<Company>'s leadership team cares about me as a human being.	45%	55%
Engagement Index	I expect to be working for <Company> three years from now.	47%	53%
Career Opportunity	I understand my possible career paths at <Company>.	48%	52%
Company	I believe <Company> has a game changing strategy and product roadmap.	49%	51%
Peers	Other teams put the collective needs of the larger organization ahead of their own.	52%	48%
Company	<Company> has a culture in which diverse perspectives are valued.	53%	47%
Peers	I leave meetings with clear decisions and actions.	57%	43%
Comp & Benefits	<Company>'s Benefits are as good as or better than the Benefits in other companies.	57%	43%
Engagement Index	I would recommend <Company> as a great place to work.	58%	42%
Company	I feel my opinions count at <Company>.	58%	42%
Career Opportunity	I see future opportunities for myself at <Company>.	59%	41%
Engagement Index	If I were offered a comparable position at another company, I would stay at <Company>.	66%	34%
Peers	I have a close friend at work.	71%	29%
Peers	The structure of my immediate team allows me to be effective in my work.	72%	28%
Engagement Index	I expect to be working for <Company> one year from now.	72%	28%
Peers	There is a clear intent around which my team rallies.	74%	26%
Peers	When things go wrong, the emphasis is on putting things right rather than placing blame.	74%	26%
Company	<Company> has a culture in which creativity is valued.	76%	24%
Job	Over the last 3 months, I knew what was expected of me at work.	77%	23%
Manager	Over the last 3 months, my manager has talked to me about my progress.	79%	21%
Manager	My manager provides clear feedback that is useful for making decisions.	81%	19%
Manager	My manager is effective.	83%	17%
Manager	My manager makes sound decisions on the basis of intellectual rigor and data.	83%	17%
Peers	My team is effective. (Team is those you work with that report to the same manager.)	85%	15%
Manager	My manager creates an environment that is conducive to 'speaking up'.	85%	15%
Peers	My team puts the collective priorities and needs of the larger organization ahead of its own.	85%	15%
Job	My job is important at <Company>.	86%	14%
Company	<Company> is creating products that improve people's lives.	87%	13%
Manager	My manager cares about me as a human being.	88%	12%
Engagement Index	I am proud to tell others that I work for <Company>.	89%	11%
Engagement Index	I would recommend <Company> products to a trusted friend or acquaintance.	92%	8%
Engagement Index	I regularly 'go above and beyond' to ensure <Company> succeeds.	94%	6%
Engagement Index	I regularly put in extra effort outside my formal job responsibilities to help my team succeed.	94%	6%

FIGURE 13-1: A complete list of employee survey items sorted from least favorable to most favorable.

Figure 13-1 may be a little difficult to see at this resolution. Figure 13-2 shows a cleaner view of just the bottom 10 and the top 10.

Figures 13-1 and 13-2 are pretty normal ways of looking at employee survey data. Percent Favorable is a calculation of the percent of people who "Agreed" or "Strongly Agreed" with the statement. Unfavorable is just the opposite. In the example, the company was going through some hard times and you can see this in the survey data. The least favorable items should be of concern to you, to say the least.

This brings us to another way of analyzing the same survey dataset: correlation. In short, correlation is a mutual relationship between two or more things. I am going to use correlation in the KDA in a moment, but I first want to show what the output of correlation looks like by itself.

Factor	Survey Items: Bottom Ten and Top Ten by Favorability	Percent Favorable	Percent unfavorable
Company	<Company> makes operational decisions based on its mission and values.	31%	69%
Company	There is a clear intent around which all of <Company> rallies.	32%	68%
Leadership	<Company>'s leadership team makes sound decisions on the basis of intellectual rigor and data.	34%	66%
Leadership	<Company>'s leadership team has provided clear information that is useful for making decisions.	35%	65%
Leadership	<Company>'s leadership team creates an environment that is conducive to 'speaking up'.	39%	61%
Comp & Benefits	<Company>'s pay is as good as or better than the pay in other companies.	42%	58%
Leadership	<Company>'s leadership team cares about me as a human being.	45%	55%
Engagement Index	I expect to be working for <Company> three years from now.	47%	53%
Career Opportunity	I understand my possible career paths at <Company>.	48%	52%
Company	I believe <Company> has a game changing strategy and product roadmap.	49%	51%
Peers	My team is effective. (Team is those you work with that report to the same manager.)	85%	15%
Manager	My manager creates an environment that is conducive to 'speaking up'.	85%	15%
Peers	My team puts the collective priorities and needs of the larger organization ahead of its own.	85%	15%
Job	My job is important at <Company>.	86%	14%
Company	<Company> is creating products that improve people's lives.	87%	13%
Manager	My manager cares about me as a human being.	88%	12%
Engagement Index	I am proud to tell others that I work for <Company>.	89%	11%
Engagement Index	I would recommend <Company> products to a trusted friend or acquaintance.	92%	8%
Engagement Index	I regularly 'go above and beyond' to ensure <Company> succeeds.	94%	6%
Engagement Index	I regularly put in extra effort outside my formal job responsibilities to help my team succeed.	94%	6%

FIGURE 13-2: Employee survey items: Bottom 10 favorable, top 10 favorable

Here's the task I've set for myself: Out of all the questions on the survey, I want to understand which ones most correlate to a measure I call *Intent to Stay*, which is a KPI measure I included on the survey. The item I use to measure *Intent to Stay* is: "I expect to be working for *<Company>* one year from now." Remember that correlation is a statistical measure of the relationship between two variables. In the case of the example in Figure 13-3 below, y= Intent to Stay, x is an item of the survey, and the correlation calculation for every item in the survey targets *Intent to Stay*.

In Figure 13-3, the number you see in bar graph to the right represents the Pearson correlation coefficient, also referred to as Pearson's r, the Pearson product-moment correlation coefficient, the bivariate correlation, r (just the lowercase letter), or just correlation coefficient. (Pearson must have been a spy; this guy had a lot of names!) The correlation coefficient is a calculated measure of the linear correlation between two variables x and y — the range between 0 and 1 indicates the extent to which two variables are linearly related.

While correlation does not indicate a causal relationship, the larger your correlation coefficient, the more the variables change together, indicating at least the possibility of a causal relationship. The smaller your correlation coefficient, the less likely that is.

Figure 13-4 is a cutout of the top correlates of Intent to Stay from this survey, with some contrasting items I have left in for perspective.

Factor	Survey item	Correlation to Intent to Stay
Engagement Index	I would recommend <Company> as a great place to work.	0.56
Career Opportunity	I see future opportunities for myself at <Company>.	0.47
Leadership	<Company>'s leadership team cares about me as a human being.	0.45
Company	<Company> has a culture in which creativity is valued.	0.42
Job	Over the last 3 months, I knew what was expected of me at work.	0.41
Leadership	<Company>'s leadership team creates an environment that is conducive to 'speaking up'.	0.40
Company	I believe <Company> has a game changing strategy and product roadmap.	0.40
Career Opportunity	I understand my possible career paths at <Company>.	0.40
Manager	My manager is effective.	0.39
Peers	I have a close friend at work.	0.39
Engagement Index	I am proud to tell others that I work for <Company>.	0.38
Company	<Company> has a culture in which diverse perspectives are valued.	0.38
Leadership	<Company>'s leadership team has provided clear information that is useful for making decisions.	0.37
Manager	My manager makes sound decisions on the basis of intellectual rigor and data.	0.36
Leadership	<Company>'s leadership team makes sound decisions on the basis of intellectual rigor and data.	0.35
Job	My job is important at <Company>.	0.35
Engagement Index	I would recommend <Company> products to a trusted friend or acquaintance.	0.30
Peers	The structure of my immediate team allows me to be effective in my work.	0.30
Company	<Company> makes operational decisions based on its mission and values.	0.28
Company	There is a clear intent around which all of <Company> rallies.	0.27
Manager	Over the last 3 months, my manager has talked to me about my progress.	0.27
Peers	There is a clear intent around which my team rallies.	0.27
Company	<Company> is creating products that improve people's lives.	0.26
Comp & Benefits	<Company>'s pay is as good as or better than the pay in other companies.	0.24
Manager	My manager provides clear feedback that is useful for making decisions.	0.22
Peers	My team is effective. (Team is those you work with that report to the same manager.)	0.22
Company	I feel my opinions count at <Company>.	0.19
Manager	My manager cares about me as a human being.	0.17
Peers	I leave meetings with clear decisions and actions.	0.16
Engagement Index	I regularly put in extra effort outside my formal job responsibilities to help my team succeed.	0.16
Manager	My manager creates an environment that is conducive to 'speaking up'.	0.16
Peers	Other teams put the collective needs of the larger organization ahead of their own.	0.16
Peers	My team puts the collective priorities and needs of the larger organization ahead of its own.	0.15
Comp & Benefits	<Company>'s Benefits are as good as or better than the Benefits in other companies.	0.14
Engagement Index	I regularly 'go above and beyond' to ensure <Company> succeeds.	0.12
Peers	When things go wrong, the emphasis is on putting things right rather than placing blame.	0.03

FIGURE 13-3: Employee survey items: Correlation of survey items to the Intent to Stay KPI.

Factor	Survey Items: Top Ten and Bottom Ten by Correlation to Intent to Stay	Correlation to Intent to Stay
Engagement Index	I would recommend <Company> as a great place to work.	0.56
Career Opportunity	I see future opportunities for myself at <Company>.	0.47
Leadership	<Company>'s leadership team cares about me as a human being.	0.45
Company	<Company> has a culture in which creativity is valued.	0.42
Job	Over the last 3 months, I knew what was expected of me at work.	0.41
Leadership	<Company>'s leadership team creates an environment that is conducive to 'speaking up'.	0.40
Company	I believe <Company> has a game changing strategy and product roadmap.	0.40
Career Opportunity	I understand my possible career paths at <Company>.	0.40
Manager	My manager is effective.	0.39
Peers	I have a close friend at work.	0.39
Company	I feel my opinions count at <Company>.	0.19
Manager	My manager cares about me as a human being.	0.17
Peers	I leave meetings with clear decisions and actions.	0.16
Engagement Index	I regularly put in extra effort outside my formal job responsibilities to help my team succeed.	0.16
Manager	My manager creates an environment that is conducive to 'speaking up'.	0.16
Peers	Other teams put the collective needs of the larger organization ahead of their own.	0.16
Peers	My team puts the collective priorities and needs of the larger organization ahead of its own.	0.15
Comp & Benefits	<Company>'s Benefits are as good as or better than the Benefits in other companies.	0.14
Engagement Index	I regularly 'go above and beyond' to ensure <Company> succeeds.	0.12
Peers	When things go wrong, the emphasis is on putting things right rather than placing blame.	0.03

FIGURE 13-4: Employee survey items: Correlation with Intent to Stay KPI — Top Items.

So, yes, "I would recommend <Company> as a great place to work" is the most highly correlated item to "I expect to be working for <Company> one year from now." That makes sense, but it's also not that enlightening. That's OK, though, because this item is followed by "I see future opportunities for myself at <Company>" and then some other stuff. Helping someone see future opportunities for themselves at <Company> is a little more practical to achieve than making the whole company better all at once. In any case, you may see many practical areas of focus at the top of this list. If your objective is to get people to stick around a little while longer (while you figure out whatever is troubling your company) you want to get good at the things at the top first.

What we can glean from the correlation results shown in Figure 13-4 is that if an employee selected a low number for one pf the top 10 items, they were also more likely to select a low number on the *Intent to Stay* measure. Alternatively, if they selected a high number on one, they were also more likely to select a high number on the other. The lower the correlation score the less that is true – there was no pattern. (That's pretty much the whole idea behind correlation, by the way.)

REMEMBER

With this report on correlation we now know the items that should be of most concern to us, if we are at all concerned about retaining employees; however, this report doesn't tell us how well the company did on the items. To know that, we need our favorability score, but that is stranded on the other report. Wouldn't it be nice to have them in one place? Yes! You got it. That's what the KDA is. We are going to get to that below.

Suffer me one more point to make. If you selected a different KPI other than *Intent To Stay* to correlate to, then you get yet another list of items in a different order. See Figure 13-9, where I define the KPI as *Team Effectiveness.*

Yes, Figure 13-5 shows a different list of important items than 13-4, but that doesn't mean that one is right and the other is wrong; it simply illustrates the point that what you have defined as your KPI matters and will necessarily *drive* (drive as in the second word of key driver analysis) what actions you take if your decisions are based on what is on these lists.

Having settled the point that what you choose as your objective will necessarily drive your priorities through key driver analysis, I'll return to the original *Intent to Stay* KPI focus and put it all together, as shown in Figure 13-6.

Figure 13-6 provides the missing consolidated view of Item Favorability and Correlation to Intent to Stay. So that you can see what I'm doing more clearly, I have trimmed the list — otherwise the list could include a ranking of all 40 items.

Factor	Survey item	Correlation to Team Effectiveness
Peers	My team puts the collective priorities and needs of the larger organization ahead of its own.	0.50
Manager	My manager is effective.	0.38
Peers	The structure of my immediate team allows me to be effective in my work.	0.37
Manager	My manager makes sound decisions on the basis of intellectual rigor and data.	0.34
Peers	There is a clear intent around which my team rallies.	0.32
Manager	My manager provides clear feedback that is useful for making decisions.	0.32
Manager	My manager creates an environment that is conducive to 'speaking up'.	0.29
Manager	Over the last 3 months, my manager has talked to me about my progress.	0.29
Peers	I leave meetings with clear decisions and actions.	0.27
Peers	When things go wrong, the emphasis is on putting things right rather than placing blame.	0.25
Job	Over the last 3 months, I knew what was expected of me at work.	0.24
Engagement Index	I would recommend <Company> as a great place to work.	0.23
Manager	My manager cares about me as a human being.	0.23
Peers	Other teams put the collective needs of the larger organization ahead of their own.	0.21
Engagement Index	If I were offered a comparable position at another company, I would stay at <Company>.	0.19
Engagement Index	I expect to be working for <Company> three years from now.	0.18
Career Opportunity	I see future opportunities for myself at <Company>.	0.18
Leadership	<Company>'s leadership team has provided clear information that is useful for making decisions.	0.17
Company	<Company> has a culture in which diverse perspectives are valued.	0.15
Leadership	<Company>'s leadership team creates an environment that is conducive to 'speaking up'.	0.15
Leadership	<Company>'s leadership team makes sound decisions on the basis of intellectual rigor and data.	0.15
Career Opportunity	I understand my possible career paths at <Company>.	0.15
Engagement Index	I expect to be working for <Company> one year from now.	0.15
Company	<Company> makes operational decisions based on its mission and values.	0.15
Leadership	<Company>'s leadership team cares about me as a human being.	0.13
Company	I believe <Company> has a game changing strategy and product roadmap.	0.13
Company	<Company> has a culture in which creativity is valued.	0.13
Engagement Index	I would recommend <Company> products to a trusted friend or acquaintance.	0.12
Company	There is a clear intent around which all of <Company> rallies.	0.12
Company	<Company> is creating products that improve people's lives.	0.12
Comp & Benefits	<Company>'s pay is as good as or better than the pay in other companies.	0.12
Engagement Index	I am proud to tell others that I work for <Company>.	0.11
Engagement Index	I regularly 'go above and beyond' to ensure <Company> succeeds.	0.10
Company	I feel my opinions count at <Company>.	0.10
Engagement Index	I regularly put in extra effort outside my formal job responsibilities to help my team succeed.	0.09
Comp & Benefits	<Company>'s Benefits are as good as or better than the Benefits in other companies.	0.09
Job	My job is important at <Company>.	0.08
Peers	I have a close friend at work.	0.08

FIGURE 13-5: Employee survey items: Correlation with Team Effectiveness– Top Items.

Factor	Survey Items: Top 10 Intent To Stay Importance vs. 10 less important examples	Percent Unfavorable	Correlation to Intent to Stay	Intent to Stay Importance
Leadership	<Company>'s leadership team cares about me as a human being.	55%	0.45	2451
Leadership	<Company>'s leadership team has provided clear information that is useful for making decisions.	65%	0.37	2432
Leadership	<Company>'s leadership team creates an environment that is conducive to 'speaking up'.	61%	0.40	2430
Engagement Index	I would recommend <Company> as a great place to work.	42%	0.56	2373
Leadership	<Company>'s leadership team makes sound decisions on the basis of intellectual rigor and data.	66%	0.35	2338
Career Opportunity	I understand my possible career paths at <Company>.	52%	0.40	2077
Company	I believe <Company> has a game changing strategy and product roadmap.	51%	0.40	2027
Company	<Company> makes operational decisions based on its mission and values.	69%	0.28	1950
Career Opportunity	I see future opportunities for myself at <Company>.	41%	0.47	1934
Company	There is a clear intent around which all of <Company> rallies.	68%	0.27	1873
Comp & Benefits	<Company>'s pay is as good as or better than the pay in other companies.	58%	0.24	1307
Company	I feel my opinions count at <Company>.	42%	0.19	776
Comp & Benefits	<Company>'s Benefits are as good as or better than the Benefits in other companies.	43%	0.14	608
Manager	Over the last 3 months, my manager has talked to me about my progress.	21%	0.27	569
Job	My job is important at <Company>.	14%	0.35	486
Manager	My manager provides clear feedback that is useful for making decisions.	19%	0.22	432
Company	<Company> is creating products that improve people's lives.	13%	0.26	358
Peers	My team is effective. (Team is those you work with that report to the same manager.)	15%	0.22	335
Peers	My team puts the collective priorities and needs of the larger organization ahead of its own.	15%	0.15	214
Manager	My manager cares about me as a human being.	12%	0.17	194

FIGURE 13-6: Employee survey items ranked by Importance.

The first column to the right of the survey item name shows the percentage of people who responded unfavorably to the item. Just to the right of that is the correlation of the item to Intent to Stay. The column furthest to the right, "Intent to Stay Importance" is a calculated metric I created to combine the favorability and the correlation in one measure. The value of the number you see there in the Importance column has no absolute meaning — it simply allows a rank ordering of items.

So what is Figure 13-6 telling us? Clearly, when it comes to employee retention, there are some serious leadership issues that require some introspection, corrective action, and communication. These issues may be what is bleeding into employees' interest in recommending the company to others. The next most actionable item on the list has to do with career opportunity and clarity about possible career paths at the company. Finally, it wouldn't hurt to build up a greater sense of camaraderie and teamwork for the company mission.

REMEMBER

The items I just described, if improved or resolved, are more likely to have an impact than items near the bottom of the list. As good as the items on the bottom of the list may seem in general, putting focus there will just distract from the issues that our data show matter most.

To close out this section, I want to circle back and spell out how I calculated the Intent to Stay Importance figure. Figure 13-7 shows the formula I used in Excel's formula bar: =(F22*100)*(E22*100). Translating from Excel-speak to the language I've been using in this chapter, you multiply the correlation coefficient by the percent unfavorable — except both are fractions, so I have to convert them into whole numbers first by multiplying both sides by 100 before carrying out the operation

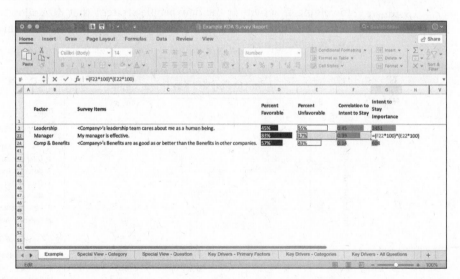

FIGURE 13-7:
How to calculate item "Importance".

Having a Look at KDA Output

Check out Figure 13-8, which shows you a typical key driver *quadrant*, the preferred method for displaying the output of a key driver analysis. This particular infographic allows you to see two intersecting information points: the correlation of a series of survey items to a chosen KPI (axis =x) and the average favorability of the company response (axis =y). Figure 13-8 also shows how you can divide survey items into three distinct categories:

» **Improve Weakness:** The high importance .37 and low favorability (35 out of 100) percent puts *Executive Communication* in the lower right quadrant of the KDA chart.

» **Leverage Great:** The high importance .39 and high favorability (89 out of 100) of *Pride in Company* can be seen in the upper right quadrant of the chart.

» **Disregard:** In other items on the survey, there is a range of favorable and unfavorable responses, but those items should be ignored because they aren't important — as they relate to Intent to stay.

REMEMBER

Broadly speaking, you want to explore a wide range of measures to uncover what is most important. (By *important*, I mean whatever influences a chosen objective outcome or KPI). Measuring your effort against influence of outcomes as opposed to volume of activity is the new people strategy that KDA allows. KDA helps you better understand where to focus your energy so that you can get the results you're looking for.

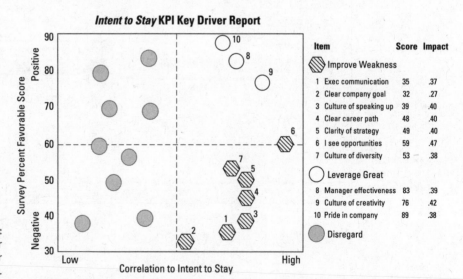

FIGURE 13-8:
Key driver quadrant for likelihood to exit.

Outlining Key Driver Analysis

OK, I've done my KDA for the day. Now it's your turn. Here's a step-by-step look at how you'd carry out your KDA:

1. **Decide what KPI you want to understand, predict, or drive**.

    Here are some examples:

    > What drives candidate attraction?
    >
    > What drives employee happiness?
    >
    > What drives employee engagement?
    >
    > What drives individual performance?
    >
    > What drives team performance?
    >
    > What drives employee commitment?
    >
    > What drives intent to stay or likelihood to exit?
    >
    > What drives employee retention or exit?

2. **Find or create a measure of what it is you want to understand, predict, or drive.**

    If it's an attitude like employee happiness, engagement, or commitment, you'll need to design a survey index. If it's something else —actual performance or exit, for example — you'll need to get that data from wherever it lives, probably in your human resources information system (HRIS).

3. **Go get the data.**

    Most KDA begins with a broad set of data collected from surveys that ask employees to express their level of agreement with a series of statements about different aspects of working for the company and attitudinal KPI measures such as satisfaction, commitment, and engagement. You can find sample survey categories and items in Appendix B.

4. **If it is not already in one dataset, bring all the data together in one dataset.**

5. **Bring the data into a statistical application (such as Minitab, R, SPSS, STATA, or STATISTICA) or Excel and run the Pearson Correlation procedure.**

6. **Correlate the response to each survey item and the KPI outcomes you want to change (increase or decrease) to derive the strength of relationship.**

The goal of correlation is to establish the strength of the relationships between potential drivers (attitudes and behaviors) and consequences (employee attrition, customer satisfaction, sales, or measures of organization citizenship and performance).

7. **Use the magnitude of the relationship to identify the factors that matter and the order in which they matter, based on the strength of the relationship.**

   You will use the correlation coefficient to plot and sort the data.

8. **While you're at it, calculate the average value or percentage of favorable responses of the measure by segment to identify the segments with the weakest measures.**

   When you analyze survey data, in some cases you may report the percentage of responses that are in a range you define as favorable. Hold on to this information, too — you will use it together with the correlation coefficient to plot and sort your data.

9. **Construct visual quadrants, models, and other tools to communicate the findings to others and plan actions to influence the intended outcomes.**

   To help you focus on those actions that will have the most impact, consider the relative strength of the relationship of each driver with key outcomes and the current level of company or segment performance on that driver.

Learning the Ins and Outs of Correlation

Whenever you first start working with a dataset, it's always helpful to first visualize the data you have so that you can see the shape of it. You can visualize data in many different ways. How you choose to do so depends on the data you're working with and the questions you're trying to answer. In key driver analysis, your objective is to understand key associations between two or more variables. Given that objective, I recommend using scatterplots to see the relationship between two variables. This section shows you how.

Visualizing associations

You can visualize the relationship between two variables by graphing them in a scatterplot. A scatterplot can be used to gain a first impression about whether a relationship exists between two variables and to observe the direction and strength of the relationship.

Figure 13-9 shows the relationship between an employee's engagement with a company and the perceived levels of support that employees feel they're getting from the company.

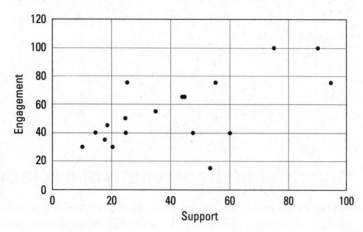

In Figure 13-9, each dot represents 1 of 183 people's summarized support-and-engagement index responses, which was captured on a multiple-question survey at the same time:

>> The horizontal axis (the *x-axis*) shows the employees' perception of support on an index from 0 to 100.

>> The vertical axis (the *y-axis*) shows the employees' engagement on an index from 0 to 100.

Figure 13-10 shows the same scatterplot with one arrow pointing to an individual with a 20 score on the Perceived Support index and a 30 score on the Engagement index (A) and another arrow pointing to an individual with a 58 score on the Perceived Support index and about an 80 score on the Engagement index (B).

As the perceptions of support increase, so does engagement: in other words, when x increases, y tends to increase; by this you can infer there is a positive correlation between the two pieces of data.

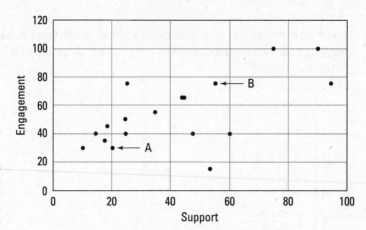

FIGURE 13-10:
Person A,
Support = 20;
Person B,
Support = 58.

Quantifying the strength of a relationship

You can numerically quantify the strength of a relationship between two measures by using something called the *Pearson product-moment correlation.* The result is a correlation coefficient that is represented by the symbol *r* (lowercase letter r). The correlation is used to quantify the association between any two measures. (For the purposes of this example, the measure I call *support* and the measure I call *engagement.*)

The correlation coefficient varies from an r of −1, which indicates a perfect negative correlation to 1, which means a perfect positive correlation. Figure 13-11 shows three examples of scatterplots that show a positive correlation, three scatterplots that show a negative correlation, and one scatterplot that shows no correlation whatsoever. (A correlation coefficient for no relationship would mean r = 0).

A *correlation* between two variables means that they move together. A correlation between two variables allows you to make a prediction about where one variable will be based on the location of the other. The further the correlation is from 1 or −1, the more error you have in predicting one variable based on the other.

Think about a couple who have been dancing together their whole lives. As one partner steps, the other knows where to go and vice versa. If the correlation is 1, the couple is moving in such a way they might as well be thought of as one and the same person. The further the correlation is from 1, the more chaotic their dance routine appears. They don't seem to go together at all.

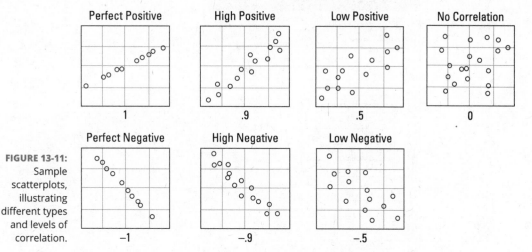

Correlations

Perfect Positive — 1

High Positive — .9

Low Positive — .5

No Correlation — 0

Perfect Negative — −1

High Negative — −.9

Low Negative — −.5

FIGURE 13-11: Sample scatterplots, illustrating different types and levels of correlation.

Computing correlation in Excel

When I was in college, we students had to compute correlations by hand — it took a lot of time, and it was prone to errors. Now people use software. Although you can find a number of affordable applications for statistics — Minitab, R, SPSS, and Stat Lab come to mind — often you can get by using only Excel. Computing a correlation coefficient with the help of the Pearson product–moment correlation is one of those times. Here's how to do it:

1. **Set up the data in rows and columns in Excel.**

Have one column for each variable and one column for the person ID. Each row should represent the same employee's data on two variables: support and engagement. Figure 13-12 shows a portion of the dataset. (You can see 21 people and the support and engagement scores for each person.)

TIP

Always use numerical ID's when working with data. If you ever want to bring in other data later or find some way back to check your facts, the ID will be instrumental. Sometimes people keep names in datasets, but names aren't as good as IDs, for a number of reasons — names are stored with variations, names change, two people can have the same name, and names are personal. People get uncomfortable with personal data associated with their personal name floating around on your computer. When I'm working with data, I want to be able to get back to the person if I need this to do my job, but I don't want my dataset to get personal or risk divulging anyone's personal secrets so I use IDs; you should too.

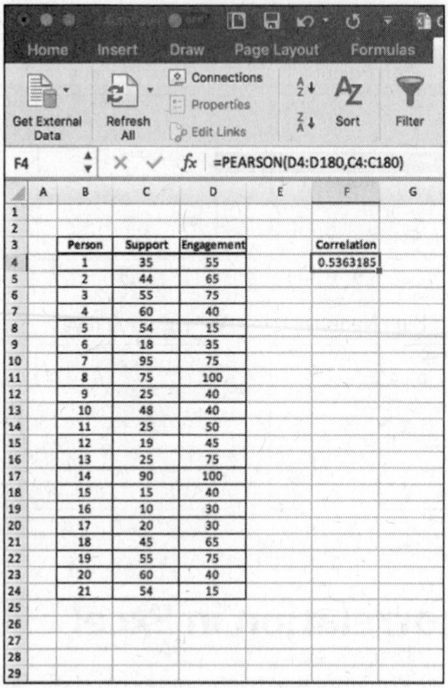

Person	Support	Engagement
1	35	55
2	44	65
3	55	75
4	60	40
5	54	15
6	18	35
7	95	75
8	75	100
9	25	40
10	48	40
11	25	50
12	19	45
13	25	75
14	90	100
15	15	40
16	10	30
17	20	30
18	45	65
19	55	75
20	60	40
21	54	15

FIGURE 13-12: Setting up the data in Excel to compute a correlation.

2. **In any cell, type** = PEARSON (
3. **Select all values for the first variable.**

   My data for support appears in column C, and the data goes from cell C4 to cell C24.

4. **Type a comma (,) and select all values for the second variable.**

   My data for engagement appears in column D, and the data goes from cell D4 to cell D24.

   Be sure to select the same number of values for both variables.

5. **Close the parenthesis and then press Enter to get the correlation.**

   The correlation for this data, between support and engagement, is .5363185. As the scatterplot back in Figure 13-9 showed, there's a positive correlation between support and engagement.

Interpreting the strength of a correlation

After you compute a correlation, you need to interpret the strength of the relationship. In other words, what does a correlation between support and engagement where r = .54 actually mean?

CORRELATION DOES NOT IMPLY CAUSALITY

You've probably heard the old saying "Correlation isn't causality." It means that just because one variable is correlated with another doesn't mean that one variable is caused by the other variable. In other words, just because you found two people at the scene of the crime doesn't mean that they're both guilty. There are various possibilities:

- The dark-haired guy is the criminal; the blonde is the victim.
- The blonde is the criminal; the dark-haired guy is the victim.
- Neither is guilty.
- Both are guilty.

It's an important part of the story that you found them at the scene of the crime together, but all parties are innocent until proven guilty.

It's not possible to determine a causal relationship with correlation alone. What correlation can do is help you see the association between the variables and point you in the right direction. To determine causation, you need other methods. See Chapter 16 to learn how to use experiments to determine causation.

Though correlations are context dependent, it can help to have some guidance on what you'll see. Researcher Jacob Cohen examined correlations in peer-reviewed behavioral science research and provided these guidelines:

>> Small: r = .10

>> Medium: r = .30

>> Large: r = .50

If you want a general guide for how to interpret a correlation coefficient, Cohen's schema is better than most.

Making associations between binary variables

Quite often in people analytics, you encounter binary data that takes the form of yes/no, high performer/other, sourced from university/other, stayer/leaver, minority/nonminority, and so on. It's possible to understand the association between binary variables just like you can understand the association between measures with bigger numbers; you just have to do it a little differently.

If you were predicting employee exit in the period 12 months from hire, for example, all employees can be classified as either meeting this condition or not, as in "Yes, they left the company in their first year" (1) or "No, they did not leave in their first year" (0). Of course, you wouldn't look at this by itself; you would also want to include other data to see how other conditions coincide. For the sake of a simple example, Figure 13-13 adds two additional prehire factors — College and Experienced — to the employee exit data. In each column example, if the candidate met the criteria, there's a (1); if not, there's a (0).

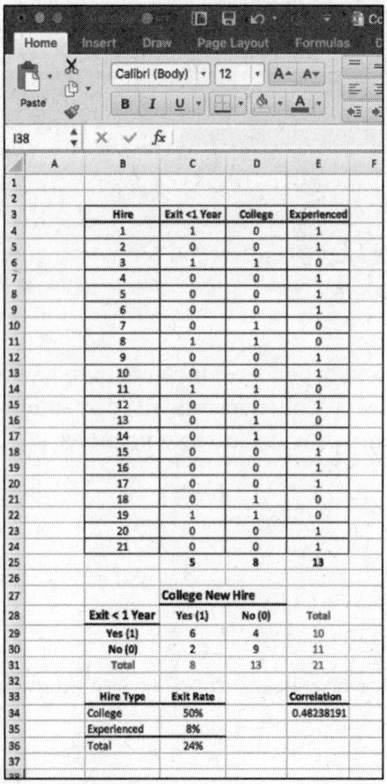

FIGURE 13-13: First-year exit and prehire characteristics.

Hire	Exit <1 Year	College	Experienced
1	1	0	1
2	0	0	1
3	1	1	0
4	0	0	1
5	0	0	1
6	0	0	1
7	0	1	0
8	1	1	0
9	0	0	1
10	0	0	1
11	1	1	0
12	0	0	1
13	0	1	0
14	0	1	0
15	0	0	1
16	0	0	1
17	0	0	1
18	0	1	0
19	1	1	0
20	0	0	1
21	0	0	1
	5	8	13

College New Hire

Exit < 1 Year	Yes (1)	No (0)	Total
Yes (1)	6	4	10
No (0)	2	9	11
Total	8	13	21

Hire Type	Exit Rate		Correlation
College	50%		0.48238191
Experienced	8%		
Total	24%		

The simplest way to analyze the association between all these variables is to leave your data in Figure 13-13 the way it is and ask Excel or your statistics application to calculate the Pearson product-moment correlation. You can interpret associations between binary numbers the same way you'd do with the Pearson correlation r for continuous variables.

To compute the association between any two characteristics or conditions the long way, follow these steps:

1. **Count the number of new hires who lasted the year and met the conditions for one of the other variables in cross-tab tables.**

   For example, in the following minitable, I have counted those new hires who exited the company in the first year *and* were hired from the college recruiting program and those who exited in the first year and were not so hired. I also calculated the same factors for those who didn't exit in the first year.

	College hire	
Exit	**Y (1)**	**N (0)**
Y (1)	6	4
N (0)	2	9

   Note where the a, b, c, and d are in this equation key:

	College hire	
Exit	**Y (1)**	**N (0)**
Y (1)	a	b

2. **To determine the correlation between two binary variables, use the numbers found in the first table, the key found in the second table, and the following formula:**

   $$\Phi = ad - bc \div \sqrt{(a+b)(c+d)(a+c)(b+d)}$$

   A correlation between binary variables is called *phi*, and it's represented by the Greek symbol Φ

   For this example, the computations would look like this:

   $$\Phi = 6(9) - (4)(2) \div \sqrt{(6+4)(2+9)(6+2)(4+9)}$$
   $$\Phi = 46 \div \sqrt{11,440} = .429$$

   In this case, the correlation between employees who exit in their first year and who were selected from the college recruiting program is .43.

Regressing to conclusions with least squares

Though there are many ways to draw lines through your data, the least squares analysis is a mathematical way that reduces the distance between the lines you draw and each dot in the scatterplot that serves as the basis for those lines. This analysis can be done by hand or by using popular statistics software such as Minitab, R, SAS, SPSS or by using Excel.

Figure 13-14 shows the least squares regression line from the scatterplot using the support data and engagement data from Figure 13-9.

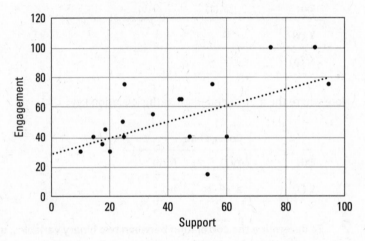

FIGURE 13-14: Least squares regression line.

The math, done by the software, can give you the equation to the regression line:

Engagement = .5395(Support) + 28.37

The regression equation takes the general form of $y = b_0 + b_1x + e$, where y is the predicted value of the dependent variable (engagement), b_0 (the *y-intercept*) is where the line would cross (or *intercept*) the y-axis, b_1 is the slope of the predicted line (how steep it is), X represents a particular value of the intendent variable (support), and e represents the inevitable error the prediction will contain.

In this example, the regression equation indicates that the predicted Engagement index is equal to $y = 28.37 + .5395$ times the support index.

Creating a regression equation in Excel

To create a regression equation using Excel, follow these steps:

1. **Insert a scatterplot graph into a blank space or sheet in an Excel file with your data.**

   You can find the scatterplot graph command on the Insert ribbon in Excel 2007 and later.

2. **Select the x-axis (horizontal) and y-axis (vertical) data and click OK.**

   Put what you want to predict in the y-axis. Engagement data is in column B, and support data is in column C. You now have a scatterplot.

3. **Right-click any of the dots on the scatterplot and select Add Trendline from the menu that appears.**

   The Format Trendline dialog box opens, as shown in Figure 13-15.

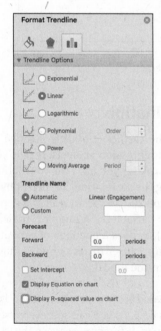

FIGURE 13-15:
Add the regression equation and r-squared value to the trendline.

4. **If necessary, click the arrow next to Trendline Options to open the submenu, and then select the Display Equation on Chart and Display R-Squared Value on Chart check boxes.**

   The Excel Add Trendline feature automatically defaults to Linear, which is good if you expect it to display a linear trendline against your data, which we do in this case. If you have some other expectations or want to experiment with non-linear forms, you can test the other options provided in the menu. (Don't worry, you won't break anything.)

You now have a scatterplot with a trendline, an equation, and an r-squared value, as shown in Figure 13-16. The regression equation is (as expected) y = .5395x + 28.37.

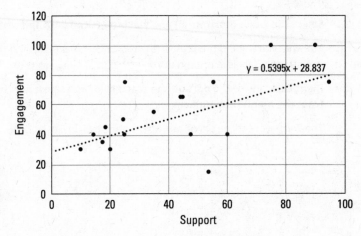

FIGURE 13-16: Scatterplot, regression line, and equation, computed in Excel.

r^2 : Coefficient of determination

r^2 ("r-squared"), also known as the *coefficient of determination*, is a calculated value that is a standard output from regression analysis. It tells you how well the best-fitting line actually fits the data. After you have the correlation coefficient, r, r^2 is calculated by simply multiplying the correlation coefficient by itself (squaring it). r^2 is interpreted as the proportion of the variance in the dependent variable that is explained by the independent variable(s). A higher r^2 indicates that differences in the independent variable(s), x, does a good job of explaining differences in the dependent variables(s) (y). An r^2 closer to zero implies that the outcome is unexplainable by the data included in the model.

For example, a correlation of r = .5 squared becomes .25. Note that r^2 is often expressed as a percentage — 25 percent, in this case. As you can see, even a strong correlation of above r = .5 still explains a minority of differences between the variables.

REMEMBER

A low r^2 likely indicates that you have missed important variables in your analysis, so it would suggest that you need to add new data or new survey items.

Though a high r^2 doesn't necessarily imply that you have measured everything that matters, it can tell you whether you have done a reasonable enough job to understand what is going on and make a decent prediction.

r^2 is used in the context of statistical models whose main purpose is either the prediction of future outcomes or the testing of hypotheses on the basis of other related information. It provides a measure of how well-observed outcomes are replicated by the model, based on the proportion of total variation of outcomes explained by the model. The equation takes predicted scores in a dataset and compares them to the actual scores. The coefficient of determinations is the square of these two.

Cautions

Watch out for the following three factors when correlating data:

>> **Range restriction:** Two variables might have a low correlation because you're measuring one of the variables in a narrower range than the other.

>> **The missing "third variable" problem:** It's often the case that another variable you aren't measuring at all is actually influencing several of the variables you are measuring to move together. The two variables you are measuring appear to be related or causing each other to move but in reality the third missing variable is what is more important. For example, crime statistics appear to be associated with ice cream consumption statistics. Before you board up the local ice cream shop, it may help to pay mind to the fact that both crime and ice cream consumption are associated to a missing third variable temperature: there is more crime in the summer. There may even be a fourth missing variable — free time of youth. This is not a book on criminology, so I will leave this to the criminologists to decide.

>> **Nonlinearity:** The relationship between variables needs to be linear — that is, it needs to follow a line somewhat. If the relationship curves downward or upward, a linear correlation or regression equation will not properly describe the relationship

Improving Your Key Driver Analysis Chops

So you have completed your first key driver analysis. Now what? Prepare to make your next one even better. Here are some ways you can make your next KDA even better:

>> **Remove items that are redundant.** Remove any items that correlate with any other item above .70 and share the same mean or percent of favorable responses.

For example, in the survey I used above, we asked employees about leadership and management in a lot of different ways. We had aspirations for specificity, but it turned out employees didn't care about the nuances. Employees simply agreed or disagreed with those statements the same way. They think the manager is good, or they don't. You are going to have to get the nuances in another way. That being the case, why ask a question in ten different ways if two would do? Feel free to remove eight.

>> **Apply multiple regression**. It's a similar idea to correlation but uses a different method. If you are not familiar with multiple regression yet, visit Chapter 14 in this book. Here is brief intro to what I'm asking you to do:

Multiple regression analysis works by examining the correlations between many x variable inputs (survey items) and one KPI (y) to identify the best combination of survey items and the relative contribution of each item to explain the selected KPI.

The idea behind multiple regression is that it provides a calculated output measure that tells you how well all of the combined x variables (call this your model) predict the y variable – calculated by adjusted r^2 and/or F statistic (sometimes called Significance F). The adjusted r^2 gives you the proportion of variance explained by your model which provides a rough indication how far you are on your journey to understand the KPI. If you have only explained 10% of the variance in y with your model, you still have a lot more work to do on your model. (You can improve your model by revising your theory and adding more survey items.) On the other hand, if you've already explained 60% or more of the variance in your KPI, then your model is doing a really good job and you might consider telling everyone this.

Last but not least, the output of multiple regression tells you how much each x contributed to your understanding of the KPI (on a relative basis) and whether or not you can be confident in the magnitude of each x variables' contribution to the KPI. Multiple regression puts all this in a neat little table for you called the *coefficients table*.

Again, you can learn more about multiple regression analysis in Chapter 14. For now, the takeaway is that you want to see whether or not each survey item is statistically significant — you want to know the p-statistic (also known as the p-value). After you have completed a multiple regression. you should replace the correlation coefficient you were using above (represented by lowercase r in correlation) with the coefficients (represented by the lowercase b) from the multiple regression coefficients table.

To make a long story short, the results from your multiple regression analysis give you an opportunity to remove any items that turn out to be not as significant as you thought they were. Now you can remove any items the multiple regression shows you are not statistically significant and at the same time replace the correlation coefficient you were using (lowercase r) with a better one (lowercase b).

Revise your theoretical model and begin to create new items to add to your next survey. Consider that, if there are a thousand possible items you could add to your survey, and the first time you ran the survey you picked 50 items, then there are 950 chances you missed an item that would have been better to include on the survey.

How do you know if you have the right items? Well, what we learned in this chapter is that the best set of items depends on the KPI you have selected, so first you need to get that in order. You have measured the KPI and you have done a KDA. The adjusted R^2 of your multiple regression analysis provides a clue if you have missed an important factor or two The larger the adjusted R^2, the closer you are to retirement. The smaller, back to the drawing board.

How do you get the right items? The ideas about what items should or should not be included on the survey reflect views that may or may not be accurate. The common assumptions about what items should be measured on surveys may or may not help the company get to the outcomes you or the leaders you support want in the end. Whether censoring of survey items is of the intentional or unintentional variety, the selection of survey items produces a bias that gets relayed into the survey analysis and into any downstream analysis that follows. Others will see things you didn't and vice versa. In one individual may, and often will, be wrong. The way you get it right is through trial and error, guided by theory, which should be made clear with a visual model and discussed with others. I encourage you to check out Chapter 10 for more on models; my discussion there might inspire you beyond the brief words I have here.

Chapter **14**

Modeling HR Data with Multiple Regression Analysis

I f you were going on a great adventure to a place where nobody had ever been before you and you could bring along one thing, what would you bring? I don't know what you would choose, but if I could only bring one thing, I'd bring *multiple regression*, a form of linear regression that is used to explain the relationship between one continuous dependent variable (Y) and two or more independent variables (x1, x2, x3 . . .).

Why put so much faith in multiple regression? Well, if people analytics is this great journey to the unknown and you need to travel light, then multiple regression is a great tool to put in your backpack. It is the machete for the jungle, the life vest for the ocean, and the fire starter for the North Pole. It may not be the only thing you need to survive in the wild, but once you get familiar with it, you will want to sleep with it close by your side at night.

Taking Baby Steps with Linear Regression

When it comes to the analysis of people, multiple regression is (in the right hands) a superior weapon to nearly all others. Multiple regression is an incredibly versatile statistical tool with a number of important advantages, not the least of which is the ability to see the influence of one variable on another variable while controlling for the influence of many other variables at the same time. People are complex and so seldom can the behavior of people be explained sufficiently by only two variables at once (x and y).

I'll start this chapter with a simple two variable regression. Why? Well, if you were to boil all linear analysis down to its essence, multiple regression analysis included, there are a few important things you need to understand, and a simple two variable linear regression will make these important things easier to see. Once you understand these important things, then you can move on to multiple regression. You must master fighting one ninja first, before you can fight 12 of them at once.

If you could stare into the distance ahead of you and calculate the movement of two ninjas swinging their swords at the same time, you could then see a number in your mind's eye that represented the exact location of each sword, which would allow you to plot the numerical intersection of the location of both swords over time on a graph, so you could then carefully draw the best line you could between all the plots you just created to try to see if the two swords are moving together — if you did all that, then you'd have the outline of a basic linear regression analysis. Maybe I am being too poetic. See Figure 14-1 to see what I described in my mind's eye in terms of a problem more suitable for people analytics.

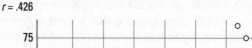

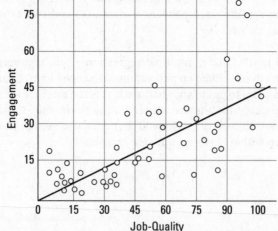

FIGURE 14-1: A graph of the correlation between employee engagement and job quality.

It can be described visually, as it is in Figure 14-1, or it can be described as an equation: $y = b_0 + b_1(x)$, where y represents the numbers on the vertical axis and x represents the numbers on the horizontal axis. As for b_0, that's the mathematically derived *y intercept* for the line formed from your plots — the point where your plotted line crosses the vertical axis. b_1 represents the mathematical *slope* of the line. Slope is just like a hill. Some hills are steeper than others and you have to go up or down depending on where you are starting from and where you are going. Visually, you see the angle of the hill (slope) on the page by travelling with your eyes from left to right. The way you see slope mathematically is to calculate the unit change in the y variable for each one unit change in the x variable. Remember you were watching those ninjas' swords move at the same time. The line is your visual summary of their joint movement, and the foundation for this particular mathematics. Recall we called it linear regression. Linear means line. Now you basically have it!

If the two things you had observed in the wild were not ninjas, but rather {job quality} and {engagement} (as shown in Figure 14-1) and you had followed the procedure I just described, you would end up with {engagement} = $b_0 + b_1$({job-quality}). The intercept, b_0 would be a number, as would b_1. To predict where engagement is at an any time, you just need to know where job-quality is and multiply job quality by the number preserved in the location of b_1 and add it to the number recorded in the location of b_0. Written as a shorthand mathematical expression, the information you went through all this effort to record becomes lighter to carry around and easier either to transfer to others or to use on your own at some later date.

REMEMBER

In the not-so-distant past, instructors or students would sit down with a sheet of paper and calculate the linear regression. Fortunately, you don't have to do that anymore; you have your trusty friend Excel or a statistics application that can calculate the linear regression for you. I bring up the graphs and the lines and a little of the math because it's helpful to know what you're trying to achieve and how it connects to the outside world so that you have a better grasp of what it all means when the statistical application spits things out.

The example I mention shows the relationship between a variable I call {Job-Quality} and one I call {Engagement} — a 2-variable linear regression, in other words. Whether your understanding of this relationship is useful depends on what you are trying to do, but before you do anything, you had to first be able to describe the relationship mathematically. If you now know the way {Engagement}and {Job-Quality} move together, you have a clue for how they work. Assume you want to move {Engagement}, your next task might be to do something to try to get {Job-Quality} to move and then see what happens to {Engagement}.

What if you knew more than just {Job-Quality} for each employee? What if you also measured what each employee has observed about her manager — {Manager-Quality}, in other words — and you also have measured what employees think about the Company {Company-Quality}? You can use that information also! If you can combine {Manager-Quality}, {Company-Quality}, and {Job-Quality} in a mathematical equation, you might have a more accurate appreciation for the location of {Engagement} than if you used the {Job-Quality} score alone. You could think of {Company-Quality} and {Job-Quality}as tools to help you predict or explain the location of {Engagement}. You won't know there is causal relationship just yet, but you can learn enough to know how they move together and go from there.

When you work with more than one independent variable, it's called *multiple regression*. If linear regression is your basic everyday knife, then multiple regression is a Swiss army knife — a utility knife made with a bunch of different blades for different situations, scissors, and maybe a toothpick, too. In multiple regression, as in linear regression, you find multiple b0 coefficients — just like you did above in the simple two ninja scenario — only now you can get the coordinates for as many of the ninjas as you want at the same time. With many independent variables, however, my visual tool breaks down because I can't show you scatterplots in so many dimensions at the same time on a two-dimensional piece of paper. The simple example I have provided requires four dimensions. I can't even imagine what that kind of ugliness would look like if I tried to draw it. So, because no one can draw persuasively in four dimensions, the convention developed by those ancient people who paid a lot for paper is to just dispense with the drawings and stick to the math instead. This way, all you need to do is write a brief equation down:

$$y' = a + b1(x1) + b2(x2) + bn(xn) \ldots$$

For the current example, the outline of the equation is

Predicted {Engagement} = a + b1{Job-Quality} + b2{Company-Quality} + b3 {Manager-Quality}.

You can measure the overall fit and measure of each of the variable's coefficients. (Coefficient is the word used to represent the funny letter/number combinations (b1, b2, b3) that stand for the multipliers used for the variables to get the unit change in the predicted {engagement} score.) I won't go through all of the mathematics for finding the coefficients in the multiple regression equation, because that gets unnecessarily boring and complicated. (I will tell you, though, that the letter b here stands for *beta* or *beta-weight*.) Instead, I go right to how to get the answers you want using either Excel or any statistics application.

Here are a few things to keep in mind before you proceed:

>> You can have any number of x-variables. I use four in my example just to keep it to a handful of columns.

>> Basic linear regression and multiple regression are built on certain important assumptions. Assumptions can feel like drudgery, but if they're broken, you get the wrong answers. I start things off in this chapter with the useful and fun "how-to" part of multiple regression, but if you have not taken a college course in statistics and if this is the first time you are using regression yourself, you should seek the counsel of a data scientist, a behavioral scientist, or a mathematics professional with a 4 to 8-year college degree that included several years of college level statistics to put you on the right path, provide advice, and certify your results.

Mastering Multiple Regression Analysis: The Bird's-Eye View

After you have constructed a dataset that includes all the variables you want to test, you can carry out the multiple regression in any statistical program (such as R, SPSS, SAS, Stata, STATISTICA) or even in Excel.

Before diving into the details of the menus native to any specific application, here's a high-level overview of how to do a multiple regression:

1. **Identify the independent variables you want to include in your model for whatever dependent variable you want to understand or predict.**

   In the example, I want you to understand the relationship between the perception of certain key employment features that I think matter and a measure of employee engagement.

2. **Use employee systems and/or surveys to collect information as quantitative measurements (data).**

   If you already have those measurements stored somewhere, "unstore" them. Do it now.

3. **Bring the data together, import it into R, SPSS, SAS, Stata, STATISTICA, Excel, or whatever other program you choose, and then select the appropriate regression procedure based on the nature of the dependent variable.**

Point the application to the dataset and tell it to go, in other words.

The application spits out some summary tables as output, including tables indicating the statistical significance of not only the overall combination of independent variables at explaining the dependent variable but also the statistical significance and magnitude of the contribution of each included independent variable.

These outputs are just like correlation coefficients, except for the fact that, unlike correlation coefficients, these *beta* coefficients (remember we talked earlier about b0, b1, b2, b3. . .) take into consideration the other variables, so they represent the independent effect of each variable in the model.

4. **After you're confident that the model works, use the beta coefficients to construct mathematical models, perceptual models, and other conceptual tools that are useful to communicate the results of your analysis to others and work with them to plan your next actions.**

It's just that simple. Well, close. Below I show you how to do this in 10 steps in Excel. Microsoft adds a few steps. Now, maybe you are the type of person who has no interest in ever doing a multiple regression in your life and in particular not in Excel. Well, that's OK. One reason why I included this chapter is so that you can see that some of the most complex people analytics anyone will ever tell you about can be performed in 4 to 10 easy steps that probably take about 5 minutes total to do in a desktop application most people have already have that costs less than $150 dollars per year. How about them apples?

After the simplicity of all this sinks in, you might be wondering, "What sort of charade am I missing here? This is it? Is this a secret to a better work life balance? Those sneaky nerds were holding out on us! What could they possibly be doing with all their time?"

Before you totally lose it, let me try to explain. The real work of people analytics is defining the problem to be solved, determine what questions when answered will shed light on the problem in question, formulate a model of what concepts you think matter, devise a way to get data to measure those specific concepts and then get it all together in one file that you can apply statistics to — only then do you get to hit Go. All the work I mention has to occur before you can even get the data into Excel (or the statistics application). The real work of people analytics is in the setting up of the data and the explanation of the result, and therefore I aim to spend a majority of my time in this book concentrating on those topics.

Multiple regression is one of the options in Excel's Analysis ToolPak add-in, but not all versions of Excel have this capability. Excel is great for accessibility and transparency in working with data, but it does lack some of the robust features included in other statistics packages. For example, the regression option in Excel can handle multiple regressions with continuous dependent variables, but it doesn't offer support for the logistic regression procedure, which is necessary for dependent variables that are binary (1,0), such as employee exit. If you were to use binary logistic regression to analyze what variables relate to employee attrition, you would make Exit your dependent variable, classifying all employees as 1 or 0. 1 = exited and 0 = didn't, or vice versa). You might be able to get by using Excel for a time, but if you're a doing a lot of work with statistics, you'll eventually need to acquire another statistical application to "up your game."

Doing a Multiple Regression in Excel

Though I like to do my more advanced statistical work in more advanced statistical applications, in this section I show how to do a multiple regression in Excel because . . . well, because I'm pretty sure you have Excel and I'm not sure you have any of the more sophisticated applications.

In any event, here's what you would need to do in Excel:

1. **Put the data you want to work with into a single Excel worksheet and label the columns with the variable names you want to use.**

   Figure 14-2 shows what such a worksheet would look like, using the {Engagement}, {Job-Quality}, {Company-Quality), and {Manager-Quality} variables.

2. **If you haven't already added the Analysis ToolPak, start by choosing Excel Add-ins from the Tools menu.**

3. **In the Add-ins dialog box that appears, select the Analysis ToolPak check box and then click OK.**

4. **Click the Ribbon's Data tab.**

   You should now see the Data Analysis button on the Ribbon's far right end. (You can also find the Data Analysis option on the Tools menu.)

5. **Select the Tool menu's Data Analysis command or click its button on the Data tab to open the Data Analysis dialog box, shown in Figure 14-3.**

6. **When Excel displays the Data Analysis dialog box, scroll through the Analysis Tools list, select Regression, and then click OK.**

   Doing so opens the Regression dialog box, shown in Figure 14-4.

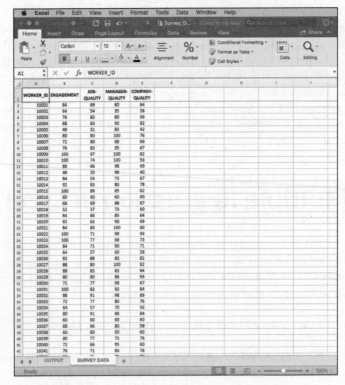

FIGURE 14-2: The {Engagement}, {Job-Quality}, {Company-Quality}, and {Manager-Quality} dataset in Excel.

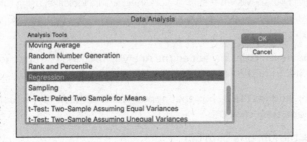

FIGURE 14-3: Excel displays the Data Analysis dialog box.

7. **After identifying the y and x values, use the Input Y Range text box to specify the worksheet range holding the dependent variables, and then use the Input X Range text box to identify the worksheet range reference holding the independent variables.**

TIP

If you include the variable names in the column headings and these column headings are part of the range of observations you have already specified, be sure to select the Labels check box.

8. **(Optional) Click any additional options in the dialog box that you want Excel to provide in the Regression output.**

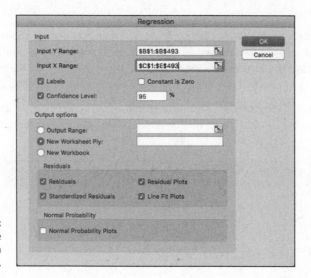

FIGURE 14-4:
Excel displays the
Regression
dialog box.

For example, if you know what you are doing with this, you can select the Confidence Level check box and enter a value, then Excel will automatically calculate the corresponding confidence level for you based on what you have entered. If you don't know what an option is or why you would fool with it, then ignore the option and proceed with the default.

9. **In the Output Options section, select a location for the regression analysis results.**

I usually just stick with the default here — New Worksheet Ply — which puts the results on a new page.

10. **Give the entire regression dialog box a quick inspection to make sure you caught all of the output options you want and when you are ready for the magic to happen, click OK.**

The Excel Regression Analysis tool automatically provides a range of summary statistics from multiple regression. Figure 14-5 shows the output of the Excel Regression Analysis tool when applied to the sample dataset.

Don't let some of these more obscure terms scare you. I provide more details on the definitions of these words and their use in the following section.

The Regression Statistics table includes the Multiple R stats, R-Squared stats, Standard Error stats, and Observations stats.

The analysis of variance (ANOVA) table includes information about the degrees of freedom, sum-of-squares value, mean square value, f-value, and significance of F.

Beneath the ANOVA table, the coefficients table supplies information about the regression line calculated from the data, including the coefficient, standard error, t-stat, and probability values (p-values) for the intercept — as well as the same information for the independent variable.

If you selected scatter charts options in the Regression dialog box, Excel also plots out some of the regression data using simple scatter graphs.

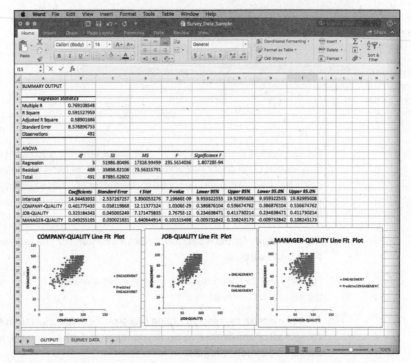

FIGURE 14-5:
Output of the Excel Regression tool.

Interpreting the Summary Output of a Multiple Regression

As I explain earlier in this chapter, multiple regression is used to understand how multiple independent variables (x1, x2, x3, . . .) are statistically related to one dependent variable (y) and to what degree. This powerful statistical tool is capable of helping you do several things at once:

>> Mathematically describe the form of the relationships between multiple variables (x1, x2, x3, . . .) and (y)

>> Mathematically determine how good the overall model is at explaining or predicting the behavior of (y)

>> Mathematically isolate the independent contribution of each variable (x1, x2, x3, . . .) to the total variance in (y)

That's what we are going for, but some of the terminology used to explain the results of multiple regression can be intimidating. To lower the intimidation level, in this section I walk you through what you can expect from a standard multiple regression output summary by defining some of the terminology and explaining some of the logic.

Regression statistics

The first thing you see in Excel output for multiple regression is the table with the header Regression Statistics. This table gives you the big picture about your analysis. Practically speaking, it allows you to answer questions such as, "How good is my model?" In more detail, it answers, "What percentage in the variation in Y is explained by the many x variables that were included in the analysis?"

Multiple R

Right off the bat, the first thing you see in the top row under Regression Statistics is Multiple R. No, this is not the introduction to a story with two pirates greeting each other. Big picture, Multiple R is telling you how good this dataset you have created is at doing its job. Technically, Multiple R is the absolute value of the correlation coefficient — basically, the correlation coefficient without the negative sign. Good pirates are never negative!

REMEMBER

A correlation coefficient is a measure of how closely two variables move in tandem with each other. In this case, the two variables that are being correlated are a) the location of the model's regression line (the line Excel drew through all the dots on the graph) compared to b) the dots Excel used to position the line. Correlation coefficients range from –1 to +1, but since Multiple R is the absolute value of the correlation coefficient, it can only range from 0 to 1. The correlation coefficient is also referred to as the Pearson correlation coefficient or Pearson's r.

The Multiple R in the case of our example, .769, indicates that our model including the variables {Company-Quality}, {Job-Quality}, and {Manager-Quality} does a good job creating a linear equation that correlates with {Engagement}. You know this because it is close to 1, which would be perfect.

R-Square

R-Squared, or R², for short (Excel, for reasons unclear to anyone, calls it "R-Square.") is sort of like the story of Santa Claus — he may be dressed differently in different places, but what he does for children is pretty much the same everywhere. R-Square, R-Squared, Coefficient of Determining, R², and Multiple R-Squared, it doesn't matter; they all mean the same thing.

R^2 is a calculated variable that indicates the proportion of variance in the dependent variable y that is explained by the x variables (x1, x2, x3, . . .). Another way of putting it is that R^2 tells you how good you would be at predicting the location of y if you know the location of the x variables. Yet another way of saying it is that R^2 indicates the percentage variation in y that is explained by the x variables. Like Multiple R, the calculated values in R^2 ranges between 0 and 1. In fact, as the name suggests, R^2 is equal to the square of Multiple R — meaning R^2 is equal to Multiple R multiplied by Multiple R. "Arr!", the pirates say.

Coming back to our example, we know that a unit change in {Engagement} will be influenced by a variety of factors, including: the job, the company, the manager, peers, pay, and maybe other things. If we knew everything that influenced {Engagement}, the R^2 would be 1, meaning if we have all the x variables that matter, we can predict the value of {Engagement} perfectly with no missing variance or error. In our example, we don't know everything that matters yet; we just know three things: {Company-Quality}, {Job-Quality}, and {Manager-Quality}. The R^2 is telling us that when these three variables are combined together in a model, they can explain roughly 60% (.59) of the variance in {Engagement}. The other 40% left behind is error or things we don't know yet that matter.

REMEMBER

R^2 ranges from between 0 and 1 — the closer R^2 is to 1, the better the x variables are at predicting the y variable. You can also say that R^2 represents the percentage of variance in y explained by the x's included in your dataset. What you consider to be a "good" R^2 will vary depending on context, but you can always say that .30 is better than zero, .50 is better than .30, .70 is better than .50, and so on.

If the R^2 value is an abstract calculated value, you can also look at the ANOVA table, which is another output of multiple regression produced by most statistics applications. Like R^2, the ANOVA table also provides statistics on the performance of the xy predictions made within a particular dataset. I tell you more about ANOVA in the later section, "Analysis of variance (ANOVA)."

Adjusted R-square

Adjusted R-square is a calculated value unique to multiple regression. When you have more than one x variable in your analysis, the computation process inflates the calculated R² accidentally. *Adjusted R-square* is an adjusted version of R² that removes the accidental inflation created by the number of variables added to the model. The adjusted R-square increases only if the new term improves the model more than would be expected by chance. It decreases when a predictor improves the model by less than expected by chance.

Going back to our example, the *Adjusted R-square* is .589, which is very close to the R² value of .591, showing there was an insubstantial amount of accidental inflation created by the number of variables in the model. Recall we only used three variables. If we added 97 other variables, the R² may be higher than it should be just by chance, inflating the R². The Adjusted R-square removes this inflation problem and so it is better to use. The statistical output provides both so you can see what is going on and then fiddle with your dataset inputs and run again if you want or need to.

Standard Error

You can find the standard error in the summary, right under *Adjusted R-square*. Standard error can also be designated simply by the letter S. Both *Adjusted R-square* and S provide an overall measure of how well the model works, but S provides the point of view of the error. S represents the average distance that the observed y values fall from the regression line or, in short, the average error of all the individual y predictions made by the model. Conveniently, S tells you how wrong the regression model is, on average, using the units of the y variable. Smaller values are better because they indicate that the real y observations are closer to the fitted line, which represents the y prediction.

In our example, as shown in Figure 14-5, the S of our prediction of {Engagement} is 8.58, meaning that each time we use a person's measures of {Company-Quality}, {Job-Quality}, and {Manager-Quality} to predict their level of {Engagement}, we are on average off by 8.6 units of {Engagement}. We measured {Engagement} on a scale of 0 to 100, so on average our prediction is off by about 9%. Some of our guesses are high, some are low, and some are right on what we would expect, but on average we are only off by about 9 units. So, if we used the three variables we know to estimate that a person's likely {Engagement} score is 70, then we are very confident their real {Engagement} score is somewhere between 61 and 79. The better our model is, the closer this range will get to the real value.

Analysis of variance (ANOVA)

In the Excel regression output, below the Regression Statistics table you find the ANOVA table next. This table gives you yet another way to think about how well the x variables you selected to be in your multiple regression model worked to explain the y variable. The analysis of variance table provides the breakdown of the total variation of the y variable (across all the individual observations in your dataset) in explained and unexplained portions.

The sum of squares regression (SS Regression) is the variation explained by the regression line; the sum of squares residual (SS Residual) is the variation of the dependent variable that is not explained.

REMEMBER

Most of the ANOVA table is firmly out there in the weeds of statistics. For your purposes, you probably don't need to know all the details. What I want you to look out for in an ANOVA table is the Significance F on the far upper right of the table. This is the summary of the entire analysis of variance in your model.

Significance F

You see Significance F to the far right in the ANOVA table; beneath this header is a calculated value. The simplest way to understand the meaning of the calculated value is to think of it as the probability that your regression model is wrong and needs to be discarded. You want the Significance F to be as small as possible. (Look carefully, because Excel uses scientific notation if the value is so large or small it exceeds 12 decimal points. If the number is less than zero, there is a minus sign before the exponent)

You can see in the example in Figure 14-5 that the Significance F is so small that Excel had to use scientific notation (1.80728E-94). The scientific notation is telling you the decimal point should be 94 places to the left of 1.8. Like this: .00000000000, . . . OK, I'll stop there. For all intents and purposes, this extremely small Significance F number indicates that the probability the result is wrong and needs to be discarded is pretty much zero. This is the part of the story where if you have been working on a model for months, you can get out the bottle of champagne. Go ahead, give a glass to each of your co-workers and your boss and make a toast.

Technically speaking, the Significance F is the probability that the *null hypothesis* can be rejected. The null hypothesis is a funny little game professors of statistics play on students to keep them on their toes. The null hypothesis is a default position that there is no relationship between the x variables and the y variable. Since in the example the probability that there is no relationship is extremely small, you can say that the model is statistically significant.

REMEMBER

Significance F is similar in interpretation to p-values, discussed in the next section. The difference is that the Significance F is the significance test of the entire model as a whole, whereas the p-value is the significance test of each variable at a time.

I am so excited about our model's significance that I'm not going to bother with anything else in the ANOVA table — I'm going to take you right down to the Coefficients table.

Coefficients Table

As you proceed through the summary, eventually you find a table that provides summary statistics on each x variable you have included in the multiple regression model. (If you used column labels for variables, you see these names as part of the table.) The coefficients table will tell you what x variables you have included in your model are statistically significant and will also tell you what independent impact they have on the y variable, while controlling for impact of other variables in your model.

As is to be expected, you will have multiple x variables in your multiple regression equation. (That's why it's called *multiple*.)

Recall the basic mathematical form of the multiple linear regression model is $y = a + b_1(x_1) + b_2(x_2) + b_3(x_3)$ . . . In the coefficients table you will find the intercept value corresponds to the a in the regression equation. You also will find the coefficient values that correspond to the b values for each x variable. If you plug in the numerical values you want or expect for each x at a point in the future into the regression equation and then do the algebra, it outputs a single number that represents the predicted future y.

The first summary statistic to look at is the coefficient. This can be found in the second column. After the Intercept value, there will be a value for each variable you have included in your model. The value found represents the unit change in the y variable from each unit change in the x variable. The larger the value in the coefficient column, the more a unit change in x will impact y. Therefore, the relative value of each x variable coefficient represents the relative impact each x variable has on the y variable compared to all the other x variables. You can rank order the x variables impact on y by their coefficient value.

REMEMBER

Everything I have stated just now about the coeffients assumes all the variables you are comparing are statistically significant. If a variable is not statistically significant, the magnitude of the coefficient does not matter. If a variable is not statistically significant, you should ignore it or remove it from your model.

A unique feature of the resulting multiple regression equation is that it can be used to predict things. After running a multiple regression analysis, you can use the x coefficients' output in a formula to predict how much a change to each x variable will likely affect the y. For the purpose of predicting y given x inputs, if you know what x variables (x_1, x_2, x_3, . . .) are significant, you can create an equation using regression coefficients (b1, b2, b3, . . .) corresponding to those X variables. After you have those details, you can simply plug the x variable data you have into the equation to make a y variable prediction.

Knowing which x variables are statistically significant

To determine which x variables are statistically significant, you should look at the p-value column. p-values are just like the F statistic I describe earlier in the chapter, except p-values reflect the statistical significance level of each variable separately, whereas the F statistic represents the statistical significance of the entire model. The p-value tells you the probability that the estimated coefficient is wrong. p-values range between 0 and 1. You want the p-value to be as small as possible because you want to keep the probability of being wrong as low as possible. Usually I consider a p-value to be statistically significant if it is less than .05 — this corresponds to a 95% confidence that the coefficient is not a result of chance. Situationally, you may decide to use some other cutoff —.1 or .01, for example — depending on how much risk you want to take based on what you are analyzing.

REMEMBER

The p-values represents each variable's *statistical* significance; whether or not the variable has any *practical* significance can be assessed by the coefficient value. The larger the coefficient, relative to other coefficients, the more a change in the x value corresponds to a change in the y value — and therefore the more practically significant it is. However, a large coefficient that is not also statistically significant should be ignored entirely because the lack of statistical significance indicates it is most likely a result of chance. In other words, bigger is not necessarily better; bigger and significant is better.

Determining what a specific correlation table can tell you

Looking back at Figure 14-5, what the multiple regression model indicates is that {Engagement} is dependent on {Company-Quality} and {Job-Quality}, while {Manager-Quality} did not have a significant impact.

If an employee has rated {Company-Quality} 50 and{Job-Quality} 50, then you can expect that employee to have an {Engagement} score of 53.94. ({Engagement} = 14.94 + .46 (50) + .32 (50))

If another employee has rated {Company-Quality} 100 and{Job-Quality} 100 then you can expect that employee to have an {Engagement} score of 92.94. ({Engagement} = 14.94 + .46 (100) + .32 (100))

If yet another employee has rated {Company-Quality} 90 and {Job-Quality} 40 then you can expect that employee to have an {Engagement} score of 69.14. ({Engagement} = 14.94 + .46 (90) + .32 (40))

Interpreting specific intercepts

The intercept of 14.94 indicates that {Engagement} will be 14.94 if an employee rates both {Company-Quality} and {Job-Quality} a zero. This is arrived at because when {Company-Quality} and {Job-Quality} are zero, their relative contribution is zero because each of the coefficient values is multiplied by zero, leaving only your intercept value of 14.94. If you drew the line for the linear equation {Engagement} = 14.94 + .46{Company-Quality} + .32{Job-Quality} then 14.94 is where the line would touch the y axis.

Interpreting specific coefficients

The coefficient .46 for {Company-Quality} indicates that every unit increase in {Company-Quality} increases {Engagement} by .46 units.

The coefficient .32 for {Job-Quality} indicates that every unit increase in {Job-Quality} increases {Engagement} by .32 units.

In the example of Figure 14-5, both statistically significant coeffients have positive values. In theory, a coefficient could have a negative value and that would mean something different. If the coefficient of the variable is negative, for every unit increase in the x variable, the {Engagement} will decrease by the value of the coefficient.

We have only three x variables in our example. If you had 20 variables in your multiple regression model, then the coefficient table would be larger, and you would see a coefficient value for every x variable in the multiple regression output. The interpretation of these coefficients will be the same.

Interpreting specific p-values

Recall, the value for the p-values is the probability that the corresponding coefficient of the x variable is not reliable; it could be zero.

{Company-Quality} has a p-value of 1.0306E-29, which is scientific notation for a very small number. Since this is scientific notation and you see the negative sign after the E, you know your decimal will move to the left the number of decimal places you find after the E. Since this very small number is less than .05 (my cutoff for statistical significance) you can reject the null hypothesis that {Company-Quality} has no impact on {Engagement}. Basically, {Company-Quality} is statistically significant.

{Job-Quality} has a p-value of 2.7675E-12, which is scientific notation for another very small number. Since this very small number is less than .05, you can reject the null hypothesis that {Job-Quality} has no impact on {Engagement}. Basically, {Job-Quality} is statistically significant.

{Manager-Quality}, on the other hand, has a p-value of .101, which is not less than .05 so you cannot reject the null hypothesis that {Manager-Quality} has no impact on {Engagement}. Basically, {Manager-Quality} is not statistically significant. This is why I excluded it from the rest of the conversation above.

Moving from Excel to a Statistics Application

You just learned how to run a multiple linear regression in Microsoft Excel! I don't know what you think about that, but I think that is pretty great that you can do something this advanced in Excel.

The upsides of Excel for statistics are that it is inexpensive, you probably already have it, there is a plethora of help for it that you can easily find online, and if you are doing other work in Excel already, it may provide a comfortable transition for you.

The downsides of Excel for statistics are that it doesn't have all of the statistical methods you may want to apply, and Excel doesn't have as many built-in functions and nifty tools designed for statistics that applications built for statistics do. Frankly, Excel is bare bones compared to other desktop applications built for statistics.

I suggest you try to use Excel for as long as you can, and only purchase a real statistics package when you exceed the capabilities of Excel for what you are trying to achieve. An example of a statistical procedure you may want to try that isn't supported by Excel is a *logistic regression*. A logistic regression is what you would use to analyze or predict a *binary outcome* — an either/or outcome, like whether someone will stay or leave over the course of the next year. You won't find a logistic regression option in Excel, but you can find it in almost any current statistics application, like R, SPSS, SAS, Stata, or JMP. Because you already learned how to do a multiple linear regression in Excel, I want to move on now to show you how to do a logistic regression in another application, and for this I choose SPSS.

REMEMBER

You can download many statistics applications for free from the Internet, as either trial software or freeware. Even the most expensive statistics applications, like SPSS cost less than $1,500 for a single-user desktop license.

CONSULTING THE ADVICE OF A STATISTICS PROFESSIONAL

When you choose to analyze data using multiple regression, it is important to check to make sure that the data you want to analyze can actually be analyzed using multiple regression. Missing important assumptions can put a wrench in what you are trying to achieve. The worst thing that can happen is that you may get it going and get a result but because an important assumption is missing, the multiple regression may cause you to be more confident about something that is not true at all — I'm not okay with that.

Checking for assumptions isn't technically difficult or time consuming; it just requires you to know the jargon of statistics and apply a lot of attention to detail. It doesn't add too much time to run a few preliminary statistical procedures, look at some scatterplots, and click a few more buttons in a statistics application after you get to the point of performing the analysis. What is difficult is that you have to know what you are looking for in the first place.

The most important decisions surrounding the type of statistical analysis you use and how to interpret the output are usually made by a data scientist, a behavioral scientist, or a mathematics professional with a 4 to 8-year college degree that included several years of college level statistics. If you aren't one of these animals, you should consult one to help you check assumptions, work through problems you run into, and check your work until you're completely comfortable on your own. If you do all the setup work and follow-up you really only need these specialists help for a few hours here and there — their advice is worth a lot more than it costs you.

Don't be surprised if, while analyzing your own data, one or more of the assumptions required isn't met. This isn't uncommon when working with real-world data. However, don't let that stop you — you can always find remedies for these problems with the assistance of statistics professionals.

Doing a Binary Logistic Regression in SPSS

The *logistic regression* is a special kind of regression tool for binary outcomes. In that sense, a logistic regression is just like a regular multiple regression, except that the y variable is a condition that is binary — either On (1) or Off (0), in other words. Another way of saying it is that a logistic regression version of regression is used to estimate the probability of a binary categorical dependent variable based on one or more independent variables, allowing for the measurement of factors that increase the odds of a given binary outcome.

An example of a binary dependent variable where the outcome can be only one of two possibilities is employee exit. The binary outcome may be determined by observing, over 12 months, whether the employee exited the company. If the employee exited the company in that 12 months, then that variable is recorded as a 1; if the employee stayed, it's recorded as a 0. The options are *binary*: For all rel-evant employees, the y variable {Exit} can be only a 1 or a 0.

Here are the steps to complete a binary logistic regression analysis in the SPSS statistical application:

1. **For setup in advance of working in SPSS, put the data you want to work with in a single Excel worksheet and label the columns with the variable names you want to use.**

The sample dataset has {Exit}, {Function}, {Job_Level}, {Tenure_Category}, and {Tenure_YRS} variables, as well as 14 other variables (Q1, Q2, Q3 . . . Q14), as shown in Figure 14-6.

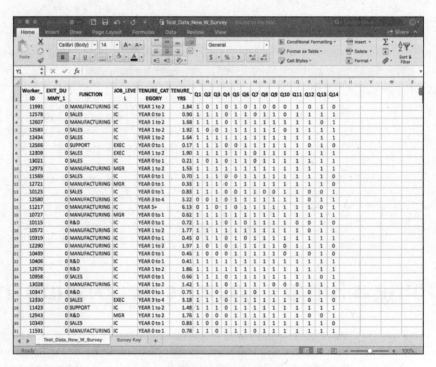

FIGURE 14-6: Labeling your columns in Excel.

2. **With SPSS open, tell it to load the Excel worksheet you put your data in, using whatever name you used to save it.**

After you open SPSS, ignore whatever windows are open and use your cursor to click on the File option on the light blue IBM SPSS Statistics application ribbon. A sub menu list will open. From this menu list, use your cursor to choose Import Data. Again, another sub menu list will open and from this list use your cursor to select Excel. Click on the Browse button. Navigate to and select the filename of the Excel file you want SPSS to use and double click it with your cursor.

After you have selected the Excel file, SPSS displays the Read Excel File dialog box (see Figure 14-7), which shows part of the dataset in the Excel worksheet you have selected as well as some options. Generally, everything here is fine, and you can just click OK, but you should give the dialog box a quick inspection to make sure everything is the way you want it to be.

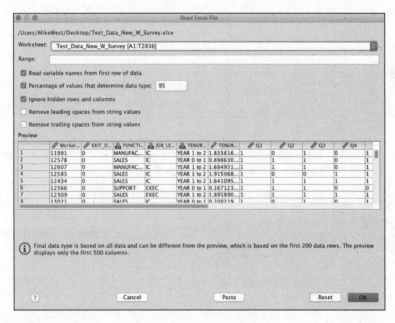

FIGURE 14-7:
The Read Excel
File dialog box in
SPSS.

3. **Click OK.**

Doing so brings up the SPSS Statistics Data Editor, as shown in Figure 14-8.

In the data editor, you should see your variable names along the top row and the data itself in the lower rows, much like it appeared in Excel. Notice on the bottom of the screen that the Data View tab is highlighted in blue. If you click the Variable View tab, you can inspect what data type SPSS thinks each of your variables is and change the data type here if you need to.

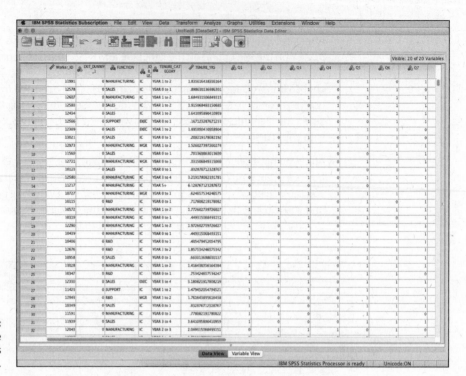

FIGURE 14-8:
SPSS displays the
SPSS Statistics
Data Editor.

4. **From the SPSS main menu, choose Analyze ⇨ Regression ⇨ Binary Logistic, as shown in Figure 14-9.**

Doing so opens the Logistic Regression dialog box, shown in Figure 14-10.

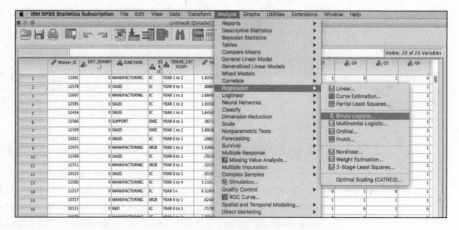

FIGURE 14-9:
From the SPSS
analysis options,
select Binary
Logistic
Regression.

5. **Using the list on the left side of the dialog box, identify your Dependent (y) and Independent (x) variable names.**

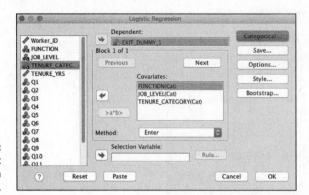

FIGURE 14-10:
The Logistic Regression dialog box.

REMEMBER

The idea here is that, after you highlight a variable (or multiple variables at the same time) in the list, you'd use the arrow icons to move the selection to the section of the dialog box where it (or they) should be.

By default, SPSS uses the Enter method for multiple regression. If you know something about the different regression methods and want to change this to something else, you can; otherwise, stay with the default setting. The same advice applies to any of the other selections in this dialog box. You aren't required to enter a selection variable. Without a selection, it defaults appropriately.

You're just about ready to run the logistic regression; however, I want to show you several of the options available from this screen that make useful modifications to the output you receive.

6. **In the Logistic Regression: Save dialog box, select the Probabilities and Group Membership check boxes.**

These options add columns to your dataset that will add a probability of the binary outcome and the most likely outcome category for each record. Though you can do many different things with this output, one of the more useful tasks is to compare the predicted outcome value with the actual value. You can use this strategy to try to identity patterns that may help explain the cases that the model is able to predict — or not able to predict, for that matter.

7. **Select the Save option.**

Doing so opens yet another dialog box — this time, the Logistic Regression: Save dialog box, shown in Figure 14-11.

While you're here, check out any of the other options that you might find interesting, depending on your level of statistical acumen. None of them is required, but it's nice to know what's available.

8. **Click Continue when you're ready to move on.**

This step takes you back to the main Logistic Regression dialog box.

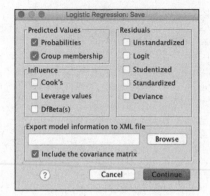

FIGURE 14-11:
The Logistic
Regression: Save
dialog box in
SPSS.

9. **Back in the Logistic Regression dialog box, click the Options button. (Refer to Figure 14-10.)**

Doing so brings up the Logistic Regression: Options dialog box, shown in Figure 14-12.

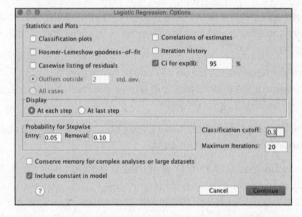

FIGURE 14-12:
SPSS displays the
Logistic
Regression:
Options
dialog box.

10. **(Optional) Look through the options and click all the additional ones that you want SPSS to provide in the regression output.**

For example, if you select the CI for exp(B) check box and enter the confidence level you want, SPSS automatically calculates a confidence level for you with the specifications you specify. (*CI* here stands for *confidence interval*, which is just another way of expressing confidence level. In the example, I selected CI for exp(B) and input 95%.)

REMEMBER

exp(B) is SPSS's word for the coefficient. Remember that the x variable coefficient is represented by the letter b, which stands for beta or beta-weight. Nothing to be afraid of – it is all the same stuff.

Look for the classification cutoff in the lower right corner of the dialog box as well. SPSS defaults to .5, or 50 percent, so the probability for the 1 categorical response to the outcome variable must be greater than 50 percent for the model to classify it as a 1. In the employee exit example, I know that the base probability of exit is 15 percent, so I set the classification cutoff to .3 to classify the value as a 1 when the odds of being a 1 are at least two times the base rate. (This is a judgment call.)

Note that the model stays about the same, but it does change where you're more willing to accept error. Do you want to error more in predicting the 1s, or do you want to error more in predicting the 0s? Changing these settings can give you different results.

11. **Identify what additional summary data you want returned, if any, and then click Continue when you're ready to move on.**

This step takes you back to the main Logistic Regression dialog box.

12. **Back in the main Logistic Regression dialog box, click OK. (Refer to Figure 14-10.)**

SPSS runs the logistic regression analysis and automatically opens a screen showing the summary statistics, as shown in Figure 14-13.

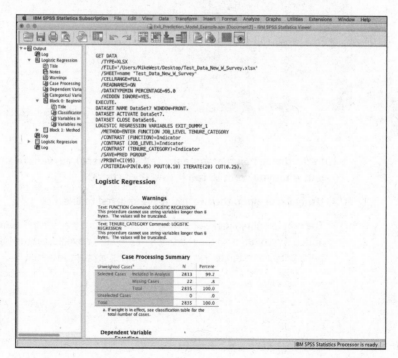

FIGURE 14-13: SPSS displays your initial view of the output of the binary logistic regression analysis.

Figure 14-13 shows the initial output of the binary logistic regression analysis. As you scroll down, you will find a variety of summary statistics and tables.

Rather than spend additional time in this chapter interpreting the output of this binary logistic regression, let me point you to Chapter 16 in this book, where I cover this topic in a practical application.

For all practical purposes, your job is complete and the answers you're seeking are in the output file.

After you have done all this work in SPSS, you may want to inspect the actual employee data with the actual exit coding (what really happened) and the predicted result (what the model predicted) together in one place. Because you selected this option earlier, you have these results also in the output file. If you want to export them to Excel, complete the following three steps.

13. **Back in the SPSS Data Editor, choose File ⇨ Export ⇨ Excel from the main menu, as shown in Figure 14-14.**

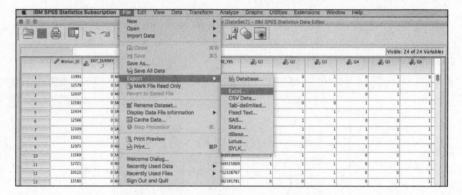

FIGURE 14-14:
Exporting data from SPSS to Excel.

14. **In the dialog box that appears, tell SPSS where you want to save the file and what you want to call it, and then click OK.**

15. **Using Excel, open the file you just exported to Excel.**

The output should look something like the output you see in Figure 14-15. SPSS added the columns to the right side of the file. I have added the highlighting, to point your attention to the predicted values versus the actual.

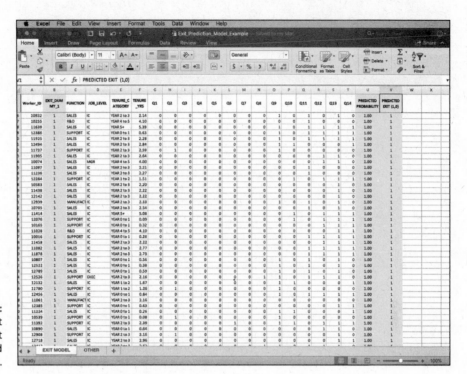

FIGURE 14-15:
The Excel output of your dataset with predicted values.

Chapter **15**

Making Better Predictions

P redictive people analytics uses people data from the past coupled with statistics to predict what will happen in the future. You reveal patterns to identify future risks and opportunities. The forward-looking orientation of prediction, coupled with analysis of what really matters (Chapter 15) and with action-oriented experiments (Chapter 16) gives you a great jab, left hook, and uppercut combination. With this combination, you can not only win more fights, you also have the power to change the future of your company.

REMEMBER

You make predictions all the time — you just do it with a limited number of observations and without checking your work with math.

Here are some examples of the kinds of predictions you have made (or are currently making) without the support of data:

» Whether this orange laundry detergent or that blue laundry detergent will do a better job

» What to wear to fit the occasion and/or weather

» Where to invest your time for the most productivity or pleasure

>> Whether you think the car in front of you will or won't stop at the next intersection

>> Whether to let this person or that person into your life as a friend or dating partner

These are just the predictions you make on the way to making other predictions that you don't even realize you're making. The truth is that we humans make so many predictions that we don't even notice we're doing it. In that sense, to predict is to be human. In the grand scheme of things, some predictions are incredibly trivial, but others are incredibly important. We make some predictions well and we make some poorly. In nearly all cases, we're using the information we have within our reach, based on our experiences and learning — you might call it *intuition* — but this intuition is rooted in some prior observations. The purpose of using data to make predictions is to expand the carefulness and number of observations into a summary that is useable for making better decisions when it matters most.

When you make predictions, you're leveraging some past experiences (consciously or not) to predict future events with a goal to make better choices. The same principle applies to prediction in organizations, human resources, and people analytics. You use past observations to predict the future with a goal of making better choices. It's just that now you have the opportunity to use a larger body of meticulously collected observations and statistical methods to be extra careful about how you interpret those observations.

Here are some examples of the kinds of predictions frequently made at the office that matter a great deal:

>> Where to look to find your next superstar employee

>> Whom to pick to be your next superstar employee

>> Which actions to take to create a happier and more productive work environment

>> Which actions you can stop doing and still obtain the same, if not better, results

>> Which pay-and-benefits combination is the right one for optimal talent attraction, retention, and group performance

>> Whom to promote or not promote and when

>> Which actions you can take to increase the longevity of key talent at your company and decrease the likelihood of key talent departures

All of these are predictions that you (or others) could be making more successfully if you had the help of people analytics. I think we can agree that important people decisions made without the scrutiny of data have most assuredly been made suboptimally. Worse, those who make decisions in this manner are disadvantaged when compared to others who have already begun to make decisions with the help of data analysis. That's why, throughout this book, I've covered which problems people analytics can solve, what people analytics needs to measure to understand those problems, and which methods can be used to collect those measures. After you have learned the letters of this language, you can learn words, and once you learn the words, you can work with others to create your future. This chapter represents a culmination of that effort, not a start.

Predicting in the Real World

Time for a game. Pick any random employee and think carefully about the following question: What is the probability that this person (and others with characteristics like her) leaves the company over the next 12 months? Think of somebody right now. Maybe you think you have an answer, or maybe you think you don't. I am certain that the cleverest among you might just go to your randomly chosen person and ask. I'm not opposed. If you do this, she may say to you, "I have no idea" or "Get out of here — you're crazy!" or she might tell you something you don't want to hear. If you asked a hundred people in this off-the-cuff manner, you'd probably get a hundred different answers, and it might be hard to see what to do with all of it. The real, generalizable answer to why and when people leave is this: It depends. If you want to get better at predicting who will leave in the next 12 months, you have to be able to answer this question: It depends on what?

Starting with no additional information and assuming that there are only two possibilities (stay or leave) and assuming that the actions of people are totally random, there's a .50 (50 percent) probability that this person leaves in the next year. By this logic, if you have 100 employees, each employee has a 50/50 chance of leaving. If you believe this to be true, you should forecast that your annual company exit rate will be equal to 50 percent. It can drift above and below 50 percent erratically for a stretch of time, but it will always stay near 50 percent year after year after year after year. Think about your company. Is this true? The good news is that your real company exit rate probably isn't 50 percent. The other good news is that, by and large, complete unpredictability of human behavior isn't the real world you live in. Lastly, the best news is that you have more information than you probably think you do. You can make a much better guess than a 50/50 coin flip, but you have to carefully identify, define, and use the information that matters in order to do so.

In the following sections, I show you how you can use the information you have right now to systematically turn the odds in favor of the final prediction you make. Then, if you want to learn how to do it even better, I point you in the direction of how to do so. Science and statistics are for improving the odds of being right. What you do with this depends on you.

Introducing the Key Concepts

Statistics is a branch of mathematics that deals with the collection, analysis, interpretation, presentation, and organization of data in order to aid deductive reasoning and further human learning. Statistics is very old, dating back at least to the fifth century BCE; however, statistics continues to advance with improvements in computer processors, software, and data storage. It has been a crucial element in the evolution of human decision-making. To not use statistics is to leave something important off the table.

If you look more closely, you can make out three distinct statistical emphases:

>> **Descriptive statistics** are used to summarize a particular set of data (using concepts like mean, standard deviation, and distribution).

>> **Inferential statistics** draw inferences about a population based on an analysis of a representative sample of that population. The results of an inferential analysis are generalized to the larger population from which the sample originates.

REMEMBER

Inferential statistics uses data from a sample of a population to make probability-derived predictions about that population, taking into consideration that each sample would turn up something different and that there always is the potential for observational error — missing data, inaccuracies (such as reporting incorrect units), imprecision, random noise, and systematic bias, for example. Specific procedures and techniques have been developed to help the analyst use imperfect data, avoid making incorrect conclusions as a result of imperfect data, and finally to interpret what is observed, despite having imperfect data. (One strategy is to randomly select samples in order to ensure that that the assumptions of the statistics can be met; only then can the inferences about the population be extended from a small sample while knowing that the next sample drawn might be randomly different.

>> **Predictive analysis** is the application of statistics to make an educated guess about the future.

TECHNICAL
STUFF

There is debate about whether today's hot topic, prediction, actually warrants a new category of statistics. Technically, prediction is an extension of inferential statistics.

Independent and dependent variables

When working with data in classic statistics and scientific research, variables are usually designated as either independent (x) or dependent (y). As the names imply, dependent variables are the ones affected when the independent variables change. You predict dependent variables with independent variables.

TECHNICAL STUFF

The names *independent* and *dependent* imply a cause-and-effect relationship. For purposes of working with data through statistics, you have temporarily assigned a causal direction to the relationship whether there really is one there or not. There is always the possibility that you have your x's and your y's reversed or that you are missing an important unmeasured x that would better explain the changes in y than the x's you are currently using. It is possible the unmeasured x explains your other x's and your y. This is why we are trained to say, "correlation does not imply causation." If you want to prove causation, then you need to run an experiment. (See Chapter 16 for more on experiments.)

Here's an example of how dependent and independent variables work: If an instructor wants to study success in a class, she might collect data for independent x variables like prior GPA (call it x1) and study time (call it x2) and use test scores (call it y) as the dependent variable y. Through an analysis of the collected data, the instructor can correlate each x variable (GPA & study time) to the y variable (test scores). If GPA and study time are highly correlated to test scores, the teacher could observe the student's GPA and study time before taking the test and just apply a little algebra to make a prediction about how well each student will score on the test. Voilà.

Here is the equation for this scenario: $Y = a + b1(x1) + b2(x2)$. Where y equals Test Score, x1 equals GPA and x2 equals Hours of Reported Study Time. (For more on what the a and b's mean and how you arrive at them, check out Chapter 13.)

After you know the prediction works, it's up to teachers and students to determine whether and how they'll use this information. If it turns out that study time matters (mathematically speaking), the instructor could use this information to encourage all students who want to have high test scores in the future to increase study time because based on her analysis she can tell you it matters. The teacher could also identify those students most at risk of low test scores because of a history of low GPA and take extra care to make sure those students study. That, in a nutshell, is how applied predictive analytics works.

Deterministic and probabilistic methods

Most of mathematics uses deterministic methods to form a quantitative description of the world. *Determinism* is based on the notion that all events are determined completely by previous existing causes — that old standby cause-and-effect.

From a deterministic standpoint, all equations should balance perfectly with no remainders. Remember the clarity of algebra, $A = B + C$, or the rock-solid certainty of geometry, $C = \sqrt{A^2 + B^2}$? Though a fantastic goal in the real world, in some subjects we have not and may never be able to achieve this type of precision.

Due to the messy world we humans live in, statistics relies on a probability-based approach to problems in order to form a quantitative description of the world — taking into consideration that our world contains uncertainty and error. Statistics is about being right more than you are wrong, despite imperfect information. We resort to this because we have to live in the real world, and in the real world, people can't wait around for perfect information.

Probability refers to the likelihood that something will happen. In statistics, a probability is represented as a decimal number between 0 and 1. Zero indicates that there is no possibility, and 1 indicates certainty.

A simple example is the tossing of a fair (unbiased) coin. Since the coin is fair, the two outcomes (heads and tails) are both equally probable; the probability of heads equals the probability of tails; and because no other outcomes are possible, the probability of either heads or tails is 1/2 (which could also be written as 0.5 or 50 percent). If you were to toss a coin 100 times, you would expect to get close to 50 heads and 50 tails.

DEPLOYING BAYES' THEOREM FOR FUN AND PROFIT

Bayes' theorem is named after Reverend Thomas Bayes (1701–1761), who first provided an equation that allows new evidence to update beliefs in his "An Essay towards solving a Problem in the Doctrine of Chances" (1763). It was further developed by Pierre-Simon Laplace, who first published the modern formulation in his 1812 "Théorie analytique des probabilités." Sir Harold Jeffreys wrote that Bayes' theorem "is to the theory of probability what the Pythagorean theorem is to geometry." That sounds pretty important to me, thank you very much.

Here's a simple example of how one would use Bayes' theorem: If cancer has in the past demonstrated a relationship to age, then, using Bayes' theorem, a person's age would be used to more accurately assess the probability that he has cancer, compared to the assessment of the probability of cancer made without knowledge of the person's age. This is just a simple example — the power of Bayes' theorem is a rational methodology to combine many estimates with varying certainty together into an overall final estimate. With Bayes' theorem, there are even ways to use subject inputs that deterministic methods would have no path to let you include in your prediction at all.

REMEMBER

Because events can randomly go on streaks, in reality you may have to throw the coin a lot more than 100 times to get a perfect 50 percent balance between heads and tails, but any large number of throws should produce close to an even balance as long as the coin is fair.

Statistics versus data science

People who work in industry (as opposed to academics) are practical and adapt their methods and language more rapidly. People who do things for a living, as opposed to study things for a living, don't like boxes (unless they work for Amazon) and they don't easily fit in them. Simply put, the origin of the word data science is the intersection of data analysis and computer science — they just put the words together and dropped the word "analysis" from "data analysis" and "computer" from "computer science". A pure data scientist is an aficionado of the application of developments in computer science to data analysis. To clarify a possible misunderstanding, in industry, very few people referred to as *data scientists* have a background in science — in the classic sense of the natural and social sciences or the scientific method. Most have instead a background in statistics and software engineering.

The main distinction between a statistician and a data scientist in practical application in industry is rooted in a different expectation regarding subject matter expertise. Statisticians are not expected to extrapolate beyond the data they have been provided. Because statisticians usually have only a limited amount of information about what is going on outside of the data they have and the methods of statistics they use, they're always forced to consult with a subject matter expert to verify the precise meaning of the elements of data provided them. Rooted more directly in the domain they study, data scientists benefit from a strong subject matter expertise in the area in which they're working. Data scientists generate deep insights and then use their domain-specific expertise to understand exactly what those insights mean with respect to the area in which they're working. People analytics is a very specific kind of data science. In people analytics, we must have at our disposal four areas of expertise: people strategy, people science, people systems, and statistics. The statistics by itself doesn't get you very far without the others.

Putting the Key Concepts to Use

I start this chapter with a little game where I ask you to pick any random employee and ask yourself how probable it is that this person (and others with characteristics like her) leaves the company over the next 12 months. I also note that, absent all other information, there are only two possibilities out there (stay or leave) and everyone has a 50 percent probability of leaving. I also quickly reassure you that, no, it's highly unlikely that you will lose half your employees over the course of the next year and that, yes, there are ways to improve your predictive capabilities. This list presents some information that you can apply from the world around you — right this very minute — to make a better prediction:

- » **US Bureau of Labor Statistics (BLS) total annual separations rate (total US population):** From the US BLS data, you can learn that the average annual US employee separation rate (Leavers ÷ Total Workers) between 2013 and 2017 is 41.8 percent. With this information, you can start out by saying that each US employee has slightly less than a 42 percent chance of leaving each year. Good to know, I guess, but also . . . so what! That's almost the same as your 50 percent estimate. Fortunately, that's not the end of your research. Taking the next step, you ask the US BLS website for the separation rate by industry, figuring it wouldn't hurt.

- » **US BLS total separation rate by industry:** Also from the US BLS system, you learn that the average annual separation rate by industry varies from between 16.5 percent (Federal Government) to 79.5 percent (Arts, Entertainment, and Recreation). That's a pretty big range, suggesting that industry seems to matter in your prediction. For the purposes of the fictitious game, let's say you're primarily operating in the Finance and Insurance industry. The average separation rate for a company in this industry is 24.5 percent. Now, with this information you can say that each of your US employees has slightly less than a 25 percent chance of leaving.

  Notice the distance you have already travelled from 50 percent just by getting more specific (looking up the separation rate by industry) and using this information in your prediction. There's a big difference between a 50 percent chance of leaving and a 25 percent chance of leaving — two times different, actually. Still, you can do even better than this by getting even more specific.

- » **Your own company data:** Using your own employee exit calculations, you learn that as a company your 2017 annual voluntary exit rate was 15.3 percent. Knowing nothing but this information, you can now make a more accurate prediction that the person you're thinking about actually has only a 15 percent chance of leaving. This means that out of 100 randomly chosen employees, you can expect 15 of them to leave — you just don't know which ones. Still, your overall leaver forecast will be much more accurate with this assumption than any of the assumptions you made before having this information.

The voluntary exit rate is calculated by dividing the number of voluntary exits in a year by average headcount in that year.

REMEMBER

WARNING

Despite the improvements you have made so far (traveling from 50 percent to 15 percent), there are still several obvious problems with this work:

>> **Exit rates change over time:** There are big-picture trends over years, and then there are quarterly and monthly ups and downs. How much consideration you should give to these fluctuations depends on where you are and what you're trying to do. (I walk you through how to decide on this later in this chapter.)

>> **The more carefully you segment, the wider range of values you find:** Industry and company are just a very broad (and crude) ways of looking at the problem. Industry and company are broad segments — to make a better prediction you need much more refined and careful segments. Even within a single company, there can be a wide range of different voluntary exit rates and associated implied individual probability of exit, depending on what ways you decide to segment. This includes (but isn't limited to) job type, job level, tenure, division, job function, performance, pay, age group, and more. (More on these factors later in this chapter as well. Stay with me.)

Understanding Your Data Just in Time

Time can be tricky, so to handle all that trickiness, we have a whole new set of terms designed to talk about time intelligently. *Time series data* is a set of data points listed in time order. *Time series analysis* compares values of a metric by itself or with others over time. Time series analyses are displayed as line charts — we call these trend reports.

A *trend report* is a graph of a metric taken at successive, equally spaced points in time or time intervals. Basic examples of commonly reported time series data in people analytics are headcount, exits and hire counts, and/or percentages. When these metrics are positioned in a trend, you can see whether they're staying the same, increasing, decreasing, or moving about erratically. Hopefully, they aren't moving about erratically — this might suggest a problem you can't understand given the information you have. If so, it suggests you should collect more information or adjust the way you are looking at the information you have.

Time series forecasting is the use of statistics to predict future values based on previously observed values. A natural extension of trend data, time series forecasting regresses past data collected over regular intervals to predict future data on the same intervals. The regression analysis observes the impact of time on a dependent variable, not taking into consideration any other information. (Be careful with terminology — we haven't gotten to multiple regression yet in this story.

Here we are regressing a single variable against itself over time.) For example, if you have data on the voluntary exit rate trended over time, you can use this information to predict a future voluntary exit rate by drawing the best line you can extend through your data at the best angle the trend suggests.

REMEMBER

A special type of regression analysis called *multiple regression* can take into consideration the influence of more than one variable on the matter you're predicting. I offer an application of multiple regression to prediction later in this chapter, but I provide all the details of how to do multiple regression in Chapter 13.

Exponential smoothing is an extension of the simple method of time-based forecasting. The smoothing process involves exponentially decreasing the weights of older observations so that recent observations are given more value.

For instance, you might forecast employee exits over the next six months using exits over the previous 24 months while still applying greater weights to the bends in the more recent data. Exponential smoothing will not be as precise or accurate as the multivariate models I describe later in this chapter, but it's simple to perform and requires a lot less data.

But enough about terminology. Let me show you how to actually do some time studies.

Predicting exits from time series data

Figure 15-1 shows the company-wide voluntary exit rates from 2013 to 2017. The idea here is that, with this data, you can use the past pattern of exits to predict what future exits will be.

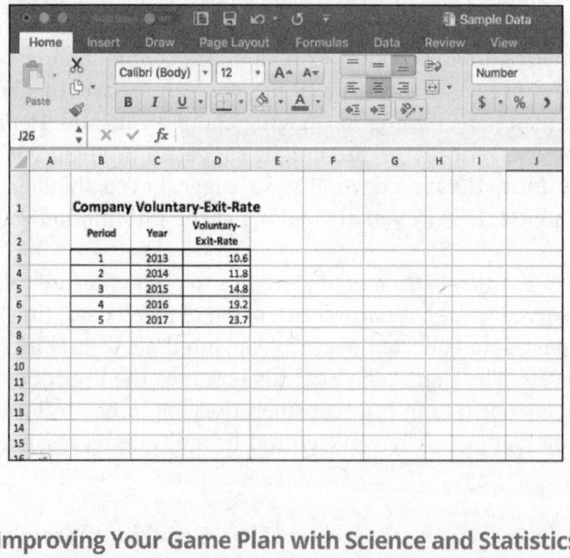

Period	Year	Voluntary-Exit-Rate
1	2013	10.6
2	2014	11.8
3	2015	14.8
4	2016	19.2
5	2017	23.7

Company Voluntary-Exit-Rate

FIGURE 15-1:
Table of the voluntary exit rate by year.

REMEMBER

The data I'm using is based on real data, but the names have been changed to protect the innocent (and the guilty as well, for that matter). For this reason, if you look carefully, you may see that I filled in data gaps or skipped over minor details for the purpose of illustrating clearly the patterns I want to show. I'm not trying to dupe you — I just can't share anyone else's real HR data. People are kind of sensitive about that.

Though you can use many applications to work with data, I try to provide as many examples as I can in Excel because of the availability, accessibility, and transparency of this nearly ubiquitous business application. Love it or hate it, nearly everybody uses it — or at least has it on their computer.

To estimate the voluntary exit rate in the future from time series data using Excel, follow these steps:

1. **Highlight the cells containing the data you want to see in a graph (in this example cells D3:D7), click on the Insert tab of the Excel ribbon, and select a 2-D line graph chart from the displayed options.**

2. **Right click with your mouse anywhere on the graph and choose Select Data.**

   Doing so brings up the Select Data Source dialog box.

3. **Click into the Horizontal (Category) axis labels box and highlight the cells containing your data labels (in this example, cells C3:C7). (See Figure 15-2.)**

4. **Click OK to create a line graph from the data you have selected in Excel.**

   From Figure 15-2, you can see that trend is going up and to the right.

5. **Right-click the data line and choose Add Trendline from the menu that appears.**

   Doing so calls up the Format Trendlines dialog box. You'll start with the default selections and add a few. Go to step 6.

6. **In the Format Trendlines dialog box, scan your eyes from top to the bottom and select both the Display Equation on Chart and the Display R-Squared Value on Chart options by clicking the check boxes, as shown in Figure 15-3.**

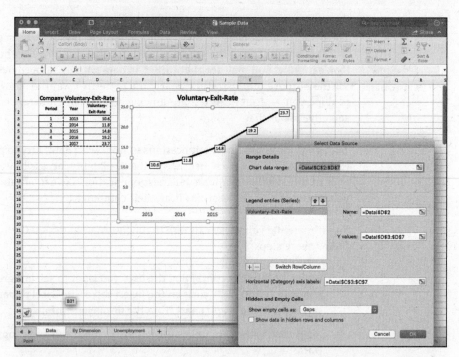

FIGURE 15-2:
Graph of the voluntary exit rate by year.

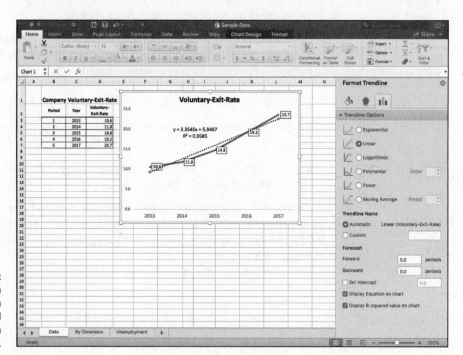

FIGURE 15-3:
Adding a trendline and an associated regression equation.

You end up with a graphical illustration of the best-fitting trendline and linear regression equation for these data. By adding a trendline and regression equation, you can see how linear the trend really is *and* predict the future voluntary exit rate (assuming that the voluntary exit rate continues to exhibit this linear pattern).

In the example provided in Figure 15-3 the equation (y = 3.3545x + 5.9467) simply expresses the dotted line in the language of mathematics. y is the voluntary exit rate, which is on the y-axis, which you can see ranges from 0 to 25. x represents the period, which ranges from 1 to 5, but you can see it labeled on the x axis as years — 2013 to 2017, to be precise. 5.9467 is the y-intercept — where the dotted line crosses the y axis. 3.3545 is the slope of the dotted line. So for each period between 1 and 5 the voluntary exit rate line increases by about 3.4.

You can see how well the best-fitting line does at describing the changes in data over time with R^2. This R^2 value in the example is .959, meaning this dotted line explains 96 percent of the variation in company voluntary exit rate over time (represented by the gray line), which is excellent.

Note that the independent variables used here are the intervals of time over five years (time intervals 1 to 5) corresponding to 2013 to 2017. The regression equation for the dependent variable voluntary-exit-rate for this 5-year period is

Voluntary-Exit-Rate = 3.3545(x) + 5.9467, where x equals time intervals 1 to 5

You can now predict the voluntary exit rate for a given year — say, 2018 — which would be the sixth data point (1-time interval into the future).

The estimated voluntary exit rate for 2018 is

Predicted 2018 Voluntary-Exit-Rate = 3.3545(**6**) + 5.9467 = 26.1%

REMEMBER

Though past performance is often the best predictor of the future that we have, the underlying mechanisms that drive what happened in the past may change, which then creates errors in your prediction of the future. If you understand the mechanics of the long-term trends, you can be sure to capture them and include them in your forecast; to do this, however, you have to identify what other longer-term variables change to drive change in the dependent variable (voluntary-exit-rate, in this case). To deal with this problem, you must capture longer-term data that includes all — or at least many of — the things that really matter. (Them's the breaks.)

Dealing with exponential (nonlinear) growth

One benefit of first graphing data is that you can examine the shape to be sure that a line does a good job of fitting it. You may find that the data you're trending looks linear over short intervals (a few years) but is exponential (growing at an increasing rate) over longer periods (for example, maybe five to ten years). If the data you are fitting to is exponential, an exponential equation line will fit your data better than a linear line and, consequently, an exponential line equation will make a better prediction.

Before you do anything else, see whether an exponential trendline better describes the voluntary exit rate data than a linear one. Here's how you do that:

1. **Going back to the example used in 15-3, right-click the data line again and again choose Add Trendline from the menu that appears.**

   The Format Trendlines dialog box makes another appearance.

2. **In the Format Trendline section, select the Exponential radio button (moving the selection from the Linear option to the Exponential option).**

   An updated trendline with an exponential regression equation is added to the chart, as shown in Figure 15-4.

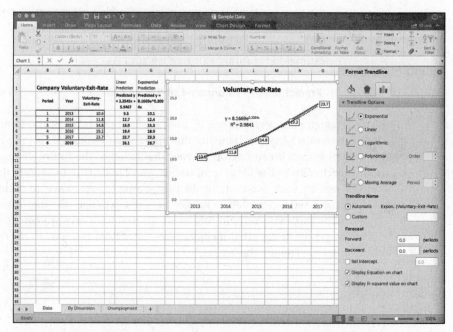

FIGURE 15-4: The exponential regression equation, added to the graph.

The figure clearly shows that an exponential trendline is a better fit for the data in the example than a linear trendline. As further evidence of this, notice that R^2 has improved from .96 to .98.

Notice that in Figure 15-4 I have added some data in columns F and G for purposes of illustrating for you what is happening when you toggle between a linear and an exponential trendline option. What I have put there is not necessary to have Excel calculate the trendline — I have added it to show the implications of the two trendline options side by side. I have noted the linear prediction equation in cell F2 and the exponential prediction equation in G2 and you can see the predicted values by period when plugging x into the equations below each. (The values clearly show the superiority of the exponential prediction.)

Checking your work with training and validation periods

A way of testing how well you have done with your prediction would entail partitioning your data into training and validation periods. In the training period, you build a regression equation on the earliest section of data (two-thirds to three-fourths of your data). You then apply the regression equation to the later part of your data in the validation period to see how well the earlier data actually predicts the later data.

REMEMBER

If excluding one quarter to one third of your data feels like you're tying one hand behind your back, it's because you are. It's worth it, though, because this allows you to see how well your predictions from former data work, which gives you a likely estimate of how they should perform in the future should nothing else change.

We don't have a lot of time intervals in the dataset example for voluntary exit rate data. For the purpose of the example, go ahead and use the first four years (2013 through 2016) as the training period and the final year 2017 as the validation period. This approach is testing the equation using data you already have, which is as close as you can get now to testing how well a prediction might perform when new data comes in later. If you are stepping through this with me on your own in Excel, what I am saying is do what you just did to create an exponential trend line but leave out the last year (2017). This will give you a slightly different equation than you arrived at when using all five years.

The regression equation for the first four years is:

Voluntary-Exit-Rate = $8.3062e^{0.2009x}$, where x equals time intervals 1 to 4

The R^2 equals .97, which shows a good fit for the exponential line. You can then use this regression equation to see how well the first four years of the dataset predict the last year of the dataset. I have reconfigured the graph to estimate the prediction based on the regression equation from the first four years, adding an estimated value for the fifth year, which is 2017. Figure 15-5 shows the predicted and actual values.

To assess how well this prediction works, I created four additional columns. Column E is the prediction using the exponential trendline equation for the first four years, whereas column F is the error from the actual number to the prediction. For example, in 2017, the prediction was short by about 1 point (22.7 minus 23.7). When communicating how much error your predicted values have, it's often easier to speak in terms of the absolute value or absolute percentage of error. Column G is the absolute value of the difference, whereas Column H contains the absolute percentage of error per period.

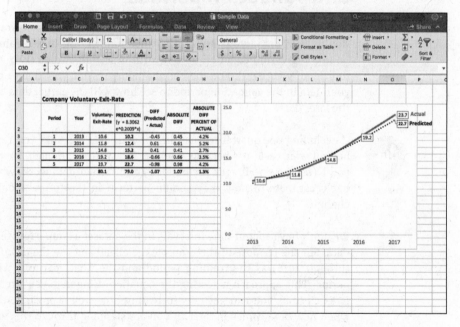

FIGURE 15-5:
Estimating 2017 using 2013 to 2016.

You can see from Column F that each year the predicted values are a little above or a little below the actual values ranging from an absolute 2.7 to 5.2 points error per year. If you look at the difference between actual and predicted values spanning the total 5-year period, the prediction is only off by about 1.3 percent. From 2013 to 2017 overall, the regression equation underpredicted by 1.1 points. This equates to 1.3 percent. The reason this isn't higher is that some years were below, and some years were above, which resulted in an overall value for this period closer to the middle. All this is summed up in the following formula:

2013 to 2017 Absolute Error = (ABS(79.0-80.1) ÷ 80.1) × 100 = 1.3%

Specifically, in 2017, the prediction was short by about 1 point (22.7 percent minus 23.7 percent), which is about a 4 percent difference:

2017 Absolute Error = (ABS(22.7-23.7) ÷ 23.7) × 100 = 4.2%

You win some and you lose some, but 4 percent error isn't bad — I'll take it any day.

Dealing with short-term trends, seasonality, and noise

My little voluntary exit rate example has a yearly period aggregation for just five years, so it doesn't show much variability. If you end up working with different time aggregations, you may end up with something that looks quite different. For example, if you look at the voluntary exit rate in shorter time period aggregations — say, a quarter or a month — you will find more variability and/or noise. If you look at it by month, week, or day, the line jumps up and down so erratically that it will become utterly uncompressible and useless to you. (Figure 15-6 shows some of the infinite variety you can expect if the same data is aggregated at different period levels.)

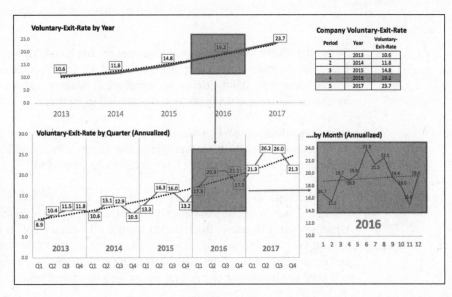

FIGURE 15-6: Comparison of the same voluntary exit rate data by year, quarter, and month aggregations.

TIP

It's worth viewing data at different levels of aggregation just to see what could be the most useful. If your graph looks like an abstract painting or a plate of spaghetti to you, go ahead and try a different level of aggregation.

Useful varies by context, but my advice is to choose a window of time to report where it's possible to understand, predict, and influence what you're measuring. If you're trying to make predictions to identify segments and individuals at greater-than-average risk over the next year, for example, an annual view may suffice. You know they're at risk and so you can take some action — you don't need a week-by-week update. If you're predicting exits just for purposes of annual headcount planning, you don't need to know that 14 exits are likely to happen in June and 7 exits in October. You just need to know how many will happen over the next year so that you can plan accordingly. However, if you're trying to forecast exits to plan hiring to hit a precise headcount target by the end of each quarter, it may be more useful to look at data by quarter. The relevant data for this includes actual headcount, hires, exits, and corresponding predictions per quarter.

TIP

For most use cases, quarters provide a useful compromise between month (too erratic and unactionable) and year (a long wait).

If your data goes up and down by quarter, month or week, how can you make any accurate predictions at all? The key is identifying a useful level of aggregation and then teasing apart the big underlying trends from the up and down variation. To do that, you can use the theory of time series, which states that the data (Yt, in this case, where Y = variance in voluntary exit rate over time) is equal to the product of the trend (Tt), the seasonal variation factors (St), and a random noise factor (Nt). Sum it up as a formula and you have

$$Yt = Tt \times St \times Nt$$

To predict future values, you need to isolate the big trend. To do that, you have to factor out the noise and seasonality so that the big trend can be extrapolated by a simple linear regression. Finally, seasonality can be factored back into the specific by-quarter or by-month prediction if you need to go there.

If the preceding equation is Greek to you, don't worry! There's a semi-complex math behind forecasting seasonal data, but fortunately, Excel has an option for doing exactly this, so you don't have to calculate it by hand:

WARNING

Some versions of Microsoft Excel, including the versions created for Apple Macintosh hardware, do not have all of the features of Excel created for Microsoft Windows. Unfortunately, the Forecast feature I describe below is available on the current Windows version of Excel, but not on the current Mac version of Excel. If you do not have a Windows based operating system on your computer, then you will need to borrow one to perform the actions described below.

1. **Starting out from a new dataset — one where each of the five years has been divided into quarters — select the data range you want to work with, select the Data tab on the main Excel Ribbon, and then click the Forecast Sheet button.**

   Doing so brings up the Create Forecast Worksheet dialog box, as shown in Figure 15-7.

   If you click the Forecast Sheet button without having chosen any data, you'll see the message "Forecasting can't be created." Just click Options in the Create Forecast Worksheet dialog box to expand the dialog box to reveal fields where you can choose the Timeline range and Values range. (See Figure 15-8, where Column A contains the timeline range and Column E contains the Values range.)

   The Confidence Interval will default to 95%, as will the selection of Seasonality, Detect Automatically.

   The Forecast Start automatically begins with your last period of data. In this example, it starts at 20. Feel free to adjust the Forecast End to include as many periods as you'd like your forecast to show.

2. **Click Create.**

   That's it. You're done! Excel reformats your data to include a few extra lines of forecasted values, including confidence bounds based on the confidence interval specified in the Options section. The forecast and its associated dataset are created on a new sheet in Excel.

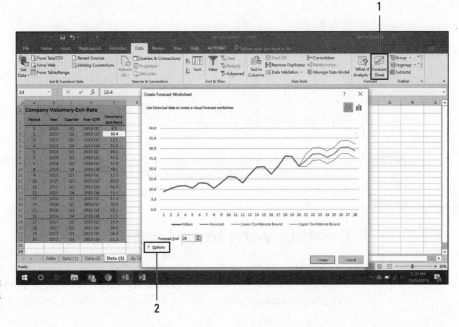

FIGURE 15-7:
Using Excel's
Forecast feature.

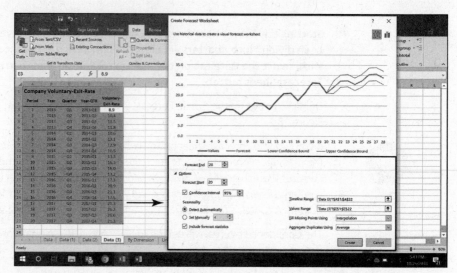

FIGURE 15-8:
Selecting options in the Create Forecast Worksheet dialog box.

At this point, Excel has done all the heavy lifting for you. Now feel free to format your dataset and graph as you see fit for your purposes. Figure 15-9 shows you what I came up with.

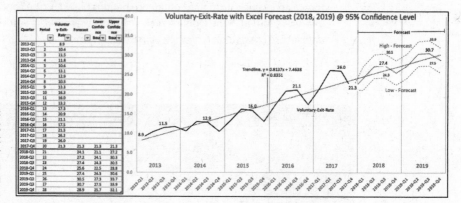

FIGURE 15-9:
Forecasting voluntary exit rate over 8 quarters with trend and seasonality.

REMEMBER

Most statistical applications have options to provide forecasts using similar or more advanced methods. Examples of statistical software that do this are R, SPSS, SAS, STATA, STAT LAB, JMP, and Minitab.

Dealing with long-term trends

It's all fine and dandy to fine-tune the predictions you have made with time series data based on a single variable (voluntary exit rate) over a 5-year period where you simply extend a best-fitting line. If you take a longer-term perspective, however, it could totally change the shape of the data and, in turn, your prediction. Why bother, then? Well, a broader time perspective often helps you see — and better take into consideration — the impact that macroeconomic (big picture) variables, like the job market or any other pattern that's difficult to spot in a short time perspective, may have on trends you're trying to predict. A majority of the time, you end up missing big-picture variables if you rely solely on short-term windows. You can't see the forest, for the trees, they say. In other words, the trees are blocking your view. These gaps in perspective become a major problem when the big-picture trends change, such as when the economy changes directions. If you haven't found a way to include important variables (big picture or small picture) into your calculations, your prediction will increasingly miss the mark — and you won't know why. To see what I mean, check out Figure 15-10, which graphically illustrates how long-term phenomenon can fundamentally change your understanding of the problem you're trying to solve.

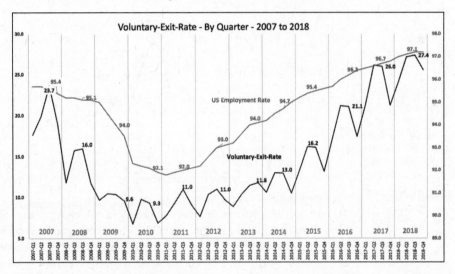

FIGURE 15-10: The voluntary exit rate over a longer time horizon.

Figure 15-10 shows the company voluntary exit rate by quarter over a much longer period. Notice how in the first five years the trend is downward and the next seven years the trend is upward. If you were to try to fit a linear line to this graph, it would go right down the middle and, consequently, wouldn't make a good prediction at any single point. So, in the context of this data, you need to know whether you're on an upward trend or downward trend, what explains these big shifts, and how to fit a better line.

I have added an additional line, US Employment Rate, which corresponds to the axis to the right. From this view, over a 12-year span it appears that the job market influences the direction of the company's voluntary exit rate, which supports the theory that voluntary exit isn't just about what you do as a company, but rather it's also mediated by external opportunity, which I am measuring (admittedly, rather bluntly) as the employment rate (1-{Unemployment-Rate}).

Using US Bureau of Labor statistics from 1949 to 2018 and the Excel Forecast feature, I'm estimating that there will be a 96 percent employment rate in 2019. However, using a 95 percent confidence interval, the actual employment rate is 95 percent likely to land anywhere from 93.9 percent to 98.1 percent. (See Figure 15-11.) This doesn't sound like a wide range, but on this dataset, that's a pretty big swing. All this suggests that the voluntary exit rate will be higher in 2017 and even higher in 2018.

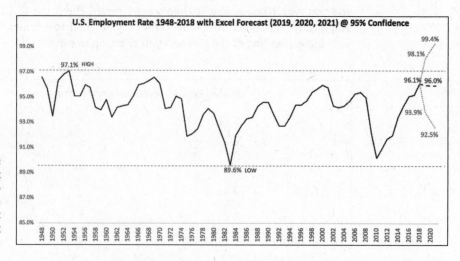

FIGURE 15-11:
US employment rate from 1948 to 2018 with an Excel forecast extending to 2019.

Figure 15-11 clearly demonstrates the wisdom of looking at the big picture. Trying to get by without that insight only reveals how little you know about what is really going on now and what may happen next. You could be climbing up a steep incline, at a plateau, or climbing down. Knowing where you currently are on this employment trend and where you're likely to be going matters a great deal. The way you deal with this problem is to include the information you have about where broad trends are likely to be next year in your own company's voluntary exit rate prediction.

So let's add statistics drawn from the macroeconomic picture to what you know about the voluntary exit rate at the company. When you do that, the strong correlation between the US employment rate and the company's voluntary exit rate immediately becomes clear. (See Figure 15-12.)

On the scatterplot in Figure 15-12, you can see that a regression of the annual US employment rate and the annual company voluntary exit rate from 2007 to 2017 yields the following formula:

$y = 237.77x - 207.89$, where y is the voluntary exit rate and x is the US employment rate.

This equation represents the best fitting line for that data we have. This equation was provided by Excel by selecting the Display Equation on Chart check box in the Format Trendline dialog box as described above. Here is how you interpret it:

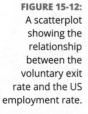

FIGURE 15-12:
A scatterplot showing the relationship between the voluntary exit rate and the US employment rate.

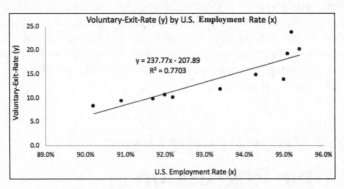

If the employment rate is 90%, then: **Voluntary exit rate prediction** = 237.77(.9) – 207.89 = 6.1%

If the employment rate is 95%, then: **Voluntary exit rate prediction** = 237.77(.95) – 207.89 = 18.0%

Notice that R^2, the coefficient of determination, is 0.77. (Recall that R^2 can range from 0 to 1.) This suggests that variation in US employment conditions (representing external opportunity) explain 77 percent of the variance in the company's voluntary exit rate. That gives us the confidence to assume, within a range of knowable error, that employment conditions data is useful for the purpose of predicting your company's future voluntary exit rate.

So, given three different employment rate scenarios, here's the range of 2018 company voluntary exit rates possibilities within the 95 percent confidence interval for US employment:

>> **93.9% employment** = 15.61% Forecasted Voluntary-Exit-Rate

>> **96% employment** = 20.4% Forecasted Voluntary-Exit-Rate

>> **98.1% employment** = 25.1% Forecasted Voluntary-Exit-Rate

Combining the historical company data and the US Bureau of Labor employment data, my new prediction is a 20.4 percent company voluntary-exit rate in 2018. Before you went on this little journey through time/time series analysis, your best guess was that your random employee would have a 15 percent probability of leaving in the next year. Now that you have seen where you are in time and have considered one of the large influences on probability of employee exit over time — external opportunity — there's better evidence to revise the probability that the employee will leave the company in the next year, up to 20.4 percent. To put this into perspective, it means that out of 100 randomly chosen employees, with this information you can expect roughly 20 of them to leave the company.

With each new piece of information you have considered, you have improved your prediction; however, your prediction is still missing a lot of important information. In the next section, you find out how to make better company forecasts, make segment forecasts, and make better predictions about individual exit risk, by considering the combined effect of multiple independent variables using a unified historical dataset.

Improving Your Predictions with Multiple Regression

This chapter is all about working with the information you have right now in order to make better predictions about what might happen in the future — more specifically, a better prediction about the probability of a randomly chosen employee leaving your company. Earlier in this chapter, I show you how to improve your prediction by looking at your company's historical voluntary exit rate and by working with time series analysis to make a prediction from the trend. However, just like taking the average voluntary exit rate of your specific company provided a much better estimate than the Bureau of Labor Statistics (BLS) information about your industry as a whole, it definitely helps to break down your work population by characteristics and segment if you want to understand the differing exit probability of specific employee types. The more you know about the characteristics of the people in your company and the relationship of these characteristics with probability to exit, the better your prediction of exits.

From the exit data illustrated in the fictitious company shown in Figure 15-13, you can see that exit probability can vary greatly by characteristic. Do note that these are just a few of the more easily accessible examples. You can use dozens, if not hundreds, of different characteristics to describe your employee population or any given employee in that population. The provided examples are a simplified variation of data that exists in every human resources information system (HRIS) or HR database.

Taking a closer look at Figure 15-13, here are some of the major data points you can determine for the fictitious company:

>> Employees in their first year of tenure have about an 11 percent probability of leaving on average, whereas employees between their second to third years of tenure have a 29 percent chance of leaving. The risk of exit between the second and third years is nearly three times the risk of exit in the first year.

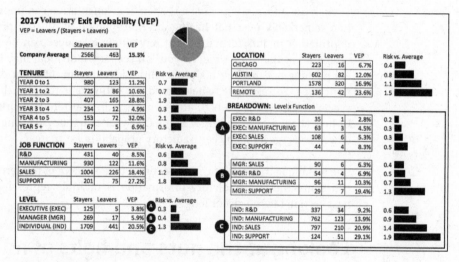

FIGURE 15-13: A fictitious company's voluntary exit probability by major segments.

>> Employees in specialized R&D roles have about half the average exit risk (9 percent versus 15 percent company average), whereas employees in common support roles have almost two times the average exit risk (27 percent versus 15 percent).

>> Executive-level employees have about one-third the average risk (4 percent versus 15 percent company average), whereas employees who don't manage other people (commonly referred to as individual contributor-level employees) on average have just a little over the company average risk (21 percent versus 15 percent).

>> If you break down the employee pool even further, you can see that there can be wide variation in exit probability even within a segment. In the Level by Type example, you can see exit probability ranging from less than one-fourth of the company average (Level = Executive, Type = R&D) to two times the company average (Level = Individual, Type = Support).

Figure 15-13 illustrates that in order to make a good prediction of an individual exit probability, it's important to know, at a minimum, what type of work people are doing, at what level, where they're located, and how long they have been at their jobs. Just like you did with larger macroeconomic measures like the US employment rate, you can use this new information to make better predictions about the future.

REMEMBER

The data strategy I am following here is tailored to my realistic — yet nevertheless fake — dataset. It may not apply at all to your company. You can certainly take my strategy as a guide, but you have to make sure it makes sense when applied to your own data.

Though the information using any specific segmentation can improve the prediction remarkably over not having any information at all, the problem with the information in this format is that any single employee can be put in multiple categories at the same time. As you can see, any individual may have forces that are pushing and pulling his probability of leaving in different directions at the same time. For example, what should you estimate is the probability of exit of a specialized individual contributor in his fourth-year tenure, working in Chicago? Or how about a sales manager in his first year of tenure, working remotely? How do you leverage so many contradictory probability estimates?

One technique that can be used to address this problem of numerous, overlapping and sometimes contradictory information is multiple regression analysis. The next section takes a closer look.

Looking at the nuts-and-bolts of multiple regression analysis

Multiple regression analysis helps you predict the value of an outcome (y) given values of multiple independent variables (x1, x2, . . .) using however much information you have. That is to say that any information you have that can be recorded as a numerical value can be included in the multiple regression. The multiple regression tells you the overall ability of the variables you have included in your dataset to predict the outcome (and also the independent contribution) of each variable.

You can perform a multiple regression analysis in a wide variety of statistics software (R, SPSS, SAS, STATA, or JMP, for example) or in some cases possibly even in Excel. After you have brought a data source into a statistics application and run the multiple regression, all the details you need in order to make predictions show up in the application's summary output.

TIP

I'm offering a bird's-eye-view of multiple regression in this chapter. For a more detailed overview of (and how-to for) multiple regression see Chapter 13.

In this chapter, working with a simulated dataset, I want to walk you through what you can learn about employee exit while using multiple regression. To get things started, I imported a dataset I had prepared in Excel into SPSS, a popular statistics program. From there, I ran a special type of multiple regression, known as a binary logistic regression, including the following variables:

Dependent variable = Leave (1) or Stay (0).

Independent variables:

Tenure Year (0–1, 1–2, 2–3 . . .)

Job Function (Manufacturing, R&D, Sales, or Support)

Job Level (Executive, Individual Contributor, or Manager)

Figure 15-14 shows the portion of the output from SPSS that summarizes how well the variables that were used actually predicted exits.

Model Summary

Step	–2 Log likelihood	Cox & Snell R Square	Nagelkerke R Square
1	1438.156[a]	.167	.334

a. Estimation terminated at iteration number 7 because parameter estimates changed by less than .001.

Classification Table[a]

			Predicted		
			EXIT_DUMMY_1		Percentage Correct
	Observed		0	1	
Step 1	EXIT_DUMMY_1	0	2252	251	90.0
		1	118	192	61.9
	Overall Percentage				86.9

a. The cut value is .250

FIGURE 15-14: Checking the overall fit of the basic employee exit prediction model.

Though you can make a variety of observations from this output, I don't want to venture too far into a complicated discussion of the mathematics here. Nor do I want to get bogged down in complicated interpretations of obscure statistic tests included in this output, like the Cox & Snell R Square, which are (unfortunately) a little different from the R^2 correlation coefficient covered earlier in this chapter. At this stage, the Cox & Snell R Square and other obscure details are neither here nor there to you — what you really want to know is how well the variables you included in the model helped you predict exit.

Notice the table at the bottom of Figure 15-14. In this table you can see that one axis shows the predicted values and that the other axis shows the actual (observed) values as found in the data. The table shows that, by using the information provided, the regression model predicts that 2370 (2252+118) people in the dataset will stay (coded as a 0) and 443 (251+192) people will leave (coded as a 1). Additionally, it shows that the model correctly classified 2252 who stayed and correctly classified 192 people who left. However, it predicted that an additional 118 people who actually left would stay and it predicted that an additional 251 people would leave who actually stayed. This breaks down to an overall accuracy of 86.9 percent; however, the model was only 61.9 percent correct at predicting the people who left.

Though 61.9 percent accuracy doesn't sound great, you should consider that, when all you knew was that 15 percent of the people would leave your company but nothing else, if you randomly picked 15 people out of 100, you would be wrong about who leaves at least 85 percent of the time. Seen in that light, 61.9 percent accuracy represents a remarkable improvement over 15 percent. What you have is a pretty good base model.

Refining your multiple regression analysis strategy

Okay, maybe 61.9 percent just isn't good enough for you. The best way to improve your prediction at this point is to obtain information that is in the minds of the employees. That means going back to your surveys. When you first put them together, you may or may not have known which questions would be useful to help you understand and predict employee exit. Fortunately, multiple regression doesn't care if you knew this or not. It tells you what works and what doesn't. Ideally, you have some good theory that pointed you to ask the right questions. In any case, you'll find out how good of a job you did after you get all that data into the multiple regression.

The following small sample of questions were asked of employees on an employee survey 12 months before this analysis. In this analysis, you want to associate the survey data to the other data you were just working with and rerun the multiple regression. Each question was measured on a 5-point Likert agreement scale: 1–Strongly Disagree, 2–Disagree, 3–Neutral, 4–Agree, and 5–Strongly Agree.

Q1	I expect to be working for *<Company>* one year from now.
Q2	I understand my possible career paths at *<Company>*.
Q3	I believe extra effort is appropriately recognized at *<Company>*.

Q4	*<Company>* makes operational decisions based on its mission and values.
Q5	Over the past three months, I knew what was expected of me at *<Company>*.
Q6	I feel a sense of personal accomplishment at *<Company>*.
Q7	*<Company>*'s executive leadership team cares about me as a human being.
Q8	I fit well into the culture of *<Company>*.
Q9	I am proud to tell others that I work for *<Company>*.
Q10	Over the past three months, someone at *<Company>* encouraged my development.
Q11	I can be myself at *<Company>*.
Q12	*<Company>*'s pay is as good as or better than the pay in other companies.
Q13	My manager at *<Company>* provides clear feedback that is useful for making decisions.
Q14	*<Company>*'s benefits are as good as or better than the benefits in other companies.

Figure 15-15 shows you what a prepared dataset based on the answers to this survey would look like in Excel.

You can see from the figure that I have already recoded the survey items — any 4 or 5 is listed as (1), representing a "favorable" response, and anything other than a 4 or 5 is listed as (0) for "unfavorable."

After you pull the completed dataset into your statistics application and run the multiple regression, you get something that looks a lot like what is shown earlier, in Figure 15-14 — but this time it includes the survey data and the prediction is noticeably better. (The new output is shown in Figure 15-16.)

Notice that, with the new survey data included, the model summary scores are larger and — most importantly — the classification table has improved dramatically. With the new data, the model is accurately predicting 99.1 percent of those employees who stay and 97.1 percent of those employees who leave for an overall prediction accuracy of 98.9 percent.

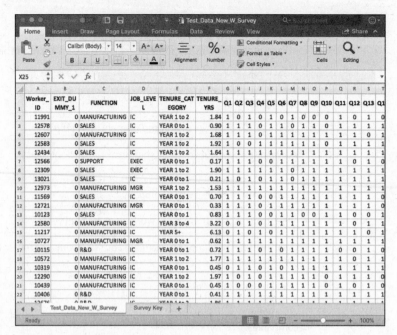

FIGURE 15-15:
An Excel file, prepared for binary logistic regression.

Model Summary

Step	−2 Log likelihood	Cox & Snell R Square	Nagelkerke R Square
1	157.631[a]	.472	.942

a. Estimation terminated at iteration number 12 because parameter estimates changed by less than .001.

Classification Table[a]

		Predicted EXIT_DUMMY_1 0	Predicted EXIT_DUMMY_1 1	Percentage Correct
Observed				
Step 1 EXIT_DUMMY_1	0	2481	22	99.1
	1	9	301	97.1
Overall Percentage				98.9

a. The cut value is .250

FIGURE 15-16:
The overall fit of a survey-enhanced employee exit prediction model.

Before you recommend me for the Nobel prize in Economics, be advised that this example has one foot in reality and one in a make-believe world, merely because I needed a safe dataset I could share for this book without getting sued. (Basically, I had to take two partial datasets, simulate a full dataset with no identities, and extrapolate.) That said, my example shows signs that it would work pretty well, given the opportunity with the right access and data. (Probably not 98.9 percent good, but good enough.) Notice that, if an exit probability exceeds 25 percent,

I classify the person as likely to exit. Employee exit is a probabilistic, not deterministic, problem, so there will be misses, but those misses outline the nature of the problem, not necessarily a problem with the methods.

Now that we're pretty confident that the variables included in our multiple regression are working well together, it's time to have a look at their independent contributions. That's covered in the next section

Interpreting the Variables in the Equation (SPSS Variable Summary Table)

As you proceed through the SPSS summary output, eventually you find a table that provides summary statistics on each x variable you have included in the multiple regression model. What you see in Figure 15-17 is a standard binary logistic regression summary output table — often called a coefficients table — much like what you would get from any statistical application. Here you find information about the specific variables you included in your dataset. To the left (in the gray column), you find each of the variables that SPSS observed in the dataset. (If you used column labels for variables, you see these names as part of the table.)

From a bird's eye view, the first thing you need to know is that the variable names on the left in Figure 15-17 represent the independent variables (x1, x2, x3, x4, . . .) in the generic multiple regression equation $y = a + b1(x1), + b2(x2) + b3(x3) \ldots$ The letter a is the constant, which represents the starting point of the line — also called the y intercept. The interaction of the y intercept and the x variables describe the best fitting line built from your historical dataset. The rest of what you see here are values calculated by SPSS that summarize the significance and importance of each independent variable on an individual's likelihood of exit, which is what we are trying to first understand and then use to predict.

To determine what x variables are statistically significant, you should look at the Sig. column. It reflects the statistical significance level of each variable, telling you the probability that the estimated coefficient is wrong. Sig. ranges between 0 and 1, but you want the Sig. to be as small as possible because you want to keep the probability of being wrong as low as possible. Usually, I consider a Sig. to be statistically significant if it is less than .05 – this corresponds to a 95% confidence that the coefficient is not a result of chance. (You may decide to use some other cutoff, for example .1 or .01 depending on how much risk you want to take based on what you are analyzing.)

FIGURE 15-17: Variables in the exit prediction model equation.

Variables in the Equation

	B	S.E.	Wald	df	Sig.	Exp(B)	95% C.I.for EXP(B) Lower	Upper
Step 1^a FUNCTION			28.561	3	.000			
FUNCTION(1)	-4.718	.911	26.839	1	.000	.009	.001	.053
FUNCTION(2)	-4.071	.984	17.110	1	.000	.017	.002	.117
FUNCTION(3)	-2.774	.748	13.761	1	.000	.062	.014	.270
JOB_LEVEL			7.734	2	.021			
JOB_LEVEL(1)	.876	1.588	.304	1	.581	2.401	.107	53.951
JOB_LEVEL(2)	2.702	1.159	5.432	1	.020	14.912	1.537	144.692
TENURE_CATEGORY			31.942	5	.000			
TENURE_CATEGORY(1)	-2.861	1.108	6.670	1	.010	.057	.007	.502
TENURE_CATEGORY(2)	-2.474	1.097	5.085	1	.024	.084	.010	.724
TENURE_CATEGORY(3)	-.299	1.026	.085	1	.771	.742	.099	5.541
TENURE_CATEGORY(4)	-2.817	1.586	3.156	1	.076	.060	.003	1.337
TENURE_CATEGORY(5)	2.194	1.406	2.436	1	.119	8.973	.570	141.162
Q1	-7.180	.874	67.529	1	.000	.001	.000	.004
Q2	-4.331	.764	32.176	1	.000	.013	.003	.059
Q3	-4.294	.705	37.143	1	.000	.014	.003	.054
Q4	-7.993	1.363	34.395	1	.000	.000	.000	.005
Q5	-6.807	1.036	43.141	1	.000	.001	.000	.008
Q6	-5.737	.967	35.201	1	.000	.003	.000	.021
Q7	-9.439	1.231	58.831	1	.000	.000	.000	.001
Q8	-4.806	.937	26.319	1	.000	.008	.001	.051
Q9	1.955	1.014	3.717	1	.054	7.064	.968	51.546
Q10	.061	.684	.008	1	.929	1.063	.278	4.060
Q11	-.077	.911	.007	1	.932	.926	.155	5.517
Q12	1.033	.621	2.764	1	.096	2.810	.831	9.496
Q13	-.669	.762	.770	1	.380	.512	.115	2.282
Q14	-1.600	.862	3.449	1	.063	.202	.037	1.093
Constant	26.703	3.574	55.819	1	.000	3.952E+11		

a. Variable(s) entered on step 1: FUNCTION, JOB_LEVEL, TENURE_CATEGORY, Q1, Q2, Q3, Q4, Q5, Q6, Q7, Q8, Q9, Q10, Q11, Q12, Q13, Q14.

The Sig. represents each variable's *statistical* significance; whether or not the variable has any *practical* value for purposes of predicting exit is another matter. The relative importance of each variable can be assessed by the B coefficient value (and/or the Exp(B) columns) — these columns represent two different ways of looking at the coefficient for logistic regression.

I don't want to get you bogged down in math theory in this book; I just want to help you use the output SPSS provides to make a better prediction. The precise meaning of the x coefficient values in terms of a unit change in y (probability of exit) is unnecessary. For practical purposes, all you need to know is that the larger the value of the x's (B) the more the x variable corresponds to the odds of the y variable state you are predicting — an employee exit, in other words. That means the larger the (B), the more impact the x variable has.

Using only the statistically significant survey variables, Table 15-1 shows how I have ordered the variables from the one that helps best explain the difference between stayers and leavers to the worst.

So which variable tops the list? The winner is . . . Question # 7, "<Company>'s executive leadership team cares about me as a human being"!

TABLE 15-1

Ranking variables in order of significance

Survey Item Number	Absolute Value of B	B	Exp (B)	Sig.
Q7	9.4	-9.4	.000	.000
Q4	8.0	-8.0	.000	.000
Q1	7.2	-7.2	.01	.000
Q5	6.8	-6.8	.001	.000
Q6	5.7	-5.7	.003	.000
Q8	4.8	-4.8	.008	.000
Q2	4.3	-4.3	.013	.000
Q3	4.3	-4.3	.014	.000

Wait, what's up with the negative coefficient B values? Here's what's up: For purposes of interpreting the output of this particular dataset there are two important things you have to keep in mind:

» **Y variable direction:** In the original dataset, I had coded the y variable Exit_Dummy_1 as 1 if the employee left the company and 0 if the employee stayed. Therefore, what the multiple regression is measuring is whether or not a unit change in each x variable increased the odds of employee exit.

» **X variable direction:** In the original dataset, I coded the survey data so that a favorable response to the survey item is 1, and an unfavorable response is 0. This coding decision is the reason why you see the negative coefficient B values. If an employee responds favorably to any of these survey items, they are less likely to exit. Inversely, if the employee responded unfavorably to the survey item, then they are more likely to exit. The logistic regression produced coefficients with negative values because I coded my x variables on a positive scale and the regression found a positive response to the survey item is inversely related to the probability exit.

TIP

Had I had thought about this dataset more carefully, I would have coded the survey questions just the opposite way. I should have coded them a 1 when they were unfavorable, as opposed to coding them a 1 when they are favorable. This would make the coefficients of the survey items easier to interpret because the presence of an unfavorable response would indicate an increased probability of exit — a positive relationship — as opposed to an inverted relationship represented by a negative value. Regardless of which way you coded the variables, the math will work the same, but you should be careful to recall how you coded variables to interpret the meaning of the coefficient values.

Applying Learning from Logistic Regression Output Summary Back to Individual Data

Just when you thought it couldn't get any better, there's one more thing that SPSS statistics application provides. You might be surprised to learn that, in addition to providing all these great summary statistics that indicate how well your overall model is performing, what variables matter, and how much, the SPSS statistics application also provides you with an output of your dataset that does all the math for you to show you what prediction it made for each person in your historical dataset given the x data the model had for each individual. The SPSS output I refer to includes the calculated probability of exit of each individual case you have included in your dataset, along with the categorical classification that indicates whether the model predicts this individual case would exit (1) or stay (0).

Since this output is probably easiest to read in Excel, I'm going to start by quickly showing you how to import the individual logistic regression prediction from SPSS into Excel:

1. **From the SPSS main menu, choose Analyze ⇨ Regression ⇨ Binary Logistic**

   Doing so opens the Logistic Regression dialog box, shown in Figure 15-18

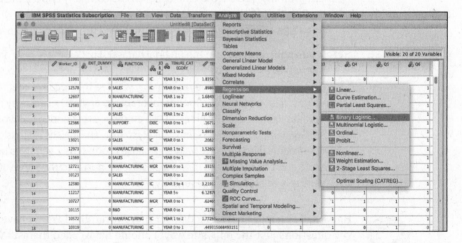

FIGURE 15-18: From the SPSS analysis options, select Binary Logistic Regression.

2. **In the Logistic Regression dialog box (see Figure 15-19, select your x (independent) variables and y (dependent) variables if you have not already done so or just confirm they are the way you want them to be if you have already been working with the Binary Logistic regression on the current dataset.**

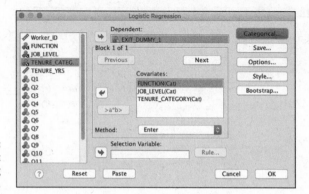

FIGURE 15-19:
The Logistic Regression dialog box in SPSS.

3. **Click Save.**

   Doing so brings up the Logistic Regression: Save dialog box, shown in Figure 15-20.

4. **In the Logistic Regression Save dialog box, select the Probabilities and Group Membership check boxes.**

   These options add columns to your dataset that will add a Probability of the Binary Outcome and the Most Likely Outcome classification category for each record.

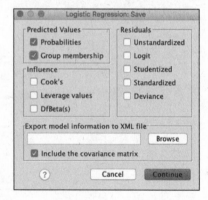

FIGURE 15-20:
The Logistic Regression: Save dialog box in SPSS.

5. **Click Continue when you're ready to move on.**

   This step takes you back to the main Logistic Regression dialog box.

6. **In the main Logistic Regression dialog box, click OK.**

7. **Back in the SPSS Data Editor, choose File ⇨ Export ⇨ Excel from the main menu, as shown in Figure 15-21.**

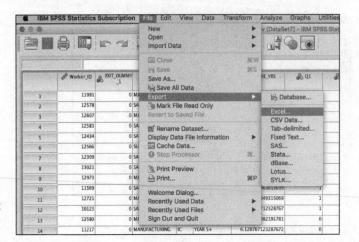

FIGURE 15-21:
Exporting
data from
SPSS to Excel.

8. **In the dialog box that appears next, tell SPSS where on your computer you want to save the file and what you want to call it, and then click OK.**

9. **Using Excel, find and open the file you just exported from SPSS.**

   The output from SPSS should look something like the output you see in Figure 15-22

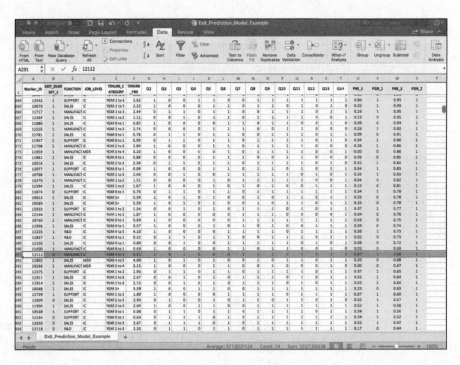

FIGURE 15-22:
The Excel output
with predicted
values.

What you can get back from the statistics application is the same dataset you so carefully prepared and started with, plus some additional columns that represent the prediction the application has made based on the data you provided. Column U represents the calculated probability of exit using the base model (excluding the survey data), and column W contains the probability estimate including the survey data (improved model). Columns V and X represent the prediction (1) leave and (0) stay. You can compare these results to column B, which contains the actual leave or stay data coded the same way.

REMEMBER

The predictions in this file are being made on the historical dataset. What the model is doing is estimating whether it predicted the Exit Dummy Variable in column B will be a 1 or 0 based on the data provided and putting the prediction in columns V and X. X represents the best prediction using the HRIS and survey data. You can compare the prediction in column X with column B.

Let's sum up where we are. We started off in a coin-toss world where everything is totally random. In that world, everyone's probability of exit would be 50 percent. Fortunately, we don't live in a coin-toss world, meaning the behavior of people isn't random. In this chapter's sample company, for example, you were able to determine that the natural probability of exit rate was 15 percent. Sounds good; however, this means when predicting the exit of any randomly chosen individual (without the benefit of any other information), you would probably be wrong 85 percent of the time. Not good. To improve your ability to predict these rare exits, you need to know something about the characteristics and conditions related to exit. To do this, you have to collect information over time in advance of exit and do this repeatedly over time until you get good at it.

In the example I provide, you have substantially improved your chances of predicting correctly who will leave (and why) using just 17 variables, 14 of which were found on a survey. Keep in mind that I had to collect the survey data and hold on to it for over a year so that I could test it to see who actually stayed and left. That sounds like a lot of work; however, after you know what works, you can use your learning about the variables that matter to predict exits in the future, and you don't have to go through all that waiting again. (Technically, you're collecting data all the time anyway, so you don't need to do anything special; you just need to hold on to your data for future use.) When you're able to determine what matters when it comes to the voluntary exit rate, you can change that rate by influencing one of the variables that matters with tiny nudges.

Chapter **16**

Learning with Experiments

If I accomplish nothing else in this chapter, I hope to at least tamp down some of the fear surrounding the word *experiment*. It's worth noting that, though the word has come to be associated with white lab coats, the logic for experiments is a natural part of human learning. The fact is, we all conduct experiments in our lives all the time — you just may not know that you're doing it. All adult skills were learned through experimentation: eating, walking, talking, riding a bicycle, driving a car, and so forth. Think about what happens when you prepare your evening meal: You add a tiny bit of seasoning, taste, add some more, taste, and so on until you get it just right.

I vividly remember learning how to cook, in about the third grade. I was making scrambled eggs, and I assumed that if a bit more salt was good, then a whole lot more salt was even better — so I dumped in a good handful of the stuff. I still remember biting into what I assumed would be the most delicious eggs ever made, before nearly choking during my search for water. Unfortunately, try as hard as I might, there was no way to get the eggs back to an edible state. The result of my earliest cooking experiment was inedible eggs. This could be considered a failure or a success, depending on how you look at it. The good news is that I have never added that much salt again. The bad news is that I wasted a couple of eggs. In the grand scheme of things, I learned a valuable lesson and little harm was done, so I consider the experiment a success.

The kind of learning arising from my salt experiment applies equally well in the professional HR world. If you think you have a great idea and apply that idea to the entire company, you might not call it an experiment, but that's exactly what it is, simply because you don't know exactly what will happen. Moreover, it's an experiment that could have considerable costs associated with it. Worse, if it goes wrong, you might not be able to undo it. When experiments are done right, they allow you to experiment and fail when it's cheap and the consequences are small. That means you can learn valuable lessons quickly, before the stakes are high. Unfortunately, before people analytics came along, the most common way that HR changes were applied was in an all-or-nothing mode: Consequently, a lot of risks were taken and — even worse — no new learning occurred.

REMEMBER

Others may make expensive company changes by pouring in all the salt, but my entire life experience suggests that this is not the best strategy. Learning is produced by patience and attention to detail: Perform small experiments, a little at a time — and taste-test before you add anything new.

Boiled down to their essence, experiments require only two actions: One is acting, and the other is observing the consequences of that action. The rest of what you do involves paying careful attention to detail so that you can properly interpret what you observe.

In this chapter, you have a chance to examine the logic, math, and science supporting people analytics experiments and the techniques you will need to carry out such experiments in real life. The first part of this chapter covers how to design controlled experiments to answer a research question; the second part covers how to create two random samples, and the third part covers how to analyze the data from the experiment to determine the answer to the question you set out to answer.

Introducing Experimental Design

Much of what people think of as analytics is actually just producing more efficient descriptions. You count things, and then you show how many things you counted. If you have seen the items counted before, the report isn't especially exciting, and not a lot of new learning is created from looking at it.

In contrast to descriptive analytics, experimentation is especially suited for exploration and production of new insight. Suppose that one of your three primary HR goals is to increase diversity and promote a culture of inclusion. (This is a popular company goal when it comes to hiring practices, so this example may strike close to home for you.) The two types of analytics described in this section depict two distinct approaches to tackling this goal — one that focuses on description and one that aims for insight.

Compare the examples in this section to see the difference between description and insight.

Analytics for description

Every year you count the number of people you have by ethnicity and gender, and you report this number by job and by level (individual contributor, manager, director, Vice President, and so on). Every year the company survey asks questions about diversity and inclusion, and every year you duly report the results by ethnicity and gender to management. The numbers aren't terrible, but they aren't great, either. The problem is that the numbers don't seem to change much. Whatever is happening just seems to continue on its own inertia. Maybe HR and Corporate Communications work together to change the pictures hanging on the wall in the break room to "reflect an environment of diversity and inclusion"; maybe they change some of the wording on the company website and in the job posting advertisements. Maybe you've also committed to a company-wide diversity training program, and the head of HR talks a lot about diversity whenever she attracts the spotlight. However, again, from an analytics perspective, year after year you count the people and you look at the survey data and not much seems to change. Even worse, people who match the diversity characteristics you're looking for don't see your communication programs as a true substitute for diversity and inclusion, and, at the same time, some of the people who don't meet the underrepresented characteristics you're promoting feel that their opportunities are shrinking. You see this predicament sometimes in anonymous communication channels, and you hear rumors. All measurable evidence indicates that your program is producing no real change, and, worse, for all you know it might even be producing cynicism. I call this a disaster; others call this diversity.

Analytics for insight

Having experienced analytics for description, as described in the preceding section, you may want to try something a little bit different. You have noticed that the company is hiring more underrepresented minorities than it did ten years ago and that no one seems to be explicitly racist; nevertheless, underrepresented minorities don't seem to be hired and promoted at the rate that a statistical review suggests they should be, which suggests prejudice. It's a bit of a paradox that you can neither find any explicit racists nor see underrepresented minorities making it through the hiring process or being promoted at the rate you think they should be. You want to understand how this could be occurring, and you want to know specifically what you can do to change it. You do a little research, you talk to some people, and you come up with three theories.

REMEMBER

A *theory* is just a fancy word for an idea that you believe explains the world around you — an idea that you intend to explore with the help of mathematical analysis and hard science. A *hypothesis* is a fancy word for a specific idea that you want to challenge with data. A hypothesis can defend or attack a theory. Hypothesis and theory are similar to the point of being synonymous. A hypothesis is a more specific version of a theory that can be exposed to immediate approval or rejection with data, whereas a theory is more far-reaching and requires more time and effort to unravel. A theory may contain many hypotheses.

So, what theories have you come up with for this particular case?

>> **Theory 1:** Underrepresented minorities are screened out before they even get to the interview stage in your recruiting funnel as a result of subconscious prejudice. The success rate of underrepresented minorities can be improved by allowing candidates to be sourced using only facts associated with validated success criteria. That means consciously not showing those who screen candidates the names of those candidates, because "ethnic-sounding" names can be triggering subconscious bias.

>> **Theory 2:** Underrepresented minorities are more likely to be selected from an onsite interview if you make hiring decisions by applying a structured interview format with a diverse, 5-person interview team and using the average scores of the five instead of either having one person make the decision.

>> **Theory 3:** All people have subconscious biases that influence their decisions, but they can grow increasingly aware of these biases and change them with the help of an adult learning group experience that couples a subconscious bias demonstration with a carefully facilitated diversity-&-inclusion group experience. (The MicroInequities program at http://insighteducationsystems.com/microinequities-the-power-of-small/ is a good example here.)

Breaking down theories into hypotheses and experiments

Theories with multiple "*and*" statements can be difficult to untangle with data. For example, Theory 1 can be broken down into several concurrent or sequential testable ideas (hypotheses) that can be approved or rejected using data. By design, a hypothesis must be falsifiable with data. (*Falsifiable* simply means that you must be able to prove it false.)

Your first test of Theory 1 can be quite simply to use data to scrutinize the assertion that "underrepresented minorities are screened out of the recruiting funnel at a rate higher than their availability in the population." This is a falsifiable statement. If you have the data and you look at it and find the answer is that underrepresented minorities *do* make it through the recruiting funnel at a rate proportional to their availability in the population, you need to stop and consider this before you proceed with any further experiments on Theory 1. The simple act of breaking up your work into steps can save you the time and money associated with testing a theory that has problems from the start. If the answer is no, the rate is not proportional, you can proceed to test the rest of the theory before moving on to other questions and theories.

To try out the three theories, you have to devise a series of experiments. Here's what they might look like:

>> **Experiment 1:** Verify a candidate's underrepresented minority status at the time of résumé submission. Using some unrelated administrative support, take 50 underrepresented minority résumés received and then the résumés of 50 white candidates, and then create candidate profiles that remove personal names and other information not pertinent to the recruiting process and any information with an unknown relationship to previously identified job success criteria. Mix them up and don't visibly associate the minority status information with the résumé content, although you should maintain a key. Have 10 different people select candidates for a prescreen from the scrubbed résumé content and 10 different people select from the normal résumé. Calculate the number of minority candidates selected from each method and compare.

Experiment 1 variation: You may also consider pairing and swapping the minority and nonminority names and calculate the pass-through levels when it comes to the white candidate's résumé with the *nonminority* name versus the white candidate's résumé with the *underrepresented minority* name.

>> **Experiment 2:** Have 20 underrepresented minority candidates and 20 white candidates complete an interview process with two different 5-person interview teams. On one of the interview teams, a diverse group of interviewers is instructed to use a particular structured interview technique, and candidates are ranked by the average score from the interview team. The other interview team operates in a manner traditional to your company. In this experiment, calculate the number of candidates recommended for hire by minority status for each of the two interview formats. Again, you compare the two interview teams that have different methods to see whether there are any differences in the number of underrepresented minorities recommended for hire.

>> **Experiment 3:** You can test Theory 3 (from the earlier section "Analytics for insight") by creating an adult learning group experience that couples a subconscious bias demonstration with a carefully facilitated diversity-&-inclusion group experience. (Again, MicroInequities: `http://insighteducationsystems.com/microinequities-the-power-of-small/`

is a good example.) You will have 50 people undergo the group experience and 50 people undergo a control experience — in other words, a typical teambuilding experience lacking any diversity-related learning. Because 50 is a large number of people in this example, these are broken into five groups of 10 people. Begin the experiment by pretesting the participants' belief systems about bias, diversity, and inclusion. Using a questionnaire, you can measure

- The degree of confidence an individual has that she's capable of making independent decisions free from bias

- The perception of the individual's own inclusion

- The perception the individual has of the inclusion of others in this company

You can compute each individual response, the group average, and the standard deviation between minority and nonminority participants. After exposing the group to the group experience, you can administer the same survey again. Responses provided in the post-test enable you to measure the later belief system for each person, the average of the group, and the standard deviation. If you discover a change during the second administration of the survey, you can conclude that the group experience likely had an impact on the belief system of the participants. The control group helps you to further isolate whether the change is related to the group experience or to something else.

REMEMBER

In statistics, the standard deviation (SD, also represented by the lower case Greek letter sigma σ or the Latin letter s) is a measure that is used to quantify the amount of variation or dispersion of a set of data values. A low standard deviation indicates that the data points tend to be close to the mean of the set, while a high standard deviation indicates that the data points are spread out over a wider range of values.

Paying attention to practical and ethical considerations

At the conclusion of each experiment, put everything back to normal and conduct the best screening/recruiting process based on what you have learned so that everyone has the fairest possible opportunity. You don't want the experiment to unnecessarily disadvantage anyone or expose a disadvantage in your traditional process and then not remedy it for everyone. If an experiment exposes a problem, it's proof that the experiment is worth completing. Given the benefits generated by the experiment, it's only fair that you make it right for the experiment's participants. Similarly, if the group experience works, you should share this group experience with more people to drive change in the company.

Designing Experiments

The examples in the earlier section "Introducing Experimental Design" may not be relevant to you or just may not be your cup of tea. Not a problem. The number of possible experiments is limited only by your creativity. Though the design of an experiment can vary considerably, most experiments have these three important components:

>> Independent and dependent variables

>> Experimental and control groups

>> Pre-measurement and post-measurement

The following sections look at each of these components in greater detail.

Using independent and dependent variables

An *experiment* examines the effect of an independent variable on a dependent variable. The independent variable takes the form of an experimental change, which is either present or absent. In the earlier example of the résumé screening, subconscious bias is the dependent variable, and removal of minority-sounding names (and other criteria not related to job performance) are the independent variables. The hypothesis is that underrepresented minorities are screened out of the recruiting process as a result of the effect that underrepresented minority-sounding names have on those who screen the candidates. The purpose of the experiment is to test the validity of this hypothesis. Removing the names is the cause; the relative proportion of minorities making it through the first stage of the recruiting funnel is the effect. What we hope to do is be able to say that a bias against underrepresented minority names is causing the underrepresented minorities to be screened out at a disproportional rate.

REMEMBER

The method of measuring both independent and dependent variables must be defined for the experiment in advance of the experiment. In the example, the dependent variable is a measurement of underrepresented minority prescreen pass-through rate, and the independent variable is either the presence or absence of access to names on the résumés.

In practice, the entire experiment can be conceived in many different ways; the independent and dependent variables can also be measured in many different ways. Often researchers intentionally conduct experiments with different experimental designs, different definitions, and under different conditions to see whether the conclusions are reliable and independently verifiable by other researchers under different conditions. For this reason, research findings sometimes contradict; however, science marches onward until the contradictions have been resolved and the matter has been settled.

REMEMBER

A variable can serve as a dependent variable in one experiment and as an independent variable in another. The independent and dependent variable and their configuration for experimentation are infinite.

Relying on pre-measurements and post-measurements

In the simplest experimental design, subjects are measured in terms of a dependent variable (pretested), exposed to a stimulus representing an independent variable, and then remeasured in terms of the dependent variable (post-tested). Differences noted between the first and last measurements on the dependent variables are then attributed to the influence of the manipulation of independent variable.

In the example of Theory 3 (from the earlier section "Analytics for insight"), you can begin by pretesting the participants' belief systems about bias, diversity, and inclusion. Using a questionnaire, you can measure

>> The degree of confidence individuals have that they are capable of making make independent decisions free from bias

>> The perception of the individual's own inclusion

>> The perception the individual has of the inclusion of others in this company.

Using the initial survey results, compute each individual response, the group average, and the standard deviation between minority and nonminority participants. After exposing the group to the group experience, administer the same survey again. Responses provided in the post-test enable you to measure the amount of change for each person, the change to the average of the group, and the change to the standard deviation. If you discover a change during the second administration of the survey, you can conclude that the group experience likely had an impact on the belief system of the participants.

WARNING

In the study of attitudes and opinions such as bias, there's a special problem related to validity: It's possible that the participants in the group experience may respond differently to the survey the second time around, even if their attitudes have remained unchanged. During the first survey, the subjects may have been unaware of its purpose. By the time they take the second survey, they will have figured out that you're interested in proving to them that everyone has bias and they may just tell you what they think the right social answer is. Thus, the experience would seem to have changed their opinion, although, in fact, it might not. This problem is well known among social scientific researchers — so well known, in fact, that someone came up with the term *Hawthorne effect* to describe it. In broad terms, the Hawthorne effect is based on the notion that the very act of studying something may change it. For this reason, the best researchers try some rather clever ways to work around this problem. In this example, a long-term before-and-after view of other diversity- and inclusion-related metrics can help to establish if in fact the group experience had any long-term impact among the groups that participated. These long-term findings (among other measurements) could help to validate or invalidate the temporary conclusions taken from the less reliable opinion data.

Working with experimental and control groups

To isolate the effect of an independent variable on the dependent variable while ruling out all other influences, randomly divide the experiment into two groups. One group receives the change in the independent variable, and the other group does not. (The group that doesn't receive the change is the *control* group.)

The control group may be given some other group activity — a day together at an amusement park, for example. Both groups are given the questionnaire beforehand and afterward. Figure 16-1 illustrates this basic experimental design.

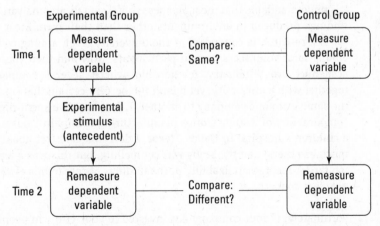

FIGURE 16-1: Diagram of experimental design.

The basic idea is illustrated in Figure 16-1, where you split the sample into two groups: an experimental group and a control group. The experimental group receives a stimulus, a change, or an antecedent, and the control group does not.

You measure the dependent variable at the beginning and end of the experiment for both the experimental group and the control group. These measurements allow you to compare the dependent variable between the experimental group and the control group to isolate the effect of the change.

A control group allows you to control for the effect of the experiment itself as well as many other potentially intervening variables. If the mere fact that the experiment was being conducted changed behavior (the dreaded Hawthorne effect) or if it was something else that changed the response of the post-test, the change should be the same in both the experimental and control groups. If the pre- and post-test responses were changed in the experimental group and not in the control group, it can be inferred that the group experience changed the attitudes or opinions of participants.

If it turns out that the group experience designed to change beliefs related to bias, diversity, and inclusion is successful relative to the control group, then after this is certain, be sure to "flip" the groups and provide the diversity-related group experience to the control group. You may conduct further testing in group batches like this, or you may be ready to apply the program broadly across the company.

Selecting Random Samples for Experiments

It's understandable that most business professionals are unaware (or skeptical) of findings produced in environments other than their own. Most published social science research is conducted at the university level, among college students or among local volunteers or paid participants. Now and then you do find a cross-academic, cross-industry relationship where several companies participate together with a university, yet it isn't 100 percent certain that conditions would be the same from one company to another. I, for one, have spent time pondering the comparability of a study from a manufacturing facility in Pakistan to one done at a children's hospital in Dallas, Texas. I don't usually fret about these things as much as others, and the study was compelling, but this was a leap that was even too far for me. Generalizability of the findings of research is always a debatable if not clear concern.

Fortunately, if your company has invested in your effort in people analytics, you have a perfect opportunity to produce learning that is highly relevant to your environment. Being able to tout this fact means that your findings should land with more credibility among the people you need to impress.

Introducing probability sampling

The purpose of *sampling* is to select a set of elements from a population in such a way that descriptions of those elements accurately portray the total population from which the elements are selected. Probability sampling enhances the likelihood of accomplishing this aim and also provides methods for estimating the degree of probable success.

The key to this process is *random sample selection,* in which each object or person has an equal chance of selection independent of any other event in the selection process. (If you need to visualize how random selection works, imagine repeatedly flipping a coin, rolling a die, or selecting random colored marbles from a jar.)

Random selection is important for two reasons:

» It eliminates the introduction of conscious or subconscious biases that might compromise the construction of the experiment and, in turn, the findings.

» It produces the conditions necessary for probability theory — conditions that are the basis for the math that's used to determine whether the findings were a result purely of chance, a result of error, or a result of the independent variable that you want to isolate and understand. The assumptions underlying the mathematics of certainty assume that the samples have been selected from the population randomly, so randomness has to happen.

When looking at other assumptions, and in order for people analytics (or any other type of analytics) to work, you must be able to isolate the variables. For that, you have only two true options:

» Collect all other variables that may influence the dependent variable (known or not known), and include them in a multiple regression or machine learning algorithm.

» Randomly select samples and apply the changes you want to measure to only one of those samples.

The first option, collecting all other variables that may influence the dependent variable, isn't practical, and it may not even be possible. The second option (random selection) is less time consuming, less expensive, and less intrusive — and it produces more mathematical and scientific confidence than any other method you could deploy. If a method is perfectly suited to people analytics, it's rapid experimentation using random samples.

Randomizing samples

Beginning with a list composed of all the people in your company, you select two random samples. The question you face is, how many people should you include in those two samples?

The larger the sample size, the easier it is to produce a statistically significant finding — meaning that there's less chance your results happened by coincidence. The more confident you want to be in the results, the larger the sample size needs to be. When selected randomly, a surprisingly small proportion of a large group can be used to predict the result of the population. However, the smaller the group you study, the larger the proportion of that group you need to sample to be certain.

All this may sound above your mathematical pay grade, but rest easy — you can use simple online calculators. Focus on understanding the big picture of what you're trying to do and why, and then take advantage of the online recommended sample size calculators as well as the statistical applications out there (Minitab, R, SAS, SPSS, or STATA, for example) or Excel to take you the rest of the way.

TIP

Looking for a great sample size calculator? Here's one at `www.qualtrics.com/blog/calculating-sample-size`.

To walk you through the basics you need in order to get the job done, here are some key terms you need to understand if you want to efficiently and effectively calculate the necessary sample size:

>> **Population:** In most cases, the population is the total number of people in your company. This is true if you're interested in research that generalizes to the entire company, but in some cases you may be interested in generalizing findings to only a segment of employees. In any event, the *population* is the entire group you want to study, whether that's the whole company or a segment of the company.

>> **Sample size:** The sample size is the number of people included in your study. It's called a sample because it represents only a portion of the population you're studying. A *random* sample is a method of choosing a sample where the members of the sample were selected entirely by chance.

>> **Representativeness:** If the two samples were selected randomly, you know (based on probability theory, mentioned earlier in this chapter) that the people selected resemble the population they were selected from and that the two samples also resemble each other. The degree to which you can be sure they resemble the population and each other is a function of the total size of the population and sample size.

>> **Mean:** the mean, also called the average, is the central value of a discrete set of numbers: specifically, the sum of the values divided by the number of values.

The true mean refers to the population mean. When you are contrasting between the mean and "the *true mean*," then the mean refers to the *sample mean* and the *true mean* refers to what the mean is if you measured everyone in the population. In the absence of the true population mean, the sample mean is the best estimate.

>> **Margin of error:** No dataset or sample is perfect, so you need to decide how much error to allow. The margin of error specifies a percentage that tells you how much you can expect your measurements of the sample to reflect the *true mean*. The smaller the margin of error, the closer you are to be sure of your findings.

>> **Confidence interval:** This figure determines how much higher or lower than the population mean you're willing to let the sample mean fall. If you've ever seen a political poll on the news, you've seen a confidence interval. It looks something like this: "58% of registered voters sampled said yes to Proposition Z, with a margin of error of +/– 5%." This means that based on the poll (a sample of the population of all registered voters) the proportion of actual registered voters expected to favor of the proposition in the actual vote could be as low as 53% and as high as 63%.

>> **Confidence level:** How confident do you want to be that the actual mean falls within your confidence interval? The most common confidence intervals are 90 percent, 95 percent, and 99 percent confident. For example, if you ran a study 100 times, an 80 percent confidence level would produce an incorrect conclusion 20 times out of 100, and a 99 percent confidence level would produce an incorrect conclusion 1 time out of 100. You choose the confidence level based on your tolerance for error. The goal should not be to produce perfect certainty, but rather to increase your odds of being right about your conclusions. If you're making a life-or-death decision, you want to get as close to perfect as you can within your budget. If it isn't a life-or-death decision, you can play the odds.

>> **Standard deviation:** How much variance do you expect in the responses? The standard deviation is a measure that is used to quantify the amount of variation or dispersion of a set of data values. A low standard deviation indicates that the data points tend to be close to the mean, while a high standard deviation indicates that the data points are spread out over a wider range of values.

Having determined the number of overall people you need to select to represent the population, your next step is to randomly select people to meet this need and to break them into two groups — one that will be exposed to the change and another that will be in the control group.

For purposes of this example, let's assume that you need 100 randomly selected people to represent your company population, which you intend to break into two samples of 50 people. One quick-and-dirty way to accomplish this task is by using Excel. Here's how:

1. **Put a list of all employees from the population you want to study into an Excel spreadsheet.**

   For example, if you have 1,000 employees, you should have a list of 1,000 employees in Excel, with one person per row. From this you want to select a random sample of 100 to be in your study, and you don't want any systematic bias — conscious or subconscious. Fortunately, Excel has a formula to generate random numbers and is a versatile spreadsheet application, so you can accomplish what you need.

2. **Add a new column just to the right of the list of employees, and name it** Random-Number.

3. **In the first cell underneath the heading row of Random-Number, type** = RAND() **and then press Enter.**

   A random number appears in the cell.

4. **Copy-and-paste this first cell into the other cells in this column, spanning the entire list of employees.**

   In Excel, you can accomplish this copy-and-paste action spanning a large range in different ways. One method is to grab the lower right corner of the cell and drag the formula down for the span of the employee list. Another method involves copying the cell with the formula, selecting the entire area where you want to paste it, and then clicking the Paste button on the Home tab.

   After each employee row contains a random number, you'll want to sort the entire table (all columns) by the Random-Number column.

5. **Start by using your cursor to select all the columns with your data in it.**

   Make sure to select all of the columns in the dataset so that you don't tell Excel to sort some columns and not others.

6. **After your entire dataset has been selected, click the Data tab on the Excel ribbon.**

   A submenu opens, displaying a number of options for handling data.

7. **Select Sort.**

   Doing so opens the Sort dialog box, which allows you to tell Excel exactly which column or columns you want to use to sort your data and precisely how you want to sort the data using those columns. By default, this menu looks like a table with one row partially populated.

Before you go any further, take this opportunity to look up to the upper right for a My List Has Headers check box. If your list has headers, be sure to check this box. This will tell Excel not to sort the first row — your header — into your list. You want to keep your column headers at the top.

8. **In the Sort dialogue box, click the blank cell beneath the Column header and select the column that has your random numbers in it. Working your way right, make sure Sort On is set to Values. Next, make sure Order is set to sort by Smallest to Largest.**

9. **When you have made all of your selections click the OK button in the bottom right of the dialogue box.**

Excel sorts your data as you have requested.

After you have sorted the table by the randomly generated numbers, the first 100 rows represent a random selection of 100 out of 1,000 employees. To determine which 50 of the 100 should be in the study sample and which should go to the control group, you could assign a new random number and repeat the process or just split them into groups of 50 from the list the way it is because they're already in random order.

Matching or producing samples that meet the needs of a quota

When selecting a statistically significant sample from a list of people, you can expect that the selected sample will represent the list. However, if the question of your study involves some characteristic (ethnicity, for example) in which some groups are minorities and therefore not a large percentage of the population, then by definition they're less likely to be selected in your random samples. In many circumstances, this may not be a problem for you; however, if you're designing group experiences that require a diverse sample (a deliberate mix of underrepresented minorities and others for purposes of study of diversity and inclusions beliefs, for example), you might need to modify your random selection technique. I explain how to do this here:

REMEMBER

What you're trying to do here is create two randomly selected groups while meeting the criteria necessary for the study to work — in this case, the need to enforce that there will be some deliberate mixture of "underrepresented minorities" and "others." The technique I suggest for this is called *stratified random sampling*, a method of sampling that involves dividing the population into smaller groups known as strata. The strata can be formed based on any variable or characteristic. In the case of my example, I am stratifying based on a classification of underrepresented minority and other.

To remain representative of the overall population, the goal is to keep both samples of 50 close to the actual distribution of underrepresented minorities and others. This may in fact happen randomly; however, because minorities are by definition a small part of your population, they may not come up in the random list. The simplest way to make sure it happens is to add columns to the spreadsheet for those characteristics you want to use to enforce a quota, populated with a value for each row labeled either Underrepresented Minority or Other. Let's say you want to have 20 percent be Underrepresented Minorities and 80 percent Other in each of the samples of 50. You still want to remain random, but you're looking for 10 underrepresented minorities to be added to each sample (20 percent of 50 is 10).

To continue the earlier example, here's how you can ensure that it happens:

1. **Populate the additional column with the necessary values (Underrepresented Minority or Other) for each employee.**

2. **Assign random numbers the same way you did a little earlier.**

3. **Sort the list in order of the random numbers.**

   Starting at the beginning of the list, put the first 40 Others in Group A and the first 10 Underrepresented Minorities in Group A. Then put the next 40 Others in Group B, and the next 10 Underrepresented Minorities in Group B.

   Now you have two samples of 50 people drawn randomly to be representative of each other and that, when combined, are representative of the population you want to study as a whole. With that behind you, you can now begin the experiment, whatever you have devised it to be.

Analyzing Data from Experiments

When tackling the data culled from your experimental work, it's always good to start out with a clear understanding of the terminology involved. For example, in scientific research intended to measure relationship between variables, variables are either independent or dependent. As their names imply, dependent variables are the variables that are affected when the independent variables change. Independent variables are labeled x and dependent variables labeled y. If there are multiple independent variables, this may be noted generically as $x_1, x_2, x_3, \ldots$ with as many (x)s as the number of independent variables you have.

Here's an example: If an instructor wants to study success in a class, she might collect data for independent variables like completion of earlier related classes, GPA, and study time and then use test scores as the dependent variable. Using the collected data, the instructor can correlate each independent variable (GPA, study time, and so on) to the dependent variable (test scores). If the Test Score variable is highly correlated with the Study Time variable, the instructor could use this information to encourage students who want to have high test scores to increase study time.

Significance is determined by the probability that a sample would show such a relationship if it didn't exist in the population as a whole. If a relationship between variables is regarded as significant, it's taken by inference to exist in the population as a whole.

The analyst must determine the critical value of the probability below which the relationship will be viewed as significant and above which it will be attributed to probable sampling error. If the desired confidence interval is set at 95 percent, then the significance value is .05 and there's only a 5 percent chance that the demonstrated relationship doesn't actually exist — that it had occurred as a result of chance, in other words.

With a confidence interval set at 95 percent, if you ran this experiment 100 times, you would likely make a wrong conclusion 5 times. Such is life when dealing with probabilities.

Statistical significance quantifies the possibility that your result is simply due to chance. *Practical significance* determines whether the difference you find is big enough to be of practical value to you. The goal of statistical significance is to represent a mathematically defensible confidence in the finding. The goal of practical significance is to figure out whether those statistical differences matter to you in the real world.

You may have a high degree of statistical confidence that there is in fact a difference between 10 cents and 20 cents; that difference, however, may not buy you anything of any practical value in the real world. The latter is practical significance.

A relationship cannot be viewed as important if it isn't significant, because there's too great a chance that it resulted from sampling error (randomness). However, a relationship that's statistically significant may or may not be important (be practically significant), because importance depends on the strength and meaning of the relationship.

With the basic vocabulary out of the way, it's time to do some analyzing. The next section gets you started.

Graphing sample data with error bars

Let's talk about a simple, rough method for judging whether an experiment might support its hypothesis. You want to know if the mean for the experimental group is in fact different from the control group or if the difference is simply a result of chance.

The *standard error of the mean* is a statistic that measures how likely the mean statistic you computed is in fact the true mean. The standard error is like a region of likelihood around the computed mean — the region around the computed mean in which the true mean probably lies. The standard error is computed by taking the standard deviation of the measurements and dividing by the square root of n — the number of measurements.

To use the standard error technique, draw a bar chart of the means for each condition, with error bars ("whiskers") stretching one standard error above and one standard error below the top of each bar. If you look at whether those error whiskers overlap or are substantially different, you can make a rough judgment about whether the true means of those conditions are likely to be different. Suppose that the error bars overlap — then it's possible that the true means for both conditions are actually the same. But if the error bars don't overlap, it's likely that the true means are different.

The error bars can also give you a sense of the reliability of your experiment. If you didn't put enough people in the samples, your error bars will be large relative to the size of the data. So the error bars may overlap even though there really is a difference between the conditions. The solution is more repetition — more people — in order to increase the precision of your understanding of the true location of the means.

Here's a step-by-step look at how to add error bars to your bar graphs in Excel:

1. **In a spreadsheet, summarize your collected data with the mean (average of all data), standard deviation (using the Excel formula =STDEV), and standard error (using the Excel formula =STDEV/SQRT(n)) for the data in your table, as shown in Figure 16-2.**

2. **Highlight your summary chart, click the Insert tab, and then click the tab's Bar icon to insert a bar chart graph of the mean.**

3. **Click the Chart Design button on the Excel ribbon, then choose Add Chart Element ⇨ Error Bars ⇨ More Error Bar Options from the menu that appears, as shown in Figure 16-3.**

4. **In the Format Error Bars pane on the right, leaving all other selections in their default position, click the Specify Value button and then use the Custom Error Bars dialog box to select the range of data containing the standard error.**

   In the example, that would mean selecting cells containing your calculated standard error from your summary chart for both the positive and negative error values. (See Figure 16-4.)

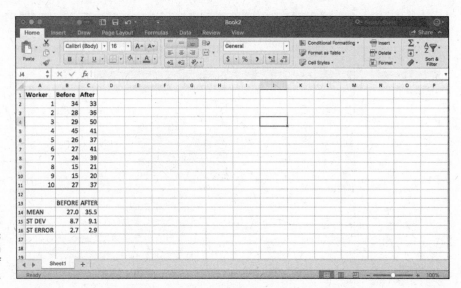

FIGURE 16-2:
Sample table with
a summary of
statistics.

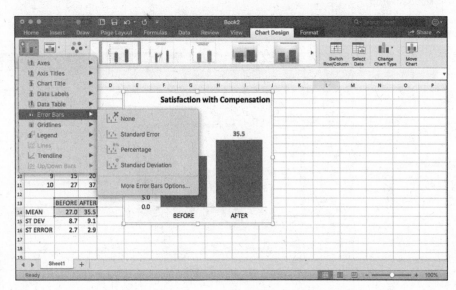

FIGURE 16-3:
Inserting error
bars.

5. **Finish formatting the graph for style. (See Figure 16-5.)**

Figure 16-5 shows the finished graph with error bars. If the error bars overlap, meaning the top of the Before whisker extends higher than the bottom of the After whisker, that implies that, even though the means represented by the bars look different, with error taken into consideration they may in fact be the same mean. If the bars don't overlap, it's unlikely they are the same mean.

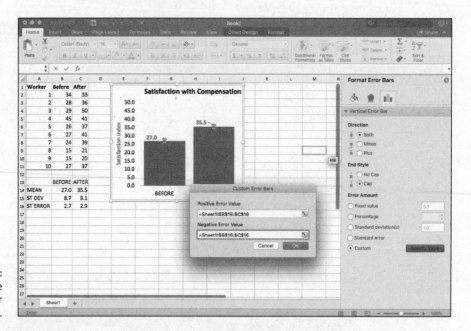

FIGURE 16-4:
Select the
standard error
range.

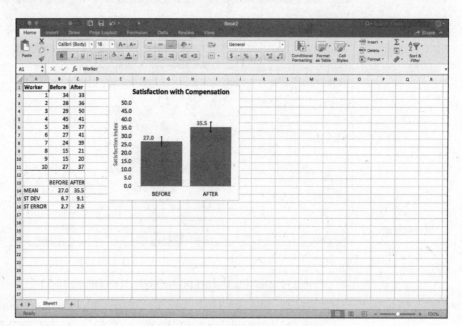

FIGURE 16-5:
The finished
graph with error
bars.

Using *t*-tests to determine statistically significant differences between means

The *t-test* is a statistical method often used in experimental design when comparing groups or samples for the purpose of determining the impact of some change. Nobody has come up with a good reason why it's called a *t*-test rather than a z-test or a p-test, but some speculate that the person who developed the *t*-test, William Sealy Gosset, simply chose the last letter of his last name. (Fun fact: Gosset, an English statistician, offered his services to the Guinness Brewery of Dublin, Ireland, where his talents were used to improve the quality of its signature stout.)

There are a few things you should know about *t*-tests before we go any further. First, I'll explain the 3 types of *t*-tests, the 2 forms of *t*-tests, and the specific descriptors you'll need to understand to complete a *t*-test in Excel.

First off, the 3 types of *t*-tests are:

>> **Unpaired (or independent samples) *t*-test:** This is the most common form of *t*-test. It will allow you to compare two sets of data. Our example below will use an unpaired *t*-test. I will compare a group who received training versus a group that did not.

>> **Paired *t*-tests:** Use a paired *t*-test when you run a *t*-test on dependent samples. For example, you would run a paired *t*-test if you collected data on the same group of people before and after a training. Comparing the same person's test scores before and after training means that you're effectively using each person as his own control. Rather than compare the test results of a sample of employees who received training versus a sample who didn't, you're comparing changes in the same group's prior sample with their own later test measurements

>> **One (or single) sample *t*-test:** This *t*-test will compare the mean of your collected sample to a known value. For example, you can use a one sample *t*-test to compare the number of sick days taken within your organization to the industry average.

Now the 2 forms of *t*-tests:

>> **Two-tailed *t*-tests:** In the more conservative, 2-tailed *t*-test, your hypothesis is merely that the means are different, so an extreme t-value, either positive or negative, counts as evidence against the null hypothesis that the means are the same.

>> **One-tailed *t*-test:** The other form is the 1-tailed test, in which your hypothesis expects the difference to go one way or the other.

Finally, here's how Excel labels each type

>> **Paired test:** Use this option when performing a paired *t*-test.

>> **Two-sample equal variance (homoscedastic):** Use this option when doing an unpaired *t*-test with equal standard deviations.

>> **Two sample unequal variance test:** Use this option when doing an unpaired *t*-test with unequal standard deviations.

Now, suppose that you want to evaluate the effect of an effort to help employees better understand all elements of their pay, including how their pay compares to the market as well as how the company makes salary decisions. As a pilot, you enroll 100 subjects into your study and then randomly assign 50 subjects to the experimental group (training class) and 50 subjects to the control group (no training class). In this case, you have two independent samples and would use the unpaired form of the *t*-test. After the training is over, the next performance review scores of the participants in the experimental group can be compared to the control (those who didn't go to training) using the *t*-test.

With a paired or unpaired *t*-test, you're using the statistical *t*-test to determine whether there's a difference in test outputs as a result of the training or whether there's no difference. Technically, you're accepting or rejecting whether the differences found (if any) are likely a result of chance or likely caused by something else. (For your research, you'll assume that the "something else" is the training program until proven otherwise.)

REMEMBER

The actual calculation of the t-statistic and the proof that it's a valid test are beyond the scope of this book. In practice, nobody computes their own t-statistic; they use a statistical package (or that jack-of-all-trades, Excel) to do the computations, which is what I recommend.

Performing a *t*-test in Excel

Taking another look at the example, you're trying to figure out whether an employee's satisfaction level in terms of his compensation improves after undergoing training designed to explain the logic behind such compensation levels. You can postulate that, yes, satisfaction levels will rise as a result of such training. To test this theory, you come up with a hypothesis suggesting that the means of the two samples — the experimental group and the control group — are not equal, meaning that there's a statistically significant difference between the satisfaction levels of both groups.

REMEMBER

Science always requires that you test the opposite of your hypothesis. If the actual hypothesis is that the means are not equal, the opposite hypothesis is that the means of two samples are equal: this is called the *null hypothesis.* If the two means are different you reject the null hypothesis (they are the same) and temporarily accept the alternative to the null — that the two means are different as a result of whatever your theory has suggested. For now, your theory holds up.

As I mention earlier in this chapter, one of the best ways to determine whether there's a significant difference between the means of two groups is to use a *t*-test. You'll want to apply a *t*-test to the before–and–after levels of satisfaction with compensation among the experimental group and then compare those values with those of the control group. A quick way to calculate this is by using the built-in Excel *t*-test function: =T.TEST({array1},{array2},{tails},{type}).

{array1} refers to the first set of data.

{array2} is the second set of data.

{tails} refers to whether you want to run a 1-tailed or 2-tailed test. In {tails}, enter a **2** for a 2-tailed test or **1** for a 1-tailed test.

{type} refers to the type of *t*-test. You have 3 options:

1 = paired test

2 = two sample equal variance test (homoscedastic)

3 = two sample unequal variance test

So, to compare Experimental Group Before to Experimental Group After, begin by entering the following syntax directly into the cell you'd like to display your result in:

=T.TEST(

Automatically, placeholders for the parameters you need appear in the cell. (Figure 16-6 shows you what I mean.)

Supply the correct parameters, shown here:

{array1}: Input **B3:B12** for Experimental Group Before.

{array2}: Input **C3:C12** for Experimental Group After.

{tails}: Enter a **2** for a 2-tailed test.

{type}: Enter a **2** for a two sample equal variance test.

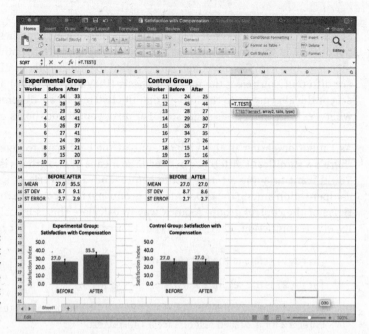

FIGURE 16-6:
For the *t*-test function, begin by entering the following syntax directly into any cell: **=T.TEST(**.

Press Enter and Excel carries out the *t*-test for you. The result here is a p-value (short for *probability value*) of 0.045. In statistical analysis, the *p-value* is the probability that the differences you observed happened purely by chance. Every run of an experiment has random noise; the p-value is the probability that the means were different only because of this random noise. Thus, if the p-value is less than 0.05, you can have 95 percent confidence that there really is a difference.

REMEMBER

A small p-value (typically ≤ 0.05) indicates strong evidence against the null hypothesis, so you reject the null hypothesis. A large p-value (> 0.05) indicates weak evidence against the null hypothesis, so you fail to reject the null hypothesis.

To compare Experimental Group After to Control Group After, re-create what you see in Figure 16-7. Begin by entering the following syntax directly into the cell you'd like to display your result in:

```
=T.TEST(
```

Replace the placeholder parameters with this information:

{array1}: Input **C3:C12** for Experimental Group After.

{array2}: Input **J3:J12** for Control Group After.

{tails}: Enter **2** for a 2-tailed test.

{type}: Enter **2** for a two sample equal variance test.

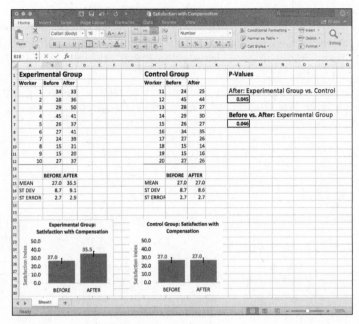

FIGURE 16-7:
The p values
returned from
these two
applications of
the *t*-test formula
are 0.045 and
0.046.

Press Enter and Excel carries out the *t*-test for you. The result here is a p-value of 0.046, as shown in Figure 16-7.

Admittedly, a full-featured statistics application will return a more complete table of summary statistics; this simple shortcut formula in Excel returns only a simple p-value. Fortunately, the p-value is the most important value for the purpose of this discussion. To interpret the p-value, you just need to know whether the p-value is less than the value you picked for the confidence level: for example, .10, .05, or .01.

For the purpose of this example, go ahead and set the confidence level to a pretty easy bar to get under — 90 percent confidence = (0.10). When you apply this standard to the p-value of both comparisons, you'll find that the p-values of both (0.045 and 0.046) are indeed below the minimum threshold you set to be confident that your means are different. This allows you to reject the null hypothesis that the means are the same and accept the alternative hypothesis that the means are different.

For now, based on the level of confidence you want to have and this experiment, there's enough evidence to support the position that Compensation Total Rewards Training helps to increase satisfaction with pay. You can now say that there's a statistically significant difference between the means.

REMEMBER

Keep in mind that statistical significance doesn't imply importance. There might be better ways to improve satisfaction with pay, or maybe satisfaction with pay has no impact on employee attrition. If that's the case, statistical significance may not matter to you. For a complete decision, you should consider what you have learned about the relative importance of factors, including pay, in a key driver analysis. (See Chapter 13 for more on key driver analysis.)

5

The Part of Tens

Chapter **17**

Ten Myths of People Analytics

P eople analytics work is different from other analytics, so knowing how to manage it can be especially difficult. Traditional ways of working and leading have inertia. Many folks you work with — some that are well-meaning and some that feel threatened by this new thing – can directly or indirectly conspire to knock you off course and derail your success. Myths abound about the nature of people analytics, and many large, very successful, and well-resourced companies have fallen prey to one or more of these myths. As a result, although they started out with high expectations, they soon discovered they had run into a wall with people analytics. Imagine how much more challenging it is if your company isn't large and well-resourced!

In this chapter, I fill you in on the most common myths standing in the way of successful people analytics and tell you how to think about it differently. These myths are tenacious – and they can be real problems for you if you're not careful. Be on the lookout for them and be ready with answers. Doing so can save your people analytics initiative, your job and, if you believe this stuff matters as much I do, the success of your entire company.

Myth 1: Slowing Down for People Analytics Will Slow You Down

Myth: Stopping your traditional human resource efforts to work on data collection and analysis for people analytics will slow you down and keep you from the results you are trying to achieve.

Truth: It is true that people analytics requires spending more time up front to define problems, develop processes to collect data, and then analyze it, but this time spent up front can save you much more over the long run. People analytics is about helping the entire team work smarter, not harder.

Stopping to collect data and analyze it seems to run counter to whatever tasks you are trying to accomplish, but people analytics is actually the quickest, most effective, and most efficient way to get impact from what you are doing in human resources.

Here is a scenario that illustrates how people analytics can help you do the same work you already do a little differently to save a lot of time and effort in the long run.

Imagine you are the head of recruiting. Your team is working as hard as it possibly can to fill open positions for your company. Recruiters are working ten to twelve-hour days trying to keep up with candidate interactions. On top of this, management wants to expand into a new market so they are asking you to do even more.

You might be thinking, "How can we possibly spare a member of our team for this people analytics thing — we are so busy!"

Now, imagine you resisted this fear and did it anyway. You discovered through analysis of resumes and recruiting process data that by screening resumes for new criteria you can reduce the number of people you push into later stages of the recruiting process that inevitably fail. A simple tweak in how you screen resumes can reduce recruiter interactions with candidates later in the process by 25%, with no reduction in the number of hires or quality of hire. By reducing the workload, the application of this insight would be like getting 25% more recruiters.

Your analysis also discovers another pattern. People that respond to a question in their interview in a certain way are more likely to stay with the company for many years, rather than turning around and leaving in the first year. By choosing for characteristics that produce longevity you can decrease need to backfill seats of people who are leaving – this amounts to an additional 25% reduction in demand for recruiters.

Adding up these two insights, you have decreased recruiter workload, achieving more with the same number of recruiters — in effect increasing the overall productivity of your recruiting team by 50%. If there are 50 working weeks in a year, the savings from the example above is equivalent to 25 work weeks. Even if you stopped your entire team to do nothing else but work on analysis for two whole weeks, you would still be 23 weeks of work ahead. That's just in one year! If the insights you produced in those two shut down weeks continued to work for the next five years, imagine the savings you have received by stopping to do analysis. That would be 115 work weeks over five years saved from just two weeks of analysis.

The example above illustrates the power of analysis — you can achieve a lot more with less input if you slow down to do analysis.

Myth 2: Systems Are the First Step

Myth: You must select and implement a new system before you can start people analytics.

Truth: The people analytics process I have found works the best doesn't even get to system implementation until the end — it is Step 8 in the process below:

1. Determine what problem is most important to work on.

2. Study what you already know about the problem.

3. Form new theories about the causes of the problem and predictions about the evidence of the problem that you'll see in the data.

4. Develop measurements to test your theories.

5. Collect the right data to perform the measurements.

6. Perform the measurements and analysis to see whether they support your theories.

7. Determine if the insight produced by this analysis is useful. If it is not useful, return to Step 1. If it is useful, go to next step.

8. If the insight produced by the analysis is useful, determine if you want it to be running continuously. If so, then implement a system to automate the analysis. If not, then return to Step 1.

   As you can see, this process doesn't require you to have any particular new systems for people analytics at the outset. In fact, starting with systems may actually take your attention away from those things that matter most. There's no need to make large up-front investments in specialized systems to start your people analytics initiative. You can start on whatever HR technology infrastructure and basic desktop business application you already have until you have proven some value from your efforts.

The systems you use are not the most important part of people analytics — the analysis is. Software developers are always making new systems that are better than the last systems and this is good, but you probably don't need a new system to get started. You can solve even the most difficult analytical puzzles with logic, experimentation, and widely available business applications that need not be sophisticated or cost a lot of money. All of the things you need to get started with people analytics can be performed in standard desktop applications like Microsoft Excel, cloud-based spreadsheet software like Google Sheets, or in open-source statistics software you can find online for free like R. Anything beyond this is just intended to make what you do better or more efficient in some way. I'm all for better and more efficient, but don't let perfect be the enemy of getting started.

There's no need to make large up-front investments in new technology systems to start your people analytics initiative.

Myth 3: More Data Is Better

Myth: The more data, metrics, reports, and dashboards you have, the better job you have done.

Truth: The more data, metrics, reports, and dashboards you have the more you (and everyone else at your company) will be overburdened and confused.

Overwhelming end users with access to every bit of data and all possible ways to slice it can stifle adoption because the end users start to see it as a tangled mess too big to unravel- — what they need may be there somewhere but finding the information they need is going to take too much work.

Moreover, collecting, storing, moving, cleaning, sharing, and viewing data costs something. Even if money isn't a limiting factor, time is. It takes time to tend to the details of all this data. Chasing a higher quantity of data without resolving what you are going to do with it can result in getting tied up in a lot of activities that in the end don't contribute to your success. Activity does not equal progress. Make sure the actions you take with data will support valuable insights that others will use.

The most important part of any data analysis is the ability to pull out insights and take action based on the findings. The data you have on hand may or may not contain the answers to your (and others') questions, but it certainly doesn't contain the questions themselves. Those have to come from you. Resolve to identify the most important questions first and work backwards. This will help you prioritize your effort and make the output of what you produce more relevant to others.

Myth 4: Data Must Be Perfect

Myth: The HR dataset has to be exhaustive and without flaw and all together in the same system before you can start.

Truth: If you look at other fields you will learn there are no perfect datasets — and yet we keep marching onward.

The more you work with data (and talk to other people who work with data) the more you will realize, there are no perfect datasets. Finance doesn't have a perfect dataset. Sales doesn't have a perfect dataset. Marketing doesn't have a perfect dataset. University researchers don't have a perfect dataset. Einstein didn't have a perfect dataset. Marie Curie didn't have a perfect dataset. Nobody has a perfect dataset.

If data isn't in the same system, it can be moved and joined. If data isn't in the right shape, it can be transformed. If data is missing, it can be filled in. These activities are normal part of the process of analysis.

Most importantly, statistical methods allow you to draw conclusions from imperfect data. Statistical methods are tolerant of error — meaning they do not require perfect datasets. Statistical methods are intended to increase certainty in an uncertain world. Most statistical procedures are about comparing if two measures are different and then deciding with math if the difference is real or a result of random chance. It is possible to have error in your data and still be able to obtain an answer with reasonable certainty.

We are looking for reasonable certainty, not perfect certainty. Perfection has a value and a cost. In the world of people analytics, it turns out that the value of perfection isn't very high — and the cost is higher if it prevents you from getting started.

Myth 5: People Analytics Responsibility Can be Performed by the IT or HRIT Team

Myth: People Analytics responsibility can be performed by the IT or Human Resource Information Technology (HRIT) teams.

Truth: Though people analytics and Human Resource Information Technology (HRIT) both have something to do with data and human resources, these trades require fundamentally different skills. Aside from this, the good folks in charge of maintaining the HR systems have responsibilities on their shoulders already.

Within the scope of HRIT you typically find that folks are responsible for system selection, integration, ETL (extract, transform, load), security and administration for the following kinds of HR systems:

>> Applicant tracking systems

>> Onboarding systems

>> Human resource information systems (the employee system of record connecting to many other systems)

>> Payroll systems

>> Compensation planning systems

>> Performance management systems

>> Learning management systems

Increasingly, systems facilitate nearly all aspects of the day-to-day work of HR. The confusion may stem from the fact that many of the systems that HR professionals use to collect data also offer direct access to data through embedded self-service dashboard interfaces, which many people will think of as synonymous with analytics, but they are not the same. The HR systems help you do many things better than you could do without the system, and they capture data, but they don't do analysis.

Good HRIS management by professionals with an IT background and an HRIT emphasis is essential. IT professionals have a lot to offer in facilitating system selection, overall system architecture, designing how data flows between systems, oversight of system security and help desk interaction with those who have day-to-day interactions with systems. As you can imagine, that is a big workload by itself, without including behavioral science, statistics and HR domain expertise — the other important aspects of people analytics which are all totally different in terms of basic knowledge, skills, and abilities. IT professionals already have plenty to learn and do without adding data analysis to their plates!

TECHNICAL STUFF

There are systems that are used to facilitate the work of people analytics. Like any other business analytics function, the traditional systems used to facilitate people analytics include systems designed specifically for one or more of the following: ETL (extract, transform, load), data workflow, data warehousing, reporting or business intelligence, statistics, DevOps, machine learning, and data visualization. On top of the regular business analytics application needs, people analytics also requires the ability to perform surveys. Increasingly, there are niche applications designed for people analytics specifically. For example, there are systems that will help you wrangle HR data from multiple source systems into a single uniform data model (OneModel), visualize HR data (Visier), check for diversity bias in pay (Syndio), and analyze the talent acquisition process (RecruitFactors).

Ultimately, HRIS management is a domain-specific IT function, and people analytics is a domain-specific data analysis function. IT and HRIT professionals define system architecture, gather requirements for systems, and manage systems implementations. People analysts perform analysis, which requires deep domain knowledge in behavioral science, statistics and human resources.

Myth 6: Artificial Intelligence Can Do People Analytics Automatically

Myth: You can implement a system that will automatically use the data you have to solve all your problems for you.

Truth: Artificial intelligence applications can be useful tools once a clear task has been defined that a computer algorithm is capable of doing on its own, but the current total of applications of artificial intelligence for people analytics are still very small.

Today's systems can grind through tasks at breakneck speed once its task is clearly defined, but today's systems still cannot define objectives, define problems, figure out the right questions to ask, define the measures you will use to answer those questions, rally people to provide the information necessary, interpret the results, or garner the enthusiasm of others for change.

People analytics requires the inputs and efforts of people with enthusiasm, curiosity, creativity, and problem-solving skills. Truly, some tasks are simply better for computer algorithms to do. However, you need a person to tell that system which task to do in the first place. You also need people to identify new data that may be beneficial to the algorithms as well as design processes, provide data, scrutinize the algorithms, and find ways to communicate and use the output. The current state of artificial intelligence still leaves a lot of work for people in people analytics!

Myth 7: People Analytics Is Just for the Nerds

Myth: People analytics is just for nerds — regular people need not apply. Nothing less than a really smart PhD data science person (or a team of them) can possibly get the job done.

Truth: People analytics is a team sport.

Though I'd never turn down a chance to get a super-genius on my team, the idea that you must hire a team full of super-geniuses to do all the work of people analytics on others' behalf is simply false. Everybody in today's rapidly evolving and competitive job market should learn how to form good data questions, how to collect good data, how to make good data-informed decisions, and how to work with a little data in a spreadsheet.

Aside from this, many of the tasks necessary for people analytics don't require a PhD or any special intelligence. 80% or more of the work of analytics falls into the category of preparing a dataset for analysis, as opposed to the analysis itself. Some examples of the work that is required:

>> Project management

>> Talking to people to find out where data is in systems

>> Getting data into databases and spreadsheets

>> Filling in data holes

>> Putting calculations into a dataset to combine things, separate things, add things, or remove things

>> Getting data fields into the right format for analysis

>> Moving the entire dataset into the right orientation for analysis

>> Creating graphs

>> Adding the graphs to presentation slides and annotating them

> » Sharing data and insights with others

> » Facilitating integration of the insight into decision-making processes

Get everyone involved! When something extremely complicated comes up, you can grab the attention of PhDs working in other areas of your company or a graduate student at a local college.

Myth 8: There are Permanent HR Insights and HR Solutions

Myth: There are permanent HR insights and HR solutions. Once you've run a successful analysis and have extracted a people analytics insight, you are done.

Truth: You are never done with people analytics.

HR insights have a shelf life and statistical models require constant care to continue being useful over time. All statistical models start with environmental, behavioral, and cognitive assumptions which require similar conditions for the results to generalize from one situation to the next. You need to reevaluate the assumptions and update statistical models with new data continually.

Even if you can manage to quash a problem entirely, the next problem is about to emerge elsewhere. The intrinsic dynamic qualities of human beings are what makes them the heart and soul of your business, but those same qualities consistently generate problems that you will never finish solving.

Rather than strive for an empty to-do list, you should measure your success by the additional results your company is achieving and the benefits the human beings in it are enjoying thanks to your effort.

Myth 9: The More Complex the Analysis, the Better the Analyst

Myth: The more complex the analysis, the better the analyst.

Truth: The best analyst answers the question in the simplest manner possible.

REMEMBER

Occam's razor (or Ockham's razor) is a principle from philosophy that states that the simplest explanation is usually the right one. Suppose there exist two explanations for an occurrence. The principle of Occam's razor suggests that the one that requires the least speculation is usually better, because it requires less assumptions. It is also easier to understand.

Of all the dangerous myths to befall people analytics, the one that is perhaps the most insidious is believing that the more complex the analysis, the better. Left to their own devices, people usually define "better" as the newest or most advanced tools. People love new toys — a new technique, a new form of analysis, a new software program. When they get a new toy, they get to play with something they haven't had before, which makes it exciting for a time. It is OK to have some excitement for your work, but this needs to be balanced against the need to solve problems that matter and picking the most efficient tool for the job. If you are not careful, you will spend all your time and money chasing the latest fad.

New tools are constantly emerging. For a few years it was predictive analytics, then it was natural language processing (NLP), then organization network analysis (ONA) and, at the time of the writing of this book, artificial intelligence (AI). If you buy into the AI fad, you might settle on the idea you should just drop "people" from the name "people analytics" and get into something else entirely. Like fad diets and exercise equipment, these shiny new objects can sometimes distract you from what you are trying to achieve and all the other options available for you to achieve it. Be careful, because often what is popular is being driven by the marketing efforts of big technology companies that are out to make a quick buck from your excitement at the expense of your time and wallet.

Take Organization Network Analysis (ONA), for example. ONA is an advanced statistical method for studying communication and socio-technical networks within a company based on social network theory. This technique creates statistical and graphical models of the people and knowledge patterns in organizational systems. Two years ago, if you were not doing something with ONA, you were old hat. According to the cool crowd if you were not doing ONA, you might as well remove "analytics" from the name "people analytics" because you are just "people" doing something or other but certainly not analytics in any serious way. I disagree. ONA is a great tool for understanding patterns of information flow and a great new approach to study diversity. If this information is useful for a question you are trying to answer and you can figure out how to use it, you should, but absent a good use, your interesting network graph isn't going to hold attention for very long. We will still be figuring out the possible applications of ONA for a while, but the buzz around ONA seems to have come and gone in a flash — the world has now moved on to AI. Again, some people might have you believe if you aren't doing AI, you might as well just give up analytics now. I don't buy it.

A carpenter cannot build a house with just the latest laser level, and you cannot fully understand a company with just organization network analysis (ONA) or whatever the newest sexy tool is. There are many different things relating to people you should measure and many different methods you can apply, but each do not fit equally to the task at hand. You need a tool box that includes an array of tools to solve a variety of different problems. It is great to have new tools, but don't get fixated on them.

Myth 10: Financial Measures are the Holy Grail

Myth: The Holy Grail of people analytics is to measure the actions relating to people through traditional financial measures like Return on Investment (ROI).

Truth: People analytics may still lack the common definitions, conventions, and oversight that finance has benefited from for hundreds of years; however, people analytics represents a new measurement system for understanding and controlling the performance of a company that is different and, in some ways, much better than traditional financial measures.

Criticisms of the finance method of analysis include:

>> Financial measures aggregate so many different actions and conditions together that you lose the ability to determine causal linkages.

>> Navigating the company based on financial measures can be like navigating your car from the rear-view mirror. Financial measures make a decent scorecard, but they don't make a great playbook.

>> Financial measures can encourage decisions that have short-term financial benefits but have devastating long-term consequences.

The idea that the old ways of accounting for business performance are the only ways to analyze a business and make decisions is incorrect. People analytics goes upstream from financial measures to provide insight and control over those things that impact the long-term health and performance of the company. People analytics incorporates the financial measures, but it offers insights that you cannot see in the financial measures by themselves.

REMEMBER

Do not expect traditional accounting methods and systems to reflect improvements accomplished through human resources immediately. Eventually, improvements in control over talent attraction, activation, and attrition will impact the bottom line, but it may take some time for the benefits to accumulate and it may be difficult, if not impossible, to isolate the impact of individual decisions or actions in financial measures. This is not to say that the impact of individual decisions or actions cannot be tested — they just have to be tested by scrutinizing causal assumptions with other measures.

Chapter **18**

Ten People Analytics Pitfalls

Over my career in people analytics, I certainly have made my share of mistakes. You don't have to learn everything the hard way, though. In this chapter, I share ten of the most common (and most serious) pitfalls I have seen people analytics efforts succumb to over the years. I hope that by reading these, you can prepare yourself and your teammates to steer clear of trouble.

Pitfall 1: Changing People is Hard

People analytics can change the entire nature of human resources — and nothing gets people stirred up quite like change. Regardless of the scope of people analytics you are implementing, it's likely that you'll encounter some level of difficulty if you are trying change the way people think, the way people make decisions, and the way people do what the they do.

Quite often I hear about resistance to change. More often I encounter ambivalence rather than resistance. Ambivalence, however, can be worse than resistance because everyone may outwardly cheer you on and yet not provide the support you need to be successful. The difficulties associated with change materialize in many different ways. Here are just a few:

>> You need someone to give you access to a system and there is a lengthy, unexplained delay.

>> You need to get others to explain data definitions to you and they claim they are too busy right now to get to it.

>> You need to talk to someone about a report you are building for them and you can't get time on their calendar.

>> You need someone to change how others are inputting data into systems and help you with data clean-up and nobody follows up with you.

You need to proactively build awareness of the benefits of change and address the difficulty of change to try to get everyone pitching in. Otherwise, what starts out as ambivalence can quickly turn into full-blow resistance, leaving your movement toward data-informed decision making in tatters.

Here are some ways you can proactively improve the probability of your success:

>> **Set up a cross-functional people analytics task force** to help you be more aware of the needs of others and create an umbrella of support. Whenever you encounter problems, talk it over at a monthly meeting. Not only will you get valuable input, but you'll also get buy-in.

>> **Build lasting relationships with IT, data-management, and human resource information technology (HRIT) folks.** You need their blessing, their input, their support, and their friendship. As with any important relationship, you usually get out what you put in.

>> **Get an important project sponsor.** When you communicate with others, you can let drop that the head honcho is closely watching the outcome of the project. That tends to get people's attention.

>> **Three words: communicate, communicate, communicate.** It is a good idea to send notes to all stakeholders periodically. Be sure to reinforce the importance of people analytics, revisit the benefits of the project, and give them updates on the project's status.

REMEMBER

In the introduction to people analytics in Chapter 1, I refer to the Four S People Analytics Framework — also referred to as the People Analytics Intersection. By this I mean people analytics is the new thing that is created at the intersection of people strategy, science, statistics, and systems. Figure 18-1 illustrates how people analytics joins the four broad people S capabilities (strategy, science, statistics, and systems) to create some new innovation that didn't exist before. Most companies will start people analytics with strengths in some S and deficiencies in one or more of the others. It is important to recognize that different strengths and deficiencies will produce different blind spots or pitfalls. It is the component that is most deficient that will define the pitfall that will materialize. It is my hope that by clarifying capability-related blind spots below you can avoid these capability-related pitfalls entirely.

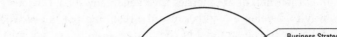

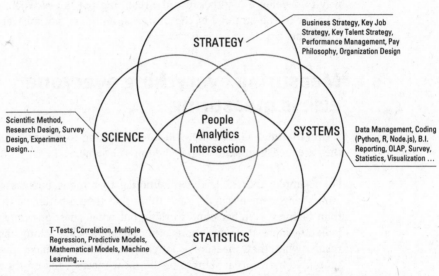

FIGURE 18-1:
People analytics is the intersection of people strategy, science, statistics and systems.

Pitfall 2: Missing the People Strategy Part of the People Analytics Intersection

People analytics is only really useful if it is aligned to your strategy and informs decision making. Anything else is just going in circles. When data analysis is not linked to strategy or determined by strategy, then the company is wasting time and money in all this activity that is never going to be used.

In the absence of a linkage of people analytics to company strategy most companies either attempt to measure everything or measure everything that everyone else is measuring, because they don't know what else to do.

Measuring everything that is easy to measure

This is by far the biggest mistake that people make — they work out what is easy to measure and measure everything that is easy to measure regardless of its relevance to the business.

HR executives will often brainstorm measures and analyses. Usually the ones they end up with will be the ones they have heard of before, read about in a management journal, or are metrics they've already seen. Obviously, this is not the best way to develop a plan because the resulting list is overwhelmingly long, is not relevant to the strategy of the business, and does not answer the most critical questions.

Measuring everything everyone else is measuring

A trap that many businesses fall into is looking to other companies to see what they are measuring and then just doing the same.

For example, the HR leader may notice that many businesses are conducting annual engagement surveys and think that they'd better do that as well. Rather than taking a step back and working out what questions they need to ask, they look elsewhere at the questions other businesses are asking and follow suit. As a result, what they measure is often just what they have always done before, prompted by external sources or the most recent book on the market. The ones they should be measuring are the ones that are directly relevant.

>> If you start with an ill-defined problem, your work turns into a fishing expedition as you cast your line into the data lake and hope something hooks itself.

>> If you start on an unimportant problem, your efforts turn into a trivial pursuit, where you might win the game but the fact that you won doesn't matter a bit when you're done.

>> If you try to start without even specifying a problem, you make yourself into an atmospheric scientist: You're analyzing the air.

The best insights come from focused projects. You need to understand the problem you're trying to solve and have a clear notion of what you need to analyze to get the results you're looking for.

Start with an idea, form a hypothesis, and look to confirm, refine, or reject the hypothesis with data.

Focus matters because, unless you have a large team and unlimited resources, you don't have the time or the money to do everything. Strategy helps drive focus.

Pitfall 3: Missing the Statistics Part of the People Analytics intersection

The are many reasons to learn about statistics, but perhaps its most important purpose is to help you make better decisions in a world of much uncertainty. Yes, the world is an uncertain place, but increasingly, the world is also a place overflowing with data. Statistics can help you make sense of data, and in so doing make more sense of the world.

People unfamiliar with statistics expect to be able to see clearly the answers to their questions in a line graph or bar chart. However, visual patterns can mislead you. Just because a line seems to increase over time doesn't mean that your conclusions about *why* it is increasing are the actual causes. Just because two bars on a graph are different sizes doesn't mean that the difference is significant or meaningful. Only very large differences among very simple comparisons present themselves obviously in visualizations. Overreliance on visualization leads to simplistic observations that are not up to the task of producing answers to complex questions. The real world is complex: many factors push and pull in different directions at the same time. These don't translate readily to visualization.

REMEMBER

Statistics can be an intimidating subject for many people, but ultimately it's a subject involving a certain logic and certain procedures that can be learned by anyone. Relationships are much more uncertain, and you manage those every day!

Pitfall 4: Missing the Science Part of the People Analytics Intersection

Popular opinion suggests that knowledge of systems that a company happens to be using (or wants to use) or other technology tools like Python, R or machine learning are the most important skills to look for in analysts hired to lead people analytics initiatives. In my experience, though, nothing could be further from the truth. About the only things in common among the best analysts I've met in people analytics are curiosity, imagination, and a knack to get to the heart of problems. Aside from this, I have also noticed that they tend to have studied some form of behavioral science, in particular psychology, sociology, operations science or economics.

Science is everywhere in today's world, so much so now that we hardly notice it. Science has impacted nearly every aspect of our daily lives, from what we eat to how we dress to how we get from point a to point b. Why not the workplace, too? Advances in technology and science are transforming our world at an incredible pace and our children's future will surely be filled with leaps we can only imagine. No one can escape the significance of science in our world, but not everyone understands the importance of science, has been taught to think critically, or been provided with the tools to analyze and test a problem in the ways people who study science have. The application of science to people at work is a new frontier of science that I'm proud to be a part of, and you can be part of this, too!

REMEMBER

The beauty of science is that it's self-correcting. Science is coming up with an idea, testing that idea, and then observing to decide if it works or if you have to throw that idea out. If an idea is wrong, you have to get rid of it to make way for a new one. Science is a way of looking at anything you want to understand and saying how does this work, why does it work, and how can you know about this?

Pitfall 5: Missing the System Part of the People Analytics Intersection

Today it goes without saying that companies have systems supporting the many transactional functions of human resources. You certainly have a system for payroll so you can pay people as well as a human resource information system and some combination of other systems to facilitate all of the specialized activities of human resources, including applicant tracking, performance management, compensation planning, employee relations, learning management, and other specialized operational HR activities or activities facilitated by HR. Systems are almost never the missing ingredient when it comes to HR — the problem is that the systems required for people analytics to operate efficiently are different.

The operational systems described in the paragraph above are designed primarily to serve the transactional needs of HR, not the reporting or analysis needs of people analytics. Sure, each system may have a front-end reporting interface to provide access to data in the systems directly; however, these interfaces leave much to be desired. In most cases, the standard reports available from transactional systems are just lists of people or facts and most of the time you have too little control over what goes into those reports. These lists of facts are necessary but not sufficient for the analyses you need. Transactional systems are not designed to perform the core tasks of analytics.

Here are just a few examples of the tasks necessary for analytics that transactional systems are generally not designed to do:

» Provide control over workflow functions like extract, transform, load (ETL) from and to other data environments — how you move data to or from other data sources and join them, in other words.

» Provide control over how you add or remove data elements on a report and how you group data.

» Provide control over what calculations you perform and how you perform calculations.

» Allow you to construct custom datasets to perform statistics operations like correlation, chi-square, multiple regression, t-tests, and so on.

» Provide control of the design of graphs for reports.

» Provide business users a central location for all of the information relevant for them to manage their teams. (Believe me, you don't want to have to tell business users they have to go to four different systems to pick up data on different topic areas.)

As a result of the reporting and analysis deficiencies of the transactional HR systems, data-minded professionals serving sub-functions of HR create makeshift reports, dashboards, and analysis in desktop tools like Tableau or Excel to serve needs not met currently by the transactional systems. For example, if the reporting needs of Recruiting have not been picked up by a centralized HR reporting team, then the Talent Acquisition team may hire their own analyst to build reports on the recruiting process. The reports the analysts in Talent Acquisition build may speak only to the data from the applicant tracking system (ATS), which serves the operational needs of the Recruiting function. The Talent Acquisition analyst may have no access to data in other HR systems and will likely have no insight or interest into how all the data from the different environments fit together.

Aside from the sub-HR-function splintering of analytics effort I describe in the paragraph above, many companies are large enough that you also find a splintering of effort between divisions of the company. For example, executives and HR professionals serving the Sales division may acquire their own analysts and the Research & Development division may form another. At another company, the split may be by geography or by business line. At a very large, complex company, the splits may be all of the above and more.

The splintering of analytics activity leads to a number of duplicative tasks being performed in different places of the company without awareness of the work being performed by others. Often the same tasks are repeated by different people that could be more efficiently handled in one common data environment and then split out for their needs or modification. Inefficiency is the problem you find if you have missed the systems part of the four S's of people analytics.

More importantly, the problems you're trying to understand and resolve with data may actually cross functional or divisional boundaries — the splintering makes it so that you cannot see the insights that cross functional boundaries. Inevitably, problems may be resolved in one part of the company and just pushed to another or a solution may remain elusive to you forever because you're not able to bring a more universal data perspective together.

REMEMBER

People analytics can be cobbled together and performed using borrowed systems and scraps of data; however, this can only be a short-term solution. If you have a lot of people performing a lot of tasks on data in an inefficient (and overall ineffective) manner, your chances of long-term success are slim. United you stand, divided you fall. This is why you should try to get your systems house in order by creating a centralized people analytics data environment that brings together multiple data sub-domains and data management functions into one common area.

Pitfall 6: Not Involving Other People in the Right Ways

What if you built a data dashboard and nobody showed up to use it? The users are what will make your data dashboard a success or failure. There are lots of reasons why users may not flock to the tools you roll out. First and foremost, if the data dashboard doesn't add value to their job, they won't use it; it may be as simple as that. It also may be that they access the information from time to time but not on a regular basis — they don't log into the system frequently enough to remember how it could be helpful to them or be comfortable operating in that environment to enjoy it.

Rather than start with data that may or may not have any value, start by getting away from your desk to understand better the world of the people you support. Ask questions about production, sales, and other processes. To help other people, you need to understand what those people do, what their pain points are, and what success looks like to them. Armed with that information, you can connect them with an analysis or a report to help them do what they do better.

While it is good to meet with end users early in the process, at the same time you must realize that you can't expect people to be able to translate their needs to you into the language of dashboard and analysis design. You should not simply walk in and ask them what they want to see on a dashboard. More often than not, they'll simply describe something they have seen before. Unfortunately, this may not be the best report or analysis to help them solve their problem — and you won't find this out until you build what they asked for and discover they aren't using it. Contemplating what went wrong you may think, "but this is what they asked me for." Absent a deliberate strategy of interaction with end users from beginning to end, this disconnect will happen a lot.

REMEMBER

People analytics is new. Despite a lot of head nodding, keep in mind that most people don't know what people analytics is (or is capable of doing), let alone what kind of analysis could help them right now. Figuring out what other people need should be your area of expertise. Your job is not to take specific report and analysis design instructions from them, and their job isn't to give you specific report and analysis design instruction. Their job is something else. Your job is to elicit from them an understanding of what their job is and what business problems they are solving right now and then design a reporting or analysis solution that will help them do it better.

After you have met with people to talk about what they do, the next thing you should do is create a prototype data analytics solution. In this context, a prototype is a subset of the total solution, where the scope is narrowed down to a few of the most important data elements and/or company segments. At its core, a prototype usually consists of a limited dashboard or analysis solution combined with a stripped-down version of one or more end-user tools that visualize the data. A prototype is a great way to get a reaction, flush out uncertainties, model the challenges that will be found in working with a particular dataset at full-scale implementation, and get people involved along the way for what's ahead.

Pitfall 7: Underfunding People Analytics

If your hired to head up people analytics and find out you have no budget, don't feel bad. You aren't the first, and you won't be the last. Whether it makes sense to quit now or ride it out and fail later depends on your own personal circumstances. One thing is certain: if you don't communicate clearly and honestly about the level of expectations others have for what they hope to achieve from people analytics versus the level of support and resources provided to you to achieve those results, then your efforts will fail.

Full-time people analytics professionals have a notoriously high incidence of burn out because people analytics crosses every department in the company, every sub-function of HR (Recruiting, Compensation, Benefits, Payroll, Employee Relations, Learning & Development, Organization Design, Diversity, and so on) and requires data from many different systems (ATS, HRIS, Compensation Planning, Performance Management, and more). Before you know it, you're getting requests from the chief human resources officer, division vice presidents, mid-level managers, head of HR sub functions, and people you haven't even heard of before.

If you can't get resources to build a scalable data environment and you can't keep up with report demand, then something is clearly out of whack. Obviously what you are doing must be important or you wouldn't be getting hit with all these report requests, and yet how then can it not be important enough to invest in the proper data, systems, and support? I have always felt that having too many people coming to you for reports is a better problem to have then not having any, but that being said you will need to navigate this situation carefully or you might just end up going under.

REMEMBER

Don't let enthusiasm for the work of people analytics get in the way of making rational decisions about what you can reasonably deliver. It is a natural tendency to get excited that others are asking for your help and say yes to everything. Resist this tendency. You should think long and hard before you take on a project. Here are some considerations:

» Does this project offer enough business value to justify the effort?

» Are you considering the relative value of this project to other projects that will inevitably receive less of your time and attention if you take on the new project?

» Do you truly have what you need to be successful for this new project?

» What is the person asking for the analysis or report from you willing to do to help you be successful?

There are some things you can do that will help you:

» Be blunt about the time and resource realities you face.

» Create a transparent prioritization system. Point to this. Use it.

» Request that the people who need something from you do something for you, too. This could be as simple as becoming an advocate for people analytics and you in the company or it could involve them becoming a project sponsor or member of the people analytics task force. Whatever it is, make sure they pay you back.

Pitfall 8: Garbage In, Garbage Out

Garbage in, garbage out (GIGO) describes the concept that flawed input data produces flawed output or "garbage". If you have questionable data feeding into your dashboards and analysis, then their output won't be worth a pile of rotten tomatoes.

If there were ever a poster child for a garbage-in-garbage-out statement, it's the realm of HR data. Data quality is an ongoing problem in all analytics but especially when there's people data involved. People and their reporting relationships are in a constant state of change; so are the data entities that represent them. That can create confusion and headaches.

For example, if you implement a data dashboard to work with the latest organization hierarchy definition, what will happen when you need to look at historical records when the company had a different organization hierarchy structure? Nothing can destroy the credibility of a reporting or analysis initiative faster than not being able to explain the numbers you get back.

Source data is not a fix-it-and-forget element. Managerial and organizational changes are not just a problem in past data. Organizational changes are constantly happening, so you have to continue to be on the lookout for changes that are occurring anywhere in the company: reorganizations, manager changes, acquisitions, divestitures, and name changes can happen at any time. How do you recognize when you are getting bad results? And if you do recognize a problem, can you trace it to its source? Imagine if one of the operational data sources feeding your data environment breaks and a field that your extract, transform and load (ETL) process uses as a primary key fails to come through. Suddenly everything is wrong on downstream reports. If there is no data check alert designed in the data process, you'll have no way of knowing that this problem is happening until someone opens up a report in a meeting and says, "this is wrong". A meeting is not a place where anyone wants to find a problem they can't explain.

REMEMBER

You might be surprised to learn this, but most executives only know the units they manage. This means they have no visibility into the complexities of the company beyond their bailiwick and no awareness of the history of changes across the units of the company for which they do not have direct responsibility. It may be that nobody before you has attempted to report on all of the units of the company as a complete, coherent picture over time. You also may find that some divisions define organization units by manager, some by financial cost centers, others by location, and others by something else entirely. You have to facilitate agreement on a method of arranging organizational structure to report on the company and its many pieces that represents how the company really operates, but that also maintains data integrity and efficient data processing as a whole.

On top of the problem of complexity and change endemic to people you also have to deal with HR system complexity. Most companies use different systems for applicant tracking, human resource information systems, performance management, compensation planning, and other transactional human resource management needs. Even if all of those transactions are performed in one system, you still likely have several payroll and benefits partners, with each one also having their own systems to contend with. Different system owners apply different business rules and often show no interest in maintaining data entry and corrections for data elements they have little need for. Since their job is transactions, they are on to the next transaction — they could not care less about the data for transactions they have completed in the past.

Piecing together the data picture as a whole — gathering the entirety of current business rules and naming conventions — is a challenging exercise. In facing this challenge, I offer the following three pieces of advice:

>> Pick a topic that really matters and start slowly. Make sure you can do a few things well before you sign up to do more things.

>> Plan ahead for confusion and change by creating visibility and flexibility in your master set of metric definitions, data hierarchies, and data relationships.

>> Whenever planning for a project, you need to include time to audit, analyze, and (if necessary) fix the data at the source if at all possible.

Perhaps the most important advice I can give you in all of this book is that you need to carefully to pick the metrics and analyses you're going to focus on based on what will offer the company the most value. If you try to mine the whole of HR data your company has, hoping to aimlessly find something of value, you are going to end up in a world of pain fast. It is just impossible to keep everything perfect all the time and even if you could do that it will be a waste because most of the data you have perfected will go unused anyway.

Pitfall 9: Skimping on New Data Development

Data is the lifeblood of people analytics. Transactional HR systems are designed to speed up operational HR processes; if they produce data on the side, that is more or less accidental. Data from transactional systems is necessary for people analytics, but data produced by these transactions is limited to only a certain range of insights. Failing to understand this fact will limit the value you can derive from people analytics. Here are a few tips that will help you create new data to crank out new insights.

>> **Budget for new data development.** Neither HR or IT (or even specialized Analytics departments) do a good job at budgeting for investment in collecting new data or in acquiring subscriptions to new external data sources. Consider having a slice of your budget set aside just for new data development. You might include sending people to conferences to look for ideas for new data sources or interview other people working in the field of people analytics about the data that have proved most valuable to them. In any event, make sure you have a budget — and use it.

>> **Never miss a chance to get important new data.** Creating data is something to keep in the back of your mind at all times. Because there are so many different ways to approach this, all I can do is throw out some examples. If you interview candidates and make some decisions about them, why not record this information in a structured way so that, over the long term, it can be analyzed as well? If you have a new hire fill out a form for some information required by rule or law, why not also collect a few pieces of information that will be valuable to you for analysis reasons? If it takes them only 30 seconds longer to provide you with a few additional details and they already had to stop what they were doing to meet the regulations, then why not? You have employee addresses for other reasons, so why not use this data in conjunction with a public data source to calculate commute time? Speaking of public data, did you know that the U.S. Department of Labor maintains a database of the number of people in a particular zip code by job classification, by ethnicity, by gender and so on? You may talk about diversity, but do you really know if the percentage of people you hire by job classification is proportional to what you can expect in the population? Did you even know that the data you need to answer this question exists? When you deliberately think about the types of data you can use in people analytics, you will find there is an endless variety of surveys, personality inventories, tests, subscription benchmark data sources, and so on, which represent new data sources that can augment your existing people analytics efforts to produce new insights.

>> **Reinvest time.** By tradition or lack of imagination, most people analytics capabilities are focused on producing more efficient outputs. For example, data warehousing tools, data management tools, and data visualization tools are all geared towards more efficiently producing insights that people have previously produced manually in rudimentary applications like Excel. The movement to more scalable and efficient analytics systems is valuable in itself, but it cannot by itself produce new insights if it is simply answering the same questions with the same data. I suggest you take some of the time or money saved by moving to more efficient tools and set it aside for new data

development. Simply look at the time people used to spend in Excel before implementing the new automated reporting environment for the same metrics. Allocate some of the time or money saved to obtain or design new data collection instruments that can produce new metrics. Deliberately putting time and money into developing new data sources to go into your people analytics effort will drive more value out of your people analytics effort in the end.

Pitfall 10: Not Getting Started at All

The list of possible pitfalls for people analytics is long, as is the list of excuses used to not getting started.

Anything worth doing requires hard work and carries a certain amount of risk. What you have to decide is whether you believe that your company can make better people-related decisions continuing with the old way or whether trying to make things better with data is more likely to give you predictable, repeatable successes.

The reality is that *both* options come with pitfalls and risk. Regardless of whether you choose to use or ignore data in your decision making, your company can't avoid making decisions. The part you can control is how well you equip yourself to make good ones. People analytics will serve you well, but to do so you must get started. So, get to it!

Index

N

natural language processing (NLP), 406

The Nature of Statistics (Wallis and Roberts), 21

Net Activated metric, calculating, 123, 213

Net Activated Percent metric, calculating, 123, 127

Net Activated Value (NAV), combining lifetime value and activation with, 126–128

Netflix, 200

90-Day On-Board survey, 151–152

NLP (natural language processing), 406

noise, 347–350

non-employee, defined, 165

nonlinear (exponential) growth, 344–345

Nonregretted Voluntary exit type, 234

null hypothesis, 391

O

observed behavior, extrapolating from, 196–198

OCAI (organizational culture assessment instrument), 216

Occam's razor, 406

Offer-Accepts, as a process metric for Talent Acquisition, 174

Offers, as a process metric for Talent Acquisition, 174

Ohmae, Keniche (author)
The Mind of the Strategist, 80

ONA (Organization Network Analysis), 406

Once-Per-Quarter Check-In survey, 152–153

Once-Per-Year Check-In survey, 153–155

one (single) sample *t*-test, 389

one-tailed *t*-test, 389

one/zero counting variable, 169

ongoing assessment, 185

online support (website), 6

operationalization, 260–261

opinions
measuring, 62
as a survey measure, 255

organization climate, 218–221

Organization Network Analysis (ONA), 406

organizational change, supporting, 130

organizational culture, 215–216

organizational culture assessment instrument (OCAI), 216

Ostermiller, Steven J. (author)
Agile Project Management For Dummies, 7

P

pay, as a sensitive topic, 90–91

Pearson product-moment correlation, 290

"peeling the onion," 32–34

people
accounting for in business results, 24–25
applying statistics to management of, 20–22
changing, 409–411
identifying problems of, 34–35
incorrectly using, 416–417
using data on in business analytics, 19–20

people analytics. *See also specific topics*
about, 11–13
business case for, 27–42
as a decision support tool, 38–40
getting executives to buy into, 29–38
myths of, 397–407
pitfalls of, 409–422
solving problems by asking questions, 14–19
underfunding, 417–418
who is it for, 404–405
who should perform it, 402–403

people strategy, 411–413

performance management, 88–91, 119–121

personality tests, 162

personality types, measuring, 62

PetSmart, 86

physical ability tests, 163

physical examinations, 163

Pierson, Lillian (author)
Data Science For Dummies, 7

value, as a survey measure, 255

vanity measure error, 273–274

variables
  binary, 293–295
  dependent, 375–376
  independent, 375–376

visualizing
  associations, 288–290
  headcount, 62–63

vocabulary, in surveys, 265

volume, measuring for Talent Acquisition, 163–172

voluntary employee attrition rate, 34

Voluntary exit type, 233

W

Wallis, Allen (author)
  The Nature of Statistics, 21

Warning icon, 3

waterfall project management, 47

websites
  CEB, 181
  Cheat Sheet, 6
  The Hackett Group, 181

MicroInequities program, 372, 373

online support, 6

organizational culture assessment instrument (OCAI), 216

PWC, 181

sample size calculator, 380

SHRM, 181

Welch, Jack (CEO), 89

What's In It For Me? (WIIFM), 271

WIIFM (What's In It For Me?), 271

win/loss ratio of hires and exits, compared to top competitors, 34

The Wisdom of Crowds: Why the Many Are Smarter Than the Few and How Collective Wisdom Shapes Business, Economies, Societies and Nations (Surowiecki), 252

X

x variables, 318

Y

y intercept, 305

Yuk, Mico (author)
  Data Visualization For Dummies, 7

About the Author

Mike West is a pioneer in the field of people analytics. He was a founding member of what we now call people analytics at Merck, PetSmart, Google, Children's Health Dallas, Jawbone, and Pure Storage. He has a dual B.S. degree in Sociology and Psychology from Northern Arizona University and a master's degree in Human Resources and Industrial Relations from the University of Minnesota. His expertise in Human Resource Information Systems (HRIS) has been developed on the job. All said, Mike has been doing innovate work at the intersection of people science, statistics, strategy and systems for over 10 companies, in over 7 industries, over 20 years.

Mike was one of a handful of early analytical hires on Google's world-renowned People Operations team, credited with using data to reinvent human resources and in the process turning Google into the talent magnet that it is today. Mike's contributions at Google included work on the first HR data reporting architecture, the first professional employee survey design, the first benefits analytics, the first employee onboarding analytics and the first work on employee attrition, which included Google's first employee exit prediction model. Since then, Google has built one of the most impressive reputations for people analytics in the world and has gone on to win the number one spot on the *Fortune 100 Best Company to Work For* list more than any other company in the awards history: 8 times and counting since Google first qualified in 2006.

In 2013, Mike started the first niche people analytics design company, PeopleAnalyst, and has partnered to found two other companies in the space: PeopleFlow LLC and People Analytics LLC. He has also served as the first Vice President of Product Strategy at OneModel INC.

Mike is an established visionary, architect, speaker, and writer of people analytics, specializing in the design and execution of data-informed talent management methods for companies whose future success is contingent upon product leadership, innovation agility, and people operations cleverness. Mike can generally be found on some node in the triangle of Austin (TX), San Francisco (CA) and Springfield (MO).

Mike invites you to connect with him on LinkedIn, where he stays in touch with others and has published over 50 articles: www.linkedin.com/in/michaelcwest

Dedication

This book is dedicated to everyone who has ever applied for a job and been passed over for a less qualified applicant, anyone who has been hired to do a job and then not been properly equipped and supported to do that job, everyone who has ever slaved with no hope under a bad manager, and anyone who has ever patiently listened to their spouse talk endlessly about frustrations at work.

In short, this book is dedicated to humanity.

Author's Acknowledgments

Nothing of lasting substance can be done without a team, and Wiley provided me with a great one for this project. Acquisitions Editor Amy Fandrei started the ball rolling and Steven Hayes picked up where she left off. Project Editor Paul Levesque got me on track, oversaw profound changes to my writing, and kept all the moving parts in motion. Copy Editor Becky Whitney tightened my writing and made the book you're holding easier to read. Technical Editor Amit Mohindra kept me honest on the technical underpinnings of the book. He did his best — I am the owner and sole proprietor of any omissions and errors that remain.

Speaking of indispensable individuals, my love to Jaimie Saratella, my partner of more than five years, who keeps loving me despite my flaws. I should also mention the many friends, colleagues, and mentors who have helped me with this project, whether they were aware of it or not. So here's to Steven Grant (Pure Storage), Maria Cespedes (Pure Storage), Rich Tobey (People Analytics), Corey Butler (People Flow), Dave Jobe (MentorTex), Chris Butler (OneModel), Steven Huang (CultureAmp), John Budd (UMN), Connie Wanberg (UMN), Rick Hou (Eyecue Lab), Laszlo Bock (Humu), John Miller (VizableHR), Alvan Santoso (Google), Adam Dorenfield (research), Craig Heyrman (German skepticism), Robert Lanning (SLOAP) and Phil Simon (who taught me how to play poker, among other vices). Others offered assistance, but I ran out of time to cash in on it.

I need to specifically call attention to Maria Cespedes for her thoughts on employee surveys, Corey Butler for his thoughts on technology, Alvan Santoso for his help assembling lists of survey items, Tim Weinzirl for creating a word cloud for me, Adam Dorenfield for countless hours mining peer-reviewed research, Ryan Hammond for picking up the pieces where I left off at Pure Storage, and Rich Tobey for everything else while I was writing.

Publisher's Acknowledgments

Acquisitions Editor: Amy Fandrei
Senior Project Editor: Paul Levesque
Copy Editor: Becky Whitney
Technical Editor: Amit Mohindra
Editorial Assistant: Matthew Lowe
Sr. Editorial Assistant: Cherie Case

Production Editor: Magesh Elangovan
Cover Image: © iLexx/iStock.com

Take dummies with you everywhere you go!

Whether you are excited about e-books, want more from the web, must have your mobile apps, or are swept up in social media, dummies makes everything easier.

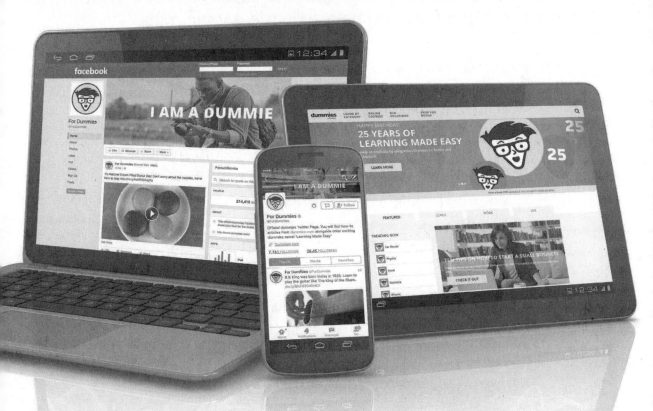

Find us online!

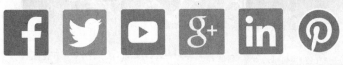

dummies.com

dummies
A Wiley Brand

Leverage the power

Dummies is the global leader in the reference category and one of the most trusted and highly regarded brands in the world. No longer just focused on books, customers now have access to the dummies content they need in the format they want. Together we'll craft a solution that engages your customers, stands out from the competition, and helps you meet your goals.

Advertising & Sponsorships

Connect with an engaged audience on a powerful multimedia site, and position your message alongside expert how-to content. Dummies.com is a one-stop shop for free, online information and know-how curated by a team of experts.

- Targeted ads
- Video
- Email Marketing
- Microsites
- Sweepstakes sponsorship

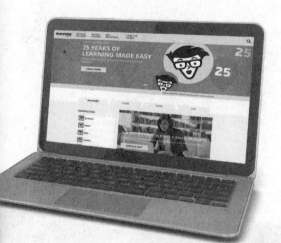

20 MILLION PAGE VIEWS
EVERY SINGLE MONTH

15 MILLION UNIQUE
VISITORS PER MONTH

43% OF ALL VISITORS ACCESS THE SITE
VIA THEIR MOBILE DEVICES

700,000 NEWSLETTER SUBSCRIPTIONS
TO THE INBOXES OF
300,000 UNIQUE INDIVIDUALS EVERY WEEK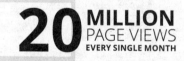

# of dummies

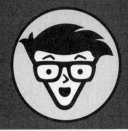

Custom Publishing

Reach a global audience in any language by creating a solution that will differentiate you from competitors, amplify your message, and encourage customers to make a buying decision.

- Apps
- Books
- eBooks
- Video
- Audio
- Webinars

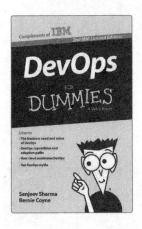
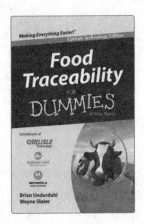
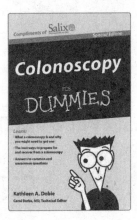
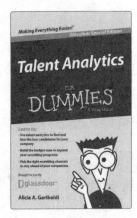

Brand Licensing & Content

Leverage the strength of the world's most popular reference brand to reach new audiences and channels of distribution.

For more information, visit dummies.com/biz

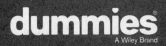

PERSONAL ENRICHMENT

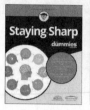
Staying Sharp
9781119187790
USA $26.00
CAN $31.99
UK £19.99

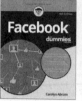
Facebook
9781119179030
USA $21.99
CAN $25.99
UK £16.99

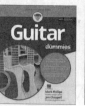
Guitar
9781119293354
USA $24.99
CAN $29.99
UK £17.99

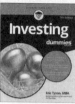
Investing
9781119293347
USA $22.99
CAN $27.99
UK £16.99

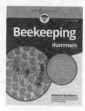
Beekeeping
9781119310068
USA $22.99
CAN $27.99
UK £16.99

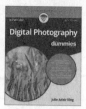
Digital Photography
9781119235606
USA $24.99
CAN $29.99
UK £17.99

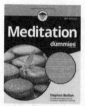
Meditation
9781119251163
USA $24.99
CAN $29.99
UK £17.99

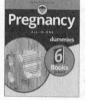
Pregnancy
9781119235491
USA $26.99
CAN $31.99
UK £19.99

Samsung Galaxy S7
9781119279952
USA $24.99
CAN $29.99
UK £17.99

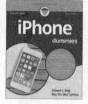
iPhone
9781119283133
USA $24.99
CAN $29.99
UK £17.99

Crocheting
9781119287117
USA $24.99
CAN $29.99
UK £16.99

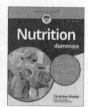
Nutrition
9781119130246
USA $22.99
CAN $27.99
UK £16.99

PROFESSIONAL DEVELOPMENT

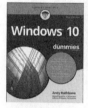
Windows 10
9781119311041
USA $24.99
CAN $29.99
UK £17.99

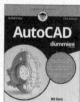
AutoCAD
9781119255796
USA $39.99
CAN $47.99
UK £27.99

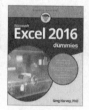
Excel 2016
9781119293439
USA $26.99
CAN $31.99
UK £19.99

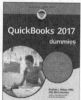
QuickBooks 2017
9781119281467
USA $26.99
CAN $31.99
UK £19.99

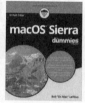
macOS Sierra
9781119280651
USA $29.99
CAN $35.99
UK £21.99

LinkedIn
9781119251132
USA $24.99
CAN $29.99
UK £17.99

Windows 10
9781119310563
USA $34.00
CAN $41.99
UK £24.99

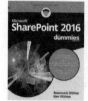
SharePoint 2016
9781119181705
USA $29.99
CAN $35.99
UK £21.99

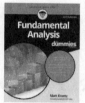
Fundamental Analysis
9781119263593
USA $26.99
CAN $31.99
UK £19.99

Networking
9781119257769
USA $29.99
CAN $35.99
UK £21.99

Office 2016
9781119293477
USA $26.99
CAN $31.99
UK £19.99

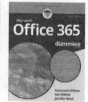
Office 365
9781119265313
USA $24.99
CAN $29.99
UK £17.99

Salesforce.com
9781119239314
USA $29.99
CAN $35.99
UK £21.99

Coding
9781119293323
USA $29.99
CAN $35.99
UK £21.99

dummies.com

dummies
A Wiley Brand

Learning Made Easy

ACADEMIC

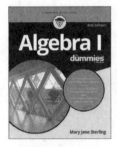

9781119293576
USA $19.99
CAN $23.99
UK £15.99

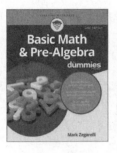

9781119293637
USA $19.99
CAN $23.99
UK £15.99

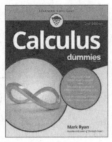

9781119293491
USA $19.99
CAN $23.99
UK £15.99

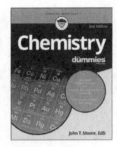

9781119293460
USA $19.99
CAN $23.99
UK £15.99

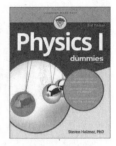

9781119293590
USA $19.99
CAN $23.99
UK £15.99

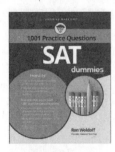

9781119215844
USA $26.99
CAN $31.99
UK £19.99

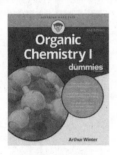

9781119293378
USA $22.99
CAN $27.99
UK £16.99

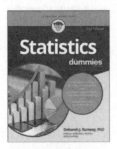

9781119293521
USA $19.99
CAN $23.99
UK £15.99

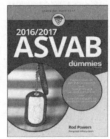

9781119239178
USA $18.99
CAN $22.99
UK £14.99

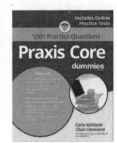

9781119263883
USA $26.99
CAN $31.99
UK £19.99

Available Everywhere Books Are Sold

dummies.com

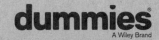

Small books for big imaginations

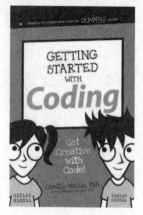

GETTING STARTED WITH Coding
Get Creative with Code!
Camille McCue, PhD

9781119177173
USA $9.99
CAN $9.99
UK £8.99

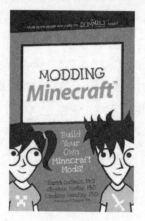

MODDING Minecraft
Build Your Own Minecraft Mods!
Sarah Guthals, PhD
Stephen Foster, PhD
Lindsey Handley, PhD

9781119177272
USA $9.99
CAN $9.99
UK £8.99

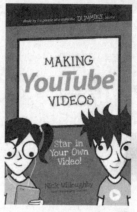

MAKING YouTube VIDEOS
Star in Your Own Video!
Nick Willoughby

9781119177241
USA $9.99
CAN $9.99
UK £8.99

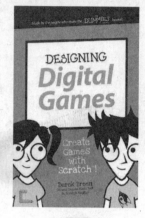

DESIGNING Digital Games
Create Games with Scratch!
Derek Breen

9781119177210
USA $9.99
CAN $9.99
UK £8.99

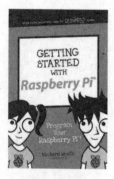

GETTING STARTED WITH Raspberry Pi
Program Your Raspberry Pi!
Richard Wentk

9781119262657
USA $9.99
CAN $9.99
UK £6.99

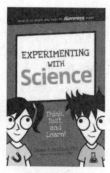

EXPERIMENTING WITH Science
Think, Test, and Learn!

9781119291336
USA $9.99
CAN $9.99
UK £6.99

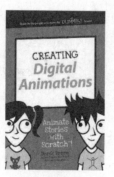

CREATING Digital Animations
Animate Stories with Scratch!
Derek Breen

9781119233527
USA $9.99
CAN $9.99
UK £6.99

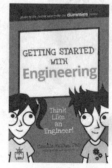

GETTING STARTED WITH Engineering
Think Like an Engineer!
Camille McCue, PhD

9781119291220
USA $9.99
CAN $9.99
UK £6.99

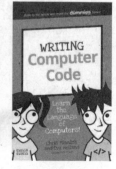

WRITING Computer Code
Learn the Language of Computers!
Chris Minnick and Eva Holland

9781119177302
USA $9.99
CAN $9.99
UK £8.99

Unleash Their Creativity